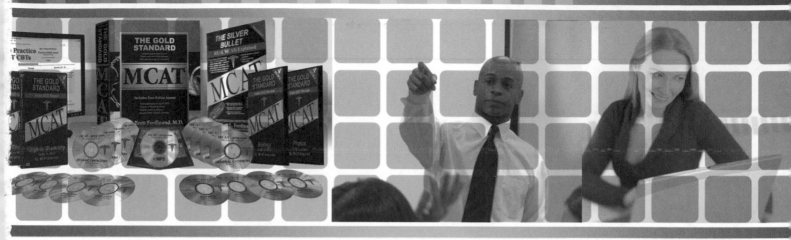
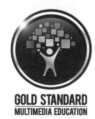
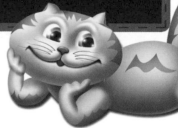

THE GOLD STANDARD

MCAT

Editor and Author

Brett Ferdinand BSc MD-CM

Contributors

Lisa Ferdinand BA MA
Sean Pierre BSc MD
Kristin Finkenzeller BSc MD
Ibrahima Diouf BSc MSc PhD
Brigitte Bigras BSc MSc PhD
Naomi Epstein BEng
Charles Haccoun BSc MD-CM

Illustrators

Daphne McCormack
Nanjing Design
 • Ren Yi, Huang Bin
 • Sun Chan, Li Xin

RuveneCo
inc

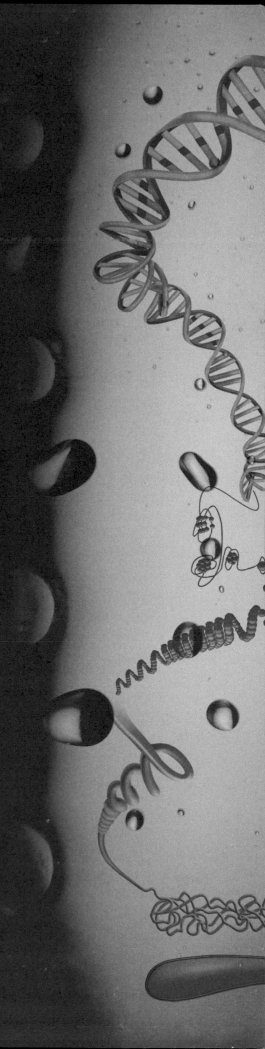

Students who own The Gold Standard textbook can get access to special online features for up to one year. To start your online access, click on FREE MCAT in the top Menu of the mcat-prep.com homepage and then you will find "Click here if you own the Gold Standard textbook". Then follow the directions provided.

Visit MCAT-prep.com's Education Center at www.mcat-prep.com.

PREFACE

Imagine that you did a practice test question and it was followed by a clear explanation. But that was not all - the explanation had a direct link to a video for background information as well as a reference to a particular chapter and section in this very book that you are reading. But that was not all - the explanation gave a difficulty ranking and a direct link to a forum thread to open or continue a discussion about that particular question. Well, that's a Gold Standard explanation.

We have integrated your learning experience. The textbook you are reading includes online chapter review questions, 10 hours of teaching videos, equation lists and an organic chemistry summary. These bonus online features also include the computer based test (CBT) versions of the longer tests, GS-1 to GS-3, at the end of the book. We have an active online forum so that you can share your learning experience with other students and ensure you are not studying too much or too little.

Study too much?

Though it is true that the MCAT covers introductory level college physics, biology, general and organic chemistry, it does not mean that everything you may have studied at that level is covered on the MCAT. Some college professors, or even poorly structured MCAT materials, may emphasize memory skills. The focus of the MCAT is concepts.

We use a multimedia approach to both teach and then expand your understanding in the subjects required for the new MCAT. At the same time, we try to limit your distractions from areas that you may have studied in 1st year university, but are simply not required for the MCAT.

Ironically, students had been using our first generation Gold Standard practice MCAT CBTs 6 years before the real MCAT became a CBT. Our innovations continue with our Complete Package, DVDs, MP3s, iPhone Apps focused on concepts not just definitions, The Silver Bullet Real MCATs Explained with Verbal Prep, our live online interactive classrooms, YouTube videos on the medical school admissions process, our free interactive study calender (MCAT-prep.com), the Platinum Program, our "Tweets," our Facebook events, and so much more to come.

Learning used to be more about the teacher, now it's about you. We can be your guide but you must choose the tools that work best for you.

Good luck!

- BF, MD

Table of Contents

Preface v
Introduction I

Part I: MEDICAL SCHOOL ADMISSIONS

1. Improving Academic Standing 5
2. The Medical School Interview 11
3. Autobiographical Materials and References 19
4. The Directory of North American Medical Schools 23

Part II: THE new MEDICAL COLLEGE ADMISSION TEST

1. The Structure of the new MCAT 43
2. The Recipe for MCAT Success 51
3. Review for Verbal Reasoning 57
4. Review for the Writing Sample 61

Part III: THE PHYSICAL SCIENCES

A. General Chemistry CHM-01

1. Stoichiometry CHM-03
2. Electronic Structure and the Periodic Table CHM-13
3. Bonding CHM-25
4. Phases and Phase Equilibria CHM-35
5. Solution Chemistry CHM-47
6. Acids and Bases CHM-57
7. Thermodynamics CHM-71
8. Enthalpy and Thermochemistry CHM-79
9. Rate Processes in Chemical Reactions CHM-89
10. Electrochemistry CHM-101

RuveneCo
inc

B.Physics PHY-01

1. Translational Motion PHY-03
2. Force, Motion, and Gravitation PHY-11
3. Particle Dynamics PHY-19
4. Equilibrium PHY-25
5. Work and Energy PHY-33
6. Fluids and Solids PHY-39
7. Wave Characteristics and Periodic Motion PHY-49
8. Sound PHY-61
9. Electrostatics and Electromagnetism PHY-67
10. Electric Circuits PHY-77
11. Light and Geometrical Optics PHY-89
12. Atomic and Nuclear Structure PHY-99

Part IV: THE BIOLOGICAL SCIENCES

A.Biology BIO-01

1. Generalized Eukaryotic Cell BIO-03
2. Microbiology BIO-21
3. Protein Synthesis BIO-29
4. Enzymes and Cellular Metabolism BIO-35
5. Specialized Eukaryotic Cells and Tissues BIO-47
6. Nervous and Endocrine Systems BIO-61
7. The Circulatory System BIO-81
8. The Immune System BIO-91
9. The Digestive System BIO-97
10. The Excretory System BIO-105
11. The Musculoskeletal System BIO-113
12. The Respiratory System BIO-121
13. The Skin as an Organ System BIO-127
14. Reproduction and Development BIO-133
15. Genetics BIO-145
16. Evolution BIO-155

B.Organic Chemistry ORG-01

1. Molecular Structure of Organic Compounds ORG-03
2. Stereochemistry ORG-13

3. Alkanes ·· ORG-21
4. Alkenes* ·· ORG-29
5. Aromatics* ··· ORG-37
6. Alcohols ·· ORG-45
7. Aldehydes and Ketones ······················ ORG-53
8. Carboxylic Acids ·································· ORG-61
9. Carboxylic Acid Derivatives ················ ORG-67
10. Ethers and Phenols* ·························· ORG-75
11. Amines ·· ORG-81
12. Biological Molecules ·························· ORG-87
13. Separations and Purifications ············· ORG-101
14. Spectroscopy ······································ ORG-107

*Review of these 3 Organic Chemistry sections is optional since they are no longer required for the new MCAT. For more information, see Organic Chemistry section 4.0

APPENDICES TO THE GOLD STANDARD TEXT

Appendix A: MCAT Math Review ················· 427
Appendix B: The Imperial and Metric Systems ······· 435
Appendix C: The Experiment ···················· 437
Appendix D: Study Aids for the MCAT ········· 439

Part V: GOLD STANDARD MCAT* EXAMS

1. The Gold Standard MCAT ···················· 443
2. Practice Test GS-1 ····························· GS1-1
3. Practice Test GS-2 ····························· GS2-1
4. Practice Test GS-3 ····························· GS3-1

Part VI: ANSWER KEYS & ANSWER DOCUMENTS

1. Cross-referenced Answer Keys ·············· AK-1
2. Answer Documents ···························· AK-7
3. Understanding GS-1 ·························· AK-37
4. Understanding GS-2 ·························· AK-83
5. Understanding GS-3 ·························· AK-123
6. Understanding The Writing Sample ········ AK-165

INTRODUCTION

As a rule, in order to maximize your chances of gaining admission to medical school you must show excellence in each of the following areas: academic standing, personal interviews, autobiographical materials, letters of reference, and the *new* Medical College Admission Test (MCAT). Each university will emphasize different aspects of these five areas. This textbook will give you strategies to excel in all aspects of the admission process.

First we will discuss how to improve your academic standing. High academic achievement is a principal criterion for further consideration for admission to most medical schools. Next we will examine strategies, preparation, and sample questions to help you plan for the often critically important medical school interview. We will then review the importance of autobiographical materials and letters of reference. Finally, we will address the new MCAT.

The *new* MCAT is a half day exam composed of four sections: (i) Verbal Reasoning, (ii) Physical Sciences (*physics and general chemistry*), (iii) Writing Sample (*two essays*), and (iv) Biological Sciences (*biology and organic chemistry*).

The *new* MCAT will be exposed section by section. Exam-taking tips for the *new* MCAT, the *Recipe for MCAT Success*, and a review for Verbal Reasoning and the Writing Sample will all be explored. After which, a comprehensive and fully illustrated science review will follow. The science review contains physics, general chemistry, biology, and organic chemistry - all in the necessary detail. Chapter review questions and 3 MCAT CBTs are online or you can use the super length practice tests in this textbook. Thus the information you learned will be put into practice. You will also have online access to 10 hours of teaching videos which most students find very helpful. Be sure to register at www.MCAT-prep.com by clicking on Free MCAT and following the directions for Gold Standard MCAT owners.

Before you begin, some words born from experience: (i) most students study too much *and* too little for the MCAT. The typical case is the student who studies way too much detail in the area of their expertise, while neglecting subjects they never liked (i.e. the biology student studies extra genetics while failing to memorize basic physics equations); (ii) some students feel they should not do a practice exam until they have studied every topic known to mankind! Remember the following when designing your study schedule: doing practice exams is a learning experience equal in importance to your science review; (iii) the learning experience includes Verbal Reasoning and the Writing Sample; (iv) and finally, there is something beautiful about learning and about challenging yourself with new goals. If you enjoy this experience, you will achieve optimal results. If you have questions about The Gold Standard then go to the Forum at www.MCAT-prep.com. Let's begin...

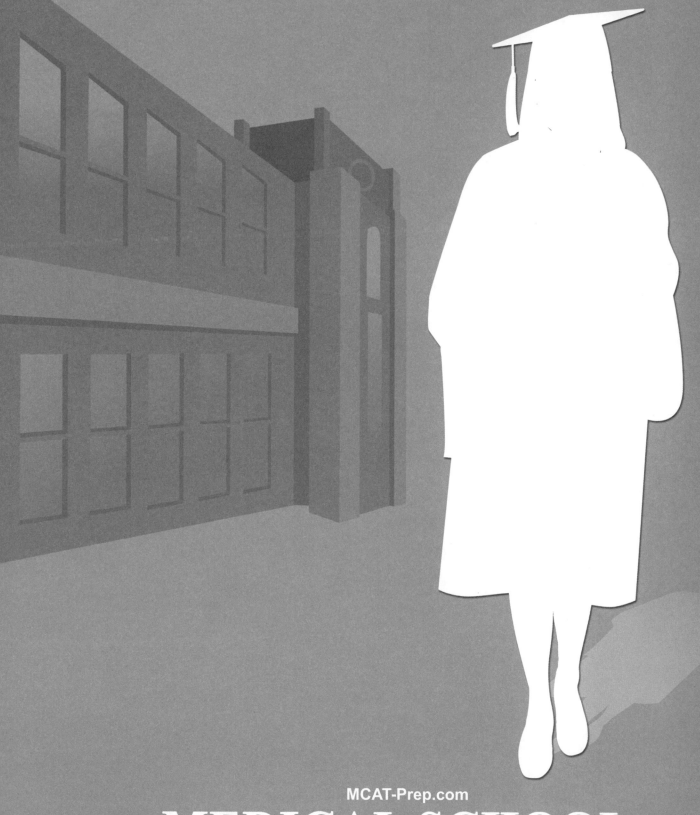

MCAT-Prep.com

MEDICAL SCHOOL ADMISSIONS

PART I

IMPROVING ACADEMIC STANDING

1.1 Lectures

Before you set foot in a classroom you should consider the value of being there. Even if you were taking a course like 'Basket-weaving 101', one way to help you do well in the course is to consider the <u>value</u> of the course to **you**. The course should have an *intrinsic* value (i.e. 'I enjoy weaving baskets'). The course will also have an *extrinsic* value (i.e. 'If I do not get good grades, I will not be accepted...'). <u>Motivation</u>, a <u>positive attitude</u>, and an <u>interest in learning</u> give you an edge before the class even begins.

Unless there is a student 'note-taking club' for your courses, your <u>attendance record</u> and the <u>quality of your notes</u> should both be as excellent as possible. Be sure to choose seating in the classroom which ensures that you will be able to hear the professor adequately and see whatever she may write. Whenever possible, do not sit close to friends!

Instead of chattering before the lecture begins, spend the idle moments quickly reviewing the previous lecture in that subject so you would have an idea of what to expect. Try to <u>take good notes</u> and <u>pay close attention</u>. The preceding may sound like a difficult combination (esp. with professors who speak and write quickly); however, with practice you can learn to do it well.

And finally, do not let the quality of teaching affect your interest in the subject nor your grades! Do not waste your time during or before lectures complaining about how the professor speaks too quickly, does not explain concepts adequately, etc... When the time comes, you can mention such issues on the appropriate evaluation forms! In the meantime, consider this: despite the good or poor quality of teaching, there is always a certain number of students who **still** perform well. You must strive to count yourself among those students.

1.2 Taking Notes

Unless your professor says otherwise, if you take excellent notes and learn them inside out, you will *ace* his course.

Your notes should always be <u>up-to-date</u>, <u>complete</u>, and <u>separate</u> from other subjects.

To be safe, you should try to write everything! You can fill in any gaps by comparing your notes with those of your friends. You can create your own shorthand symbols or use standard ones. The following represents some useful symbols:

$|\cdot|$	*between*
=	*the same as*
≠	*not the same as*
∴	*therefore*
cf.	*compare*
Δ	*difference, change in*
$\bar{c}$ or w	*with*
$\bar{c}$out or w/o	*without*
esp.	*especially*
∵	*because*
i.e.	*that is*
e.g.	*for example*

Many students rewrite their notes at home. Should you decide to rewrite your notes, your time will be used efficiently if you are paying close attention to the information you are rewriting. In fact, a more useful technique is the following: during class, write your notes only on the right side of your binder. Later, rewrite the information from class in a complete but condensed form on the left side of the binder (*this condensed form should include* **mnemonics** *which we will discuss later*).

Some students find it valuable to use different color pens. Juggling pens in class may distract you from the content of the lecture. Different color pens would be more useful in the context of rewriting one's notes.

1.3 The Principles of Studying Efficiently

If you study efficiently, you will have enough time for extracurricular activities, movies, etc. The bottom line is that your time must be used efficiently and effectively.

During the average school day, time can be found during breaks, between classes, and after school to quickly review notes in a library or any other quiet place you can find on campus. Simply by using the available time in your school day, you can keep up to date with recent information.

You should design an individual study schedule to meet your particular needs. However, as a rule, a certain amount of time every evening should be set aside for more in depth studying. Weekends can be set aside for special projects and reviewing notes from the beginning.

On the surface, the idea of regularly reviewing notes from the beginning may sound like an insurmountable task which would take forever! The reality is just the opposite. After all, if you continually study the information, by the time mid-terms approach you would have seen the first lecture so many times that it would take only moments to review it again. On the other hand, had you not been reviewing regularly, it would be like reading that lecture for the first time!

You should study wherever you are <u>comfortable</u> and <u>effective</u> studying (i.e. library, at home, etc.). Should you prefer studying at home, be sure to create an environment which is conducive to studying.

Studying should be an active process to <u>memorize</u> and <u>understand</u> a given set of material. Memorization and comprehension are best achieved by the **elaboration** of course material, **attention, repetition,** and practising **retrieval** of the information. All these principles are borne out in the following techniques.

1.4 Studying from Notes and Texts

Successful studying from either class notes or textbooks can be accomplished in three simple steps:

* **Preview the material**: read all the relevant headings, titles, and sub-titles to give you a general idea of what you are about to learn. You should never embark on a trip without knowing where you are going!

* **Read while questioning**: <u>passive studying</u> is when you sit in front of a book and just read. This can lead to boredom, lack of concentration, or even worse - difficulty remembering what you just read! <u>Active studying</u> involves reading while actively questioning yourself. For example: how does this fit in with the 'big picture'? How does this relate to what we learned last week? What cues about these words or lists will make it easy for me to memorize them? What type of question would my professor ask me? If I was asked a question on this material, how would I answer? Etc...

* **Recite and consider**: put the notes or text away while you attempt to <u>recall</u> the main facts. Once you are able to recite the important information, <u>consider</u> how it relates to the entire subject.

<u>N.B.</u> if you ever sit down to study and you are not quite sure with which subject to begin, always start with either the most difficult subject or the subject you like least (usually they are one in the same!).

1.5 Study Aids

The most effective study aids include practice exams, mnemonics and audio MP3s.

Practice exams (*exams from previous semesters*) are often available from the library, upper level students, or sometimes from the professor. They can be used like maps which guide you through your semester. They give you a good indication as to what information you should emphasize when you study; what question types and exam format you can expect; and what your level of progress is.

One practice exam should be set aside to do one week before 'the real thing.' You should time yourself and do the exam in an environment free from distractions. This provides an ideal way to uncover unexpected weak points.

Mnemonics are an effective way of memorizing lists of information. Usually a word, phrase, or sentence is constructed to symbolize a greater amount of information (i.e. LEO is A GERC = Lose Electrons is Oxidation is Anode, Gain Electrons is Reduction at Cathode). An effective study aid to active studying is the creation of your own mnemonics.

Audio MP3s can be used as effective tools to repeat information and to use your time efficiently. Information from the left side of your notes (*see 1.2 Taking Notes*) including mnemonics, can be dictated and recorded. Often, an entire semester of work can be summarized into one 90 minute recording.

Now you can listen to the recording on an iPod while waiting in line at the bank, or in a bus or with a car stereo on the way to school, work, etc. You can also listen to recorded information when you go to sleep and listen to another one first thing in the morning. You are probably familiar with the situation of having heard a song early in the morning and then having difficulty, for the rest of the day, getting it out of your mind! Well, imagine if the first thing you heard in the morning was: "Hair is a modified keratinized structure produced by the cylindrical down growth of epithelium..."! Thus MP3s become an effective study aid since they are an extra source of repetition.

Some students like to **record lectures**. Though it may be helpful to fill in missing notes, it is not an efficient way to repeat information.

Some students like to use **study cards** (flashcards) on which they may write either a summary of information they must memorize or relevant questions to consider. Then the cards are used throughout the day to quickly flash information to promote thought on course material.

1.5.1 Falling Behind

Imagine yourself as a marathon runner who has run 25.5 km of a 26 km race. The finishing line is now in view. However, you have fallen behind some of the other runners. The most difficult aspect of the race is still ahead.

In such a scenario some interesting questions can be asked: Is now the time to drop out of the race because 0.5 km suddenly seems like a long distance? Is now the time to reevaluate whether or not you should have competed? Or is now the time to remain faithful to your goals and give 100%?

Imagine one morning in mid-semester you wake up realizing you have fallen behind in your studies. What do you do? Where do you start? Is it too late?

Like a doctor being presented with an urgent matter, you should see the situation as one of life's challenges. Now is the worst time for doubts, rather, it is the time for action. A clear line of action should be formulated such that it could be followed.

For example, one might begin by gathering all pertinent study materials like a complete set of study notes, relevant text(s), sample exams, etc. As a rule, to get back into the thick of things, notes and sample exams take precedence. Studying at this point should take a three pronged approach: i) a regular, consistent review of the information from your notes from the beginning of the section for which you are responsible (i.e. *starting with the first class*); ii) a regular, consistent review of course material as you are learning it from the lectures (*this is the most efficient way to study*); iii) regular testing using questions given in class or those contained in sample exams. Using such questions will clarify the extent of your progress.

It is also of value, as time allows, to engage in extracurricular activities which you find helpful in reducing stress (i.e. sports, piano, creative writing, etc.).

THE MEDICAL SCHOOL INTERVIEW

2.1 Introduction

The application process to most medical schools includes interviews. Only a select number of students from the applicant pool will be given an offer to be interviewed. The medical school interview is, as a rule, something that you *achieve*. In other words, after your school grades, MCAT scores and/or references and autobiographical materials have been reviewed, you are offered the ultimate opportunity to put your foot forward: a personalized interview.

Depending on the medical school, you may be interviewed by one, two or several interviewers. You may be the only interviewee or there may be others (i.e., *a group interview*). There may be one or more interviews lasting from 20 minutes to two hours. Despite the variations among the technical aspects of the interview, in terms of substance, most medical schools have similar objectives. These objectives can be arbitrarily categorized into three general assessments: (i) your personality traits, (ii) social skills, and (iii) knowledge of medicine.

Personality traits such as maturity, integrity, compassion, sincerity, honesty, originality, curiosity, self-directed learning, intellectual capacity, confidence (*not arrogance!*), and motivation are all components of the ideal applicant. These traits will be exposed by the process of the interview, your mannerisms, and the substance of what you choose to discuss when given an ambiguous question. For instance, bringing up *specific* examples of academic achievement related to school and related to self-directed learning would score well in the categories of intellectual capacity and curiosity, respectively.

Motivation is a personality trait which may make the difference between a high and a low or moderate score in an interview. A student must clearly demonstrate that they have the enthusiasm, desire, energy, and interest to survive (typically) four long years of medical school and beyond! If you are naturally shy or soft-spoken, you will have to give special attention to this category.

Social skills such as leadership, ease of communication, ability to relate to others and work effectively in groups, volunteer work, cultural and social interests, all constitute skills which are often viewed as critical for future physicians. It is not sufficient to say in an interview: "I have good social skills"! You must display such skills via your interaction with the interviewer(s) and by discussing specific examples of situations which clearly demonstrate your social skills.

Knowledge of medicine includes <u>at least</u> a general understanding of what the field of medicine involves, the curriculum you are applying to, and a knowledge of popular medical issues like abortion, euthanasia, AIDS, the health care system, etc. It is striking to see the number of students who apply to medical school each year whose knowledge of medicine is limited to headlines and popular TV shows! It is not logical for someone to dedicate their lives to a profession they know little about.

Doing volunteer work in a hospital is a good start. Alternatively, getting a part-time job in a hospital or having a relative who is a physician can help expose you to the daily goings-on in a hospital setting. An even better strategy to be informed is the following: (i) keep up-to-date with the details of medically related controversies in the news. You should also be able to develop and support opinions of your own; (ii) skim through a medical journal at least once; (iii) read the medical section of a popular science magazine (i.e. Scientific American, Discover, etc.); (iv) keep abreast of changes in medical school curricula in general and specific to the programs to which you have applied. You can access such information at most university libraries and by writing individual medical schools for information on their programs; (v) do a First-Aid course.

2.2 Preparing for the Interview

If you devote an adequate amount of time for interview preparation, the actual interview will be less tense for you and <u>you</u> will be able to control most of the content of the interview.

Reading from the various sources mentioned in the preceding sections would be helpful. Also, read over your curriculum vitae and/or any autobiographical materials you may have prepared. Note highlights in your life or specific examples that demonstrate the aforementioned personality traits, social skills or your knowledge of medicine. Zero in on qualities or stories which are either important, memorable, interesting, amusing, informative or "all of the above"! Once in the interview room, you will be given the opportunity to elaborate on the qualities you believe are important about yourself.

Call the medical school and ask them about the structure of the interview (i.e., one-on-one, group, etc.) and ask them if they can tell you who will interview you. Many schools have no qualms volunteering such information. Now you can determine the person's expertise by either asking or looking through staff members of the different faculties or medical specialties at that university or college. A cardiac surgeon, a volunteer from the community, and a medical ethicist all have different areas of expertise and will likely orient their interviews differently. Thus you may want to read from a source which will give you a general understanding of their specialty.

Choose appropriate clothes for the interview. Every year some students dress for a medical school interview as if they were going out to dance! Medicine is still considered a conservative profession, you should dress and groom yourself likewise. First impressions are very important. Your objective is to make it as easy as possible for your interviewer(s) to imagine you as a physician.

Do practice interviews with people you respect but who can also maintain their objectivity. Let them read this entire chapter on medical school interviews. They must understand that you are to be evaluated *only* on the basis of the interview. On that basis alone, one should be able to imagine the ideal candidate as a future physician.

2.3 Strategies for Answering Questions

Always remember that the interviewer controls the *direction* of the interview by his questions; you control the *content* of the interview through your answers. In other words, once given the opportunity, you should speak about the topics that are important to you; conversely, you should avoid volunteering information which renders you uncomfortable. You can enhance the atmosphere in which the answers are delivered by being polite, sincere, tactful, well-organized, outwardly oriented and maintaining eye contact. Motivation, enthusiasm, and a positive attitude must all be evident.

As a rule, there are no right or wrong answers. However, the way in which you justify your opinions, the topics you choose to discuss, your mannerisms and your composure all play important roles. It is normal to be nervous. It would be to your advantage to channel your nervous energy into a positive quality, like enthusiasm.

Do not spew forth answers! Take your time - it is not a contest to see how fast you can answer. Answering with haste can lead to disastrous consequences as happened to a student I interviewed:

Q: *Have you ever doubted your interest in medicine as a career?*
A: *No!*
    Well,...ah...I guess so. Ah ... I guess everyone doubts something at some point or the other...

Retractions like that are a bad signal but it illustrates an important point: there are usually no right or wrong answers in an interview; however, there are right or wrong ways of answering. Through the example we can conclude the following: listen carefully to the question, try to relax, and think before you answer!

Do not sit on the fence! If you avoid giving your opinions on controversial topics, it will be interpreted as indecision which is a negative trait for a prospective physician. You have a right to your opinions. However, you must be prepared to defend your point of view in an objective, rational, and informative fashion. It is also important to show that, despite your opinion, you understand both sides of the argument. If you have an extreme or unconventional perspective and if you believe your perspective will not interfere with your practice of medicine, you must let your interviewer know that.

For example, imagine a student who was against abortion under *any* circumstance. If asked about her opinion on abortion, she should clearly state her opinion objectively, show she understands the opposing viewpoint, and then use data to reinforce her position. If she felt that her opinion would not interfere with her objectivity when practising medicine, she might volunteer: "If I were in a position where my perspective might interfere with an objective management of a patient, I would refer that patient to another physician."

Carefully note the reactions of the interviewer in response to your answers. Whether the interviewer is sitting on the edge of her seat wide-eyed or slumping in her chair while yawning, you should take such cues to help you determine when to continue, change the subject, or when to stop talking. Also, note the more subtle cues. For example, gauge which topic makes the interviewer frown, give eye contact, take notes, etc.

Lighten up the interview with a well-timed story. A conservative joke, a good analogy, or anecdote may help you relax and make the interviewer sustain his interest. If it is done correctly, it can turn a routine interview into a memorable and friendly interaction.

It should be noted that because the system is not standardized, a small number of interviewers may ask overly personal questions (i.e., about relationships, religion, etc.) or even questions which carry sexist tones (i.e., *What would you do if you got pregnant while attending medical school?*). Some questions may be frankly illegal. If you do not want to answer a question, simply maintain your composure, express your position diplomatically, and address the interviewers real concern (i.e. *Does this person have the potential to be a good doctor?*). For example, you might say in a non-confrontational tone of voice: "I would rather not answer such a question. However, I can assure you that whatever my answer may have been, it would in no way affect either my prospective studies in medicine nor any prerequisite objectivity I should have to be a good physician."

2.4 Sample Questions

There are an infinite number of questions and many different categories of questions. Different medical schools will emphasize different categories of questions. Arbitrarily, ten categories of questions can be defined: ambiguous, medically related, academic, social, stress-type, problem situations, personality oriented, based on autobiographical material, miscellaneous, and ending questions. We will examine each category in terms of sample questions and general comments.

Ambiguous Questions:

* *   *Tell me about yourself.*
       How do you want me to remember you?
       What are your goals?
       There are hundreds if not thousands of applicants, why should we choose you?
       Convince me that you would make a good doctor.
       Why do you want to study medicine?

COMMENTS: These questions present nightmares for the unprepared student who walks into the interview room and is immediately asked: "Tell me about yourself." Where do you start? If you are prepared as previously discussed, you will be able to take control of the interview by highlighting your qualities or objectives in an informative and interesting manner.

Medically Related Questions:

What are the pros and cons to our health care system?
If you had the power, what changes would you make to our health care system?
Do doctors make too much money?
Is it ethical for doctors to strike?
What is the Hippocratic Oath?
Should fetal tissue be used to treat disease (i.e. Parkinson's)?
If you were a doctor and an under age girl asked you for the Pill (or an abortion) and she did not want to tell her parents, what would you do?
Should doctors be allowed to 'pull the plug' on terminally ill patients?
If a patient is dying from a bleed, would you transfuse blood if you knew they would not approve (i.e. Jehovah Witness)?

COMMENTS: The health care system, euthanasia, cloning, abortion, and other ethical issues are very popular topics in this era of technological advances, skyrocketing health care costs, and ethical uncertainty. A well-informed opinion can set you apart from most of the other interviewees.

Questions Related to Academics:

Why did you choose your present course of studies?

What is your favorite subject in your present course of studies? Why?

Would you consider a career in your present course of studies?

Can you convince me that you can cope with the workload in medical school?

How do you study/prepare for exams?

Do you engage in self-directed learning?

COMMENTS: Medical schools like to see applicants who are well-disciplined, committed to medicine as a career, and who exhibit self-directed learning (i.e. such a level of desire for knowledge that the student may seek to study information independent of any organized infrastructure). Beware of any glitches in your academic record. You may be asked to give reasons for any grades they may deem substandard. On the other hand, you should volunteer any information regarding academic achievement (i.e. prizes, awards, scholarships, particularly high grades in one subject or the other, etc.).

Questions Related to Social Skills or Interests:

Give evidence that you relate well with others.

Give an example of a leadership role you have assumed.

Have you done any volunteer work?

What would you do as President of the United States with respect to the trade imbalance with Japan?

How would you address Canada's constitutional crisis?

What are the prospects for a lasting peace in Afghanistan? Eastern Europe? the Sudan? the Middle-East?

What do you think of the free-trade agreement between Canada, the United States and Mexico?

COMMENTS: Questions concerning social skills should be simple for the prepared student. If you are asked a question that you cannot answer, say so. If you pretend to know something about a topic in which you are completely uninformed, you will make a bad situation worse.

Stress-Type Questions:

How do you handle stress?

What was the most stressful event in your life? How did you handle it?

The night before your final exam, your father has a heart-attack and is admitted to a hospital, what do you do?

COMMENTS: The ideal physician has positive coping methods to deal with the inevitable stressors of a medical practice. Stress-type questions are a legitimate means of determining if you possess the raw material necessary to cope with medical school and medicine as a career. Some interviewers go one step further. They may decide to introduce stress into the interview and see how you handle it. For example, they may decide to ask you a confrontational question or try to back you into a corner (i.e. *You do not know anything about medicine, do you?*). Alternatively, the interviewer might use silence to introduce stress into the interview. If you have completely and confidently answered a question and silence falls in the room, do not retract previous statements, mutter, or fidget. Simply wait for the next question. If the silence becomes unbearable, you may consider asking an intelligent question (i.e. a specific question regarding their curriculum).

Questions on Problem Situations:

A 68 year-old married woman has a newly discovered cancer. Her life expectancy is 6 months. How would you inform her?
A 34 year-old man presents with AIDS and tells you, as his physician, that he does not want to tell his wife. What would you do?
You are playing tennis with your best friend and the ball hits your friend in the eye. What do you do?

COMMENTS: As for the other questions, listen carefully and take your time to consider the best possible response. Keep in mind that the ideal physician is not only knowledgeable, but is also compassionate, empathetic, and is objective enough to understand both sides of a dilemma. Be sure such qualities are clearly demonstrated.

Personality-Oriented Questions:

If you could change one thing about yourself, what would it be?
How would your friends describe you?
What do you do with your spare time?
What is the most important event that has occurred to you in the last five years?
If you had three magical wishes, what would they be?
What are your best attributes?

COMMENTS: Of course, most questions will assess your personality to one degree or the other. However, these questions are quite direct in their approach. Forewarned is forearmed!

Question Based on Autobiographical Materials:

COMMENTS: Any autobiographical materials you may have provided to the medical schools is fair game for questioning. You may be asked to discuss or elaborate on any point the interviewer may feel is interesting or questionable.

Miscellaneous Questions:

Should the federal government reinstate the death penalty? Explain.
What do you expect to be doing 10 years from now?

How would you attract physicians to rural areas?
Why do you want to attend our medical school?
What other medical schools have you applied to?
Have you been to other interviews?

COMMENTS: You will do fine in this grab-bag category as long as you stick to the strategies previously iterated.

Ending Questions:

What would you do if you were not accepted to a medical school?
How do you think you did in this interview?
Do you have any questions?

COMMENTS: The only thing more important than a good first impression is a good finish in order to leave a positive lasting impression. They are looking for students who are so committed to medicine that they will not only re-apply to medical school if not accepted, but they would also strive to improve on those aspects of their application which prevented them from being accepted in the first attempt. All these questions should be answered with a quiet confidence. If you are given an opportunity to ask questions, though you should not flaunt your knowledge, you should establish that you are well-informed. For example: "I have read that you have changed your curriculum to a more patient-oriented and self-directed learning approach. I was wondering how the medical students are getting along with these new changes." Be sure, however, not to ask a question unless you are genuinely interested in the answer.

2.5 Interview Feedback

Many students wish to have access to specific interview questions at the institutions to which they have applied for admission. This information is now available online at www. studentdoctor.net. In the near future, you will be able to access similar information at www.medschool-prep.com.

AUTOBIOGRAPHICAL MATERIALS AND REFERENCES

3.1 Autobiographical Materials

Most medical schools require autobiographical materials as important components of the application process. Autobiographical materials include essays, letters, sketches, or questionnaires where you are given the opportunity to write about yourself. Autobiographical materials are a sort of *written interview*. Thus the same objectives, preparation, and strategies apply as previously mentioned for interviews. However, there are some unique factors.

For example, you can begin writing long in advance of the deadline. The ideal way to prepare is to have a few sheets of paper at home which you continually write any accomplishments or interesting experiences you have had anytime in your life! By starting this process early, months later you should, hopefully(!), have a long list from which to choose information appropriate for the autobiographical materials. Your resume or curriculum vitae may also be of value.

Be sure to write rough drafts and have qualified individuals proofread it for you. Spelling and grammatical errors should not exist.

The document should be written on the appropriate paper and/or in the format as stated in the directions. Do not surpass your word and/or space limit. Ideally, the document would be prepared on a word processor and then laser printed. The document should be so pretty that your parents should want to frame it and hang it in the living room! Handwritten or typed material with 'liquid paper' or 'white-out' is simply not impressive.

Your document must be clearly organized. If you are given directive questions then organization should not be a problem. However, if you are given open-ended questions or if you are told, for example, to write a 1000 word essay about yourself, adequate organization is key. There are two general ways you can organize such a response: *chronological* or *thematic*. However, they are not mutually exclusive.

In a **chronological** response, you are organized by doing a systematic review of important events through time. In writing an essay or letter, one could start with an interesting or amusing story from childhood and then highlight important events chronologically and in concordance with the instructions.

In the **thematic** approach a general theme is presented from the outset and then verified through examples at any time in your life. For example, imagine the following statement somewhere in the introduction of an autobiographical letter/essay:

My concept of the good physician is one who has a solid intellectual capacity, extensive social skills, and a creative ability. I have strived to attain and demonstrate such skills.

Following such an introduction to a thematic response, the essayist can link events from anytime to the general theme of the essay. Each theme would thus be examined in turn.

And finally, keep in mind the advice given for interviews since much of it applies here as well. For example, the appropriate use of an amusing story, anecdote, or an interesting analogy can make your document an interesting one to read. And, as for interviews, specific examples are more memorable than overly generalized statements.

3.2 Letters of Reference

Letters of reference (a.k.a. *assessments* which are written by *referees*) are required by most medical schools. It provides an opportunity for an admissions committee to see what other people think of you. Consequently, it is often viewed as an important aspect of your application package.

Choose the people who will submit your letter of reference in accordance with instructions from the medical schools to which you are applying. If no such instructions are given, then construct a list of possible referees. Choose from this list individuals who: (i) you can trust; (ii) are reliable; (iii) can write, at least, reasonably well; (iv) understand the importance of your application; and (v) can present with some confidence attributes you have which are consistent with those of a good physician.

Often students either want or are told to have someone as a referee who they do not know well (i.e. a professor). In such a case choose your referee prudently. If they agree to give you a recommendation, give them your resume, curriculum vitae, or any other autobiographical materials you may have. Alternatively, you may ask to arrange a mini-interview. Either way, you would have armed your referee with information which can be used in a specific and personal manner in the letter of reference.

People are not paid to write you a

letter of reference! Therefore, make it as easy as possible for them. Give them an ample amount of time before the deadline for submission. Also, supply them with a stamped envelope with the appropriate address inscribed. Besides being the polite thing to do, they may also be impressed by your organization. And finally, once the letter of reference has been sent, do not forget to send a "Thank-you" card to your referee.

THE DIRECTORY OF NORTH AMERICAN MEDICAL SCHOOLS

4.1 Overview

The ideal way to get an adequate amount of information about medical schools and their admission policies is to call or write the individual medical schools to which you would like to apply. Subsequently, they may send you letters responding to your questions, pamphlets or other documents which will enlighten your knowledge of each specific school. Visiting the internet sites of medical schools that interest you can also provide significant information regarding their programs and admission policies. The best way to access the various medical school internet sites is through www.aamc.org.

If it is important to you how a medical school rates worldwide, you can consult the *Gourman Report* which is available at most large university libraries. Special editions of the *U.S. News and World Report* and *Maclean's Magazine* (in Canada) also rate university programs. If you want statistical information on the medical schools and admissions in the United States and Canada, the latest edition of *Medical School Admission Requirements* may be helpful. It is available from the AAMC (*see Section 1.5 for the address*). In Canada, such information is detailed in *The Black Book on Canadian Medical Schools* (*see* Bookstore at www.MCAT-prep.com).

4.1.1 Application Services

Application services for the admission process help to filter and standardize information for the participating medical schools. Application services do not render admission decisions; rather, they provide a processing service. In the U.S., approximately 110 of the 126 medical schools participate in the American Medical College Application Service (AMCAS). AMCAS application materials may be obtained from premedical advisors, participating medical schools or you may write or make contact online:

AMCAS, Section for Student Services
Association of American Medical Colleges
2501 M Street, N.W., Lbby-26
Washington, D.C. 20037-1300
Phone: (202) 828-0600
Web site: www.aamc.org

There is also an application service

in Canada. However, eleven of the sixteen Canadian medical schools have individualized application procedures. The five medical schools in the Province of Ontario participate in the Ontario Medical School Application Service (OMSAS). OMSAS application materials may be obtained from participating medical schools or you may write or make contact online:

OMSAS
P.O. Box 1328
650 Woodlawn Rd. West
Guelph, Ontario

Canada, N1H 7P4
Web site: www.ouac.on.ca

Some medical schools that participate in application services may *also* have their own applications to fill out. Thus despite the existence of application services, nothing can replace the importance of contacting specific medical schools to be informed about their programs, policies, tuition, admission requirements, application procedures, etc. For any medical school that may interest you, *as early as possible* you should write and clarify, among other issues, their application procedures.

4.2 The Medical Schools in North America

American Medical Schools
Alphabetized by State

Office of Medical Student Services/ Admissions
University of Alabama at Birmingham School of Medicine
VH-100, Birmingham, AL   35294
205-934-2330; 205-934-0333 (FAX)
http://www.uab.edu/uasom/

Office of Admissions, University of South Alabama College of Medicine
307 University Boulevard, Mobile, AL 36688-0002
334-460-7176; 334-460-6761 (FAX)
http://southmed.usouthal.edu/index.html

Office of Student Admissions, Slot 551
University of Arkansas for Medical Sciences, College of Medicine
4301 West Markham Street, Little Rock, AR 72205-7199
501-686-5354; 501-686-5873 (FAX)
http://www.uams.edu

Admissions Office, University of Arizona College of Medicine
Tucson, AZ   85721
520-626-6214; 520-626-7382 (FAX)
http://www.ahsc.arizona.edu/com.shtlm/

Admissions Office, University of California, Davis School of Medicine
Davis, CA   95616
530-752-2717; 916-752-1532 (FAX)
http://www-med.ucdavis.edu/

Office of Student Affairs, Division of Admissions, University of California, Los Angeles
UCLA School of Medicine, Center for Health Sciences
405 Hilgard Avenue, Los Angeles, CA 90095
310-825-6081; 310-825-4955 (FAX)
http://www.medsch.ucla.edu/

Office of Admissions, 0621, Medical Teaching Facility
University of California, San Diego School of Medicine
9500 Gilman Drive, La Jolla, CA 92093-5003
619-534-3880; 619-822-0084 (FAX)
http://medicine.ucsd.edu/

Office of Admissions, University of California, Irvine College of Medicine
118 Med Surge I, Irvine, CA 92717-3952
949-824-5388; 800-824-5388; 949-824-2083 (FAX)
http://meded.com.uci.edu/

Associate Dean for Admissions, Loma Linda University School of Medicine
Loma Linda, CA 92350
909-824-4467; 909-824-4146 (FAX)
http://www.llu.edu/llu/medicine/

Office of Admissions, Stanford University School of Medicine
851 Welch Road, Room 154, Stanford, CA 94305-9991
650-723-6861; 415-723-7796 (FAX)
http://www.med.stanford.edu/school/

Admissions, University of California, San Francisco School of Medicine
C-200, Box 0408, San Francisco, CA 94143
415-476-2342; 415-476-1734 (FAX)

Office of Admissions, University of Southern California School of Medicine
University Park Campus, 1975 Zonal Avenue, Los Angeles, CA 90089
323-342-6444; 213-342-6442 (FAX)

Office of Admissions and Records, University of Colorado Health Sciences Center School of Medicine
4200 East 9th Avenue, Denver, CO 80262
303-315-7565; 303-315-8494 (FAX)
http://www.uchsc.edu/sm/sm/

Office of Admissions and Student Affairs, University of Connecticut Health Center School of Medicine
263 Farmington Avenue, Farmington, CT 06030
860-679-2413; 860-679-1282 (FAX)
http://www.uchc.edu/

Office of Admissions, Yale University School of Medicine
367 Cedar Street, New Haven, CT 06520
203-785-4672; 203-785-7437 (FAX)
http://info.med.yale.edu/medical/

Office of Admissions, The George Washington University School of Medicine and Health Sciences
2300 Eye Street, Washington, DC 20052
202-994-3727; 202-994-0926 (FAX)
http://www.gwumc.edu/edu

Admissions Office, Howard University College of Medicine
520 W Street, NW, Washington, DC   20059
202-806-6270; 202-806-7934 (FAX)
http://www.med.howard.edu/

Office of Admissions, Georgetown University School of Medicine
3900 Reservoir Road, NW, Washington, DC 20007
202-687-1612

Office of Admissions, University of Miami School of Medicine
PO Box 016159, Coral Gables, FL   33101
305-243-6791; 305-243-4888 (FAX)
http://www.med.miami.edu/

Chairman, Medical Selection Committee, University of Florida College of Medicine
PO Box 118140, 302 Little Hall, Gainesville, FL   32611-8140
352-392-4569; 352-392-6482 (FAX)
http://www.med.ufl.edu/

Office of Admissions, University of South Florida College of Medicine
4202 East Fowler Avenue, Tampa, FL 33620-9951
813-974-4181; 813-974-3886 (FAX)
http://www.med.usf.edu/

Admissions and Student Affairs, Morehouse School of Medicine
720 Westview Drive, SW, Atlanta, GA 30310-1495
404-752-1650; 404-752-1512 (FAX)
http://www.msm.edu/

Medical School Admissions, Emory University School of Medicine
Woodruff Health Sciences Center, Room 303, Atlanta, GA   30322
404-727-5660; 404-727-0473 (FAX)
http://www.emory.edu/WHSC/MED

Associate Dean for Admissions, Medical College of Georgia School of Medicine
AA-2040, 1120 Fifteenth Street, Augusta, GA 30912-1003
706-721-3186; 706-721-0959 (FAX)
http://www.mcg.edu
sclmed.stdadmin@mail.mcg.edu

Office of Admissions and Student Affairs, Mercer University School of Medicine
1550 College Street, Macon, GA 31207-0003
912-752-2524; 912-752-2547 (FAX)
http://gain.mercer.edu/musm

Office of Admissions, University of Hawaii John A. Burns School of Medicine
2444 Dole Street, Honolulu, HI   96822
808-956-5446; 808-956-5506 (FAX)
http://medworld.biomed.hawaii.edu

Director of Admissions, The University of Iowa College of Medicine
100 CMAB, Iowa City, IA   52242
319-335-8052; 319-335-8049 (FAX)
http://www.medicine.uiowa.edu
medical-admissions@uiowa.edu

Office of Admissions, Rush University Medical College
600 South Paulina Street, Chicago, IL

60612
312-942-6913; 312-942-2333 (FAX)
medcol@rush.edu

Associate Dean for Admissions,
Northwestern University Medical School
303 East Chicago Avenue, Chicago, IL
60611
312-503-8206; 312-503-7757 (FAX)
http://www.nums.nwu.edu/

Office of the Dean of Students, University of
Chicago Pritzker School of Medicine
924 East 57th Street, Chicago, IL   60637
312-702-1939; 312-702-2598 (FAX)

Office of Admissions, Finch University of
Health Sciences/The Chicago Medical
School
3333 Green Bay Road, North Chicago, IL
60064
847-578-3206; 847-578-3284 (FAX)
http://www.finchcms.edu/

Office of Student and Alumni Affairs,
Southern Illinois University at Carbondale
School of Medicine
PO Box 19230, Springfield, IL   62794-9230
217-524-0326; 217-785-5538 (FAX)
http://www.siumed.edu/

Office of Admissions, Loyola University
Chicago Stritch School of Medicine
820 North Michigan Avenue, Chicago, IL
60611-2196
708-216-3229; 708-216-4305 (FAX)
http://www.meddean.luc.edu/

Office of Medical College Admissions,
University of Illinois at Chicago College of
Medicine
Room 165 CME M/C 783, 808 South Wood
Street, Chicago, IL   60680
312-996-5636; 312-996-6693 (FAX)
http://www.uic.edu/depts/mcam/

Admissions Office, Indiana University School
of Medicine
Fesler Hall 213, 1120 South Drive,
Indianapolis, IN   46202-5113
317-274-3772; 317-274-8439 (FAX)
http://www.iupui.edu/it/medschl/home.html
inmedadm@iupui.edu

Associate Dean for Admissions, University of
Kansas School of Medicine
3901 Rainbow Boulevard, Kansas City, KS
66160-7301
913-588-5245; 913-588-5259 (FAX)
http://www.kumc.edu/som/som.html

Admissions, Room MN-104, Office of
Education, University of Kentucky College of
Medicine
Chandler Medical Center, 800 Rose Street,
Lexington, KY   40536-0084
606-323-6161; 606-323-2076 (FAX)
http://www.comed.uky.edu/medicine/
welcome.html

Office of Admissions, University of Louisville
School of Medicine
Abell Administration Center, 323 East
Chestnut, Louisville, KY   40202-3866
502-852-5193; 502-852-6849 (FAX)
http://www.louisville.edu.medschool

medadm@ulkyvm.louisville.edu
Admissions Office, Louisiana State University School of Medicine in New Orleans
1901 Perdido Street, Box P3-4, New Orleans, LA 70112-1393
504-568-6262; 504-568-7701 (FAX)
http://www.medschool.lsumc.edu/

Office of Admissions, Tulane University School of Medicine
SL 67, 1430 Tulane Avenue, New Orleans, LA 70118-2699
504-588-5187; 504-584-2945 (FAX)
http://www.mcl.tulane.edu/
medsch@tmcpop.tmc.tulane.edu

Office of Student Admissions, Louisiana State University School of Medicine in Shreveport
PO Box 33932, Shreveport, LA 71130-3932
318-674-5190; 318-674-5244 (FAX)
http://www.sh.lsumc.edu/
shvadm@lsumc.edu

Admissions Office, Boston University School of Medicine
Building L, Room 124, 80 East Concord Street, Boston, MA 02218
617-638-4630; 617-638-5258 (FAX)
http://med-amsa.bu.edu/BUSM/

Office of the Committee on Admissions, Harvard University Medical School
25 Shattuck Street, Cambridge, MA 02115
617-432-1550; 617-432-3307 (FAX)
http://www.med.harvard.edu/
HMSADM@warren.med.harvard.edu

Director of Admissions, University of Massachusetts Medical School
55 Lake Avenue North, Worcester, MA 01655-0115
508-856-2323; 508-856-8181 (FAX)
http://www.umassmed.edu

Office of Admissions, Tufts University School of Medicine
136 Harrison Avenue, Stearns 1, Boston, MA 02111
617-636-6571; 617-636-0375 (FAX)
http://www.tufts.edu/med/
medadmissions@infonet.tufts.edu

Committee on Admissions, Johns Hopkins University School of Medicine
3400 North Charles Street, Baltimore, MD 21218-2699
410-955-3182; 410-955-0889 (FAX)
http://infonet.welch.jhu.edu/som/

Committee on Admissions, University of Maryland School of Medicine
655 West Baltimore Street, Baltimore, MD 21201-1559
410-706-7478
kalascio@schmedol.ab.umd.edu

Admissions Office, Uniformed Services University of the Health Sciences
F. Edward Hérbert School of Medicine
4301 Jones Bridge Road, Bethesda, MD 20814-4799
301-295-3101; 800-772-1743; 301-295-3545 (FAX)
http://www.usuhs.mil/

Director of Admissions, Wayne State University School of Medicine
540 East Canfield, Detroit, MI   48201
313-577-1466; 313-577-8777 (FAX)
http://www.wayne.edu/med.htm/

Admissions Office, University of Michigan Medical School
M4130 Medical Science Building I, Ann Arbor, MI   48109-0611
734-936-1508; 313-763-4936 (FAX)
http://www.med.umich.edu/medschool/grad/

Office of Admissions, Michigan State University College of Human Medicine
A-239 Life Sciences, East Lansing, MI 48824-1317
517-353-9620; 517-432-1051 (FAX)
http://www.chm.msu.edu/
mdadmissions@msu.edu

Office of Admissions and Student Affairs University of Minnesota-Twin Cities Campus Medical School-Minneapolis
Box 293-UHMC, 3-100 Owre Hall, 420 Delaware Street, Minneapolis, MN 55455-0310
612-624-1188; 612-626-4200 (FAX)
http://www.med.umn.edu
meded@tc.umn.edu

Admissions Committee, Mayo Medical School
200 First Street, SW, Rochester, MN   55905
507-284-3671; 507-284-2634 (FAX)

Office of Admissions, University of Minnesota-Duluth School of Medicine
10 University Drive, Duluth, MN   55812-2496
218-726-8511; 218-726-6235 (FAX)
http://www.d.umn.edu/medweb/

Admissions Committee, Saint Louis University School of Medicine
221 North Grand Boulevard, St. Louis, MO 63103-2097
314-577-8205; 314-577-8214 (FAX)
http://medschool.slu.edu

Council on Selection, University of Missouri-Kansas City School of Medicine
2411 Holmes, Kansas City, MO   64108
816-235-1870; 816-235-5277 (FAX)

Office of Admissions, University of Missouri-Columbia School of Medicine
MA202 Medical Sciences Building, One Hospital Dr., Columbia, MO   65212
573-882-2923; 573-884-4808 (FAX)
http://www.muhealth.org
Shari_L._Swindell@muccmail.missouri.edu

Office of Admissions, Washington University in St. Louis School of Medicine
660 South Euclid Avenue, Box 8107, St. Louis, MO   63110
314-362-6858; 314-367-6666 (FAX)
http://medschool.wustl.edu/
wumscoa@msnotes.wustl.edu

Chairman, Admissions Committee, University of Mississippi Medical Center School of Medicine
2500 North State Street, Jackson, MS 39216-4505
601-984-5010; 601-984-5008 (FAX)
http://umc.edu/

Committee on Admissions, Duke University School of Medicine
PO Box 3710, Durham, NC 27710
919-684-2985; 919-681-8893 (FAX)
http://www2.mc.duke.edu/som/

Office of Admissions, East Carolina University School of Medicine
East Fifth Street, Greenville, NC 27858-4354
252-816-2202; 919-816-3192 (FAX)
http://www.med.ecu.edu/

Admissions Office, University of North Carolina at Chapel Hill School of Medicine
CB #7000 MacNider Hall, Chapel Hill, NC 27599-7000
919-962-8331; 919-966-9930 (FAX)
http://www.med.unc.edu/

Office of Medical School Admissions, Wake Forest University Bowman Gray School of Medicine
Medical Center Boulevard, Winston-Salem, NC 27157-1090
336-716-4264; 336-716-5807 (FAX)
http://www.bgsm.edu

Secretary, Committee on Admissions, University of North Dakota School of Medicine
501 North Columbia Road, Grand Forks, ND 58202-9037
701-777-4221; 701-777-4942 (FAX)
http://www.med.und.nodak.edu/

Office of Academic Affairs, University of Nebraska Medical Center College of Medicine
Conkling Hall, Room 4004, 600 South 42nd Street, Omaha, NE 68198-4430
402-559-2259; 402-559-4148 (FAX)
http://www.unmc.edu

Admissions Office, Creighton University School of Medicine
2500 California Plaza, Omaha, NE 68178-0001
402-280-2799; 402-280-1241 (FAX)
http://medicine.creighton.edu/

Office of Admissions, Dartmouth College Medical School
7020 Remsen, Room 306, Hanover, NH 03755-3833
603-650-1505; 603-650-1614 (FAX)
http://www.dartmouth.edu/dms/

Office of Admissions, University of Medicine and Dentistry of New Jersey
Robert Wood Johnson Medical School, 675 Hoes Lane, Piscataway, NJ 08854
732-235-4576; 732-235-6315 (FAX)
http://www2.umdnj.edu/admrweb/

Director of Admissions, University of Medicine and Dentistry of New Jersey
New Jersey Medical School, 185 South Orange Avenue, Newark, NJ   07103
973-972-4631; 201-972-7986 (FAX)
http://www.umdnj.edu
njmsadmissumdnj.edu

Office of Admissions, University of New Mexico School of Medicine
Basic Sciences Medical Building, Room 107, Albuquerque, NM   87131-5166
505-277-4766; 505-277-2755 (FAX)

Office of Admissions and Student Affairs, University of Nevada School of Medicine
MS 357, Reno, NV   89557
702-784-6063; 702-784-6096 (FAX)
http://www.unr.edu/med/index.html

Office of Admissions, New York Medical College
Room 127, Valhalla, NY   10595
914-594-4507; 914-594-4145 (FAX)
http://www.nymc.edu/

Director of Admissions, University of Rochester School of Medicine and Dentistry
Medical Center Box 601, Rochester, NY 14642
716-275-4539; 716-256-1016 (FAX)
http://www.urmc.rochester.edu/smd/
mdaedmish@urmc.rochester.edu

Office of Medical Admissions, State University of New York at Buffalo School of Medicine
40 Biomedical Education Building, 3425 Main Street, Buffalo, NY   14214-3013
716-829-3467

Committee on Admissions, State University of New York at Stony Brook School of Medicine
Health Sciences Center, Level 4, Room 147, Stony Brook, NY   11794-8434
516-444-2113; 516-444-2202 (FAX)
http://www.uhmc.sunysb.edu/som/

Office of Admissions, New York University School of Medicine
PO Box 1924, New York, NY   10016
212-263-5290

Admissions Committee
State University of New York Health Science Center at Syracuse College of Medicine
155 Elizabeth Blackwell Street, Syracuse, NY   13210-2334
315-464-4570; 315-464-8867 (FAX)
http://www2.ec.hscsyr.edu/
Office of Admissions, Albany Medical College
47 New Scotland Avenue, Albany, NY   12208
518-262-5523; 518-262-5887 (FAX)
http://www.amc.edu/html/medical_college.html

Admissions Office, Columbia University College of Physicians and Surgeons
630 West 168th Street, New York, NY 10032
212-305-3595; 212-305-3545 (FAX)
http://cpmcnet.columbia.edu/dept/ps/

Director of Admissions
State University of New York Health Science Center at Brooklyn College of Medicine
450 Clarkson Avenue, Brooklyn, NY 11203-2098
718-270-2446; 718-270-4074 (FAX)
http://www.hscbklyn.edu/

Office for Admissions
Mount Sinai School of Medicine of the City University of New York
Annenberg Building, Room 5-04, Box 1002, One Gustave L. Levy Place
New York, NY   10029
212-241-6696; 212-410-6111 (FAX)
http://www.mssm.edu
admissions@mssm.edu

Office of Admissions
Yeshiva University Albert Einstein College of Medicine, Jack and Pearl Resnick Campus
1300 Morris Park Avenue, New York, NY 10461
718-430-2106; 718-430-8825 (FAX)
http://www.aecom.yu.edu
admissions@aecom.ye.edu

Office of Admissions, Cornell University Weill Medical College
445 East 69th Street, New York, NY   10021
212-746-1067; 212-746-8424 (FAX)
http://www.med.cornell.edu/
cumc-admiss@mail.med.cornell.edu

Admissions Committee, The Ohio State University College of Medicine and Public Health
370 West 9th Avenue, Columbus, OH 43210-1238
614-292-7137; 614-292-1544 (FAX)
http://www.med.ohio-state.edu/

Office of Student Affairs and Admissions, Wright State University School of Medicine
PO Box 1751, Dayton, OH   45401
937-775-2934; 937-775-3672 (FAX)
http://www.med.wright.edu

Office of Admissions and Educational Research
Northeastern Ohio Universities College of Medicine College of Medicine
4209 State Route 44, PO Box 95, Rootstown, OH   44272-0095
330-325-6270; 330-325-8372 (FAX)
http://www.neoucom.edu/

Office of Admissions, University of Cincinnati College of Medicine
231 Bethesda Avenue, PO Box 670552, Cincinnati, OH   45267-0552
513-558-7314; 513-558-1165 (FAX)
http://www.med.uc.edu/htdocs/medicine/uccom.htm

Associate Dean for Admissions and Student Affairs
Case Western Reserve University School of Medicine
2109 Adelbert Road, Cleveland, OH   44109
216-368-3450; 216-368-4621 (FAX)
http://mediswww.meds.cwru.edu/

Admissions Office, Medical College of Ohio
School of Medicine
PO Box 10008, Toledo, OH   43699-0008
419-381-4229; 419-381-4005 (FAX)
http://www.mco.edu

Director for Student Affairs, University of
Oklahoma Health Sciences Center College
of Medicine
PO Box 26901, Oklahoma City, OK   73190
405-271-2331; 405-271-3032 (FAX)
http://w3.uokhsc.edu/home/college/
medicine.html

Office of Education and Student Affairs,
Oregon Health Sciences University School
of Medicine
L102, 3181 SW Sam Jackson Park Road,
Portland, OR   97201-3098
503-494-4499; 503-494-3400 (FAX)
http://www.ohsu.edu/som

Office of Student Affairs, Pennsylvania State
University Milton S. Hershey
Medical Center College of Medicine, PO
Box 850, 500 University Drive, Hershey, PA
17033
717-531-8755; 717-531-5351 (FAX)
http://www.hmc.psu.edu

Admissions Office, Temple University School
of Medicine, Student Faculty Center
Suite 305, Broad and Ontario Streets,
Philadelphia, PA   19140
215-707-3656; 215-707-6932 (FAX)
http://www.temple.edu/medschool/
admission.html

Associate Dean for Student Affairs and
Admissions, Allegheny University of the
Health Sciences MCP
Hahnemann School of Medicine, 2900
Queen Lane, Philadelphia, PA   19129
215-991-8100; 215-843-1766 (FAX)
http://www.auhs.edu/homepage.html
admis@auhs.edu

Associate Dean for Admissions, Thomas
Jefferson University Jefferson Medical
College 1025 Walnut Street, Philadelphia,
PA   19107
215-955-6983; 215-923-6939 (FAX)
http://www.tju.edu
jmc.admissions@mail.tju.edu

Office of Admissions, University of Pittsburgh
School of Medicine
518 Scaife Hall, Pittsburgh, PA   15261
412-648-9891; 412-648-8768 (FAX)
http://www.dean-med.pitt.edu/

Director of Admissions and Financial
Aid, University of Pennsylvania School of
Medicine
Edward J. Stemmler Hall, Suite 100,
Philadelphia, PA   19104-6056
215898-8001; 215-898-0833 (FAX)
http://www.med.upenn.edu/

Office of Admissions, Universidad Central
del Caribe School of Medicine
Call Box 60-327, Bayamon, PR   00960-6032
787-740-1611; 787-269-7550 (FAX)

Admissions Office, Ponce School of Medicine
PO Box 7004, Ponce, PR   00732
787-840-2511; 787-840-9756 (FAX)

Central Admissions Office, University of Puerto Rico School of Medicine
PO Box 365067, San Juan, PR   00936-5067
787-758-2525 Ext. 1810;   787-756-8475 (FAX)
http://www.upr.clu.edu/index.html

Office of Admissions and Financial Aid, Brown University School of Medicine
Box G A212, 97 Waterman Street, Providence, RI   02912-9706
401-863-2149; 401-863-2660 (FAX)
http://biomed.brown.edu/Medicine.html
medschooladmissoins@brown.edu

Associate Dean for Student Services, University of South Carolina School of Medicine
Columbia, SC   29208
803-733-3325; 803-733-3328 (FAX)
http://www.med.sc.edu/

University Registrar and Director of Admissions, Medical University of South Carolina
College of Medicine, 171 Ashley Avenue, Charleston, SC   29425-0002
843-792-3281; 843-792-3764 (FAX)
http://www.musc.edu

Office of Student Affairs, University of South Dakota School of Medicine
Room 105, 414 East Clark Street, Vermillion, SD   57069-2390
605-677-5233; 605-677-5109 (FAX)
http://www.usd.edu/med/

Director, Admissions and Records, Meharry Medical College School of Medicine
1005 Dr. D B Todd Jr. Boulevard, Nashville, TN   37208-9989
615-327-6204; 615-327-6568 (FAX)
http://www.mmc.edu/sofm.htm
meharrysom@ccvax.mmc.edu

Admissions Office, University of Tennessee, Memphis College of Medicine
Room 307, 790 Madison Avenue, Memphis, TN   38163-2166
901-448-5559; 901-448-7255 (FAX)
http://utmgopher.utmem.edu/medicine/

Office of Admissions, Vanderbilt University School of Medicine
209 Light Hall, Nashville, TN   37232-0685
615-322-2145; 615-343-8397 (FAX)
http://www.mc.vanderbilt.edu/medschool/

Assistant Dean for Admissions and Records East Tennessee State University James H. Quillen College of Medicine
PO Box 70580, Johnson City, TN 37614-0580
423-929-6221; 423-439-6433 (FAX)
http://qcom.etsu.edu/
sacom@etsu.edu

Assistant Dean for Admissions, Texas A&M University Health Science Center College of Medicine
159 Joe H. Reynolds Medical Building, College Station, TX   77843-1114
409-845-7743; 409-847-8663 (FAX)
http://hsc.tamu.edu/
med-stu-aff@tamu.edu

Office of Admissions, Baylor College of Medicine
One Baylor Plaza, Houston, TX   77030
713-798-4842; 713-798-8522 (FAX)
http://www.bcm.tmc.edu/
melodym@bcm.tmc.edu

Medical School Admissions, Registrar's Office
University of Texas Health Science Center at San Antonio, Medical School
7703 Floyd Curl Drive, San Antonio, TX 78284-6200
210-567-2665; 210-567-2685 (FAX)
http://www.uthscsa.edu/

Office of Admissions, Room G-024, University of Texas Health Sciences Center Medical School
PO Box 20708, Houston, TX   77225-0036
713-792-4711; 713-794-4238 (FAX)
http://www.uthouston.edu/

Office of Admissions, University of Texas Medical School at Galveston
Ashbel Smith Building, G.210, Galveston, TX 77555-1317
409-772-3517; 409-772-5753 (FAX)
http://www.utmb.edu

Office of Admissions, Texas Tech University Health Sciences Center
School of Medicine, Texas Tech Health Sciences Center, Lubbock, TX   79430
806-743-3005; 806-743-3021 (FAX)
http://www.ttuhsc.edu

Office of the Register
University of Texas-Southwestern Medical Center at Dallas Southwestern Medical School
5323 Harry Hines Boulevard, Dallas, TX 75235-9002
214-648-2670; 214-648-3289 (FAX)
http://www.swmed.edu/

Medical School Admissions, University of Utah School of Medicine
10 North Medical Drive, Salt Lake City, UT 84132
801-581-7498; 801-585-3300 (FAX)
http://www.utah.edu/som
deans.admissions@hsc.utah.edu

Office of Admissions, Eastern Virginia Medical School
721 Fairfax Avenue, Norfolk, VA   23507
757-446-5812; 757-446-5817 (FAX)
http://www.evms.edu/

Director of Admissions, University of Virginia School of Medicine
Box 235, Charlottesville, VA   22908
804-924-5571; 804-982-2586 (FAX)
http://www.virginia.edu
bab7g@virginia.edu

Medical School Admissions
Virginia Commonwealth University Medical College of Virginia School of Medicine
MCV Station, Box 980565, Richmond, VA 23298-0565
804-828-9629; 804-828-7628 (FAX)
http://views.vcu.edu/html/schofmed.html

Admissions Office, University of Vermont College of Medicine
E-109 Given Building, Burlington, VT 05405-0160
802-656-2150; 802-656-8577 (FAX)
http://salus.med.uvm.edu/

Admissions Office (SC-64), University of Washington School of Medicine
Health Sciences Center, A-100, Box 356340, Seattle, WA 98195
206-543-7212; 206-685-8767 (FAX)
http://www.washington.edu/medical/som/
askuwsom@u.washington.edu

Office of Admissions, Medical College of Wisconsin
8701 Watertown Plank Road, Milwaukee, WI 53226
414-456-8246; 414-456-6505 (FAX)
http://www.mcw.edu

Admissions Committee, University of Wisconsin-Madison Medical School
Medical Sciences Center, Room 1205
1300 University Avenue, Milwaukee, WI 53706
608-263-4925; 608-262-2327 (FAX)
http://medsch.wisc.edu/homepage.html

Admissions Office, Marshall University School of Medicine
1542 Spring Valley Drive, Huntington, WV 25704
304-696-7312; 800-544-8514; 304-696-7243 (FAX)
http://musom.marshall.edu/

Office of Admissions and Records, West Virginia University School of Medicine
Health Sciences Center, PO Box 9815, Morgantown, WV 26506
304-293-3521; 304-293-4973 (FAX)
http://www.hsc.wvu.edu/som/

Canadian Medical Schools
Alphabetized by Province

Admissions Officer, University of Alberta Faculty of Medicine and Oral Health Sciences
2-45 Medical Science Building, Edmonton, AB T6G 2H7
406-492-6350; 403-492-9531 (FAX)
http://www.med.ualberta.ca/
admissions@med.ualberta.edu

Office of Admissions, The University of Calgary Faculty of Medicine
3330 Hospital Drive, NW, Calgary, AB T2N 4N1
403-220-6849; 403-283-4740 (FAX)
http://www.acs.ucalgary.ca/~medgrad/

Associate Dean of Admissions, University of British Columbia Faculty of Medicine
317-2194 Health Sciences Mall, Vancouver, BC V6T 1Z3

604-822-4482; 604-822-6061 (FAX)
http://www.medicine.ubc.ca/

The Dean's Office, University of Manitoba
Faculty of Medicine
A101 Chown Building, 753 McDermot
Avenue, Winnipeg, MB   R3T 0W3
204-789-3569; 204-789-3569 (FAX)
http://www.umanitoba.ca/
admissions@umanitoba.ca

Admissions Office, Memorial University of
Newfoundland Faculty of Medicine
Room 1751, Health Sciences Center, St.
John's, NF   A1B 3V6
709-737-6615; 709-737-5186 (FAX)
http://aorta.library.mun.ca/med/
munmed@morgan.ucs.mun.ca

Admissions Coordinator, Dalhousie
University Faculty of Medicine
Room C-23 Lower Level, Clinical Research
Center,
5849 University Avenue, Halifax, NS   B3H
4H7
902-494-1874; 902-494-8884 (FAX)
http://www.mcms.dal.ca/

Admissions and Records
McMaster University Undergraduate Medical
Programme, School of Medicine
1200 Main Street West, Hamilton, ON   L8N
3Z5
905-525-9140 Ext. 22114; 905-546-0800
(FAX)
http://www-fhs.mcmaster.ca/

Undergraduate Medical Education Building,
University of Western Ontario Faculty of
Medicine
Medical Sciences Building, Room 100,
London, ON N6A 5C1
519-661-3744; 519-661-4043 (FAX)
http://www.med.uwo.ca

Admissions Coordinator, University of
Toronto Faculty of Medicine
Toronto, ON   M5S 1A8
416-978-2717; 416-971-2163 (FAX)
http://utl1.library.utoronto.ca/www/medicine/
index.htm
medicine.admiss@utoronto.ca

Admissions Office, Queen's University
Faculty of Medicine
Kingston, ON   K7L 3N6
613-545-2542; 613-545-6884 (FAX)
http://meds-ss10.meds.queensu.ca/
medicine/
jeb8@post.queensu.ca

Admissions, University of Ottawa Faculty of
Medicine
451 Smyth Road, Room 2045, Ottawa, ON
K1H 8M5
613-562-5409; 613-562-5420 (FAX)
admissmd@uottawa.ca

Admissions Office, McGill University Faculty
of Medicine
3655 Drummond Street, Montréal, PQ   H3G
1Y6
514-398-3517; 514-398-4631 (FAX)
http://www.med.mcgill.ca/

Secretary, Admissions Committee, Université
Laval Faculty of Medicine
Cite Universitaire, Sainte-Foy, PQ   G1K 7P4
418-646-2492; 418-656-2733 (FAX)
http://www.fmed.ulaval.ca/

Committee on Admissions, Université de
Montréal Faculty of Medicine
CP 6128, Succursale Centre-ville, Montréal,
PQ   H3C 3J7
514-343-6265; 514-343-6629 (FAX)
http://www.med.umontreal.ca/

Admissions Office, University of Sherbrooke
Faculty of Medicine
Sherbrooke, PQ   J1H 5N4
819-564-5208; 819-564-5378 (FAX)
http://www.usherb.ca/

Admissions Office, University of
Saskatchewan College of Medicine
B 103 Health Sciences Building, Saskatoon,
SK   S7N 0W0
306-966-8554; 306-966-6164 (FAX)
http://www.usask.ca/medicine/
lobergh@admin.usask.ca

$$A + B = ?$$

MCAT-Prep.com

THE NEW MEDICAL COLLEGE ADMISSIONS TEST

PART II

THE NEW MEDICAL COLLEGE ADMISSION TEST

THE STRUCTURE OF THE *new* MCAT

1.1 Introduction

The *new* Medical College Admission Test (MCAT) is a prerequisite for admission to nearly all the medical schools in North America. Each year, over 50,000 applicants to American and Canadian medical schools submit MCAT test results. While the actual weight given to MCAT scores in the admissions process varies from school to school, often they are regarded in a similar manner to your college/university CGPA (i.e. your academic standing).

In applying for medicine at some medical schools, for example, the MCAT score is as important as your four years of undergraduate study! On the other hand, some universities will set a minimum level of performance on the MCAT and then analyze school grades to decide who will be invited to the interviews. Either way, doing well is imperative for most applicants.

The MCAT is administered on a Saturday or a weekday, up to 22 times per year. To register for the MCAT, you should consult your undergraduate adviser or register online:

MCAT Program
P.O. Box 4056
Iowa City, Iowa, 52243
Phone: (319) 337-1357
Web site: www.aamc.org

1.2 The Format of the *new* MCAT

The MCAT will not only test your scientific knowledge in biology, physics, inorganic and organic chemistry, but will also measure your problem-solving, critical thinking and writing skills. The exam is divided into four sections. All questions, save the Writing Sample, are multiple choice with four choices per question.

The MCAT is about 5 hours long (breaks are optional). It is a Computer Based Test (CBT) held at specific testing centers authorized by the AAMC. This is the schedule for the test day:

- Physical Sciences: 70 minutes
  Break (optional):   (10 minutes)

- Verbal Reasoning: 60 minutes
  Break (optional):   (10 minutes)

- Writing Sample: 60 minutes
  Break (optional):   (10 minutes)

- Biological Sciences: 70 minutes

1.3 How the MCAT is Scored

The MCAT is scored for each of the four sections individually. The sections consisting of multiple choice questions are first scored right or wrong resulting in a raw score. Note that wrong answers are worth the same as unanswered questions so ALWAYS ANSWER ALL THE QUESTIONS even if you are not sure of certain answers. The raw score is then converted to a scaled score ranging from 1 (lowest) to 15 (highest). The scores are scaled to ensure that the same proportion of individual marks within each section (i.e. 1-15) are given year to year.

The essay is scored by two readers on a scale of 1 (lowest) to 6 (highest). The combined scores from the two essays (2 to 12 out of 12) are then converted to a scale ranging from J (lowest) to T (highest):

The scores for each section are reported to you, the schools you designate and, with your permission, to your undergraduate advisor.

Every MCAT includes a small number of questions which will not be scored. These questions are either used to calibrate the exam or were found to be either too ambiguous or too difficult to be counted. So if you see a question that you think is off the wall, unanswerable or inappropriate, it could well be one of these questions so never panic!

2	3	4	5	6	7	8	9	10	11	12
J	K	L	M	N	O	P	Q	R	S	T

1.4 The *new* MCAT: A Closer Look

• <u>Physical Sciences</u> (70 minutes)

This section is made up of 52 multiple choice questions divided half and half between general chemistry and physics. Questions in groups of 4 to 8, based on a 250-word passage will account for about 85% of the questions. The remaining 15% of the questions will be independent of one another and of any passage. All the questions test your knowledge and understanding of concepts and your scientific problem-solving skills in chemistry and physics. You are not expected to memorize extensive amounts of material for this section of the MCAT.

An important part of the Physical Sciences section is the testing of your ability to read data presented in tabular and in graphical forms. You should therefore be familiar with the basic principles used in the presentation of data. You should also be able to identify trends and tendencies, as well as relationships in the data presented. Furthermore, you may be asked to identify the best way of presenting a particular set of data.

The concepts in chemistry and physics tested on the MCAT are those generally taught in introductory level college/university courses. While the passages may present advanced concepts, the questions accompanying the passage will only require a knowledge of basic principles. Thus, more advanced chemistry and physics courses are not required for this test. You should know the constants and formulae associated with elementary work as presented in this manual and listed in the AAMC manual. Other equations and constants will be provided in the actual MCAT exam, along with a periodic table of the elements. Finally, some basic mathematical knowledge is expected as calculators are <u>not allowed</u> for this test.

• <u>Mathematics Needed for the MCAT</u>

For the MCAT you should:

1> Be able to perform arithmetic calculations such as additions, subtractions, multiplications and divisions as well as be able to use proportions, percentages, ratios and estimations of square roots. If you have difficulty with basic arithmetic, you should include time in your review to practice. For the MCAT, you must be <u>accurate and quick.</u>

2> Be familiar with metric units and how to convert between metric and imperial units using given conversion factors. Know how to balance equations containing physical units.

3> Understand logarithms, scientific notation, quadratic and simultaneous equations, and graphical representations of data in various scales at the level of advanced high school algebra.

4>   Know how to calculate an arithmetic mean and to determine the range for a given set of data. An understanding of the general concepts associated with statistics (correlation, association, etc.) is expected, but no calculations of standard deviations and correlation coefficients are required.

5>   Be able to calculate at an elementary level the mathematical probability of an event.

6>   Be familiar with the basic concepts of trigonometry and know the value of the cosine, sine and tangent of 0, 90 and 180 degrees, as well as the relationships between the lengths of the sides of a right triangle containing angles of 45 or 30 and 60 degrees. This is essential for certain physics problems.

7>   Understand the concept of experimental error and be able to calculate it using the appropriate number of significant figures.

8>   Be familiar with vector additions and subtractions. Be able to use the right hand rule. You do not need to know how to calculate the dot or cross product of vectors.

Also:

*   No knowledge of calculus is required.

*   Time is a problem for most people taking the MCAT. You should be able to

perform the mathematics included in the MCAT quickly. If you have problems with some of the concepts described above, review them. You do not want to have something as elementary as mathematics stop you from doing well.

*   The math review in this manual is usually presented throughout the science review sections and especially during the Physics and Chemistry reviews. Otherwise, math information can be found in the appendix.

*   Please remember the following: if you practice for the MCAT using a calculator then you have not practiced for the MCAT.

● Verbal Reasoning (60 minutes)

This section is designed to measure your ability to read, understand, evaluate and apply information presented in prose texts. The passages are about 500 to 600 words long and are taken from the humanities, social sciences as well as from the natural sciences. Each passage will be followed by six to ten multiple choice questions which will not test you on specific knowledge about a subject. There are a total of 40 questions. All that you need to know to answer the questions will be included in the passage.

● Writing Sample (60 minutes)

Medical schools have noted some deficiencies in the communication skills of their graduates. In response to this problem, an experimental essay writing section was included in the 1991 format of the MCAT. The new MCAT includes a writing sample in which you will be asked to write two essays, one in each of two separated half-hour slots. The first essay cannot be returned to you once the second half-hour slot has begun.

The Writing Sample questions consist of a statement which is followed by <u>three</u> writing tasks. The statement will express an opinion, discuss a philosophy or present a policy in a field of general interest. It will not concern an emotionally-charged issue like abortion or religion, or the medical school admission process or your reasons for studying medicine.

The Writing Sample will be scored by two readers who will give your essay a mark from 1 to 6 (best). The mark given will be holistic. If the two marks differ by more than one point, a third reader will be employed to determine the final essay score. The Writing Sample will measure your ability to develop a central idea, to synthesize concepts and to present points clearly and coherently using the accepted rules of grammar, spelling and punctuation.

- <u>Biological Sciences</u> (70 minutes)

The Biological Sciences section is composed of 52 multiple choice questions. There are about 85% of the questions in sets of 4 to 8 questions each following a 250-word long passage, and about 15% independent questions. The questions concern biology and organic chemistry. Usually, the latter comprises no more than about one quarter to one third of the 52 questions.

As for the Physical Sciences section, some of the questions will assess your ability to read information found in tables, graphs or figures. The biology section of the exam will not test your ability to memorize the names of the 206 bones in the human body or any other highly memory-dependent feat. Rather, it will test your knowledge and understanding of the concepts and principles applicable to the biological sciences, and your problem-solving skills.

Also as in the Physical Sciences section, the questions in the Biological Sciences section cover material learned in elementary level college/university courses. While the passages may present advanced level topics, higher level courses in biology or organic chemistry are not required to take this test. You should know the vocabulary, constants and equations commonly presented in elementary courses. Logic and understanding are emphasized, not memorization. While the amount of material you are responsible for is huge, the actual amount of information you need to know to do well is much more manageable.

1.5 The AAMC

The Association of American Medical Colleges (AAMC) is involved in the development and administration of the *new* MCAT. The AAMC publishes several important sets of materials, particularly online: i) the *Official Guide to the MCAT Exam*; ii) *MCAT Practice Tests* which are released operational test forms from past *new* MCAT administrations. These materials can be obtained by online or by calling or writing:

Membership and Publication Orders
Association of American Medical Colleges
2450 N Street, N.W.
Washington, D.C. 20037-1126
Phone: (202) 828-0416
Web site: www.aamc.org

Some students purchase commercially available simulated MCAT exams without ever having seen the materials from the AAMC. This is often a serious mistake. If you are looking to write an actual past exam, you go to the source. The source of the MCAT is the AAMC. In this manner, you can feel confident in your preparedness. Dr. Ferdinand has prepared explanations to the answers to actual past MCAT exams, including cross-references to The Gold Standard text, in **The Silver Bullet: Real MCATs Explained**, which is available at your local university bookstore or at the Bookstore at www.MCAT-bookstore.com.

THE RECIPE FOR MCAT SUCCESS

2.1 The Important Ingredients

- Time
- Motivation
- At least 3 of the 4 basic MCAT sciences (introductory level) at college/university

- **MCAT-Specific Information**
  - The Gold Standard for Medical School Admissions
  - *optional*: The Gold Standard DVDs, MP3s or online programs (mcatstore.com)
  - *optional*: college texts or notes for topics not well understood

- • *optional*: essay writing or speed reading course if necessary

MCAT-Specific Problems
- The Gold Standard MCAT Practice Exams (GS-1, 2 and 3)
- Official AAMC practice materials and exams (e-mcat.com)
- The rest of the Gold Standard practice MCAT CBTs
- *optional*: The Silver Bullet: Real MCATs Explained

2.2 The Proper Mix

1) **Study regularly and start early.** There is a lot of material to cover and you will need sufficient time to review it all adequately. Creating a study schedule is often effective. Starting early will reduce your stress level in the weeks leading up to the exam and may make your studying easier.

2) **Keep focused and enjoy** the material you are learning. Forget all past negative learning experiences so you can open your mind to the information with a positive attitude. Given an open mind and some time to consider what you are learning, you will find most of the information tremendously interesting. Motivation can be derived from a sincere interest in learning and by keeping in mind your long term goals.

3) **Biological and Physical Sciences preparation:** *The Gold Standard* is not associated with the AAMC in any way; however, contained herein is each and every topic that you are responsible for in the Biological and Physical Sciences, as iterated by the AAMC. Thus the most directed and efficient study plan is to begin by reviewing

the science sections in this manual. {Remember the warning in the "Introduction": don't study too little, nor too much!}

As you are incorporating the information from the science review, do the Biological and Physical Sciences problems in the Official MCAT guide (AAMC) and the free chapter review questions online at MCAT-prep.com. This is the best way to more clearly define the depth of your understanding *and* to get you accustomed to the types of questions you can expect on the MCAT.

Verbal Reasoning and Writing Sample preparation: Begin by reading the advice given in Chapters 3 and 4 in this manual. Then take the Verbal Reasoning and Writing Sample Practice Items in the AAMC Guide, *always time yourself*, and practice, practice, practice.

For Verbal Reasoning, you should be sure to understand each and every mistake you make as to ensure there will be improvement. For the Writing Sample, you should have someone who has good writing skills read, correct, and comment on your essays. Have the person read Chapter 4 for guidance on what they should be evaluating. And finally, The Gold Standard, MCAT-prep.com, and *The AAMC Practice Test III* all contain corrected essays which give an indication as to the standard of writing that is expected of you.

Do practice exams. Ideally, you would finish your science review in *The Gold Standard* and AAMC guide at least one month prior to the exam date. Then each week you can do 1 or 2 practice exams and <u>thoroughly review each exam after completion</u>. Scores in practice exams should improve over time. Success depends on what you do between the first and the last exam. Start with The Gold Standard exams GS-1 to GS-3 which will lead you into the *Practice Tests*. **The Silver Bullet: Real MCATs Explained** contains explanations to actual past MCATs with cross-references to *The Gold Standard* and is available at your local university bookstore or at the Bookstore at www.MCAT-bookstore.com.

You should do practice exams as you would the actual test: in one sitting within the expected time limits and as a Computer Based Test (CBT). Doing practice exams will increase your confidence and allow you to see what is expected of you. It will make you realize the constraints imposed by time limits in completing the entire test. It will also allow you to identify the areas in which you may be lacking.

Big on concepts, small on memorization: Remember that the *new* MCAT will primarily test your understanding of concepts. The *new* MCAT is not designed to measure your ability to memorize tons of scientific facts and trivia, but both your knowledge and understanding of concepts are critical. In fact, only 15% of the science sections on the MCAT <u>directly</u> test your ability to memorize!

Evidently, some material in this manual must be memorized; for example, practically all the science equations, absorption spectra of major functional groups, rules of logarithms, trigonometric functions, the phases in mitosis and meiosis, and other basic facts. Nonetheless, for the most part, your objective should be to try to *understand*, rather than memorize the biology, physics and chemistry material you review. This may appear vague now, but as you write practice material, you will more clearly understand what is expected of you.

Relax once in a while! While the MCAT requires a lot of preparation, you should not forsake all your other activities to study. Try to keep exercising, maintain a social life and do things you enjoy. If you balance work with things which relax you, you will work more effectively overall.

2.3 It's MCAT Time!

1)   On the night before the exam, try to get a good night sleep. The MCAT is physically draining and it is in your best interest to be well rested when you take it.

2)   Avoid last minute cramming. On the morning of the exam, do not begin studying *ad hoc*. You will not learn anything effectively, and noticing something you do not know or will not remember might reduce your confidence and lower your score unnecessarily. Just get up, eat a good breakfast, consult your equation list and go do the exam.

3)   Eat breakfast! It will make it possible for you to have the food energy needed to go through the first two parts of the exam.

4)   Pack a light lunch. Avoid greasy food that will make you drowsy. You do not want to feel sleepy for the afternoon sections. Avoid sugar-packed snacks as they will cause a 'sugar low' eventually and will also make you drowsy. A chocolate bar or other sweet highly caloric food could, however, be very useful in the last section (*Biological Sciences*) when you may be tired. The 'sugar low' will hit you only after you *have* completed the exam when you do not have to be awake!

5)   Make sure you answer all the questions! You do not get penalized for incorrect answers, so always choose something even if you have to guess. If you run out of time, pick a letter and use it to answer all the remaining questions.

6)   Pace yourself. Do not get bogged down trying to answer a difficult question. If the question is very difficult, make a mark beside it and answer it later.

7)   Remember that some of the questions will be thrown out as inappropriate or used

solely to calibrate the test. If you find that you cannot answer some of the questions, do not despair. It is possible they could be questions used for these purposes.

8) Do not let others psyche you out! Some people will be saying between exam sections, 'It went great. What a joke!' Ignore them. Often these types may just be trying to boost their own confidence or to make themselves look good in front of their friends. Just focus on what you have to do and tune out the other examinees.

9) Do not study at lunch. You need the time to recuperate and rest. Eat, avoid the people discussing the test sections and relax! Lunch is optional for the new MCAT.

10) Before reading the text of the problem, some students find it more efficient to quickly read the questions first. In this way, as soon as you read something in the text which brings to mind a question you have read, you can answer immediately (*this is especially helpful for Verbal Reasoning*). Otherwise, if you read the text first and then the questions, you may end up wasting time searching through the text for answers. In fact, sometimes in the Physical Sciences and Biological Sciences sections you will be able to answer questions without having read the passage!

11) Read the text and questions carefully! Often students leave out a word or two while reading, which can completely change the sense of the problem. Pay special attention to words in *italics*, CAPS, **bolded**, or underlined. Highlight anything you believe might be important in the passage (there is an on screen highlighter for this MCAT CBT).

12) Do independent questions first! Some students have difficulty finishing the MCAT (esp. Physical Sciences). The worst scenario is getting bogged down in a passage when there were independent questions which you knew the answer to, but never had the time to answer.

13) Skip the questions which you find too difficult or too time consuming and come back to them when you are finished the other questions. You must be both diligent and careful with the way you fill out your answer document because you will not be given extra time to either check it or fill it in.

14) If you run out of time, just do the questions. In other words, only read the part of the passage which your question specifically requires in order for you to get the correct answer. As you do practice exams you will notice that many MCAT questions can be correctly answered without reading the preceding passage.

15) Expel any relevant equation onto your scratch paper! Even if the question is of a theoretical nature, often equations contain the answers and they are much more objective than the reasoning of a nervous pre-medical student! In physics, it is often helpful to draw a picture or diagram. Arrows are valuable in representing vectors.

16) Solving the problem may involve algebraic manipulation of equations and/or numerical calculations. Be sure that you know what all the variables in the equation stand for and that you are using the equation in the appropriate circumstance.

In chemistry and physics, the use of **dimensional analysis** will help you keep track of units <u>and</u> solve some problems where you might have forgotten the relevant equations. Dimensional analysis relies on the manipulation of units. For example, if you are asked for the energy involved in maintaining a 60 watt bulb lit for two minutes you can pull out the appropriate equations <u>or</u> : i) recognize that your objective (unknown = energy) is in joules; ii) recall that a watt is a joule per second; iii) convert minutes into seconds. {note that minutes and seconds cancel leaving joules as an answer}

$$60 \ \frac{joules}{second} \ \ X \ 2 \ minutes \ \ X \ 60 \ \frac{seconds}{minutes}$$

$$= 7200 \ \ joules \ \ or \ \ 7.2 \ kilojoules$$

17) The final step in problem solving is to ask yourself: *is my answer reasonable*? For example, if you would have done the preceding problem and your answer was 7200 kilojoules, intuitively this should strike you as an exorbitant amount of energy for an everyday light bulb to remain lit for two minutes! It would then be of value to recheck your calculations. {*'intuition' in science is often learned through the experience of doing many problems*}

18) Whenever doing calculations, the following will increase your speed: (i) manipulate variables but plug in values only when necessary; (ii) avoid decimals, use fractions wherever possible; (iii) square roots or cube roots can be converted to the power (*exponent*) of 1/2 or 1/3, respectively; (iv) before calculating, check to see if the possible answers are sufficiently far apart such that your values can be approximated (i.e. $19.2 \approx 20$, $185 \approx 200$). In fact, occasionally the MCAT will provide gravity as "given g = 9.8 m/s^2" but the answers are calculated based on g = 10 m/s^2!

REVIEW FOR VERBAL REASONING

3.1 Overview

The Verbal Reasoning section of the MCAT is, for many applicants, the most difficult section to do well. This can be explained by the absence of an overall set of facts to study in order to prepare. Some applicants, due to the lack of review material, neglect to prepare for this section. While the best preparation is regular reading from a variety of sources throughout your high school and undergraduate studies, it is also possible to improve your ability to do well in this section as you approach the test date. You should not neglect to prepare for this section as it accounts for one third of your final MCAT numerical scores!

3.2 How to Improve your Verbal Reasoning Score

1)   Read carefully and annotate. The test is yours. You paid for it so do not be afraid to highlight, strike out or to use any of the features of this computer based test. Even with the MCAT CBT, you can highlight, annotate anywhere within the passage and strike out answers.

2)   Always try to identify the main points of each paragraph, the idea behind the text and the structure of the passage as you read. Doing this will make it easier for you to answer the questions.

3)   Write practice materials as described in Section 2.2 points #4 and #5. The people who designed the MCAT have a particular style of questions they ask. It is in your own best interest to familiarize yourself with the type of questions you will be asked.

4)   The "Questions First, Passage Once Technique": some applicants like to quickly scan the questions prior to reading the text. Then they read the passage and answer questions as they read the information (usu. the questions are placed in the same order as you would find the answers in the passage). You may find it more efficient to work in that way. Try one of the practice exams this way and, if you find it easier to answer the questions correctly, you should use this method on the actual MCAT.

5)   Pace yourself. A major problem in this section is that test takers run out of time.

Read at a reasonable speed. This seems vague, but once you have taken a few practice tests, you will have a good idea as to how fast you will need to work. You want to read carefully but quickly.

Do not skim the passage. Ideally, you only want to read the passage once to answer the questions correctly such that you are able to finish in the allotted time.

As always, when a question is too difficult, mark it and skip to the next one. If you have time, you can come back to it. Also, although you cannot 'study' Verbal Reasoning, you CAN improve your score through practice.

6)   It is extremely rare to score more than 13 in Verbal Reasoning.

7)   The passages will be from a variety of sources, so reading diverse material in the period leading up to the exam will be useful.

8)   Warning: the Verbal Reasoning tests in the Gold Standard MCAT Practice Exams (GS-1 to GS-3) are tough! Some students find the questions more difficult or more subtle than the actual test. These same students say that they learned a lot from practicing with the GS exams and it allowed them to find the actual test easier. Some techniques for answering are reviewed in the "Understanding" sections at the back of the book which you can put to use after you have finished your first test.

3.2.1 Question and Answer Techniques

1)   Process of Elimination (PoE): cross out any answers that are obviously wrong.

2)   Beware of the Extreme: words such as *always, never, perfect, totally*, and *completely* are often (but not always) clues that the answer choice is incorrect.

3)   Comfortable Words: moderate words such as *normally, often, at times,* and *ordinarily* are often included in answer choices that are correct.

4)   Mean Statements: mean or politically incorrect statements are highly unlikely to be included in a correct answer choice. For example, if you see any of the following statements in an answer choice, you can pretty much guarantee that it is not the correct answer:
Parents should abuse their children.
Poor people are lazy.
Religion is socially destructive.
Torture is usually necessary.

5)   Never lose sight of the question. By the time students read answer choices **C.** and **D.**, some have forgotten the question

and are simply looking for "true" sounding statements; you can then fall into the next trap:

True but False and False but True: for example,

Answer Choice D.: Most people are of average height. $\longrightarrow$ This is a true statement.

However, the question was: What is the weight of most people?

Therefore, the true statement becomes the incorrect answer!
Continually check the question and check or cross out right and wrong answers.

3.3 Style of Questions

i> Comprehension: Identify key concepts and/or facts in a passage either directly taken from the text or inferred from it.

ii> Evaluation. Consider the validity, accuracy, value, etc. of ideas and facts presented.

iii> Application: Use the information presented in the passage to solve new problems described in the questions.

iv> Incorporation of new information: Reevaluate the passage based on new facts associated with the questions.

3.4 Online Help

You can get help online including additional Verbal Reasoning tests and speed reading programs at www. MCATverbalreasoning.com or MCAT-prep. com (MCAT CBT format). You can find general advice for written verbal skills at About.com.

REVIEW FOR THE WRITING SAMPLE

4.1 Overview

The *new* MCAT includes two separately timed thirty minute essays. You will be assigned a topic and will have thirty minutes to complete an essay related to that topic following specific instructions. To do well, you must explicitly address the tasks specified in the instructions. The AAMC has made available a list of topics which are very similar to the question that you will have on your MCAT. You can view these at the AAMC's website at www.aamc.org/stuapps/admiss/mcat/wsitems.htm. Using these writing sample topics to write practice essays is an excellent way to prepare for the writing sample. You can submit practice essays for marking and advice, as well as view essays that others have submitted at www.futuredoctor.net or www.MCATwritingsample.com.

Why write an essay?

The essay was included in the *new* MCAT following complaints from the deans of various medical schools concerning the communication skills of medical students. The AAMC responded by including a writing sample in a revised MCAT. Medical school admission committees attach varying value to the scores obtained for the Writing Sample. The distribution of marks in this section is usually very narrow with the great majority of students receiving an N, O or P.

The Writing Sample will measure your ability to:

1> develop a central idea
2> synthesize ideas and concepts
3> express ideas in a logical and cohesive way
4> write clearly, using standard English and appropriate grammar, spelling and punctuation.

You are not expected to type a short polished essay of final draft quality. The people grading your exam are aware that you only had 30 minutes to write the essay. Nevertheless, you will be expected to write a 'good' essay. Please refer to Section 4.3 for a scoring key. You may also consult the websites mentioned above, the Official AAMC Guidet or *Practice Test III* for examples of what a 'good' essay is in the eyes of the markers.

4.1.1 The Statement

Your essay will be based on a statement which can be an opinion, a widely-held belief, or an assertion regarding policy in areas such as history, business, ethics, art or political science. The statement will not be about your reasons for entering medical school, the application process, emotionally-charged religious or ethical issues i.e. abortion, or technical or scientific issues.

While you do not need any specific knowledge to do well in this section, you may want to start reading a popular news magazine to familiarize yourself with current political and social concerns.

4.1.2 The Instructions

You will be asked to complete three tasks. These tasks will be worded differently every time, but essentially can be summarized as follows:

1> Provide an explanation or an interpretation of the statement.

2> Give an example, real or hypothetical, that demonstrates a point of view opposite to the one presented or implied by the statement.

3> Explain a way the conflict between the viewpoint expressed in the statement and the one presented by addressing the second task, might be reconciled.

These three tasks should keep you quite busy for the 30 minutes you have to write the essay. The tasks, however, once you are familiar with them, will help you by structuring your essay for you.

4.1.3 General Pointers for the Writing Sample

You are expected to write a first draft quality essay. A few grammatical, punctuation or spelling errors will not affect your mark greatly. However, a large number of such errors will harm you. If you have difficulty with grammar, spelling or punctuation, you may want to consult a grammar or style text to improve your writing.

You are allowed to cross out words, sentences or passages. Do not try to recopy your essay. You are not expected to and will not have the time to do this. You do not have to follow a set format in your essay writing, but, if you are familiar with a standard style format, by all means, use it. Just make sure you address all three tasks.

Finally, a word about typing. While typing will not be graded on the essay (!!), clearly you must be comfortable typing quickly, efficiently with a minimal number of errors. If your typing is a problem for you then you should practice to improve before your official exam.

4.1.4 The Power of Quotations

"I quote others only in order to better express myself," DeMontaigne once said. A properly placed quotation can have a powerful effect on your Writing Sample. If used improperly, you will have inadvertently confirmed that you misunderstood the statement provided.

You can choose to use a quotation to support your position or to provide the opposite point of view. But remember: a quote is *word for word*. They will not be impressed if you misquote John F. Kennedy or The Constitution. If you only forgot the name of someone whose is not well known, you can get away with saying something like: "It has been said that . . ."

The following quotes relate to topics which are often found in the Writing Sample. The first twenty are the most important.

Those who make peaceful revolution impossible will make violent revolution inevitable.
John F. Kennedy

We hold these truths to be self-evident: that all men are created equal; that they are endowed by their creator with inherent and inalienable rights; that among these are life, liberty, and the pursuit of happiness.
Thomas Jefferson

Injustice anywhere is a threat to justice everywhere.
Martin Luther King, Jr.

...government of the people, by the people, for the people, shall not perish from the earth.
Abraham Lincoln

In the long-run every Government is the exact symbol of its People, with their wisdom and unwisdom.
Thomas Carlyle

The cost of liberty is less than the price of repression.
W. E. B. Du Bois

I have to follow them, I am their leader.
Alexandre-Auguste Ledru-Rollin

I would rather be exposed to the inconveniences attending too much liberty than those attending too small a degree of it.
Thomas Jefferson

Those who expect to reap the blessings of freedom, must, like men, undergo the fatigues of supporting it.
Thomas Jefferson

The only way to make sure people you agree with can speak is to support the rights of people you don't agree with.
Eleanor Holmes Norton

I detest what you write, but I would give my life to make it possible for you to continue to write.
Voltaire

I disapprove of what you say, but I will defend to the death your right to say it.
Voltaire

He that would make his own liberty secure must guard even his enemy from oppression.
Thomas Paine

War settles nothing.
Dwight D. Eisenhower

You can't hold a man down without staying down with him.
Booker T. Washington

Men prize the thing ungained, more than it is.
Shakespeare

Nothing is politically right which is morally wrong.
Daniel O'Connell

When a man assumes a public trust, he should consider himself public property.
Thomas Jefferson

If there is no struggle there is no progress.
John Adams

President means chief servant.
Mahatma Gandhi

One can resist the invasion of armies, but not the invasion of ideas.
Victor Hugo

All of us do not have equal talent, but all of us should have an equal opportunity to develop our talents.
John F. Kennedy

I have a dream that my four little children will one day live in a nation where they will not be judged by the color of their skin but by the content of their character. I have a dream today.
Martin Luther King, Jr.

All animals are created equal, but some animals are more equal than others.
George Orwell

It is better that ten guilty persons escape than that one innocent suffer.
William Blackstone

It is better to risk saving a guilty person than to condemn an innocent one.
Voltaire

I say that justice is truth in action.
Benjamin Disraeli

A jury consists of twelve persons chosen to decide who has the better lawyer.
Robert Frost

The right to be heard does not automatically include the right to be taken seriously.
Hubert H. Humphrey

A right is not what someone gives you; it's what no one can take from you.
Ramsey Clark

"Freedom from fear" could be said to sum up the whole philosophy of human rights.
Dag Hammarskjold

I am the interior of any man whose rights I trample under foot.
Robert G. Ingersoll

The simplest schoolboy is now familiar with truths for which Archimedes would have sacrificed his life.
Ernest Renan

All they that take the sword, shall perish with the sword.
Bible

It is better to be violent, if there is violence in our hearts, than to put on the cloak of nonviolence to cover impotence.
Mohandas K. Gandhi

We live in a moment of history where change is so speeded up that we begin to see the present only when it is already disappearing.
R. D. Laing

The love of money is the root of all evil.
Bible

Money is like a sixth sense without which you cannot make a complete use of the other five.
W. Somerset Maugham

When written in Chinese the word crisis is composed of two characters. One represents danger and the other represents opportunity.
John F. Kennedy

For unto whomsoever much is given, of him shall be much required.
Bible

The Buck Stops Here.
Harry S. Truman

And so, my fellow Americans; ask not what your country can do for you - ask what you can do for your country. My fellow citizens of the world: ask not what America will do for you, but what together we can do for the freedom of man.
John F. Kennedy

A little rebellion, now and then, is a good thing, and as necessary in the political world as storms in the physical.
Thomas Jefferson

Uneasy lies the head that wears a crown.
Shakespeare

Laws too gentle are seldom obeyed; too severe, seldom executed.
Benjamin Franklin

There are not enough jails, not enough policemen, not enough courts to enforce a law not supported by the people.
Hubert H. Humphrey

That's one small step for a man, and one giant leap for mankind.
Neil Armstrong

He who is unable to live in society, or who has no need because he is sufficient for himself, must be either a beast or a god.
Aristotle

A government which robs Peter to pay Paul can always depend on the support of Paul.
George Bernard Shaw

It is perfectly true that that government is best which governs least. It is equally true that that government is best which provides most.
Walter Lippmann

To be prepared for War is one of the most effectual means of preserving peace.
George Washington

Beauty is in the eye of the beholder.
Margaret Wolfe Hungerford

It is amazing how complete is the delusion that beauty is goodness.
Leo Tolstoy

A journey of a thousand miles must begin with a single step.
Lao-Tzu

War is nothing but the continuation of politics with the admixture of other means.
Karl Von Clausewitz

The first casualty when war comes is truth.
Hiram Warren Johnson

It is well that war is so terrible, or we should grow too fond of it.
Robert E. Lee

That man is the richest whose pleasures are the cheapest.
Henry David Thoreau

In this world nothing is certain but death and taxes.
Benjamin Franklin

The more things change, the more they remain the same.
Alphonse Karr

All things change; nothing perishes.
Ovid

Truth is the glue that holds governments together. Compromise is the oil that makes governments go.
Gerald R. Ford

What is a cynic? A man who knows the price of everything, and the value of nothing.
Oscar Wilde

In this world there are only two tragedies. One is not getting what one wants, and the other is getting it.
Oscar Wilde

All diplomacy is a continuation of war by other means.
Chou En-Lai

Let us never negotiate out of fear. But let us never fear to negotiate.
John F. Kennedy

The Nation that destroys its soil destroys itself.
Franklin D. Roosevelt

4.2 The Five Minute, Five Step Plan

Normally, an essay would be written over a considerable period of time. You would think about your essay, plan what you would write, write, correct and polish your essay, and perhaps rewrite sections. However, a timed essay is not normal. It is a situation where your thoughts have to be ordered, structured and organized straight out of your head! You have to plan what you will write quickly and efficiently. You have 30 minutes to write an essay, but if you spend a few minutes planning first, your essay should greatly improve. It is possible to write a structured complete essay in 30 minutes, but for most students, it requires practice.

The objective of the Five Minute, Five Step Plan is to take 5 minutes to prepare and 5 steps to complete the essay.

Step 1: Read the statement and the instructions.

This may seem obvious, but you would be surprised by the number of students who misread or misinterpret what is expected of them. You should carefully read the statement and underline the terms you will want to discuss. You should also carefully read the instructions and number the three tasks. This step is essential to even getting an average grade.

Example:
The government is best that governs least.

Write a comprehensive essay in which you accomplish the following objectives. Explain what you think the statement means. Describe a specific example in which the government's powers should be increased. Discuss the basis for increasing or decreasing the government's powers.

Step 2: Prewrite the three tasks.

You should jot down notes that will help you complete all three tasks:

Task 1 : Usually, you will have to explain a statement which will not be simply factual or self-evident. For example, the statement, "The government is best which governs least," has to be explained and terms have to be defined. Make notes as the information comes to mind:

Ex.: Government: -federal,state, provincial, municipal
-authority, power
-a ruling body

Governs: -rules, delegates, guides
-creates laws
-exerts control, authority

When it comes time to write (Step 4), you will formulate a statement which clearly addresses Task 1: "Explain what you think the statement means." You should choose one clear definition from amongst the possibilities. You may also want to use an example to further illustrate the point of view you are presenting:

The ideal ruling body would strive to maintain, at a minimum, its exertion of authority over the population. Clearly, a government representing the people should not have the right to indiscriminately curb the freedom of an individual. The consequence would be a contradiction of democratic principles. Thus a government should avoid extending its powers; rather, government should use its authority prudently.

There are many different interpretations and examples which can be used to explain what the statement means. One possibility is to suggest that 'big' government produces excessive 'red tape' or bureaucracy which eventually may lead to higher taxes and a greater deficit. Also consider using a quotation about government (i.e. from John F. Kennedy).

Another possibility would be to mention that 'big' government leads to too much power, and "absolute power corrupts absolutely." There are an endless number of possibilities. The key is to choose one line of thinking and present it in a clear manner.{Note how the structure and length of the sentences vary in the example}

Task 2 : Follow a similar approach for tasks two and three. Write down any points you may want to include in your essay which contradict the statement even if you completely agree with it (yes, the CBT comes will scratch paper). You should be able to see the other side. If you cannot think of something to challenge the statement, try to think what someone who actively disagrees with the statement would say.

Ex.: i> *Rights of one person begins where another person's rights end: government ensures that happens.*
ii> *National crisis*
iii> *War/draft*

Choose one specific example and elaborate. Take (iii) as a case in point. The writer may use World War II as a specific example. The fact that the U.S. government increased its powers by legislating that certain members of the population must go to war (= *draft*) could be explored. The war prevented the Nazi government from becoming an even greater destructive force and its reign of terror ended. Thus the U.S. government expanded its powers for the greater good.

Task 3 : For the third task, look back at the ideas you wrote down to address the first two tasks. You should then be able to reconcile the two opposing views. Write down what you think is the key component of your answer to the third task. Remember that you are not expected to solve all the problems in the world. Simply try to find the best way you know to solve the dilemma outlined by the first two tasks. There are no right or wrong answers for this assignment. What is being graded is your reasoning and your ability to express your thoughts.

Ex.: i> *When the survival of the community is endangered*
ii> *Government should govern for the benefit of its citizens*

Prewriting the tasks is not like writing a formal outline. It is simply a way to structure your ideas in order to enable you to write a well-organized essay in 30 minutes. While prewriting might seem like a waste of time, it is the key to helping you complete all three tasks in the time allowed.

Step 3: Organize your notes

Once you have completed the three tasks, you will want to organize and clarify your ideas. This will allow you to review your ideas before you write and to see how they fit together. You may want to remove some ideas and reformulate others. At this stage, you will decide in which order you will address the three tasks. Once you have done this, you will be ready to write the essay. At this point, you will have spent five or six minutes prewriting the tasks. In doing so, you will have created a structure for your essay which will make writing it much easier.

Step 4: Write

When you write, pace yourself. This will be much easier as your notes will provide a framework to work with in writing. You will want to ensure you have a few (about five) minutes to review your masterpiece! Make sure that your essay flows. Use transition words and phrases between your paragraphs. Pay attention to your spelling, punctuation and grammar. Be sure to vary the *structure* and *length* of the sentences in your text.

Do not assume that the reader can read your mind! Be explicit in your presentation. Furthermore, when you are asked to be specific, be *specific*. And finally, be sure to not digress from the theme of your essay.

Step 5: Proofread

Reread your text. You want to spend your last five minutes proofreading your essay. Look for and correct mistakes and ensure you followed the plan you established as you prewrote the tasks. At this point you want to simply polish your essay.

By following these five steps, you should be able to write an essay which successfully addresses all three tasks in the time allowed. This should ensure you get an acceptable mark.

4.3 The Scoring Key

Your essay will be scored from one to six before being converted to a letter grade. Here is what is expected for each mark out of six:

6   Thorough exploration of the topic and fully addressed tasks are features of six point essays. These essays show depth, structure, excellent vocabulary and sentence control as well as coherent focused organization.

5   All tasks are addressed by the essay. The treatment of the subject is substantial but not as thorough as for a six point essay. While some depth, structure and good vocabulary and sentence control is exhibited, this is at a lower level than for a six point essay.

4   All three tasks are addressed but the topic is given only a moderate exploration. Clarity of thought is present but some digression is seen although the text is structured. The quality of the vocabulary and of the sentence structure is adequate.

3   The essay distorts or neglects one of the three tasks. The issue may be only minimally treated. The essay demonstrates basic control of sentence structure and vocabulary, but the language may not serve to adequately forward the writer's thoughts. The essay may show organization but may be classified as simplistic.

2   The essay completely fails to address adequately one or more of the tasks. There may be recurring mechanical errors (i.e. spelling and grammar). Problems with analysis and organization are typical.

1   Problems with organization and mechanics in these essays make it very difficult for the reader to follow them. The essay may fail to address the topic entirely.

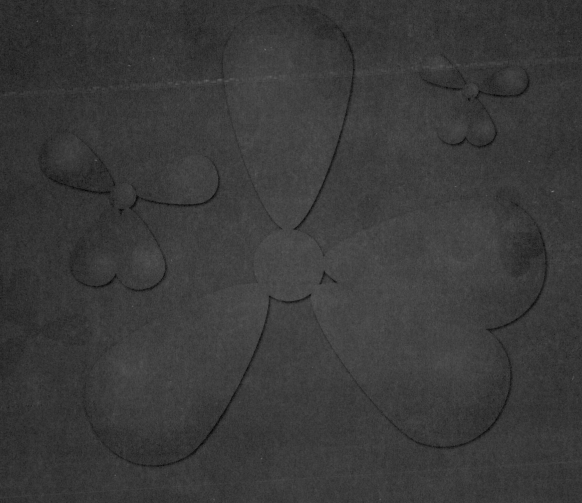

GENERAL
CHEMISTRY

PART III.A: PHYSICAL SCIENCES

STOICHIOMETRY

Chapter 1

Memorize	Understand	Not Required*
* Composition of air * Define: molecular weight * Define: empirical/molecular formula * Avogadro's number * Rules for oxidation numbers	* Composition by % mass * Mole concept, limiting reactants * Calculate theoretical yield * Basic types of reactions * Calculation of ox. numbers	* Advanced level college info * Balancing complex equations * Stoichiometric coefficients, competing reactions

MCAT-Prep.com

Introduction

Stoichiometry is simply the math behind the chemistry involving products and reactants. The math is quite simple, in part, because of the law of conservation of mass that states that the mass of a closed system will remain constant throughout a chemical reaction.

Additional Resources

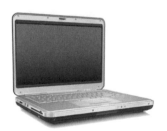

Free Online Q & A

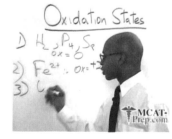

Video: Online or DVD 1, 4

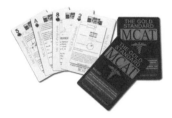

Flashcards

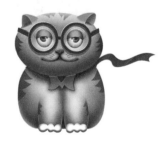

Special Guest

1.1 Generalities

Most substances known to us are mixtures of pure compounds. Air, for instance, contains the pure compounds nitrogen (~78%), oxygen (~21%), water vapor and many other gases (~1%). The compositional ratio of air or any other mixture may vary from one location to another. Each pure compound is made up of molecules which are composed of smaller units: the *atoms*. Atoms combine in very specific ratios to form molecules. During a chemical reaction molecules break down into individual or fragments of atoms which then recombine to form new compounds. Stoichiometry establishes relationships between the above-mentioned specific ratios for individual molecules or for molecules involved in a given chemical reaction.

1.2 Empirical Formula vs. Molecular Formula

The molecules of oxygen are made up of two atoms of the same element. Water molecules on the other hand are composed of two different elements: hydrogen and oxygen in the specific ratio 2:1. Note that water is not a mixture of hydrogen and oxygen since this ratio is specific and does not vary with the location or the experimental conditions. The *empirical formula* of a pure compound is the simplest whole number ratio between the numbers of atoms of the different elements making up the compound. For instance, the empirical formula of water is H_2O (2:1 ratio) while the empirical formula of hydrogen peroxide is HO (1:1 ratio). The *molecular formula* of a given molecule states the exact number of the different atoms that make up this molecule. The empirical formula of water is identical to its molecular formula, i.e. H_2O; however, the molecular formula of hydrogen peroxide, H_2O_2, is different from its empirical formula (both correspond to a 1:1 ratio).

1.3 Mole - Atomic and Molecular Weights

Because of the small size of atoms and molecules chemists have to consider collections of a large number of these particles to bring chemical problems to our macroscopic scale. Collections of tens or dozens of atoms are still too small to achieve this practical purpose. For various reasons the number 6.02×10^{23} (Avogadro's number: N_A) was chosen. It is the number of atoms in 12 grams of the most abundant *isotope* of carbon (isotopes are elements which are identical chemically since the number of protons are the same; their masses differ slightly since the number of neutrons differ). A mole of atoms or molecules (or in fact any particles in general) contains an Avogadro number of these particles. The weight in grams of a mole of atoms of a given element is the gram-atomic weight, GAW, of that element (sometimes weight is measured in atomic mass units - *see Physics section 12.2, 12.3*). Along the same lines, the weight in grams of a mole of molecules of a given compound is its gram-molecular weight, GMW. Here are some equations relating these concepts in a way that will help you solve some of the stoichiometry problems:

For an element:
moles = (weight of sample in grams)
                        GAW

For a compound:
moles = (weight of sample in grams)
                        GMW

The GAW of a given element is not to be confused with the mass of a single atom of this element. For instance the mass of a single atom of carbon-12 (GAW = 12 g) is $12/N_A = 1.66051 \times 10^{-24}$ grams. Atomic weights are dimensionless numbers defined as follows:

$$\frac{\text{mass of an atom of X}}{\text{mass of an atom of Y}} = \frac{\text{atomic weight of element X}}{\text{atomic weight of element Y}}$$

Clearly if the reference element Y is chosen to be carbon-12 (which is the case in standard periodic tables) the GAW of any element X is numerically equal to its atomic weight. The molecular weight of a given molecule is equal to the sum of the atomic weights of the atoms that make up the molecule.

1.4 Composition of a Compound by Percent Mass

The percentage composition of a compound is the percent of the total mass of a given element in that compound. For instance, the chemical analysis of a 100 g sample of pure vitamin C demontrates that there are 40.9 g of carbon, 4.58 g of hydrogen and 54.5 g of oxygen. The composition of pure vitamin C is:

%C = 40.9; %H = 4.58; %O = 54.5

The composition of a compound by percent mass is closely related to its empirical formula. For instance, in the case of vitamin C, the determination of the number of moles of atoms of C, H or O in a 100 g of vitamin C is rather straightforward:

moles of atoms of C in a 100 g of vitamin C = 40.9/12.0= 3.41

moles of atoms of H in a 100 g of vitamin C = 4.58/1.01= 4.53

moles of atoms of O in a 100 g of vitamin C = 54.5/16.0= 3.41

[GAW can be determined from the periodic table in Chapter 2]

To deduce the smallest ratio between the numbers above, one follows the simple procedure:

(i) divide each one of the previously obtained numbers of moles by the smallest one of them (3.41 in our case):

for C: 3.41/3.41 = 1.00

for H: 4.53/3.41 = 1.33

for O: 3.41/3.41 = 1.00

(ii) multiply the numbers obtained in the previous step by a small number to obtain a whole number ratio. In our case we need to multiply by 3 (in most cases this factor is between 1 and 5) so that :

for C: 1.00 × 3 = 3; for H: 1.33 × 3 = 4 and for O: 1.00 × 3 = 3

Therefore, in this example, the simplest whole number ratio is 3C:4H:3O and we conclude that the empirical formula for vitamin C is : $C_3H_4O_3$.

In the previous example, instead of giving the composition of vitamin C by percent weight we could have provided the raw chemical analysis data and asked for the determination of that composition. For instance, this data would be that the burning of a 4.00 mg sample of pure vitamin C yields 6.00 mg of CO_2 and 1.632 mg of H_2O. Since there are 12.0 g of carbon in 44.0 g of CO_2 the number of milligrams of carbon in 6.00 mg of CO_2 (which corresponds to the number of mg of carbon in 4.00 mg of vitamin C) is simply:

6.00 × (12.0/44.0) = 1.636 mg of C in 6.00 mg of CO_2 or 4.00 mg of vitamin C

To convert this number into a percent mass is then trivial. Similarly, the percent mass of hydrogen is obtained from the previous data and bearing in mind that there are 2.02 g of hydrogen (and not 1.01 g) in 18.0 g of water.

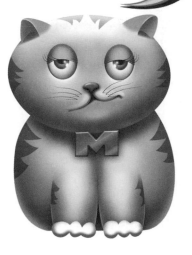

How many moles are in guacamole? Avocado's number.

1.5 Description of Reactions by Chemical Equations

The convention for writing chemical equations is as follows: compounds which initially combine or <u>react</u> in a chemical reaction are called *reactants*; they are always written on the left-hand side of the chemical equation. The compounds which are <u>produced</u> during the same process are referred to as the *products* of the chemical reaction; they always appear on the right-hand side of the chemical equation. In the chemical equation:

$$2\, BiCl_3 \;+\; 3\, H_2O \longrightarrow Bi_2O_3 \;+\; 6\, HCl$$

the coefficients represent the relative number of moles of reactants that combine to form the corresponding relative number of moles of products: they are the <u>stoichiometric coefficients</u> of the balanced chemical equation. The law of conservation of mass requires that the number of atoms of a given element remains constant during the process of a chemical reaction. Balancing a chemical equation is putting this general principle into practice. It is always easier to balance elements that appear only in one compound on each side of the equation; therefore, as a general rule, always balance those elements first and then deal with those which appear in more than one compound last.

Given the preceding chemical reaction, if H_2O is present in excessive quantity, then $BiCl_3$ would be considered the **limiting** **reactant.** In other words, since the amount of $BiCl_3$ is relatively small, it is the $BiCl_3$ which determines how much product will be formed. Thus if you were given 316 grams of $BiCl_3$ in *excess* H_2O and you needed to determine the quantity of HCl produced (theoretical yield), you would proceed as follows:

▶ Determine the number of moles of $BiCl_3$ (*see* CHM 1.3) given Bi = 209 g/mol and Cl = 35.5 g/mol, thus $BiCl_3$ = (1 × 209) + (3 × 35.5) = 315.5 or approximately 316 g/mol:

moles $BiCl_3$ = (316 g)/(316 g/mol) = 1.0 mole of $BiCl_3$.

▶ From the stoichiometric coefficients of the balanced equation:

2 moles of $BiCl_3$: 6 moles of HCl; therefore, 1 mole of $BiCl_3$: 3 moles of HCl

▶ Given H = 1 g/mol, thus HCl = 36.5 g/mol, we get:

3 moles × 36.5 g/mol = 110 g of HCl (approx.).

1.5.1 Categories of Chemical Reactions

Throughout the chapters in General Chemistry we will explore many different types of chemicals and some of their reactions. The following represents some balanced chemical equations as examples:

Substitution Reaction (CHM 9.4)
$CH_4 + Cl_2 \longrightarrow CH_3Cl + HCl$

Neutralization Reaction (CHM 6.9.1)
$2HCl + Ba(OH)_2 \longrightarrow Ba^{2+} + 2Cl^- + H_2O$

Redox Reaction (CHM 1.6,10.1)
$H_2SO_4 + Fe \longrightarrow FeSO_4 + H_2$

Disproportionation Reaction (CHM 1.6)
$2CO \longrightarrow C + CO_2$

Double Replacement Reaction
$CaCl_2 + Na_2CO_3 \longrightarrow CaCO_3 + 2NaCl$

In a disproportionation reaction, the chemical (CO in our example) is simultaneously reduced and oxidized (cf. NaCl in CHM 1.6) forming 2 differerent products. A double replacement reaction involves ions (CHM 5.2) which change partners.

1.6 Oxidation Numbers, Redox Reactions, Oxidizing vs. Reducing Agents

A special class of reactions known as *redox* reactions are better balanced using the concept of <u>oxidation state</u>. This section deals with these reactions in which electrons are transferred from one atom (or a group of atoms) to another.

First of all, it is very important to understand the difference between the ionic charge and the oxidation state of an element. For this let us consider the two compounds sodium chloride (NaCl) and water (H_2O). NaCl is made up of the charged species or ions: Na^+ and Cl^-. During the formation of this molecule, one electron is transferred from the Na atom to the Cl atom. It is possible to verify this fact experimentally and determine that the charge of sodium in NaCl is indeed +1 and that the one for chlorine is -1. The elements in the periodic table tend to lose or gain electrons to different extents. Therefore, even in non-ionic compounds electrons are always transferred, to different degrees, from one atom to another during the formation of a molecule of the compound. The actual partial charges that result from these partial transfers of electrons can also be determined experimentally. The oxidation state is not equal to such partial charges. It is rather an artificial concept that is used to perform some kind of "electron bookkeeping."

In a molecule like H_2O, since oxygen tends to attract electrons more than hydrogen, one can predict that the electrons that allow bonding to occur between hydrogen and oxygen will be displaced towards the oxygen atom. For the sake of "electron bookkeeping" we assign these electrons to the oxygen atom. The charge that the oxygen atom would have in this artificial process would be -2: this defines the oxidation state of oxygen in the H_2O molecule. In the same line of reasoning one defines the oxidation state of hydrogen in the water molecule as +1. The actual partial charges of hydrogen and oxygen are in fact smaller; but, as we will see later, the concept of oxidation state is very useful in stoichiometry.

Here are the general rules one needs to follow to assign oxidation numbers to different elements in different compounds:

1. In elementary substances, the oxidation number of an element is zero. This is, for instance, the case for N in N_2 or Na in sodium element, O in O_2,or S in S_8.

2. In monoatomic ions the oxidation number of the element that make up this ion is equal to the charge of the ion. This is the case for Na in Na^+ (+1) or Cl in Cl^- (-1) or Fe in Fe^{3+} (+3). Clearly, monoatomic ions are the only species for which atomic charges and oxidation numbers coincide.

3. In a neutral molecule the sum of the oxidation numbers of all the elements that make up the molecule is zero. In a polyatomic ion (e.g. SO_4^{2-}) the sum of the oxidation numbers of the elements that make up this ion is equal to the charge of the ion.

4. Some useful oxidation numbers to memorize:

For H: +1, except in metal hydrides (general formula XH where X is from the first two columns of the periodic table) where it is equal to -1.

For O: -2 in most compounds. In peroxides (e.g. in H_2O_2) the oxidation number for O is -1, it is +2 in OF_2 and -1/2 in superoxides (e.g. potassium superoxide: KO_2 which contains the O_2^- ion as opposed to the O^{2-} ion).

For alkali metals (first column in the periodic table): +1.

For alkaline earth metals (second column): +2.

Aluminium always has an oxidation number of +3 in all its compounds. (i.e. clorides $AlCl_3$, nitrites $Al(NO_2)_3$, etc.)

An element is said to have been *reduced* during a reaction if its oxidation number decreased during this reaction, it is said to have been oxidized if its *oxidation number* increased. A simple example is:

$$Zn(s) + CuSO_4(aq) \longrightarrow$$

Oxid.#:   0   +2

$$ZnSO_4(aq) + Cu(s)$$

Oxid.#:   +2   0

During this reaction Cu is reduced (oxidation number decreases from +2 to 0) while Zn is oxidized (oxidation number increases from 0 to +2). Since, in a sense, Cu is reduced by Zn, Zn can be referred to as the <u>reducing agent</u>. Similarly, Cu is the <u>oxidizing agent</u>.

The redox titrations will be dealt with in the section on titrations (CHM 6.10). Many of the redox agents in the table below will be explored in the chapters on Organic Chemistry.

Common Redox Agents	
Reducing Agents	**Oxidizing Agents**
* Lithium aluminium hydride ($LiAlH_4$) * Sodium borohydride ($NaBH_4$) * Metals * Ferrous ion (Fe^{2+})	* Iodine (I_2) and other halogens * Permanganate (MnO_4) salts * Peroxide compounds (i.e. H_2O_2) * Ozone (O_3); osmium tetroxide (OsO_4) * Nitric acid (HNO_3); nitrous oxide (N_2O)

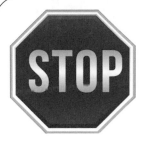

Reminder: Chapter review questions are available online for the owner of this textbook. Doing practice questions will help clarify concepts and ensure that you study in a targeted way. After you login to mcat-prep.com as a Gold Standard Owner*, click on Lessons in the Menu. Your access continues for one full year. Please note that the MCAT is expected to change in 2015 and so access will not continue after the MCAT has changed.

*To become a Gold Standard Owner, you will need to click on FREE MCAT in the top Menu of the mcat-prep.com homepage and then you will find "Click here if you own a Gold Standard textbook". Then follow the directions provided.

Memorize	Understand	Not Required*
* Definitions of quantum numbers * Shapes of s, p orbitals * Order for filling atomic orbitals * Equation for max. # of shell electrons	* Conventional notation, Pauli, Hund's * Box diagrams, IP, electronegativity * Valence, half-filled d orbitals, EA * Variation in shells, atomic size *Trends in the periodic table	* Advanced level college info * Memorizing Schroedinger's equation * Memorizing data from the periodic table * IUPAC's systematic element names (gen. chem.)

MCAT-Prep.com

Introduction

The periodic table of the elements provides data and abbreviations for the names of elements in a tabular layout. The purpose of the table is to illustrate recurring (periodic) trends and to classify and compare the different types of chemical behavior. To do so, we must first better understand the atom.

Additional Resources

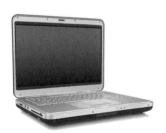
Free Online Q & A

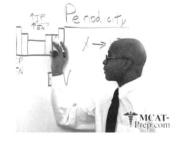
Video: Online or DVD 1

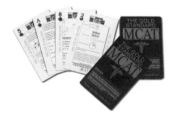
Flashcards

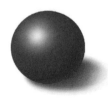
Special Guest

2.1 Electronic Structure of an Atom

The modern view of the structure of atoms is based on a series of discoveries and complicated theories that were put forth at the turn of this century. We will only present the main ideas behind these findings that shaped our understanding of atomic structure.

The first important idea is that electrons (as well as any microscopic particles) are in fact <u>waves as well as particles</u>; this concept is often referred to in textbooks as the <u>dual nature of matter</u>.

Contrary to classical mechanics, in this modern view of matter information on particles is not derived from the knowledge of their position and momentum at a given time but by the knowledge of the wave function (mathematical expression of the above-mentioned wave) and their energy. Mathematically, such information can be derived, in principle, by solving the master equation of quantum mechanics known as the <u>Schroedinger equation</u>. In the case of the hydrogen atom, this equation can be solved exactly. It yields the possible states of energy in which the electron can be found within the hydrogen atom and the wave functions associated with these states. The <u>square of the wave function</u> associated with a given state of energy <u>gives</u> the <u>probability to find the electron</u>, which is in that same state of energy, at any given point in space at any given time. These <u>wave functions</u> as well as their geometrical representations are referred to as the *atomic orbitals*. We shall explain further below the significance of these geometrical representations.

Even for a hydrogen atom there is a large number of possible states in which its single electron can be found (when it is subjected to different external perturbations). A labelling of these states is therefore necessary. This is done using the *quantum numbers*. These are:

(i) n: *the principal quantum number*. This number takes the integer values 1,2,3,4,5... The higher the value of n the higher the energy of the state labelled by this n. This number defines the atomic shells K (n=1), L (n=2), M (n=3) etc...

(ii) *l*: *the angular momentum quantum number*. It defines the shape of the atomic orbital in a way which we will discuss further below. For a given electronic state of energy defined by n, *l* takes all possible integer values between 0 and n-1. For instance for a state with n=0 there is only one possible shape of orbital, it is defined by *l*=0. For a state defined by n=3 there are 3 possible orbital shapes with *l*=0,1 and 2.

All orbitals with *l*=0 are called "s", all with *l*=1 are "p", those with *l*=2 or 3 are "d" or "f" respectively. The important shapes to remember are: i) s = spherical, ii) p = 2 lobes or "dumbbell" (*see the following diagrams*). For values of *l* larger than 3, which occur with an n greater or equal to 4, the corresponding series of atomic orbitals follows the alphabetical order h,i,j,...

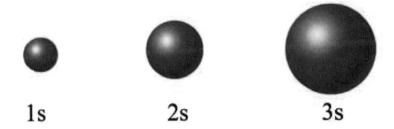

1s   2s   3s

Figure III.A.2.1: Atomic orbitals where $l = 0$. Notice that the orbitals do not reveal the precise location (position) or momentum of the fast moving electron at any point in time (Heisenberg's Uncertainty Principle). Instead, we are left with a 90% chance of finding the electron somewhere within the shapes described as orbitals.

(iii) m_l: *the magnetic quantum number*. It defines the orientation of the orbital of a given shape. For a given value of l (given shape), m_l can take any of the $2l+1$ integer values between $-l$ and $+l$. For instance for a state with n=3 and l=1 (3p orbital in notation explained in the previous paragraph) there are three possible values for m_l: -1,0 and 1. These 3 orbitals are oriented along x, y or the z axis of a coordinate system with its origin on the nucleus of the atom: they are denoted as $3p_x$, $3p_y$ and 3pz. The diagrams show the representation of an orbital corresponding to an electron in a state ns, np_x, np_y, and np_z. These are the 3D volumes where there is 90% chance to find an electron which is in a state ns, np_x, np_y, or np_z, respectively. This type of diagram constitutes the most common geometrical representation of the atomic orbitals.

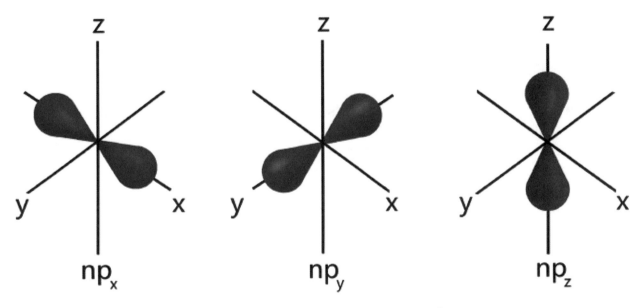

Figure III.A.2.2: Atomic orbitals where $l = 1$.

(iv) m_s: *the spin quantum number*. This number takes the values +1/2 or -1/2 for the electron. Some textbooks present the intuitive, albeit wrong, explanation that the spin angular momentum arises from the spinning of the electron around itself, the opposite signs for the spin quantum number would correspond to the two opposite rotational directions. We do have to resort to such an intuitive presentation because the spin angular moment has, in fact, no classical equivalent and, as a result, the physics behind the correct approach is too complex to be dealt with in introductory courses.

2.2 Conventional Notation for Electronic Structure

The state of an electron in an atom is completely defined by a set of quantum numbers (n, l, m_l, m_s). If two electrons in an atom share the same n, l and m_l numbers their m_s have to be of opposite signs: this is known as Pauli's exclusion principle. This principle along with a rule known as Hund's rule constitutes the basis for the procedure that one needs to follow to assign the possible (n, l, m_l, m_s) states to the electrons of a polyelectronic atom. Orbitals are "filled" in sequence, according to an example below. When filling a set of orbitals with the same n and l (e.g. the three 2p orbitals: $2p_x$, $2p_y$ and $2p_z$ which differ by their m_l's) electrons are assigned to orbitals with different m_l's first with parallel spins (same sign for their m_s), until each orbital of the given group is filled with one electron, then, electrons are paired in the same orbital with antiparallel spins (opposite signs for m_s). This procedure is illustrated in an example which follows. The electronic configuration which results from orbitals filled in accordance with the previous set of rules corresponds to the atom being in its lowest overall state of energy. This state of lowest energy is referred to as the ground state of the atom.

The restrictions related to the previous set of rules lead to the fact that only a certain number of electrons is allowed for each quantum number:

for a given n (given shell): the maximum number of electrons allowed is $2n^2$.

for a given l (s,p,d,f...): this number is $4l+2$.

for a given m_l (given orbital orientation): a maximum of 2 electrons is allowed.

There is a **conventional notation** for the electronic structure of an atom:

(i) orbitals are listed in the order they are filled

(ii) generally, in this conventional notation, no distinction is made between electrons in states defined by the same n and l but which do not share the same m_l.

For instance the ground state electronic configuration of oxygen is written as:

$$1s^2\ 2s^2\ 2p^4$$

When writing the electronic configuration of a polyelectronic atom orbitals are filled (with two electrons) in order of increasing energy: 1s 2s 2p 3s 3p 4s 3d ... according to the following figure:

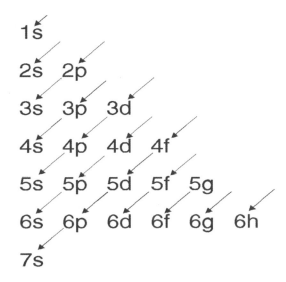

follow the direction of successive arrows moving from top to bottom

Figure III.A.2.3: The order for filling atomic orbitals.

Another illustrative notation is also often used. In this alternate notation orbitals are represented by boxes (hence the referring to this representation as "box diagrams"). Orbitals with the same l are grouped together and electrons are represented by vertical ascending or descending arrows (for the two opposite signs of m_s).

For instance for the series H, He, Li, Be, B, C we have the following electronic configurations:

H: $1s^1$ box diagram: ☐

He: $1s^2$ box diagram: ☐ and not ☐ (rejected by Pauli's exclusion principle)

Li: $1s^2$ $2s^1$

Be: $1s^2$ $2s^2$

B: $1s^2$ $2s^2$ $2p^1$

C: $1s^2$ $2s^2$ $2p^2$

(to satisfy Hund's rule of maximum spin)

To satisfy Hund's rule the next electron is put into a separate 2p "box". The 4th 2p electron (for oxygen) is put in the first box with an opposite spin.

Finally, we should point out that electrons can be promoted to higher unoccupied (or partially occupied) orbitals when the atom is subjected to some external perturbation which inputs energy into the atom. The resulting electronic configuration is called an <u>excited state configuration</u>.

2.3 Elements, Chemical Properties and The Periodic Table

Since most chemical properties of the atom are related to their outermost electrons (valence electrons), it is the orbital occupation of these electrons which is most relevant in the complete electronic configuration. The periodic table (see the end of this chapter; one is supplied in the MCAT exam) can be used to derive such information in the following way:

(i) the row or period number gives the "n" of the valence electrons of any given element of the period.

(ii) the first two columns or groups and helium (He) are referred to as the "s" block. The valence electrons of elements in these groups are "s" electrons.

(iii) groups 3A to 8A (13th to 18th columns) are the "p" group. Elements belonging to these groups have their ground state electronic configurations ending with "p" electrons.

(iv) Elements in groups 3B to 2B (columns 3 to 12) are called transition elements. Their electronic configurations end with ns^2 $(n-1)d^x$ where n is the period number and x=1 for column 3, 2 for column 4, 3 for column 5, etc... Note that these elements sometimes have unexpected or unusual valence shell electronic configurations.

This set of rules should make the writing of the ground-state valence shell electronic configuration very easy. For instance: Sc being an element of the "d" group on the 4th period should have a ground-state valence shell electronic configuration of the form: $4s^2$ $3d^x$. Since it belongs to group 3B (column 3) x=1; therefore, the actual configuration is simply: $4s^2$ $3d^1$. However, half-filled (i.e. Cr) and filled (i.e. Cu, Ag, Au) d orbitals have remarkable stability. This stability makes for unusual configurations (i.e. by the rules Cr=$4s^2$ $3d^4$, but in reality Cr=$4s^1$ $3d^5$ creating a half-filled d orbital). Some metal ions form colored solutions due to the transition energies of the d-electrons.

A number of physical and chemical properties of the elements are periodic, i.e. they vary in a regular fashion with atomic numbers. We will define some of these properties and explain their trends:

(i) First ionization energy or potential (1st IE or IP): the energy required to remove one of the outermost electrons from an atom in its gaseous state. The ionization potential increases from left to right in a period and decreases from the top to the bottom of a group or column in the periodic chart. The 1st IP drops sharply when we move from the last element of a period (inert gas) to the first element of the next period. These are general trends, elements located after an element with a half-filled shell, for instance, have a lower 1st IP than expected by these trends.

(ii) Second ionization energy or potential (2nd IE or IP): the previous trends can be used if one remembers the relationship between 1st and 2nd ionization processes of an atom of element X:

$$X + energy \longrightarrow X^+ + 1\,e^-$$
1st ionization of X

$$X^+ + energy \longrightarrow X^{2+} + 1\,e^-$$
2nd ionization of X

The second ionization process of X can be viewed as the 1st ionization of X^+. With this in mind it is very easy to predict trends of 2nd IP's. For instance, let us compare the 2nd IP's of the elements Na and Al. This is equivalent to comparing the 1st IP's of Na^+ and Al^+. These, in turn, have the same valence shell electronic configurations as Ne and Mg, respectively. Applying the previous general principles on Ne and Mg we arrive at the following conclusions:
  * the 1st IP of Ne is greater than the 1st IP of Mg

  * the 1st IP of Na^+ is therefore expected to be greater than the 1st IP of Al^+

  * the latter statement is equivalent to the final conclusion that the 2nd IP of Na is greater than the 2nd IP of Al.

(iii) Electron affinity (EA) is the energy change that accompanies the following process for an atom of element X:

$$X(gas) + 1\,e^- \longrightarrow X^-(gas)$$

This property measures the ability of an atom to accept an electron. Halogen atoms (F, Cl, Br...) have a very negative EA because they have a great tendency to form negative ions. On the other hand, alkaline earth metals which tend to form positive rather than negative ions have very large positive EA's. The overall tendency is that EA's become more negative as we move from left to right across a period, they are more negative (less positive) for non-metals than for metals and they do not change considerably within a group or column.

(iv) Atomic radius generally decreases from left to right across a period and increases when we move down a group.

(v) Electronegativity is a parameter that measures the ability of an atom, when engaged in a molecular bond, to pull or repel the bond electrons. This parameter is determined from the 1st IE and the EA of a given atom. Electronegativity follows the same general trends as the 1st IE.

2.3.1 Bond Strength

When there is a big difference in electronegativity between two atoms sharing a covalent bond then the bond is generally weaker as compared to two atoms with little electronegativity difference. This is because in the latter case, the bond is shared more equally and is thus more stable.

Bond strength is inversely proportional to bond length. Thus, all things being equal, a stronger bond would be shorter. Bonds and bond strength is further discussed in ORG 1.3-1.5.1.

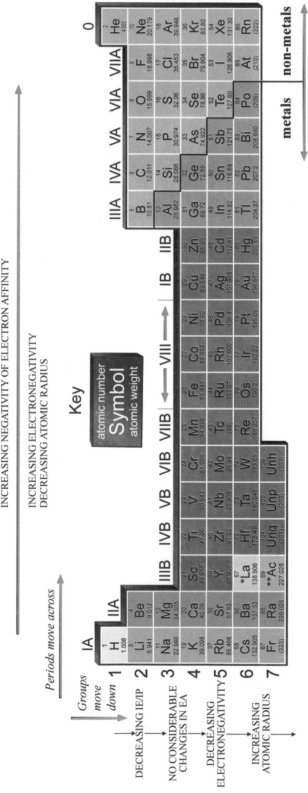

PERIODIC TABLE OF THE ELEMENTS

INCREASING IONIZATION ENERGY OR IONIZATION POTENTIAL
INCREASING NEGATIVITY OF ELECTRON AFFINITY

INCREASING ELECTRONEGATIVITY
DECREASING ATOMIC RADIUS

Key

atomic number
Symbol
atomic weight

Periods move across

Groups move down

DECREASING IE/IP
NO CONSIDERABLE CHANGES IN EA
DECREASING ELECTRONEGATIVITY
INCREASING ATOMIC RADIUS

non-metals

metals

Element	Symbol	Atomic Number
Actinium	Ac	89
Aluminum	Al	13
Americium	Am	95
Antimony	Sb	51
Argon	Ar	18
Arsenic	As	33
Astatine	At	85
Barium	Ba	56
Berkelium	Bk	97
Beryllium	Be	4
Bismuth	Bi	83
Boron	B	5
Bromine	Br	35
Cadmium	Cd	48
Calcium	Ca	20
Californium	Cf	98
Carbon	C	6
Cerium	Ce	58
Cesium	Cs	55
Chlorine	Cl	17
Chromium	Cr	24
Cobalt	Co	27
Copper	Cu	29
Curium	Cm	96
Dysprosium	Dy	66
Einsteinium	Es	99
Erbium	Er	68
Europium	Eu	63
Fermium	Fm	100
Fluorine	F	9
Francium	Fr	87
Gadolinium	Gd	64
Gallium	Ga	31

Element	Symbol	Atomic Number
Germanium	Ge	32
Gold	Au	79
Hafnium	Hf	72
Helium	He	2
Holmium	Ho	67
Hydrogen	H	1
Indium	In	49
Iodine	I	53
Iridium	Ir	77
Iron	Fe	26
Krypton	Kr	36
Lanthanum	La	57
Lawrencium	Lr	103
Lead	Pb	82
Lithium	Li	3
Lutetium	Lu	71
Magnesium	Mg	12
Manganese	Mn	25
Mendelevium	Md	101
Mercury	Hg	80
Molybdenum	Mo	42
Neodymium	Nd	60
Neon	Ne	10
Neptunium	Np	93
Nickel	Ni	28
Niobium	Nb	41
Nitrogen	N	7
Nobelium	No	102
Osmium	Os	76
Oxygen	O	8
Palladium	Pd	46
Phosphorous	P	15
Platinum	Pt	78

Plutonium	Pu	94	Tantalum	Ta	73
Polonium	Po	84	Technetium	Tc	43
Potassium	K	19	Tellurium	Te	52
Praseodymium	Pr	59	Terbium	Tb	65
Promethium	Pm	61	Thallium	Tl	81
Protactinium	Pa	91	Thorium	Th	90
Radium	Ra	88	Thulium	Tm	69
Radon	Rn	86	Tin	Sn	50
Rhenium	Re	75	Titanium	Ti	22
Rhodium	Rh	45	Tungsten	W	74
Rubidium	Rb	37	(Unnilhexium)	(Unh)	106
Ruthenium	Ru	44	(Unnilpentium)	(Unp)	105
Samarium	Sm	62	(Unnilquadium)	(Unq)	104
Scandium	Sc	21	Uranium	U	92
Selenium	Se	34	Vanadium	V	23
Silicon	Si	14	Xenon	Xe	54
Silver	Ag	47	Ytterbium	Yb	70
Sodium	Na	11	Yttrium	Y	39
Strontium	Sr	38	Zinc	Zn	30
Sulfur	S	16	Zirconium	Zr	40

Memorize	Understand	Not Required*
* Hybrid orbitals, shapes * Define Lewis: structure, acid, base * Define: octet rule, formal charge	* Ionic, covalent bonds * VSEPR, Resonance * Dipole, covalent polar bonds * Trends in the periodic table	* Advanced level college info * Details of VSEPR * Memorizing hybrids with d, f

MCAT-Prep.com

Introduction

Attractive interactions between atoms and molecules involve a physical process called chemical bonding. In general, strong chemical bonding is associated with the sharing or transfer of electrons between atoms. Molecules, crystals and diatomic gases are held together by chemical bonds which makes up most of the matter around us.

Additional Resources

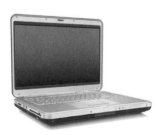

Free Online Q & A

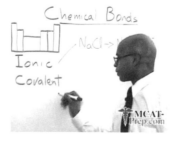

Video: Online or DVD 1, 2

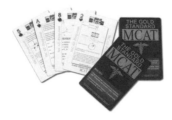

Flashcards

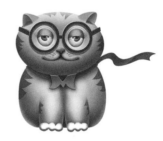

Special Guest

3.1 The Ionic Bond

When an element X with a low ionization potential is combined with an element Y with a large negative electron affinity one or more electrons are transferred from the atoms of X to the atoms of Y. This leads to the formation of cations X^{n+} and anions Y^{m-}. These ions of opposite charges are then attracted to each other through electrostatic forces. The bonds that hold these ions together are called ionic bonds. Ionic bonding favors the formation of large stable spatial arrangements of ions: crystalline solids. In our general example, note that to maintain electrical neutrality the empirical formula of this ionic compound has to be of the general form: X_mY_n (the total positive charge: $n \times m$ is equal to the total negative charge: $m \times n$ in a unit formula). For instance, since aluminium tends to form the cation Al^{3+} and oxygen the anion O^{2-} the empirical formula for aluminium oxide is Al_2O_3.

3.2 The Covalent Bond

Atoms are held together in non-ionic molecules by covalent bonds. In this type of bonding two valence electrons are shared by two atoms. A Lewis structure is a representation of covalent bonding in which shared electrons are shown either as lines or as pairs of dots between two atoms. For instance, let us consider the H_2O molecule. The valence shell electronic configurations of the atoms that constitute this molecule are:

O: $2s^2 2p^4$
H: $1s^1$

Since hydrogen has only one electron to share with oxygen there is only one possible covalent bond that can be formed between the oxygen atom and each of the hydrogen atoms. 4 of the valence electrons of the oxygen atom do not participate in this covalent bonding, these are called non-bonding electrons or lone pairs. The Lewis structure of the water molecule is:

$$H \!:\! \overset{\displaystyle ..}{\underset{\displaystyle ..}{O}} \!:\! H \quad \text{or} \quad H\text{-}\overset{\displaystyle ..}{\underset{\displaystyle ..}{O}}\text{-}H$$

Lewis formulated the following general rule known as the octet rule concerning these representations: atoms tend to form covalent bonds until they are surrounded by 8 electrons (except for hydrogen which can be surrounded by a maximum of only 2 electrons). To satisfy this rule (and if there is a sufficient number of valence electrons), two atoms may share more than one pair of electrons thus forming more than one covalent bond at a time. In such instances the bond between these atoms is referred to as a double or a triple bond depending on whether there are two or three pairs of shared electrons, respectively.

Some molecules cannot fully be described by a single Lewis structure. For instance, for the carbonate ion: CO_3^{2-}, the octet rule is satisfied for the central carbon atom if one of the C...O bonds is double (*see* ORG 1.5). While this leads us to thinking that the three C...O bonds are not equivalent, every experimental evidence concerning this molecule show that the three bonds are the same (same length, same polarity, etc...). This suggests that in such instances a molecule cannot be described fully by a single Lewis structure. Indeed, since there is no particular reason to choose one oxygen atom over another we can write three equivalent Lewis structures for the previous ion. These three structures are called resonance structures. It is the full set of resonance structures that describe such a molecule. In this picture, the C...O bonds are neither double nor single, they have both a single and a double bond character. It is often interesting to compare the number of valence electrons that an atom possesses when it is isolated and when it is engaged in a covalent bond within a given molecule. This is often quantitatively described by the concept of formal charge. This concept is defined as follows:

total # of valence e-'s in the free atom
- total # of non-bonding e-'s in the molecule
- 1/2 (total # bonding e-'s) in the molecule
_____

=formal charge

Let us apply this definition to the two previous examples: H_2O and CO_3^{2-}. This process is fairly straightforward in the case of the water molecule:

total # of valence e-'s in free O: 6
- total # of non-bonding e-'s on O in H_2O: 4
- 1/2 (total # of bonding e-'s) on O in H_2O: 2
_____

Formal charge of O in H_2O =   0

The case of CO_3^{2-} ion is not as obvious. If we consider one of the equivalent resonance forms, for the oxygen with a double bond we have:

total # of valence e-'s in free O: 6
- total # of non-bonding e-'s on O in the ion:
                                             4
- 1/2 (total # of bonding e-) on O in the ion:
                                             2
_____

Formal charge of O of C=O in the ion = 0

Similarly, the calculation of the formal charge for O of C-O in the same ion leads to the following: 6-6-1/2(2)= -1. Considering that CO_3^{2-} is represented by three resonance forms, the actual formal charge of the oxygen atom is 1/3 (-1-1+0)= -2/3. This number formally reflects the idea that the oxygen atoms are equivalent and that any one of them has a -1 charge in 2 out of three of the resonance forms of this ion. Here are some simple rules to remember about formal charges:

(i)   For neutral molecules, the

formal charges of all the atoms should add up to zero.

(ii)   For an ion, the sum of the formal charges must equal the ion's charge.

The following rules should help you select a plausible Lewis structure:

(i)   If you can write more than one Lewis structure for a given neutral molecule; the most plausible one is the one in which the formal charges of the individual atoms are zero.

(ii)   Lewis stuctures with the smallest formal charges on each individual atom are more plausible than the ones that involve large formal charges.

(iii)   Out of a range of possible Lewis structures for a given molecule, the most plausible ones are the ones in which negative formal charges are found on the most electronegative atoms and positive charges on the most electropositive ones.

In addition to these rules, remember that some elements have a tendency to form molecules that do not satisfy the octet rule:

(i)   When sulfur is the central atom in a molecule or a polyatomic ion it almost invariably does not fulfill the octet rule. The number of electrons around S in these compounds is usually 12 (e.g. SF_6, SO_4^{2-}). This situation (expanded octets) also occurs in other elements in and beyond the third period.

(ii)   Molecules that have an element from the 3A group (B, Al..) as their central atom do not generally obey the octet rule. In these molecules there are less than 8 electrons around the central atom (e.g. AlI_3 and BF_3).

(iii)   Some molecules with an odd number of electrons can clearly not obey the octet rule (e.g. NO and NO_2).

3.3 Partial Ionic Character

Except for homonuclear molecules (molecules made of atoms of the same element, e.g. H_2, O_3, etc...), bonding electrons are not equally shared by the bonded atoms. Thus a diatomic (= *two atoms*) compound like Cl_2 shares its bonding electrons equally; whereas, a binary (= *two different elements*) compound like CaO (calcium ox_ide_) or NaCl (sodium chloride) does not. Indeed, for the great majority of molecules, one of the two atoms between which the covalent bond occurs is necessarily more electronegative than the other. This atom will attract the bonding electrons to a larger extent. Although this phenomenon does not lead to the formation of two separate ionic species, it does result in a molecule in which there are partial charges on these particular atoms: the corresponding covalent bond is said to possess partial ionic character. This polar bond will also have a dipole moment given by:

$$D = q \cdot d$$

where q is the absolute value of the partial charge on the most electronegative or the most electropositive bonded atom and d is the distance between these two atoms. To obtain the total dipole moment of a molecule one must add the individual dipole moment vectors present on each one of its bonds. Since this is a vector addition, the overall result may be zero even if the individual dipole moment vectors are very large.

Non-polar bonds are generally stronger than polar covalent and ionic bonds, with ionic bonds being the weakest. However, in compounds with ionic bonding, there is generally a large number of bonds between molecules and this makes the compound as a whole very strong. For instance, although the ionic bonds in one compound are weaker than the non-polar covalent bonds in another compound, the ionic compound's melting point will be higher than the melting point of the covalent compound. Polar covalent bonds have a partially ionic character, and thus the bond strength is usually intermediate between that of ionic and that of non-polar covalent bonds. The strength of bonds generally decreases with increasing ionic character.

3.4 Lewis Acids and Lewis Bases

In the previous section we pointed out some exceptions to Lewis' octet rule. Among these were molecules that had a deficiency of electrons around the central atom (e.g. BF_3). When such a molecule is put in contact with a molecule with lone pairs (e.g. NH_3) a reaction occurs. Such a reaction can be interpreted as a donation of a pair of electrons from the second type of molecule to the first, or alternately by an acceptance of a pair of electrons by the first type of molecule. Molecules such as BF_3 are referred to as Lewis acids while molecules such as NH_3 are Lewis bases. {LEwis Acids: Electron Acceptors}

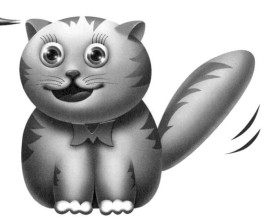

What is the name of 007's northern cousin? Polar Bond.

3.5 Valence Shell Electronic Pair Repulsions (VSEPR Models)

One of the shortcommings of Lewis structures is that they cannot be used to predict molecular geometries. In this context a model known as the valence-shell electronic pair repulsion or VSEPR model is very useful. In this model, the geometrical arrangement of atoms or groups of atoms bound to a central atom A is determined by the number of pairs of valence electrons around A. VSEPR procedure is based on the principle that these electronic pairs around the central atom are arranged in such a way that the repulsions between them are minimized. The general VSEPR procedure starts with the determination of the number of electronic pairs around A:

> \# of valence electrons in a free atom of A
> + \# of sigma bonds involving A
> - \# of pi bonds involving A
>
> _____
>
> =(total # of electrons around A)

The division of this total number by 2 yields the total number of electron pairs around A. Note the following important points:

(i) A single bond counts for 1 sigma bond, a double bond for 1 sigma bond and 1 pi bond and a triple bond for 1 sigma and two pi bonds.

(ii) The general calculation presented above is performed for the purposes of VSEPR modelling; its result can be quite different from the one obtained in the corresponding Lewis structure.

(iii) For all practical purposes, one always assigns a double bond (i.e. 1 sigma bond and one pi bond) to a terminal oxygen (an oxygen which is not a central atom and is not attached to any other atom besides the central atom).

(iv) A terminal halogen is always assigned a single bond.

Once the number of pairs around the central atom is determined, the next step is to use Figure III.A.3.1 to predict the arrangement of these pairs around the central atom.

The next step is to consider the previous arrangement of the electronic pairs and place the atoms or groups of atoms that are attached to the central atom in accordance with such an arrangement. The pairs which are not involved in the bonding between these atoms and the central atom are lone pairs. If we substract the number of lone pairs from the total number of pairs we readily obtain the number of bonding pairs. It is the number of bonding pairs which ultimately determines the molecular geometry in the VSEPR model according to Table III.A.3.1. Let us consider three examples: CH_4, H_2O and CO_2.

1 - CH4:

	# of valence electrons on C:		4
+	# of sigma bonds:	+	4
-	# of pi bonds:	-	0

$$= 8/2 = 4 \text{ pairs}$$

According to Figure III.A.3.1 this corresponds to a tetrahedral arrangement. All of these pairs correspond to an H atom attached to the central atom of carbon. Therefore, the 4 pairs are bonding pairs and the molecular geometry is also tetrahedral.

2 - H_2O:

	# of valence electrons on O:		6
+	# of sigma bonds on the central O:	+	2
-	# of pi bonds on the central O:	-	0

$$= 8 / 2 = 4 \text{ pairs}$$

3 - CO_2:

	# of valence electrons on C:		4
+	# of sigma bonds for terminal O's:	+	2
-	# of pi bonds for terminal O's:	-	2

$$= 4 / 2 = 2 \text{ pairs}$$

This total number of pairs corresponds to a linear arrangement. Since both of these pairs are used to connect the central C atom to the terminal O's there are no lone pairs left on C. Therefore, the number of bonding pairs is also 2 and the molecular geometry is also linear.

Here are some additional rules when applying the VSEPR model:

(i)   When dealing with a cation (underline positive ion) subtract the charge of the ion from the total number of electrons.

(ii)   When dealing with an anion (underline negative ion) add the charge of the ion to the total number of electrons.

(iii)   A lone pair repels another lone pair or a bonding pair very strongly. This causes some deformation in bond angles. For instance, the H-O-H angle is smaller than 109.5°.

(iv)   The previous rule also holds for a double bond. Note that in one of our previous examples (CO_2), the angle is still 180° since there are two double bonds and no lone pairs. Indeed, in this geometry, the strong repulsions between the two double bonds are symmetrical.

(v)   The VSEPR model can be applied to polyatomic molecules. The procedure is the same as above except that one can only determine the arrangements of groups of atoms around one given central atom at a time. For instance, you could apply the VSEPR model to determine the geometrical arrangements of atoms around C or around O in methanol (CH_3OH). In the first case the molecule is treated as CH_3-X (where -X is -OH) and in the second it is treated as HO-Y (where -Y is -CH_3). The geometrical arrangement is tetrahedral in the first case which gives HCX or HCH angles close to 109°. The second case corresponds to a bent arrangement (with two lone pairs on the oxygen) and gives an HOY angle close to 109° as well.

Table III.A.3.1: Geometry of simple molecule in which the central atom A has one or more lone pairs of electrons (= e-).

Total number of e-pairs	Number of lone pairs	Number of bonding pairs	Arrangement of e-pairs	Geometry	Examples
3	1	2	Trigonal planar	Bent (sp^2)	SO_2
4	1	3	Tetrahedral	Trigonal pyramidal (sp^3)	NH_3
4	2	2	Tetrahedral	Bent (sp^3)	H_2O
5	1	4	Trigonal bipyramidal	Distorted tetrahedron (dsp^3)	SF_4
5	2	3	Trigonal bipyramidal	T-shaped (dsp^3)	ClF_3

Note: dotted lines only represent the overall molecular shape and not molecular bonds. In brackets under "Geometry" is the hybridization, to be discussed in ORG 1.2.

This also corresponds to a tetrahedral arrangement, however only two of these pairs are bonding pairs (connecting the H atoms to the central oxygen atom); therefore, the actual geometry according to Table III.A.3.1 is bent or V-shape geometry.

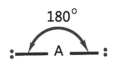

linear arrangement of
2 electron pairs around
central atom A

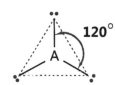

trigonal planar arrangement
of 3 electron pairs
around central atom A

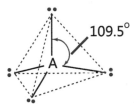

tetrahedral arrangement
of 4 electron pairs
around central atom A

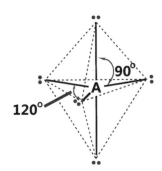

trigonal bipyramidal arrangement
of 5 electron pairs
around central atom A

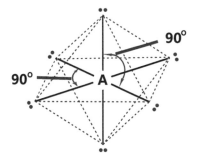

octahedral arrangement
of 6 electron pairs
around central atom A

Figure III.A.3.1: Molecular arrangement of electron pairs around a central atom A. Dotted lines only represent the overall molecular shape and not molecular bonds.

Memorize	Understand	Not Required*
* Define: temp. (C, K), gas P and weight * Define: STP, ideal gas, deviation * Equations: ideal gas/Charles'/Boyle's * Define: H bonds, dipole forces	* Kinetic molecular theory of gases * Maxwell distribution plot, H bonds, dipole F. * Deviation from ideal gas behavior * Partial Press., mole fraction, Dalton's * Intermolecular forces, phase change/diagrams	* Advanced level college info * Memorizing Van der Waals' equation * Memorizing the gas constant R * Memorizing values: triple point of H_2O

MCAT-Prep.com

Introduction ▪▪▪▪

A phase, or state of matter, is a uniform, distinct and usually separable region of material. For example, for a glass of water: the ice cubes are one phase (solid), the water is a second phase (liquid), and the humid air over the water is the third phase (gas = vapor). The temperature and pressure at which all 3 phases of a substance can coexist is called the triple point.

Additional Resources

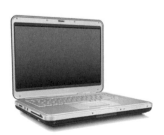

Free Online Q & A

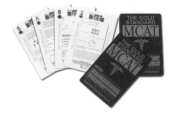

Video: Online or DVD 2

Flashcards

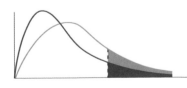

Special Guest

Elements and compounds exist in one of three states: the gaseous state, the liquid state or the solid state.

4.1 The Gas Phase

A substance in the gaseous state has neither fixed volume nor fixed shape: it spreads itself uniformly throughout any container in which it is placed.

4.1.1 Standard Temperature and Pressure, Standard Molar Volume

Any given gas can be described in terms of four fundamental properties: mass, volume, temperature and pressure. To simplify comparisons, the volume of a gas is normally reported at 0 $^{\circ}$C (273.15 K) and 1 atm (101.33 kPa = 760 mmHg = 760 torr); these conditions are known as the standard temperature and pressure (STP).

The volume occupied by one mole of any gas at STP is referred to as the standard molar volume and is equal to 22.4 l.

4.1.2 Kinetic Molecular Theory of Gases

The kinetic molecular theory of gases describes the behavior of matter in the gaseous state. A gas that fits this theory exactly is called an ideal gas. The essential points of the theory are as follows:

1.   Gases are composed of extremely small molecules separated by distances that are relatively large in comparison with the diameters of the molecules.

2.   Molecules of gas are in constant motion, except when they collide with one another.

3.   Molecules of an ideal gas exert no attractive or repulsive force on one another.

4.   The collisions experienced by gas molecules do not, on the average, slow

them down; rather, they cause a <u>change</u> in the direction in which the molecules are moving. If one molecule loses energy as a result of a collision, the energy is gained by the molecule with which it collides. <u>Collisions</u> of the molecules of an ideal gas with the walls of the container <u>result in no loss of energy.</u>

5. The <u>average kinetic energy</u> of the molecules (KE = 1/2 mv^2) <u>increases in direct proportion to the temperature</u> of the gas (KE = 3/2 kT) when the temperature is measured on an absolute scale (i.e. the Kelvin scale) and k is a constant (the Boltzmann constant).

The plot of the distribution of collision energies of gases is similar to that of liquids. However, molecules in liquids require a

minimum escape kinetic energy in order to enter the vapor phase.

The properties of gases can be explained in terms of the kinetic molecular theory of ideal gases.

Experimentally, we can measure four properties of a gas:

1. The <u>weight</u> of the gas, from which we can calculate the <u>number (N) of molecules</u> of the gas present;

2. The <u>pressure (P)</u>, exerted by the gas on the walls of the container in which this gas is placed (N.B.: a <u>vacuum</u> is completely devoid of particles and thus has *no* pressure);

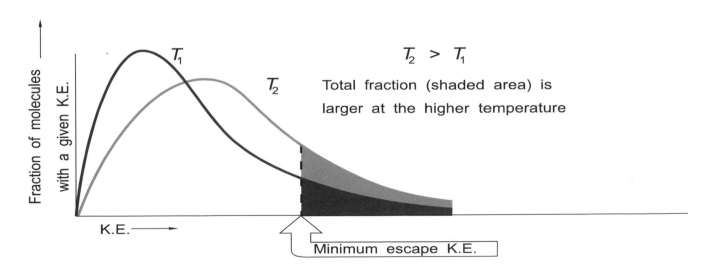

Figure III.A.4.1: The Maxwell Distribution Plot.

3.   The volume (_V_), occupied by the gas;

4.   The temperature (_T_) of the gas.

In fact, if we know any three of these properties, we can calculate the fourth. So the minimum number of these properties required to fully describe the state of an ideal gas is three.

4.1.3 Charles' Law

The volume (_V_) of a gas is directly proportional to the absolute temperature (expressed in Kelvins) when _P_ and _N_ are kept constant.

$V = $ Constant $\times T$ or $V_1/V_2 = T_1/T_2$

4.1.4 Boyle's Law

The volume (_V_) of a fixed weight of gas held at constant temperature (_T_) varies inversely with the pressure (_P_).

$V = $ Constant $\times 1/P$ or $P_1V_1 = P_2V_2$

4.1.5 Combined Gas Law

For a given mass of gas the product of its pressure and volume divided by its Kelvin temperature is a constant.

$$\frac{P_1V_1}{T_1} = \frac{P_2V_2}{T_2}$$

(at constant mass)

4.1.6 Ideal Gas Law

The combination of Boyle's law and Charles' law yields the ideal gas law:

$$PV = nRT$$

where R is the universal gas constant and n is the number moles of gas molecules.

R = 0.0821 L-atm/K-mole = 8.31 kPa-dm^3/K-mole

A typical ideal gas problem is: an ideal gas at 27 °C and 380 torr occupies a volume of 492 cm3. What is the number of moles of gas?

Ideal Gas Law problems often amount to mere exercises of unit conversions. The easiest way to do them is to convert the units of the values given to the units of the R gas constant.

P = 380 torr = 380 torr/(760 torr/atm) = 0.500 atm

T = 27 °C = 273 + 27 °C = 300 K
V = 492 cm^3 = 492 cm^3 × (1 liter/1000cm^3) = 0.492 liter
$PV = nRT$
$n = PV/RT$
n = (0.500 atm × 0.492 L)/(0.0821 L-atm/K-mole × 300 K)
n = 0.0100 mole

Also note that the ideal gas law could be used in the following alternate ways (Mwt = molecular weight):

(i)   since n = (mass m of gas sample)/(Mwt M of the gas)

$$PV = (m/M)\,R\,T$$

(ii)   since m/V is the density d of the gas :

$$P = \frac{d\,R\,T}{M}$$

4.1.7 Partial Pressure and Dalton's Law

In a mixture of unreactive gases, each gas distributes evenly throughout the container. All molecules exert the same pressure on the walls of the container with equal force. If we consider a mixture of gases occupying a total volume (V) at a temperature (T) the term partial pressure is used to refer to the pressure exerted by one component of the gas mixture if it were occupying the entire volume (V) at the temperature (T).

Dalton's law states that the total pressure observed for a mixture of gases is equal to the sum of the pressures that each individual component would exert were it alone in the container.

$$P_T = P_1 + P_2 + ... + P_i$$

where P_T is the total pressure and P_i is the partial pressure of any component (i).

The mole fraction (X_i) of any one gas present in a mixture is defined as follows:

$$X_i = n_i / n_{(total)}$$

where n_i = moles of that gas present in the mixture and $n_{(total)}$ = sum of the moles of all gases present in the mixture.

Of course, the sum of all mole fractions in a mixture must equal one:

$$\Sigma X_i = 1$$

The partial pressure (Pi) of a component of a gas mixture is equal to:

$$P_i = X_i P_T$$

The ideal gas law applies to any component of the mixture:

$$P_i V = n_i RT$$

4.1.8 Deviation of Real Gas Behavior from the Ideal Gas Law

The molecules of an ideal gas have zero volume and no inter-molecular forces. It obeys the ideal gas law. Its molecules behave as though they were moving points exerting no attraction on one another and occupying no space. Real gases deviate from ideal gas behavior as follows:

1. They do not obey $PV = nRT$. We can calculate n, P, V and T for a real gas on the assumption that it behaves like an ideal gas but the calculated values will not agree with the observed values.

2. Their molecules are subject to van der Waal attraction forces which are themselves independent of temperature. But the deviations they cause are more pronounced at low temperatures because they are less effectively opposed by the slower motion of molecules at lower temperatures. Similarly, an increase in pressure at constant temperature will crowd the molecules closer together and reduce the average distance between them. This will increase the attractive force between the molecules and the stronger these forces, the more the behavior of the real gas will deviate from that of an ideal gas. Thus, a real gas will act less like an ideal gas at

higher pressures than at lower pressures. {Mnemonic: an ideal Plow and Thigh = an ideal gas exists when **P**ressure is **low** and **T**emperature is **high**}

3.   The particles (i.e. molecules or atoms) occupy space. When a real gas is subjected to high pressures at ordinary temperatures, the fraction of the total volume occupied by the molecules increases. Under these conditions, the real gas deviates appreciably from ideal gas behavior.

4.   Their size and mass also affect the speed at which they move. At constant temperature, the kinetic energy ($KE = 1/2\ mv^2$) of all molecules - light or heavy - is nearly the same. This means that the heavier molecules must be moving more slowly than the lighter ones and that the attractive forces between the heavier molecules must be exercising a greater influence on their behavior. The greater speed of light molecules, however, tends to counteract the attractive forces between them, thus producing a slighter deviation from ideal gas behavior. Thus, a heavier molecule will deviate more widely from ideal gas behavior than a lighter molecule. {The preceding is given by Graham's law, where the rate of movement of a gas (*diffusion* or streaming through a fine hole - *effusion*) is inversely proportional to the square root of the molecular weight of the gas.}

4.2 Liquid Phase (Intra- and Intermolecular Forces)

The most striking properties of a liquid are its viscosity and surface tension (*see Physics section 6.1*). Liquids also distinguish themselves from gases in that they are relatively incompressible. The molecules of a liquid are also subject to forces strong enough to hold them together. These forces are intermolecular and they are weak attractive forces, that is they are effective over short distances only. They are also called Van der Waal forces. The most important ones are:

1.   Dipole-dipole forces which depend on the orientation as well as on the distance between the molecules; they are inversely proportional to the fourth power of the distance. In addition to the forces between permanent dipoles, a dipolar molecule induces in a neighboring molecule an electron distribution that results in another attractive force, the dipole-induced dipole force, which is inversely proportional to the seventh power of the distance and which is relatively independent of orientation.

2.   London forces are attractive forces acting between nonpolar molecules. They are due to the unsymmetrical instantaneous electron distribution which induces a dipole in neighboring molecules with a resultant attractive force.

3.   Hydrogen bonds occur

whenever hydrogen is covalently bonded to an atom such as O, N or F that attract electrons strongly. Because of the differences in electronegativity between H and O or N or F, the electrons that constitute the covalent bond are closer to the O, N or F nucleus than to the H nucleus leaving the latter relatively unshielded. The unshielded proton is strongly attracted to the O, N or F atoms of neighboring molecules since these form the negative end of a strong dipole. Hydrogen bonding is a special case of dipole-dipole interaction.

4.3 Phase Equilibria (Solids, Liquids and Gases)

4.3.1 Phase Changes

Elements and compounds can undergo transitions between the solid, liquid and gaseous states. They can exist in different <u>phases</u> and undergo <u>phase changes</u> which need not involve chemical reactions. A phase is a homogeneous, physically distinct and mechanically separable part of a system. Each phase is separated from other phases by a physical boundary.

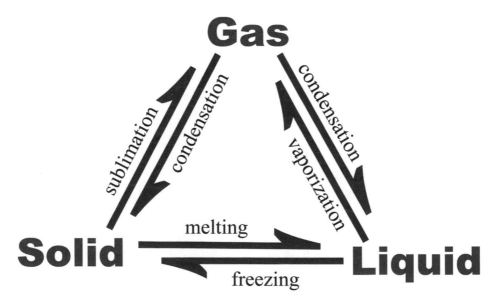

Figure III.A.4.2: Phase Changes

A few examples:

1.   Ice/liquid water/water vapor (3 phases)
2.   Any number of gases mix in all proportions and therefore constitute just one phase.
3.   The system $CaCO_3 \longrightarrow CaO + CO_2$ (2 phases, i.e. 2 solids: $CaCO_3$ and CaO and a gas: CO_2)
4.   A saturated salt solution (3 phases: solution, undissolved salt, vapor)

An example of phase change is the vaporization of water into its vapor state. A system is considered <u>homogeneous</u> when it is uniform throughout its volume so that its properties are the same in all parts. This does not imply a single molecular species: a solution of sodium chloride is homogeneous provided its concentration is the same throughout.

4.3.2 Freezing Point, Melting Point, Boiling Point

The conversion of a liquid to a gas is called <u>vaporization</u>.   We can increase the rate of vaporization of a liquid by i) increasing the temperature ii) reducing the pressure, or iii) both. Molecules escape from a liquid because, even though their average kinetic energy is constant, not all of them move at the same speed (*see Figure III.A.4.1*). A fast-moving molecule can break away from the attraction of the others and pass into the vapor state. When a tight lid is placed on a vessel containing a liquid, the vapor molecules can not escape and some revert back to the liquid state. The number of molecules leaving the liquid at any given time equals the number of molecules returning. Equilibrium is reached and the number of molecules in the fixed volume above the liquid remains constant. These molecules exert a constant pressure at a fixed temperature which is called the <u>vapor pressure</u> of the liquid.

Boiling and evaporation are similar processes but they differ as follows: the vapor from a boiling liquid escapes with sufficient pressure to push back any other gas present, rather than diffusing through it. The <u>boiling point</u> of a liquid is the temperature at which the vapor pressure of the liquid equals the opposing pressure (atmospheric, thus it is usually air). Under a lower pressure, the boiling point is reached at a lower temperature. Increased intermolecular interactions (i.e. H_2O *see* CHM 4.2, alcohol *see* ORG 6.1, etc.) will decrease the vapor pressure thus raising the boiling point. Other factors being equal, as a molecule becomes heavier (increasing molecular weight), it becomes more difficult to push the molecule into the atmosphere thus the boiling point increases (i.e. alkanes *see* ORG 3.1.1). The <u>freezing point</u> of a liquid is the temperature at which the vapor pressure of the solid equals the vapor pressure of the liquid. Increases in the prevailing atmospheric pressure decreases the melting point and increases the boiling point.

When a solid is heated, the kinetic energy of the components increases steadily. Finally, the kinetic energy becomes great enough to overcome the forces holding the components together and the solid changes to a liquid. For pure crystalline solids, there is a fixed temperature at which this transition from solid to liquid occurs. This temperature is called the melting point. Pure solids melt completely at one temperature. Impure solids begin to melt at one temperature but become completely liquid at a higher temperature.

4.3.3 Phase Diagrams

The temperatures at which phase transitions occur are functions of the pressure of the system. The behavior of a given substance over a wide range of temperature and pressure can be summarized in a phase diagram, such as the one shown for the water system (Fig. III. A.4.3).

The diagram is divided into three areas labelled **solid** (ice), **liquid** (water) and **vapor** in each of which only one phase exists. In these areas, P and T can be independently varied without a second phase appearing. These areas are bounded by curves AC, AD and AB. At any point on these curves, two phases are in equilibrium. Thus on AC, at a given T, the saturated vapor pressure of water has a fixed value. The boiling point of water (N) can be found on this curve, 100 $^{\circ}$C at 760 mmHg pressure. The curve only extends as far as C, the critical point, where the vapor and liquid are indistinguishable.

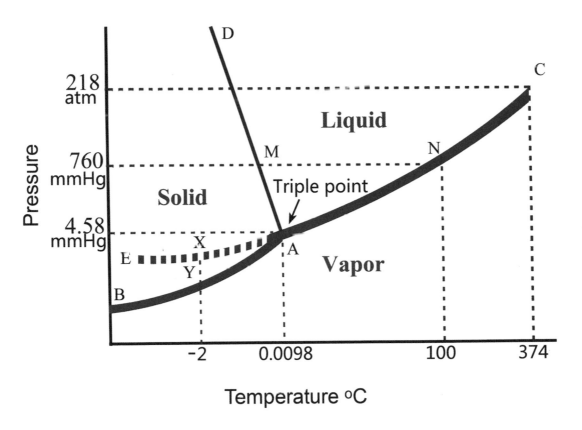

Figure III.A.4.3: Phase diagram for H_2O.

The extension of the curve CA to E represents the metastable equilibrium (*meta* = beyond) between supercooled water and its vapor. If the temperature is slightly raised at point X, a little of the liquid will vaporize until a new equilibrium is established at that higher temperature. Curve AB is the vapor pressure curve for ice. Its equilibria are of lower energy than those of AE and thus more stable.

The slope of line AD shows that an increase in P will lower the melting point of ice. This property is almost unique to water. Most substances *increase* their melting points with increased pressure. Thus the line AD slants to the right for almost all substances. Point M represents the true melting point of ice, 0.0023 $^{\circ}$C at 760 mmHg of pressure. (The 0 $^{\circ}$C standard refers to the freezing point of water saturated with air at 760 mmHg). At point A, solid, liquid and vapor are in equilibrium. At this one temperature, ice and water have the same fixed vapor pressure. This is the triple point, 0.0098 $^{\circ}$C at 4.58 mmHg pressure.

GOLD NOTES

Memorize	Understand	Not Required*
* Equations: Raoult, bp/fp up and down * Define saturated, supersatured, nonvolatile * Common anions and cations in solution * Units of concentration * Define electrolytes with examples	* Colligative properties, Raoult's law * Phase diagram change due to coll. properties * Bp elevation, fp depression * Osmotic press, equation * Solubility product, common-ion effect	* Advanced level college info * % solubility of glucose in water

MCAT-Prep.com

Introduction

A solution is a homogeneous mixture composed of two or more substances. For example, a solute (salt) dissolved in a solvent (water) making a solution (salt water). Solutions can involve gases in liquids (i.e. oxygen in water) or even solids in solids (i.e. alloys). Two substances are immiscible if they can't mix to make a solution. Solutions can be distinguished from non-homogeneous mixtures like colloids and suspensions.

Additional Resources

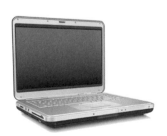

Free Online Q & A

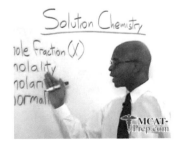

Video: Online or DVD 2, 3

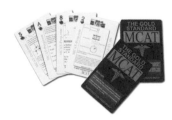

Flashcards

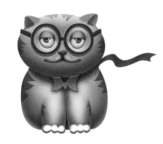

Special Guest

5.1 Colligative Properties

The previous section refers to a one-component system, i.e. a pure substance, H_2O. Pure substances are often mixed together to form solutions. A solution is a sample of matter that is homogeneous but, unlike a pure substance, the composition of a solution can vary within relatively wide limits. Ethanol and water each have a fixed composition, C_2H_5OH and H_2O, but mixtures of the two can vary continuously in composition from almost 100% ethanol to almost 100% water. Solutions of sucrose in water, however, are limited to a maximum percentage of sucrose - the solubility - which is 67% at $20^\circ C$, thus the solution is saturated. If the solution is heated, a higher concentration of glucose can be achieved (i.e. 70%). Slowly cooling down to $20^\circ C$ creates a supersaturated solution which may precipitate with any perturbation.

Generally the component of a solution that is stable in the same phase as the solution is called the solvent. If both components of a solution are in the same phase, the component present in the larger amount is called the solvent and the other is called the solute. Many properties of solutions are dependent only on the relative number of molecules (or ions) of the solute and of the solvent. Properties that depend **only** on the number of particles present are called colligative properties. The most important ones follow.

5.1.1 Vapor-Pressure Lowering (Raoult's Law)

The vapor pressure of the components of an ideal solution behaves as follows:

$$p_i = X_i \, (p_i)_{pure}$$

where p_i = vapor pressure of component i in equilibrium with the solution
$(p_i)_{pure}$ = vapor pressure of pure component i at the same T
X_i = mole fraction of component i in the liquid.

Thus the vapor pressure of any component of a mixture is lowered by the presence of the other components. Experimentally, it can be observed that when dissolving a solute which cannot evaporate (= *nonvolatile*) in a solvent, the vapor pressure of the resulting solution is lower than that of the pure solvent. The extent to which the vapor pressure is lowered is determined by the mole fraction of the solvent in solution (X):

$$P = P^o \, X$$

where P = vapor pressure of solution
P^o = vapor pressure of pure solvent (at the same temperature as P).

When rearranged this way, Raoult's law states that the lowering of the vapor pressure of the solvent is proportional to the mole fraction of solvent and independent of the chemical nature of the solute.

5.1.2 Boiling-Point Elevation and Freezing-Point Depression

When the vapor-pressure curve of a dilute solution and the vapor-pressure curve of the pure solvent are plotted on a phase diagram, it can be seen that the freezing point and boiling point of a solution must be different from those of the pure liquid.

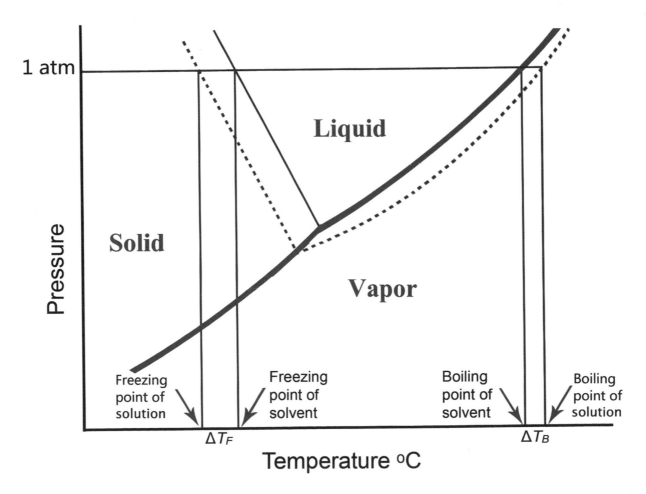

Figure III.A.5.1: Phase diagram of water demonstrating the effect of the addition of a solute.

The boiling point is higher for the solution than for the pure liquid. The freezing point is lower for the solution than for the pure liquid. Since the decrease in vapor pressure is proportional to the mole fraction of solute, the boiling point elevation (ΔT_B) is also proportional to the mole fraction of solute and:

$$\Delta T_B = K_B' X_B = K_B m$$

where K_B' = boiling point elevation constant for the solvent
   X_B = mole fraction of solute
   m = molality (moles solute per kilogram of solvent)
   K_B is related to K_B' through a change of units.

Similarly, for the freezing point depression (ΔT_F):

$$\Delta T_F = K_F' X_B = K_F m$$

where K_F' = freezing point depression constant for the solvent.

If K_F or K_B is known, it is possible to determine the molality of a dilute solution simply by measuring the freezing point or the boiling point. These constants can be determined by measuring the freezing point and boiling point of a solution of known molality. If the mass concentration of a solute (in kg solute per kg of solvent) is known and the molality is determined from the freezing point of the solution, the mass of 1 mole of solute can be calculated.

It is important to note that for a solution of strong electrolyte such as NaCl which dissociates to give positive and negative ions, the right hand side is multiplied by a factor "n" equal to the number of ionic species generated per mole of solute. For NaCl n=2 but for $MgCl_2$ n=3. {Remember: colligative properties depend on the **number** of particles present}

5.1.3 Osmotic Pressure

The osmotic pressure (Π) of a solution describes the equilibrium distribution of solvent across membranes. When a solvent and solution are separated by a membrane permeable only to molecules of solvent (a semipermeable membrane), solvent spontaneously migrates into the solution. The semipermeable membrane allows the solvent to pass but not the solute. The solvent migrates into the solution across the membrane until a sufficient hydrostatic pressure develops to prevent further migration of solvent. The pressure required to prevent migration of the solvent is defined as the osmotic pressure of the solution and is equal to:

$$\Pi = CRT$$

where R = gas constant per mole, T = temperature in degrees K and C = concentration of solute (mole/liter).

5.2 Ions in Solution

An important area of solution chemistry involves aqueous solutions. Water has a property that causes many substances to split apart into charged species, that is, to dissociate and form ions. Ions that are positively charged are called cations and negatively charged ions are called anions. {Mnemonic: anions are negative ions} As a rule, highly charged species (i.e. $AlPO_4$, Al^{3+}/ PO_4^{3-}) have a greater force of attraction thus are much less soluble in water than species with little charge (i.e. NaCl, Na^+/Cl^-).

Common Anions:

F^-	Fluoride	OH^-	Hydroxide
Cl^-	Chloride	NO_3^-	Nitrate
Br^-	Bromide	ClO_4^-	Perchlorate
I^-	Iodide	CO_3^{2-}	Carbonate
O^{2-}	Oxide	SO_4^{2-}	Sulfate
S^{2-}	Sulfide	PO_4^{3-}	Phosphate
N^{3-}	Nitride	$CH_3CO_2^-$	Acetate

Common Cations:

Na^+	Sodium	H^+	Hydrogen
Li^+	Lithium	Ca^{2+}	Calcium
K^+	Potassium	Mg^{2+}	Magnesium
NH_4^+	Ammonium	Fe^{2+}	Iron (II)
H_3O^+	Hydronium	Fe^{3+}	Iron (III)

5.3 Solubility

5.3.1 Units of Concentration

There are a number of ways in which solution concentrations may be expressed.

Molarity (M):   A one-molar solution is defined as one mole of substance in each liter of solution: M = moles of solute/liter of solution.

Normality (N):   A one-normal solution contains one equivalent per liter. An equivalent is a mole multiplied by the number of reacting units for each molecule or atom: the equivalent weight is the formula weight divided by the number of reacting units.

     # of Equiv.   = mass (in g) / eq. wt. (in g/equiv.)

          =Normality (in equiv./liter) $\times$ Volume (in liters)

For example, sulfuric acid, H_2SO_4, has two reacting units of protons, that is, there are two equivalents of protons in each mole. Thus:

     eq. wt. = 98.08 g/mole/2 equiv./mole
          = 49.04 g/equiv.

and the normality of a sulfuric acid solution is twice its molarity. Generally speaking:

$$N = n\,M$$

where N is the normality, M the molarity, n the number of equivalents per unit formula.

Thus for 1.2 M H_2SO_4:

1.2 moles/L $\times$ 2 eq/mole = 2.4 eq/L = 2.4 N.

Molality (m):   A one-molal solution contains one mole/1000g of solvent.
     m = moles of solute/kg of solvent.

Molal concentrations are not temperature-dependent as molar and normal concentrations are (since the solvent volume is temperature-dependent).

Density (ρ):   Mass per unit volume at the specified temperature, usually g/ml or g/cm^3 at 20°C.

Osmole (Osm):   The number of moles of particles (molecules or ions) that contribute to the osmotic pressure of a solution.

Osmolarity: A one-osmolar solution is defined as one osmole in each liter of solution. Osmolarity is measured in osmoles/liter of solution (Osm/L).

For example, a 0.001 M solution of sodium chloride has an osmolarity of 0.002 Osm/L (twice the molarity), because each NaCl molecule ionizes in water to form two ions (Na^+ and Cl^-) that both contribute to the osmotic pressure.

Osmolality: A one-osmolal solution is defined as one osmole in each kilogram of solution.

Osmolality is measured in osmoles/kilogram of solution (Osm/kg).

For example, the osmolality of a 0.01 molal solution of Na_2SO_4 is 0.03 Osm/kg because each molecule of Na_2SO_4 ionizes in water to give three ions (2 Na^+ and 1 SO_4^{2-}) that contribute to the osmotic pressure.

5.3.2 Solubility Product Constant, the Equilibrium Expression

Any solute that dissolves in water to give a solution that contains ions, and thus can conduct electricity, is an *electrolyte*. The solid (s) that dissociates into separate ions surrounded by water is <u>hydrated</u>, thus the ions are aqueous (*aq*).

If dissociation is extensive, we have a <u>strong</u> electrolyte:

$$NaCl\ (s) \longrightarrow Na^+\ (aq) + Cl^-\ (aq)$$

If dissociation is incomplete, we have a <u>weak</u> electrolyte:

$$CH_3COOH\ (aq) \rightleftharpoons CH_3COO^-\ (aq) + H^+\ (aq)$$

Strong electrolytes: salts (NaCl), strong acids (HCl), strong bases (NaOH).

Weak electrolytes: weak acids (CH_3COOH), weak bases (NH_3), complexes ($Fe[CN]_6$), water, soluble organic compounds (sugar), highly charged species (CHM 5.2; $AlPO_4$, $BaSO_4$, *exception*: AgCl).

When substances have limited solubility and their solubility is exceeded, the ions of the dissolved portion exist in equilibrium with the solid material. When a compound is referred to as insoluble, it is not completely insoluble, but is slightly soluble.

For example, if solid AgCl is added to water, a small portion will dissolve:

$$AgCl\ (s) \rightleftharpoons Ag^+\ (aq) + Cl^-\ (aq)$$

The precipitate will have a definite solubility (i.e. a definite amount in g/liter or moles/liter that will dissolve at a given temperature). An overall equilibrium constant can be written for the above equilibrium, called the <u>solubility product</u>, K_{sp}, given by the following equilibrium expression:

$$K_{sp} = [Ag^+][Cl^-]$$

The preceding relationship holds regardless of the presence of any undissociated intermediate. In general, each concentration must be raised to the power of that ion's coefficient in the dissolving equation (in our example = 1). A different example would be Ag_2S which would have the following solubility product expression: $K_{sp} = [Ag^+]^2[S^{2-}]$. The calculation of solubility s in mol/L for AgCl would simply be: $K_{sp} = [s][s] = s^2$. On the other hand, the expression for Ag_2S would become: $K_{sp} = [2s]^2[s] = 4s^3$. Knowing K_{sp} at a specified temperature, the solubility of compounds can be calculated under various conditions. The amount of slightly soluble salt that dissolves does not depend on the amount of the solid in equilibrium with the solution, as long as there is enough to saturate the solution. Rather, it depends on the volume of solvent. {Note: a low K_{sp} value means little product therefore low solubility and vice-versa}

5.3.3 Common-ion Effect

If there is an excess of one ion over the other, the concentration of the other is suppressed. This is called the <u>common ion effect</u>. The solubility of the precipitate is decreased and the concentration can still be calculated from the K_{sp}.

For example, Cl^- ion can be precipitated out of a solution of AgCl by adding a slight excess of $AgNO_3$. If a stoichiometric amount of $AgNO_3$ is added, $[Ag^+] = [Cl^-]$. If excess $AgNO_3$ is added, $[Ag^+] > [Cl^-]$ but K_{sp} remains constant. Therefore, $[Cl^-]$ decreases if $[Ag^+]$ is increased. Because the K_{sp} product always holds, precipitation will not take place unless the product of $[Ag^+]$ and $[Cl^-]$ exceeds the K_{sp}. If the product is just equal to K_{sp}, all the Ag^+ and Cl^- ions would remain in solution.

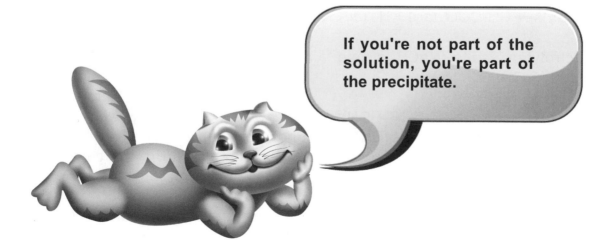

If you're not part of the solution, you're part of the precipitate.

Memorize	Understand	Not Required*
* Define: Bronsted acid, base, pH * Examples of strong/weak acids/bases * K_w at STP, neutral H_2O pH, conjugate acid/base, zwitterions * Equations: K_a, K_b, pK_a, pK_b, K_w, pH, pOH * Equivalence point, indicator, rules of logarithms	* Calculation of K_a, K_b, pK_a, pK_b, K_w, pH, pOH * Calculations involving strong/weak acids/bases * Salts of weak acids/bases, buffers; indicators * Henderson-Hasselbach equation * Acid-Base titration/curve, redox titration	* Advanced level college info * Specific values for K_a and/or K_b * Memorizing the quadratic formula or the Henderson-Hasselbach equation

MCAT-Prep.com

Introduction ▎▎▎▎

Acids are compounds that, when dissolved in water, gives a solution with a hydrogen ion concentration greater than that of pure water. Acids turn litmus paper (an indicator) red. Examples include acetic acid (in vinegar) and sulfuric acid (in car batteries). Bases may have [H+] less than pure water and turns litmus blue. Examples include sodium hydroxide (= lye, caustic soda) and ammonia (used in many cleaning products).

Additional Resources

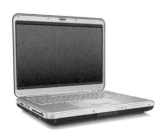

Free Online Q & A

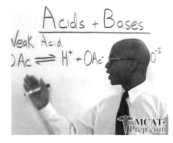

Video: Online or DVD 3

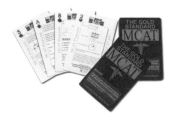

Flashcards

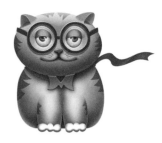

Special Guest

6.1 Acids

A useful definition is given by Bronsted and Lowry: an acid is a proton (i.e. hydrogen ion) donor (cf. Lewis acids and bases, *see* CHM 3.4). A substance such as HF is an acid because it can donate a proton to a substance capable of accepting it. In aqueous solution, water is always available as a proton acceptor, so that the ionization of an acid, HA, can be written as:

$$HA + H_2O \rightleftharpoons H_3O^+ + A^-$$

or: $$HA \rightleftharpoons H^+ + A^-.$$

The equilibrium constant is:

$$K_a = [H^+][A^-]/[HA].$$

Examples of ionization of acids are:

$$HCl \rightleftharpoons H^+ + Cl^- \quad K_a = \text{infinity}$$

$$HF \rightleftharpoons H^+ + F^- \quad K_a = 6.7 \times 10^{-4}$$

$$HCN \rightleftharpoons H^+ + CN^- \quad K_a = 7.2 \times 10^{-10}$$

Table III.A.6.1: Examples of strong and weak acids.

STRONG	WEAK
Perchloric $HClO_4$	Hydrocyanic HCN
Chloric $HClO_3$	Hypochlorous HClO
Nitric HNO_3	Nitrous HNO_2
Hydrochloric HCl	Hydrofluoric HF
Sulfuric H_2SO_4	Sulfurous H_2SO_3
Hydrobromic HBr	Hydrogen Sulfide H_2S
Hydriodic HI	Phosphoric H_3PO_4
Hydronium Ion H_3O^+	Benzoic, Acetic and other Carboxylic acids

Note that a diprotic acid (*two protons*, i.e. H_2SO_4) would have K_a values for each of its two ionizable protons: K_{a1} for the first and K_{a2} for the second.

6.2 Bases

A base is defined as a proton acceptor. In aqueous solution, water is always available to donate a proton to a base, so the ionization of a base B, can be written as:

$$B + H_2O \rightleftharpoons HB^+ + OH^-$$

The equilibrium constant is: $K_b = [HB^+][OH^-]/[B]$

Examples of ionization of bases are:

$$CN^- + H_2O \rightleftharpoons HCN + OH^- \quad K_b = 1.4 \times 10^{-5}$$

$$NH_3 + H_2O \rightleftharpoons NH_4^+ + OH^- \quad K_b = 1.8 \times 10^{-5}$$

$$F^- + H_2O \rightleftharpoons HF + OH^- \quad K_b = 1.5 \times 10^{-11}$$

Strong bases include any hydroxide of the group 1A metals. The most common weak bases are ammonia and any organic amine.

6.3 Conjugate Acid-Base Pairs

The strength of an acid or base is related to the extent that the dissociation proceeds to the right, or to the magnitude of K_a or K_b; the larger the dissociation constant, the stronger the acid or the base. From the preceding K_a values, we see that HCl is the strongest acid (almost 100% ionized), followed by HF and HCN. From the K_b's given, NH_3 is the strongest base listed, followed by CN^- and F^-. Clearly, when an acid ionizes, it produces a base. The acid, HA, and the base produced when it ionizes, A^-, are called a conjugate acid-base pair, so that the couples HF, F^- and HCN, CN^- are conjugate acids and bases.

Another example of conjugate acid-base pairs is amino acids. Amino acids bear at least 2 ionizable weak acid groups, a carboxyl (-COOH) and an amino ($-NH_3^+$) which act as follows:

$$R\text{-}COOH \rightleftharpoons R\text{-}COO^- + H^+$$

$$R\text{-}NH_3^+ \rightleftharpoons R\text{-}NH_2 + H^+$$

R-COO⁻ and R-NH₂ are the conjugate bases (i.e. proton acceptors) of the corresponding acids. The carboxyl group is thousands of times more acidic than the amino group. Thus in blood plasma (pH ≈ 7.4) the predominant forms are the carboxylate anions (R-COO⁻) and the protonated amino group (R-NH₃⁺). This form is called a *zwitterion* as demonstrated by the amino acid alanine at a pH near 7:

$$CH_3\text{-}CH\text{-}COO^-$$
$$|$$
$$NH_3^+$$

The zwitterion bears no net charge.

6.4 Water Dissociation

Water itself can ionize:

$$H_2O + H_2O \rightleftharpoons H_3O^+ + OH^-$$

or: $$H_2O \rightleftharpoons H^+ + OH^-$$

At STP, $K_w = [H^+][OH^-] = 1.0 \times 10^{-14}$ = ion product constant for water. It increases with temperature and in a neutral solution, $[H^+] = [OH^-] = 10^{-7}$ M. Note that $[H_2O]$ is not included in the equilibrium expression because it is a large constant ($[H_2O]$ is incorporated in K_w).

6.5 The pH Scale

The pH of a solution is a convenient way of expressing the concentration of hydrogen ions [H+] in solution, to avoid the use of large negative powers of 10. It is defined as:

$$pH = -\log_{10}[H^+]$$

Thus, the pH of a neutral solution of pure water where $[H^+] = 10^{-7}$ is 7.

A similar definition is used for the hydroxyl ion concentration:

$$pOH = -\log_{10}[OH^-]$$

And $pH + pOH = pK_w$.

At 25 °C, $pH + pOH = 14$

A pH of 7 is neutral. Values of pH that are greater than 7 are alkaline (basic) and values that are lower are <u>acidic</u>. The pH can be measured precisely with a pH meter (quantitative) or globally with indicator paper which will have a different color over different pH ranges (qualitative). For example, *litmus paper* (very common) becomes <u>b</u>lue in <u>b</u>asic solutions and re<u>d</u> in aci<u>d</u>ic solutions; whereas, *phenolphthalein* is colorless in acid and pink in base.

6.5.1 Properties of Logarithms

To facilitate the calculation of pH it is important to remember the following properties:

1) $\log_a a = 1$
2) $\log_a M^k = k \log_a M$
3) $\log_a(MN) = \log_a M + \log_a N$
4) $\log_a(M/N) = \log_a M - \log_a N$
5) $10^{\log_{10} M} = M$

For example, let us calculate the pH of 0.001 M HCl. Since HCl is a strong acid, it will completely dissociate into H^+ and Cl^-, thus :

$[H^+] = 0.001$
$-\log[H^+] = -\log(0.001)$
pH $= -\log(10^{-3})$
pH $= 3 \log 10$ (rule #2)
pH $= 3$ (rule #1, a=10)

6.6 Weak Acids and Bases

Weak acids and bases are only <u>partially ionized</u>. The ionization constant can be used to calculate the amount ionized, and from this, the pH.

Example: Calculate the pH and pOH of a 10^{-3} M solution of acetic acid. K_a of acetic acid at 25°C = 1.75×10^{-5}.

$$HOAc \rightleftharpoons H^+ + OAc^-$$

The concentrations are:

	[HOAc]	[H⁺]	[OAc⁻]
Initial	10^{-3}	0	0
Change	-x	+x	+x
Equilibrium	10^{-3}-x	x	x

$K_a = [H^+][OAc^-]/[HOAc] = 1.75 \times 10^{-5}$
   $= (x)(x)/(10^{-3}-x)$

The solution is a quadratic equation which may be simplified if <u>less than 15%</u> of the acid is ionized by neglecting x compared to the concentration (10^{-3} in this case). We then have:

$x^2/10^{-3} = 1.75 \times 10^{-5}$
$x = 1.32 \times 10^{-4}$ M = $[H^+]$
And   pH = -log 1.32×10^{-4} = 3.88
       pOH = 14.00 - 3.88 = 10.12

Similar calculations hold for weak bases.

6.6.1 Determining pH with the Quadratic Formula

The solutions of the quadratic equation

$$ax^2 + bx + c = 0$$

are given by the formula

$$x = [-b \pm (b^2 - 4ac)^{1/2}]/2a$$

The problem in Section 6.6 reduced to

$$K_a = (x)(x)/(10^{-3} - x) = 1.75 \times 10^{-5}$$
or
$$x^2 + (1.75 \times 10^{-5})x + (-1.75 \times 10^{-8}) = 0.$$

Using the quadratic formula where a = 1, b = 1.75×10^{-5}, c = $- 1.75 \times 10^{-8}$, and doing the appropriate multiplications we get:

$$x = [-1.75 \times 10^{-5} \pm (3.06 \times 10^{-10} + 7.0 \times 10^{-8})^{1/2}]/2$$

thus
$$x = [-1.75 \times 10^{-5} \pm (7.03 \times 10^{-8})^{1/2}]/2 = [-1.75 \times 10^{-5} \pm 2.65 \times 10^{-4}]/2$$

hence the two possible solutions are

$$x = [-1.75 \times 10^{-5} - 2.65 \times 10^{-4}]/2$$
$$= -1.41 \times 10^{-4}$$

or
$$x = [-1.75 \times 10^{-5} + 2.65 \times 10^{-4}]/2$$
$$= 1.24 \times 10^{-4}.$$

The first solution is a negative number which is physically impossible for $[H^+]$, therefore
$$pH = -log (1.24 \times 10^{-4}) = 3.91.$$

Our estimate in Section 6.6 (pH = 3.88) was valid as it is less than 1% different from the more precise calculation using the quadratic formula.

Given a multiple choice question with the following choices: 2.5, 3.9, 4.3 and 6.8 - the answer can be easily deduced.

$$-log (1.24 \times 10^{-4}) = -log 1.24 - log 10^{-4} = 4 - log 1.24$$

however

$$0 = log 10^0 = log 1 < log 1.24 << log 10 = 1$$

Thus a number slightly greater than 0 but significantly less than 1 is substracted from 4. The answer could only be 3.9.

6.7 Salts of Weak Acids and Bases

A *salt* is an ionic compound in which the anion is not OH^- or O^{2-} and the cation is not H^+. Typically, an acid plus a base produces a salt and a neutral compound (i.e. CHM 6.9.1/2). The salt of a weak acid is a Bronsted base, which will accept protons. For example,

$$Na^+ OAc^- + H_2O \rightleftharpoons HOAc + Na^+ OH^-$$

The HOAc here is undissociated and therefore does not contribute to the pH. This ionization is known as hydrolysis of the salt ion. Because it hydrolyzes, sodium acetate is a weak base (the conjugate base of acetic acid). The ionization constant is equal to the basicity constant of the salt. The weaker the conjugate acid, the stronger the conjugate base, that is, the more strongly the salt will combine with a proton.

$$K_H = K_b = [HOAc][OH^-]/[OAc^-]$$

K_H is the hydrolysis constant of the salt. The product of K_a of any weak acid and K_b of its conjugate base is always equal to K_w.

$$K_a \times K_b = K_w$$

For any salt of a weak acid, HA, that ionizes in water:

$$A^- + H_2O \rightleftharpoons HA + OH^-$$

$$[HA][OH^-]/[A^-] = K_w/K_a.$$

The pH of such a salt is calculated in the same manner as for any other weak base.

Similar equations are derived for the salts of weak bases. They hydrolyze in water as follows:

$$BH^+ + H_2O \rightleftharpoons B + H_3O^+$$

B is undissociated and does not contribute to the pH.

And
$$K_H = K_a = [B][H_3O^+]/[BH^+]$$

$$[B][H_3O^+]/[BH^+] = K_w/K_b.$$

6.8 Buffers

A buffer is defined as a solution that resists change in pH when a small amount of an acid or base is added or when a solution is diluted. A buffer solution consists of a mixture of a weak acid and its salt or of a weak base and its salt.

For example, consider the acetic acid-acetate buffer. The acid equilibrium that governs this system is:

$$HOAc \rightleftharpoons H^+ + OAc^-$$

If we were to add acetate ions into the system (i.e. from the salt), the H^+ ion concentration is no longer equal to the acetate ion concentration. The hydrogen ion concentration is:

$$[H^+] = K_a \, ([HOAc]/[OAc^-])$$

Taking the negative logarithm of each side, where $-\log K_a = pK_a$, yields:

$$pH = pK_a - \log \, ([HOAc]/[OAc^-])$$

or

$$pH = pKa + \log \, ([OAc^-]/[HOAc])$$

This equation is referred to as the Henderson-Hasselbach equation. It is useful for calculating the pH of a weak acid solution containing its salt. A general form can be written for a weak acid, HA, that dissociates into its salt, A^- and H^+:

$$HA \rightleftharpoons H^+ + A^-$$

$$pH = pK_a + \log \, ([salt]/[acid])$$

The amount of acid or base that can be added without causing a large change in pH is governed by the buffering capacity of the solution. This is determined by the concentrations of HA and A^-. The higher their concentrations, the more acid or base the solution can tolerate. The buffering capacity is also governed by the ratios of HA to A^-. It is maximum when the ratio is equal to 1, i.e. when $pH = pK_a$.

Similar calculations can be made for mixtures of a weak base and its salt:

$$B + H_2O \rightleftharpoons BH^+ + OH^-$$

And

$$pOH = pK_b + \log \, ([salt]/[base])$$

Many biological reactions of interest occur between pH 6 and 8. One useful series of buffers is that of phosphate buffers. By choosing appropriate mixtures of $H_3PO_4/H_2PO_4^-$, $H_2PO_4^-/HPO_4^{2-}$ or HPO_4^{2-}/PO_4^{3-}, buffer solutions covering a wide pH range can be prepared. Another useful clinical buffer is the one prepared from tris(hydroxymethyl) aminomethane and its conjugate acid, abbreviated Tris buffer.

6.9 Acid-base Titrations

The purpose of a titration is usually the determination of concentration of a given sample of acid or base (the analyte) which is reacted with an equivalent amount of a strong base or acid of known concentration (the titrant). The end point or equivalence point is reached when a stoichiometric amount of titrant has been added. This end point is usually detected with the use of an <u>indicator</u> which changes color when this point is reached. The end point is determined precisely by measuring the pH at different points of the titration. The curve pH=f(V) where V is the volume of titrant added is called a titration curve. An indicator for an acid-base titration is a weak acid or base. The weak acid and its conjugate base should have two different colors in solution. Most indicators require a <u>pH transition range</u> during the titration of about two pH units. An indicator is chosen so that its pK_a is close to the pH of the equivalence point.

6.9.1 Strong Acid versus Strong Base

In the case of a strong acid versus a strong base, both the titrant and the analyte are completely ionized. For example, the titration of hydrochloric acid with sodium hydroxide:

$$H^+ + Cl^- + Na^+ + OH^- \longrightarrow H_2O + Na^+ + Cl^-$$

The H^+ and OH^- combine to form H_2O and the other ions remain unchanged, so the net result is the conversion of the HCl to a neutral solution of NaCl. A typical strong-acid-strong base titration curve is shown in Fig. III.A.6.1 (case where the titrant is a base).

If the analyte is an acid the pH is initially acidic and increases very slowly. When the equivalent volume is reached the pH sharply increases. Midway between this transition jump is the equivalence point. In the case of strong acid-strong base titration the equivalence point corresponds to a neutral pH (because the salt formed does not react with water). If more titrant is added the pH increases and corresponds to the pH of a solution of gradually increasing concentration of the titrant base. This curve is simply reversed if the titrant is an acid.

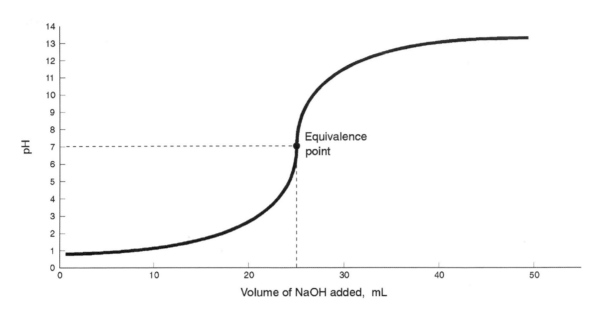

Figure III.A.6.1: Titration curve of a strong acid versus a strong base.

6.9.2 Weak Acid versus Strong Base

The titration of acetic acid with sodium hydroxide involves the following reaction:

$$HOAc + Na^+ + OH^- \longrightarrow H_2O + Na^+ + OAc^-$$

The acetic acid is only a few percent ionized. It is neutralized to water and an equivalent amount of the salt, sodium acetate. Before the titration is started, the pH is calculated as described for weak acids. As soon as the titration is started, some of the HOAc is converted to NaOAc and a buffer system is set up. As the titration proceeds, the pH slowly increases as the ratio [OAc⁻] /[HOAc] changes. At the midpoint of the titration, [OAC⁻] = [HOAC] and the pH is equal to pK_a. At the

equivalence point, we have a solution of NaOAc. Since it hydrolyzes, the pH at the equivalence point will be alkaline. The pH will depend on the concentration of NaOAc. The greater the concentration, the higher the pH. As excess NaOH is added, the ionization of the base, OAc⁻, is suppressed and the pH is determined only by the concentration of excess OH⁻. Therefore, the titration curve beyond the equivalence point follows that for the titration of a strong acid. The typical titration curve in this case is:

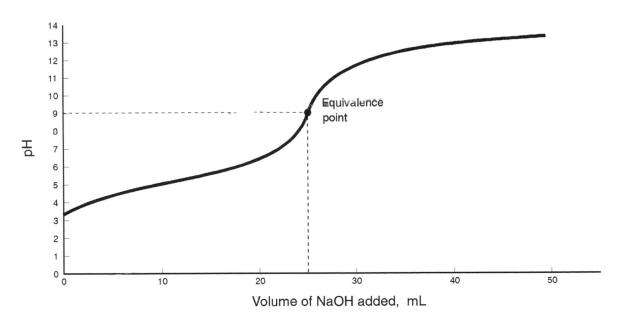

Figure III.A.6.2: Titration curve of a weak acid versus a strong base. N.B. the equivalence point is basic.

6.9.3 Weak Base versus Strong Acid

The titration of a weak base with a strong acid is analogous to the previous case except that the pH is initially basic and gradually decreases as the acid is added (curve in preceding diagram is reversed). Consider ammonia titrated with hydrochloric acid:

$$NH_3 + H^+ + Cl^- \longrightarrow NH_4^+ + Cl^-$$

At the beginning, we have NH_3 and the pH is calculated as for weak bases. As soon as some acid is added, some of the NH_3 is converted to NH_4^+ and we are in the buffer region. At the <u>midpoint of the titration</u>, $[NH_4^+]$ = $[NH_3]$ and the pH is equal to $(14 - pK_b)$. <u>At</u> <u>the equivalence point</u>, we have a solution of NH_4Cl, a weak acid which hydrolyzes to give an acid solution. Again, the pH will depend on concentration: the greater the concentration, the lower the pH. Beyond the equivalence point, the free H^+ suppresses the ionization and the pH is determined by the concentration of H^+ added in excess. Therefore, the <u>titration curve beyond the</u> <u>equivalence point will be similar to that of the</u> <u>titration of a strong base</u>. {The midpoint of the titration is the equivalence point of the titration curve}

6.10 Redox Titrations

The most useful oxidizing agent for titrations is potassium permanganate - $KMnO_4$. Solutions of this salt are colorful since they contain the purple MnO_4^- ion. On the other hand, the more reduced form, Mn^{++}, is nearly colorless. So here is how this redox titration works: $KMnO_4$ is added to a reaction mixture with a reducing agent (i.e. Fe^{++}). MnO_4^- is quickly reduced to Mn^{++} so the color fades immediately. This will continue until there is no more reducing agent in the mixture. When the last bit of reducing agent has been oxidized (i.e. all the Fe^{++} is converted to Fe^{+3}), the next drop of $KMnO_4$ will make the solution colorful since the MnO_4- will have nothing with which to react. Thus if the amount of reducing agent was unknown, it can be calculated using stoichiometry guided by the amount of potassium permanganate used in the reaction.

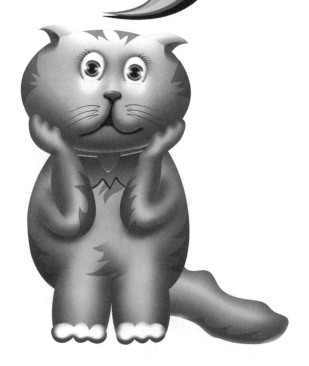

Little Jenny V. was a chemist
Little Jenny V. is no more
What she thought was H_2O
Was H_2SO_4

Memorize	Understand	Not Required*
* Equation: 1st Law of Thermodynamics * Temperature scales * Define: state function * Conversion: thermal to mechanical E.	* System vs. surroundings * Law of conservation of energy * Heat transfer * Conduction, convection, radiation	* Advanced level college info

MCAT-Prep.com

Introduction ▌▌▌▌

Thermodynamics, in chemistry, refers to the relationship of heat with chemical reactions or with the physical state. Thermodynamic processes can be analyzed by studying energy and topics we will review in the next chapter including entropy, volume, temperature and pressure.

Additional Resources

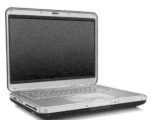

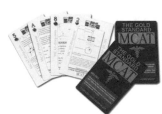

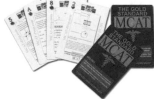

Free Online Q & A   Video: Online or DVD 4   Flashcards   Special Guest

7.1 Generalities

Thermodynamics deals with fundamental questions concerning energy transfers. One difficulty you will have to overcome is the terminology used. For instance, remember that heat and temperature have more specific meanings than the ones attributed to them in every day life. A thermodynamic transformation can be as simple as a gas leaking out of a tank or a piece of metal melting at high temperature or as complicated as the synthesis of proteins by a biological cell. To solve some problems in thermodynamics we need to define a "system" and its "surroundings." The system is simply the object experiencing the thermodynamic transformation. The gas would be considered as the system in the first example of transformations. Once the system is defined any part of the universe in direct contact with the system is considered as its surroundings. For instance if the piece of metal is melted in a high temperature oven: the system is the piece of metal and the oven constitutes its surroundings. In other instances the limit between the system and its surroundings is more arbitrary, for example if one considers the energy exchanges when an ice cube melts in a thermos bottle filled with orange juice; the inside walls of the thermos bottle could be considered as part of "the system" or as part of the surroundings. In the first case one would carry out all calculations as though the entire system (ice cube + orange juice + inside walls) is isolated from its surroundings (rest of the universe) and all the energy exchanges take place within the system. In the second case the system (ice cube + orange juice) is not isolated from the surroundings (walls) unless we consider that the heat exchanges with the walls are negligible. There is also no need to include any other part of the universe in the latter case since all exchanges take place within the system or between the system and the inside walls of the thermos bottle.

7.2 The First Law of Thermodynamics

Heat, internal energy and work are the first concepts introduced in thermodynamics. Work should be a familiar concept from reading Physics section 5.1. Heat is thermal energy (a dynamic property defined during a transformation only), it is not to be confused with temperature (a static property defined for each state of the system). Internal energy is basically the average total mechanical energy (kinetic + potential) of the particles that make up the system. The first law of thermodynamics is often expressed as follows: when a system absorbs an amount of heat Q from the surroundings and does a quantity of work W on the the same surroundings its internal energy changes by the amount:

$$\Delta E = Q - W$$

This law is basically the law of conservation of energy for an isolated system. Indeed, it states that if a system does not exchange any energy with its surroundings its internal energy should not vary. If on the other hand a system does exchange energy with its surroundings, its internal energy should change by an amount corresponding to the energy it takes in from the surroundings.

The sign convention related to the previous mathematical expression of the first law of thermodynamics is:

- heat absorbed by the system: $Q > 0$
- heat released by the system: $Q < 0$

- work done by the system on its surroundings: $W > 0$
- work done by the surroundings on the system: $W < 0$

Caution: Some textbooks prefer a different sign convention: any energy (Q or W) flowing from the system to the surroundings (lost by the system) is negative and any energy flowing from the surroundings to the system (gained by the system) is positive. Within such a sign convention the first law is expressed as:

$$\Delta E = Q + W$$

i.e. the negative sign in the previous equation is incorporated in W.

7.3 Equivalence of Mechanical, Chemical and Thermal Energy Units

The previous equation does more than express mathematically the law of conservation of energy, it establishes a relationship between thermal energy and mechanical energy. Historically thermal energy was always expressed in calories (abbreviated as cal.) defined as the amount of thermal energy required to raise the temperature of water by 1 degree Celsius. The standard unit used for mechanical work is the "Joule" (J). This unit eventually became the standard unit for any form of energy. The conversion factor between the two units is:

Chemists often refer the amount of energies exchanged between the system and its surroundings to the mole, i.e., quantities of energy are expressed in J/mol or cal/mol. To obtain the energy per particle (atom or molecule), you should divide the energy expressed in J or cal/mol by Avogadro's number.

$$1 \text{ cal} = 4.184 \text{ J}$$

7.4 Temperature Scales

There are three temperature scales in use in science textbooks. The Celsius scale, the absolute temperature or Kelvin scale, and the Farenheit scale. In the Celsius scale the freezing point and the boiling point of water are arbitrarily defined as 0 $^{\circ}$C and 100 $^{\circ}$C, respectively. The scale is then divided into equal 1/100th intervals to define the degree Celsius or centigrade (from latin centi = 100). The absolute temperature or Kelvin scale is derived from the centigrade scale, i.e., an <u>interval of 1 degree Celsius</u> is equal to an <u>interval</u> of 1 degree Kelvin. The difference between the two scales is in their definitions of the zero point:

$$0 \text{ K} = -273.13 \ ^{\circ}\text{C}.$$

Theoretically, this temperature can be approached but never achieved, it corresponds to the point where all motion is frozen out and matter is destroyed. The Farenheit scale used in English speaking countries has the disadvantage of not being divided into 100 degrees between its two reference points: the freezing point of water is 32 $^{\circ}$F and its boiling point is 212 $^{\circ}$F. To convert Farenheit degrees into Celsius degrees you have to perform the following transformation:

$$(X \ ^{\circ}F - 32) \times 5/9 = Y \ ^{\circ}C$$

or

$$^{\circ}F = 9/5 \ ^{\circ}C + 32.$$

7.5 Heat Transfer

There are three ways in which heat can be transferred between the system and its surroundings:

  (a) heat transfer by conduction
  (b) heat transfer by convection
  (c) heat transfer by radiation

In the first case (a) there is an intimate contact between the system and its surroundings and heat propagates through the entire system from the heated part to the unheated parts. A good example is the heating of a metal rod on a flame. Heat is initially transmitted directly from the flame to one end of the rod through the contact between the metal and the flame. When carrying out such an experiment you would notice at some point that the part of the rod which is not in direct contact with the flame becomes hot as well.

In the second case (b), heat is transferred to the entire system by the circulation of a hot liquid or a gas through it. The difference between this mode of transfer and the previous one is that the entire system or a major part of it is heated up directly by the surroundings and not by propagation of the thermal energy from the parts of the system which are in direct contact with the heating source and the parts which are not.

In the third case (c) there is no contact between the heating source and the system. Heat is transported by radiation. The perfect example is the microwave oven where the water inside the food is heated by the microwave source. Most heat transfers are carried out by at least two of the above processes at the same time.

Note that when a metal is heated it expands at a rate which is proportional to the change in temperature it experiences. For a definition of the coefficient of expansion see Physics section 6.3.

7.6 State Functions

As we mentioned above, the first law of thermodynamics introduces three fundamental energy functions, i.e., the internal energy E, heat Q, and work W. Let us consider a transformation that takes the system from an initial state (I) to a final state (F) (which can differ by a number of variables such as temperature, pressure and volume). The change in the internal energy during this transformation depends only on the properties of the initial state (I) and the final state (F). In other words, suppose that to go from (I) to (F) the system is first subjected to an intermediate transformation that temporarily takes it from state (I) to an intermediate state (Int.) and then to another transformation that brings it from (Int.) to (F), the change in internal energy between the initial state (I) and the final state (F) are independent of the properties of the intermediate state (Int.). The internal energy is said to be a path-independent function or a state function. This is not the case for W and Q. In fact, this is quite conceivable

since the amount of W or Q can be imposed by the external operator who subjects the system to a given transformation from (I) to (F). For instance, Q can be fixed at zero if the operator uses an appropriate thermal insulator between the system and its surroundings. In which case the change in the internal energy is due entirely to the work w (ΔE = -w). It is easy to understand that the same result [transformation from (I) to (F)] could be achieved by supplying a small quantity of heat q while letting the system do more work W on the surroundings so that q-W is equal to -w. In which case we have:

	Work	Heat	Change in internal energy
1st transf.	w	0	$-w$
2nd transf.	$W=w+q$	$\underline{q}$	$-w$

and yet in both cases the system is going from (I) to (F).

W and Q are not state functions. They depend on the path taken to go from (I) to (F). If you remember the exact definition of the internal energy you will understand that a system changes its internal energy to respond to an input of Q and W. In other words, contrary to Q and W, the internal energy cannot be directly imposed on the system.

The fact that the internal energy is a state function can be used in two other equivalent ways:

(i)   If the changes in the internal energy during the intermediate transformation are known, they can be used to calculate the change for the entire process from (I) to (F): the latter is equal to the sum of the changes in the internal energy for all the intermediate steps.

(ii)   If the change in the internal energy to go from a state (I) to a state (F) is $E_{I\text{->}F}$ the change in the internal energy for an opposite transformation that would take the system from (F) to (I) is:

$$\Delta E_{F\text{->}I} = -\Delta E_{I\text{->}F}$$

(iii)   If we start from (I) and go back to (I) through a series of intermediate transformations the change in the internal energy for the entire process is zero.

W can be determined experimentally by calculating the area under a pressure-volume curve. The mathematical relation is presented in CHM 8.1.

Memorize	Understand	Not Required*
* Define: endo/exothermic, Hess's law * Equations Hess's law, calorimetry * Conditions for standard enthalpies * Equations: calorimetry, free E. * Specific heat of water	* Area under curve: PV diagram * Equations for enthalpy, Hess's law, free E. * Calculation: Hess, calorimetry, Bond diss. E. * 2nd law of thermodynamics * Entropy, free E. and spontaneity	* Advanced level college info * Memorizing constants for latent heats

MCAT-Prep.com

Introduction ▪▪▪▪

Thermochemistry is the study of energy absorbed or released in chemical reactions or in any physical transformation (i.e. phase change like melting and boiling). Thermochemistry for the MCAT includes understanding and/or calculating quantities such as enthalpy, heat capacity, heat of combustion, heat of formation, and free energy.

Additional Resources

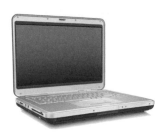

Free Online Q & A

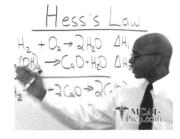

Video: Online or DVD 4

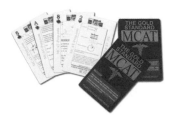

Flashcards

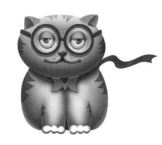

Special Guest

* The real MCAT may have advanced level information presented (ie. in a passage) but previous knowledge of said information is not required to answer the questions that would follow. Practice AAMC and GS practice MCAT CBTs can help you clarify this point.

8.1 Enthalpy as a Measure of Heat

The application of the general laws of thermodynamics to chemistry lead to some simplifications and adaptations because of the specificities of the problems that are dealt with in this field. For instance, in chemistry it is critical, if only for safety reasons, to know in advance what amounts of heat are going to be generated or absorbed during a reaction. In contrast, chemists are generally not interested in generating mechanical work and carry out most of their chemical reactions at constant pressure. For these reasons, although internal energy is a fundamental function its use is not very adequate in thermochemistry. Instead, chemists prefer to use another function derived from the internal energy: the enthalpy (H). This function is mathematically defined as:

$$\Delta H = \Delta E + P \times V$$

where P and V are respectively the pressure and the volume of the system. You may wonder about the use of artificially introducing another energy function when internal energy is well defined and directly related to kinetic and potential energy of the particles that make up the system. To answer this legitimate question you need to consider the case of the majority of the chemical reactions where P is constant and where the only type of work that can possibly be done by the system is of a mechanical nature. In this case, since $W = P \cdot V$ the change in enthalpy during a chemical reaction reduces to:

$$\Delta H = \Delta E + P \times V = (Q - W) + P \times V = Q$$

In other words, the change of enthalpy is a direct measure of the heat that evolves or is absorbed during a reaction carried out at constant pressure.

8.2 Heat of Reaction: Basic Principles

A reaction during which <u>heat</u> is <u>released</u> is said to be *exothermic* (ΔH is negative). If a <u>reaction</u> requires the supply of a certain amount of <u>heat</u> it is *endothermic* (ΔH is positive).

Besides the basic principle behind the introduction of enthalpy there is a more fundamental advantage for the use of this function in thermochemistry: it is a state function. This is a very practical property. For instance, consider two chemical

reactions related in the following way:

reaction 1: $A + B \rightarrow C$
reaction 2: $C \rightarrow D$

If these two reactions are carried out consecutively they lead to the same result as the following reaction:

overall reaction: $A + B \rightarrow D$

Because H is a state function we can apply the same arguments here as the ones we previously used for E. The initial state (I) corresponding to A + B , the intermediate state (Int.) to C, and the final state (F) to the final product D. If we know the changes in the enthalpy of the system for reactions 1 and 2, the change in the enthalpy during the overall reaction is:

$$\Delta H_{OVERALL} = \Delta H_1 + \Delta H_2$$

This is known as Hess's law. Remember that Hess's law is a simple application of the fact that H is a state function.

8.3 Hess's Law

Hess's law can be applied in several equivalent ways which we will illustrate with several examples:

Assume that we know the following enthalpy changes:

$$2 H_2(g) + O_2(g) \rightarrow 2H_2O(l)$$
$$\Delta H_1 = -136.6 \text{ kcal : R1}$$

$$Ca(OH)_2(s) \rightarrow CaO(s) + H_2O(l)$$
$$\Delta H_2 = 15.3 \text{ kcal : R2}$$

$$2 CaO(s) \rightarrow 2 Ca(s) + O_2(g)$$
$$\Delta H_3 = +303.6 \text{ kcal : R3}$$

and are asked to compute the enthalpy change for the following reaction:

$$Ca(s) + H_2(g) + O_2(g) \rightarrow Ca(OH)_2(s) : R$$

It is easy to see that reaction (R) can be obtained by the combination of reactions (R$_1$), (R$_2$) and (R$_3$) in the following way:

- 1/2 (R3): $Ca(s) + 1/2 O_2(g) \rightarrow CaO(s)$

+ 1/2 (R1): $H_2(g) + 1/2 O_2(g) \rightarrow H_2O(l)$

- (R2): $CaO(s) + H_2O(l) \rightarrow Ca(OH)_2(s)$

$$Ca(s) + H_2(g) + O_2(g) \rightarrow Ca(OH)_2(s)$$

As we previously explained, since H is a state function the enthalpy change for (R) will be given by:
$$\Delta H = -1/2\Delta H_3 + 1/2\Delta H_1 - \Delta H_2$$

There are no general rules that would allow you to determine which reaction to use first and by what factor it needs to be multiplied. It is important to proceed systematically and follow some simple ground rules:

(i)   For instance, you could start by writing the overall reaction that you want to obtain through a series of reaction additions.

(ii)   Number all your reactions.

(iii)   Keep in mind as you go along that the reactants of the overall reaction should always appear on the left-hand side and that the products should always appear on the right-hand side.

(iv)   Circle or underline the first reactant of the overall reaction. Find a reaction in your list that involves this reactant (as a reactant or a product). Use that reaction first and write it in such a way that this reactant appears on the left-hand side with the appropriate stoichiometric coefficient (i.e., if this reactant appears as a product of a reaction on your list you should reverse the reaction).

(v)   Suppose that in (iv) you had to use the second reaction on your list and that you had to reverse and multiply this reaction by a factor of 3 to satisfy the preceding rule. In your addition, next to this reaction or on top of the arrow write $-3 \times \Delta H_2$.

(vi)   Repeat the process for the other reactants and products of the overall reaction until your addition yields the overall reaction. As you continue this process, make sure to cross out the compounds that appear on the right and left-hand sides at the same time.

8.4 Standard Enthalpies

Hess's law has a very practical use in chemistry. Indeed, the enthalpy change for a given chemical reaction can be computed from simple combinations of known enthalpy changes of other reactions. Because enthalpy changes depend on the conditions under which reactions are carried out it is important to define standard conditions:

(i)   Standard pressure: 1 atmosphere pressure.

(ii)   Standard temperature for the purposes of the calculation of the standard enthalpy change: generally 25 °C. The convention is that if the temperature of the standard state is not mentioned then

it is assumed to be 25 °C, the standard temperature needs to be specified in all other instances.

(iii)   Standard physical state of an element: it is defined as the "natural" physical state of an element under the above standard pressure and temperature. For instance, the standard physical state of water under the standard temperature and pressure of 1 atm and 25 °C is the liquid state. Under the same conditions oxygen is a gas.

Naturally, the standard enthalpy change (notation: ΔH^o) for a given reaction is defined as the enthalpy change that accompanies the reaction when it is carried out under standard pressure and temperature with all reactants and products in their standard physical state.

Note that the standard temperature defined here is <u>different from the standard temperature for an ideal gas</u> which is: $0\,^{\circ}C$.

8.5 Enthalpies of Formation

The enthalpy of formation of a given compound is defined as the enthalpy change that accompanies the formation of the compound from its constituting elements. For instance, the enthalpy of formation of water is the $\Delta H_f^{\,o}$ for the following reaction:

$$H_2 + 1/2\ O_2\ \rightarrow\ H_2O$$

To be more specific the standard enthalpy of formation of water $\Delta H_f^{\,o}$ is the enthalpy change during the reaction:

$$H_2(g) + 1/2\ O_2(g) \xrightarrow[\text{1 atm}]{25^{\circ}C} H_2O(l)$$

where the reactants are in their natural physical state under standard temperature and pressure.

Note that according to these definitions, several of the reactions considered in the previous sections were in fact examples of reactions of formation. For instance, in section 8.3 on Hess's law, reaction (R1) is the reaction of formation of two moles of water, if reversed reaction (R3) would be the reaction of formation of two moles of CaO

and the overall reaction (R) is the reaction of formation of 1 mole $Ca(OH)_2$. Also note that although one could use the reverse of reaction (R2) to form $Ca(OH)_2$, this reaction, even reversed, is not the reaction of formation of $Ca(OH)_2$. The reason is that the constitutive elements of this molecule are: calcium (Ca), hydrogen (H_2) and oxygen (O_2) and not CaO and H_2O. Enthalpies of formation are also referred to as heats of formation. As previously explained, if the reaction of formation is carried out at constant pressure, the change in the enthalpy represents the amount of heat released or absorbed during the reaction.

8.6 Bond Dissociation Energies and Heats of Formation

The bond dissociation energy (also called bond energy) is defined as the change in enthalpy when a particular bond is broken in the diatomic molecules of 1 mole of gas, i.e. it is the ΔH° which corresponds to the process:

homo-nuclear diatomic molecules:
$$X_2(g) \rightarrow 2\,X(g)$$

hetero-nuclear diatomic molecules:
$$XY(g) \rightarrow X(g) + Y(g)$$

The difficulty in defining bond dissociation energies in polyatomic molecules is that the amounts of energy required to break a given bond (say an O---H bond) in two different polyatomic molecules (H_2O and CH_3OH, for instance) are different. Bond dissociation energies in polyatomic molecules are approximated to an average value for molecules of the same nature. Within the framework of this commonly made approximation we can calculate the enthalpy change of any reaction using the *sum* of bond energies of the reactants and the products in the following way:

$$\Delta H^{\circ} \text{ (reaction)} = \Sigma\, BE \text{ (reactants)} - \Sigma\, BE \text{ (products)}$$

where BE stands for bond energies.

Standard enthalpy changes of chemical reactions can also be computed using enthalpies of formation in the following way:

$$\Delta H^{\circ} \text{ (reaction)} = \Sigma\, \Delta H^{\circ}_{form.} \text{(products)} - \Sigma\, H^{\circ}_{form.} \text{ (reactants)}$$

Note how this equation is similar but not identical to the one making use of bond energies. This comes from the fact that a bond energy is defined as the energy required to <u>break</u> (and not to form) a given bond. Also note that the standard enthalpy of formation of a mole of any **element** is zero.

8.7 Calorimetry

Measurements of changes of temperature within a reaction mixture allow the experimental determination of heat absorbed or released during the corresponding chemical reaction. Indeed the amount of heat required to change the temperature of any substance X from T_1 to T_2 is proportional to $(T_2 - T_1)$ and the quantity of X:

$$Q = m\, C\, (T_2 - T_1)$$
or
$$Q = n\, c\, (T_2 - T_1)$$

where m is the mass of X, n the number of moles. The constant C or c is called the <u>heat capacity</u>. The standard units for C and c are, respectively, the $J\ kg^{-1}\ K^{-1}$ and the

$J\ mol^{-1}\ K^{-1}$. C which is the heat capacity per <u>unit mass</u> is also referred to as the <u>specific heat capacity</u>. If you refer back to the definition of the calorie (*see section 7.3*) you will understand that the specific heat of water is necessarily: $1\ cal\ g^{-1}\ {}^{\circ}C^{-1}$.

Note that heat can be absorbed or released without a change in temperature. In fact this situation occurs whenever a phase change takes place for a pure compound. For instance, ice melts at a constant temperature of $0\ ^{\circ}C$ in order to break the forces that keep the water molecules in a crystal of ice we need to supply an amount of heat of 6.01 kJ/mol. There is no direct way of calculating the heat

corresponding to a phase change. Heats of phase changes (heat of fusion, heat of vaporization, heat of sublimation) are generally tabulated and indirectly determined in calorimetric experiment. For instance, if a block of ice is allowed to melt in a bucket of warm water, we can determine the heat of fusion of ice by measuring the temperature drop in the bucket of water and applying the law of conservation of energy. The relevant equation is:

$$Q = m\,L$$

where L is the latent heat which is a constant.

8.8 The Second Law of Thermodynamics

The first law of thermodynamics allows us to calculate energy transfers during a given transformation of the system. It does not allow us to predict whether a transformation can or cannot occur spontaneously. Yet our daily observations tell us that certain transformations always occur in a given direction. For instance, heat flows from a hot source to a cold source.

We cannot spontaneously transfer heat in the other direction to make the hot source hotter and the cold source colder. <u>The second law of thermodynamics allows the determination of the preferred direction of a given transformation</u>. Transformations which require the smallest amount of energy and lead to the largest disorder of the system are the most spontaneous.

8.9 Entropy

Entropy S is the state function which measures the degree of "disorder" in a

system. For instance, the entropy of ice is lower than the entropy of liquid water since ice corresponds to an organized crystalline structure (virtually no disorder). In fact generally speaking the entropy increases as we go from a solid to a liquid to a gas. For similar reasons: the entropy decreases when an elastic band is stretched. Indeed, in the "unstretched" elastic band the molecules of the rubber polymer are coiled up and form a disorganized structure. As the rubber is stretched these molecules will tend to line up with each other and adopt a more organized structure. The second law of thermodynamics can be expressed in the alternate form: a spontaneous transformation corresponds to an increase in the entropy of an isolated system. The stretching of an elastic band is not a spontaneous process, on the other hand if an elastic band is stretched it will spontaneously return to its normal length if no external force holds it back.

8.10 Free Energy

The Gibbs free energy G is another state function which can be used as a criterion for spontaneity. This function is defined as:

$$G = H - T \cdot S$$

where: H is the enthalpy of the system in a given state,

    T is the temperature,

and   S is the entropy of the system.

For a reaction carried out at constant temperature we can write that the change in the Gibbs free energy is :

$$\Delta G = \Delta H - T \Delta S$$

A reaction carried out at constant pressure is spontaneous if

$$\Delta G < 0$$

It is not spontaneous if:
$$\Delta G > 0$$

and it is in a state of equilibrium (reaction spontaneous in both directions) if:

$$\Delta G = 0.$$

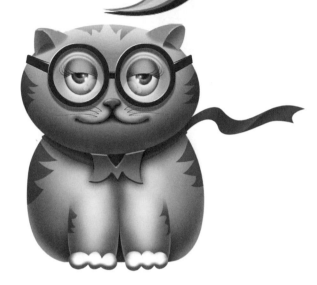

Memorize	Understand	Not Required*
* Reaction order; equations: rate law, K_{eq} * Define: rate determining step * Generalized potential energy diagrams * Define: activation energy, catalysis * Define: saturation kinetics, substrate	* Reaction rates, rate law, determine exponents * Reaction mechanism for free radicals * Rate constant equation; apply Le Chatelier's * Kinetic vs. thermodynamic control * Law of mass action, equations for Gibbs free E.	* Advanced level college info * Memorizing the rate constant equation

MCAT-Prep.com

Introduction ▌▌▌▌

Rate processes involve the study of the velocity (speed) and mechanisms of chemical reactions. **Reaction rate** (= *velocity*) tells us how fast the concentrations of reactants change with time. **Reaction mechanisms** show the sequence of steps to get to the overall change. Experiments show that 4 important factors generally influence reaction rates: (1) the nature of the reactants, (2) their concentration, (3) temperature, and (4) catalysis.

Additional Resources

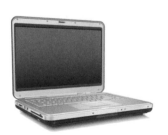

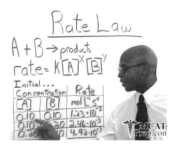

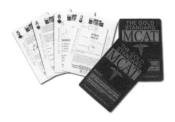

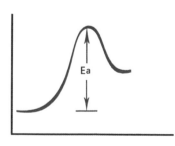

| Free Online Q & A | Video: Online or DVD 4 | Flashcards | Special Guest |

9.1 Reaction Rate

Consider a general reaction

$$2A + 3B \longrightarrow C + D$$

The rate at which this reaction proceeds can be expressed by one of the following:

(i) rate of disappearance of A :
- $\Delta[A] / \Delta t$

(ii) rate of disappearance of B:
- $\Delta[B] / \Delta t$

(iii) rate of appearance or formation of C: $\Delta[C] / \Delta t$

(iv) rate of appearance or formation of D: $\Delta[D] / \Delta t$

Where [ ] denotes the concentration of a reactant or a product in moles/liter.

Since A and B are disappearing in this reaction, [A] and [B] are decreasing with time, i.e. $\Delta[A] / \Delta t$ and $\Delta[B] / \Delta t$ are negative quantities. On the other hand, the quantities $\Delta[C] / \Delta t$ and $\Delta[D] / \Delta t$ are positive since both C and D are being formed during the process of this reaction. By convention: rates of reactions are expressed as positive numbers; as a result, a negative sign is necessary in the first two expressions.

Suppose that A disappears at a rate of 6 (moles/liter)/s. In the same time interval (1s), in a total volume of 1L we have:

$(3/2) \times 6 = 9$ moles of B disappearing

$(1/2) \times 6 = 3$ moles of C being formed

$(1/2) \times 6 = 3$ moles of D being formed

Therefore individual rates of formation or disappearance are not convenient ways to express the rate of a reaction. Indeed, depending on the reactant or product considered the rate will be given by a different numerical value unless the stoichiometric coefficients are equal (e.g. for C and D in our case). A more convenient expression of the rate of a reaction is the overall rate. This rate is simply obtained by dividing the rate of formation or disappearance of a given reactant or product by the corresponding stoichiometric coefficient, i.e.:

overall rate = $-(1/2) \Delta[A] / \Delta t$, or $-(1/3) \Delta[B] / \Delta t$,

or $\Delta[C] / \Delta t$, or $\Delta[D] / \Delta t$.

A simple verification on our example will show you that these expressions all lead to the same numerical value for the overall rate: 3 (moles/L)/s.

Whenever the term "rate" is used (with no other specification) it refers to the "overall rate" unless individual and overall rates are equal.

9.2 Dependence of Reaction Rates on Concentration of Reactants

The rate of a reaction (given in moles per liter per second) can be expressed as a function of the concentration of the reactants. In the previous chemical reaction we would have:

$$rate = k\,[A]^m\,[B]^n$$

where [ ] is the concentration of the corresponding reactant in moles per liter

k is referred to as the rate constant

m is the order of the reaction with respect to A

n is the order of the reaction with respect to B

m+n is the overall reaction order.

According to the rate law above, the reaction is said to be an (m+n)th order reaction, or, an mth order reaction with respect to A, or, an nth order reaction with respect to B.

9.3 Determining Exponents of the Rate Law

The only way to determine the exponents with certainty is via experimentation. Consider the following five experiments varying the concentrations of reactants A and B with resulting rates of reaction:

$$A + B \longrightarrow products$$

Exp. #	Initial Concentration		Initial Rate (mol L^{-1} s^{-1})
	[A]	[B]	
1	0.10	0.10	0.20
2	0.20	0.10	0.40
3	0.30	0.10	0.60
4	0.30	0.20	2.40
5	0.30	0.30	5.40

In the first three experiments the concentration of A changes but B remains the same. Thus the resultant changes in rate only depend on the concentration of A. Note that when [A] doubles (exp. 1,2) the reaction rate doubles, and when [A] triples (exp. 1,3) the reaction rate triples. Because it is directly proportional, the exponent of [A] must be 1. Thus the rate of reaction is first order with respect to A.

In the final three sets of experiments, [B] changes while [A] remains the same. When [B] doubles (exp. 3,4) the rate increases by a factor of 4 (= 2^2). When [B] triples (exp. 3,5) the rate increases by a factor of 9 (= 3^2). Thus the relation is exponential where the exponent of [B] is 2. The rate of reaction is second order with respect to B.

$$\text{rate} = k\,[A]^1\,[B]^2$$

The overall rate of reaction (n+m) is third order. The value of the rate constant k can be easily calculated by substituting the results from any of the five experiments. For example, using experiment #1:

$$k = \frac{\text{rate}}{[A]^1\,[B]^2}$$

$$k = \frac{0.20 \text{ mol } L^{-1} \text{ s}^{-1}}{(0.10 \text{ mol } L^{-1})(0.10 \text{ mol } L^{-1})^2}$$

$$= 2.0 \times 10^2 \text{ L}^2\text{mol}^{-2}\text{s}^{-1}$$

k is the rate constant for the reaction which includes all five experiments.

9.4 Reaction Mechanism - Rate-determining Step

Chemical equations fail to describe the detailed process through which the reactants are transformed into the products. For instance, consider the reaction of formation of hydrogen chloride from hydrogen and chlorine:

$$Cl_2(g) + H_2(g) \rightarrow 2 \text{ HCl}(g)$$

The equation above fails to mention that in fact this reaction is the result of a chain of reactions proceeding in three steps:

Initiation step: formation of chlorine atoms (= *radicals*, the mechanism will be

discussed in organic chemistry):

$$1/2 \text{ Cl}_2 \rightleftharpoons \text{Cl}\cdot$$

The double arrow indicates that in fact some of the Cl atoms recombine to form chlorine molecules, the whole process eventually reaches a state of equilibrium where the following ratio is constant:

$$K = [Cl\cdot] / [Cl_2]^{1/2}$$

The determination of such a constant will be dealt with in the sub-section on "equilibrium constants."

Propagation step: formation of reactive hydrogen atoms and reaction between hydrogen atoms and hydrogen molecules:

$$Cl\cdot + H_2 \rightarrow HCl + H\cdot$$

$$H\cdot + Cl_2 \rightarrow HCl + Cl\cdot$$

Termination step:

$$H\cdot + Cl\cdot \rightarrow HCl$$

The detailed chain reaction process above is called the mechanism of the reaction. Each individual reaction in a detailed mechanism is called an elementary process. Any reaction proceeds through some mechanism which is generally impossible to predict from its chemical equation. Such mechanisms are usually determined through an experimental procedure. Generally speaking each step proceeds at its own rate. The rate of the overall reaction is naturally limited by the the slowest step; therefore, the rate-determining step in the mechanism of a reaction is the slowest step. In other words, the overall rate law of a reaction is basically equal to the rate law of the slowest step. The faster processes have an indirect influence on the rate: they regulate the concentrations of the reactants and products. The chemical equation of an elementary step reflects the exact molecular process that transforms its reactants into its products. For this reason its rate law can be predicted from its chemical equation: in an elementary process, the orders with respect to the reactants are equal to the corresponding stoichiometric coefficients.

In our example experiments show that the rate-determining step is the reaction between chlorine atoms and hydrogen molecules, all the other steps are much faster. According to the principles above, the rate law of the overall reaction is equal to the rate law of this rate-determining step. Therefore, the rate of the overall reaction is proportional to the concentration of hydrogen molecules and chlorine atoms but is not directly proportional to the concentration of chlorine molecules. However since the ratio of concentrations Cl and Cl_2 is regulated by the initiation step concentration it can be shown that according to the mechanism above the rate law is:

$$rate = k\,[H_2] \cdot [Cl_2]^{1/2}$$

it is important to note that the individual orders of a reaction are generally not equal to the stoichiometric coefficients.

9.5 Dependence of Reaction Rates upon Temperature

From the collision theory of chemical kinetics it was established that the rate constant of a reaction can be expressed as follows:

$$k = A\,e^{-Ea/RT}$$

where: A is a constant related to the frequency of the collisions leading to a given reaction, it is referred to as Arrhenius' constant or the frequency factor,

e is the base of natural logarithms,

Ea is the activation energy, it is the energy required to get a reaction started, i.e., if two molecules of reactants have a total kinetic energy below Ea collide with each other, their collision will not lead to the formation of the product(s).

R is the ideal gas constant (1.99 cal $mol^{-1}\,K^{-1}$)

T is the absolute temperature.

The species formed during an efficient collision, before the reactants transform into the final product(s) is called the activated complex or the transition state.

Within the framework of this theory, when a single step reaction proceeds the energy of the system varies according to Figure III.A.9.1.

The change in enthalpy (ΔH) during the reaction is the difference between the total energy of the products and the reactants. In the diagram on the left the total energy of the reactants is higher than the total energy of the products: this is obviously the case for an exothermic reaction. The diagram on the right shows the profile of an endothermic reaction. Also note than the bigger the difference between the total energy of the reactants and the activated complex, i.e. the activation energy Ea, the slower the reaction.

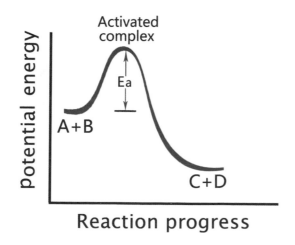
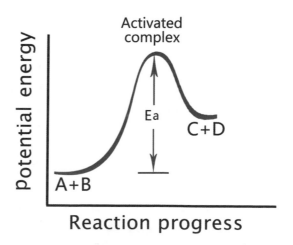

Figure III.A.9.1: Potential energy diagrams: exothermic vs. endothermic reactions.

If a reaction proceeds through several steps one can construct a diagram for each step and combine the single-step diagrams to obtain the energy profile of the overall reaction.

9.6 Kinetic Control vs. Thermodynamic Control

Consider the case where two molecules A and B can react to form either products C or D. Suppose that C has the lowest Gibbs free energy (i.e. the most thermodynamically stable product). Also suppose that product D requires the smallest activation energy and is therefore formed faster than C. If it is product C which is exclusively observed when the reaction is actually performed the reaction is said to be thermodynamically controlled (i.e. out of a list of possible pathways the reactants choose the one leading to the most stable product). If on the other hand the reactants choose the pathway leading to the product which is produced more quickly it is said to be kinetically controlled.

9.7 Catalysis

A catalyst is a compound that does not directly participate in a reaction (the initial number of moles of this compound in the reaction mixture is equal to the number of moles of this compound once the reaction is completed). Catalysts help lower the activation energy of a reaction and help the reaction to proceed. Enzymes are the typical biological catalysts. They are protein molecules with very large molar masses containing one or more active sites. Enzymes are very specialized catalysts. They are generally specific and operate only on certain biological reactants called substrates. They also generally increase the rate of reactions by large factors. The general mechanism of operation of enzymes is as follows:

Enzyme (E) + Substrate (S) $\rightarrow$ ES (complex)

ES $\rightarrow$ Product (P) + Enzyme (E)

If we were to compare the energy profile of a reaction performed with the appropriate enzyme to that of the same reaction performed in the absence of an enzyme we would obtain Figure III.A.9.2.

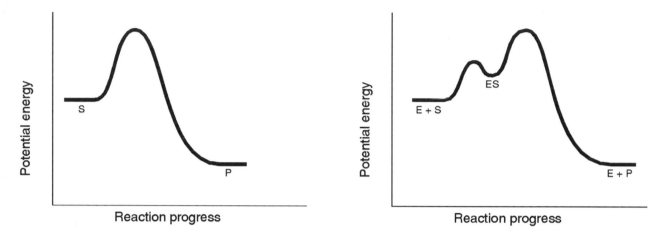

Figure III.A.9.2: Potential energy diagrams: with and without a catalyst.

As you can see from the diagram the reaction from the substrate to the product is facilitated by the presence of the enzyme because the reaction proceeds in two fast steps (low Ea's). Generally the rate of an enzyme-catalysed reaction is :

rate = k [ES]

The plot of the rate of formation of the product $\Delta [P] / \Delta t$ vs. the concentration of the substrate [S] yields a plot as in Figure III.A.9.3.

When the concentration of the substrate is large enough for the substrate to occupy all the available active sites on the enzyme, any further increase would have no effect on the rate of the reaction. This is called *saturation kinetics*.

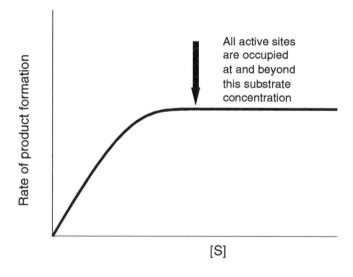

Figure III.A.9.3: Saturation kinetics.

9.8 Equilibrium in Reversible Chemical Reactions

In most chemical reactions once the product is formed it reacts in such a way to yield back the initial reactants. Eventually, the system reaches a state where there are as many molecules of products being formed as there are molecules of reactants being generated through the reverse reaction. This state is called a state of equilibrium. It is characterized by a constant K:

$$aA + bB \rightleftharpoons cC + dD$$

where a, b, c and d are the corresponding stoichiometric coefficients:

$$K = \frac{[C]^c\ [D]^d}{[A]^a\ [B]^b}$$

The <u>equilibrium constant K</u> (sometimes symbolized as K_{eq}) has a given value at a given temperature. If the temperature changes the value of K changes. At a given temperature, if we change the concentration of A, B, C or D, the system evolves in such a way as to re-establish the value of K. This is called the <u>law of mass action</u>. {Note: catalysts speed up the rate of reaction without affecting K_{eq}}

9.9 Le Chatelier's Principle

Le Chatelier's principle states that whenever a perturbation is applied to a system at equilibrium, the system evolves in such a way as to compensate for the applied perturbation. For instance, consider the following equilibrium:

$$N_2 + 3 H_2 \rightleftharpoons 2 NH_3$$

If we introduce some more hydrogen in the reaction mixture at equilibrium, i.e. if we increase the concentration of hydrogen, the system will evolve in the direction that will decrease the concentration of hydrogen (from left to right). If more ammonia is introduced the equilibrium shifts from the

right-hand side to the left-hand side, while the removal of ammonia from the reaction vessel would do the opposite (i.e. shifts equilibrium from the left-hand side to the right-hand side).

In a similar fashion, an <u>increase in total pressure (decrease in volume) favors the direction which decreases the total number of compressible (i.e. gases) moles</u> (from the left-hand side where there are 4 moles to the right-hand side where there are 2 moles). It can also be said that when there are different forms of a substance, an increase in total pressure (decrease in volume) favors the form with the greatest density, and a decrease in total pressure (increase in volume) favors the form with the lowest density.

Finally, if the <u>temperature</u> of a reaction mixture at equilibrium is increased, the equilibrium evolves in the <u>direction of the endothermic reaction</u>. For instance, the forward reaction of the equilibrium:

$$N_2O_4(g) \rightleftharpoons 2\,NO_2(g)$$

is endothermic; therefore, an increase in temperature favors the forward reaction over the backward reaction. In other words, the dissociation of N2O4 increases with temperature.

9.10 Relationship between the Equilibrium Constant and the Change in the Gibbs Free Energy

In the "thermodynamics" section we defined the Gibbs free energy. The *standard* Gibbs free energy (G^0) is determined at 25 °C (298 K) and 1 atm. The change in the standard Gibbs free energy for a given reaction can be calculated from the change in the standard enthalpy and entropy of the reaction using:

$$\Delta G^{\,o} = \Delta H - T\,\Delta S^{\,o}$$

where T is the temperature at which the reaction is carried out. If this reaction happens to be the forward reaction of an equilibrium, the equilibrium constant associated with this equilibrium is simply given by:

$$\Delta G^{\,o} = -\,R\,T\,\mathrm{Ln}\,K_{eq}$$

where R is the ideal gas constant (1.99 cal $\mathrm{mol}^{-1}\,\mathrm{K}^{-1}$) and Ln is the natural logarithm (i.e. log to the base e).

Memorize	Understand	Not Required*
* Define: anode, cathode, anion, cation * Define: standard half-cell potentials * Define: strong/weak oxidizing/reducing agents	* Electrolytic cell, electrolysis * Calculation involving Faraday's law * Galvanic (voltaic) cell, purpose of salt bridge * Half reaction, reduction potentials * Direction of electron flow	* Advanced level college info * Memorizing the value of a faraday * Nernst equation, Frost diagram

MCAT-Prep.com

Introduction ▮▮▮▮

Electrochemistry links chemistry with electricity (the movement of electrons through a conductor). If a chemical reaction produces electricity (i.e. a battery or galvanic/voltaic cell) then it is an **electrochemical cell**. If electricity is applied externally to drive the chemical reaction then it is **electrolysis**. In general, oxidation/reduction reactions occur and are separated in space or time, connected by an external circuit.

Additional Resources

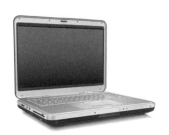

Free Online Q & A

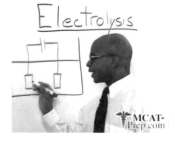

Video: Online or DVD 4

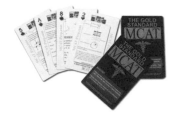

Flashcards

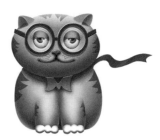

Special Guest

10.1 Generalities

Electrochemistry is based on oxidation-reduction or redox reactions in which one or more electrons are transferred from one ionic species to another. Before you read this section you should review the rules that allow the determination of the oxidation state of an element in a polyatomic molecule or ion and the definition of oxidation and reduction processes. We had previously applied the rules for the determination of oxidation numbers in the case of the following overall reaction (*see Section 1.6*):

$$CuSO_4(aq) + Zn(s) \rightleftharpoons$$

Oxid.#: +2   0

$$Cu(s) + ZnSO4(aq)$$

Oxid.#:   0   +2

The reduction and oxidation half-reactions of the forward process are:

reduction half-reaction:
$$Cu^{2+}(aq) + 2e^- \rightarrow Cu(s)$$

oxidation half-reaction:
$$Zn(s) \rightarrow Zn^{2+}(aq) + 2e^-$$

To determine the number and the side on which to put the electrons one follows the simple rules:

(i)   The electrons are always on the left-hand side of a reduction half-reaction.

(ii)   The electrons are always on the right-hand side of an oxidation half-reaction.

(iii)   For a reduction half-reaction:

# of electrons required = initial oxidation # - final oxidation #

(iv)   For an oxidation half-reaction:
# of electrons required = final oxidation # - initial oxidation #

The next step is to balance each half-reaction, i.e. the charges and the number of atoms of all the elements involved have to be equal on both sides. The preceding example is very simple since the number of electrons required in the two half-reactions is the same. Consider the following more complicated example:

reduction: $Sn^{2+}(aq) + 2e^- \rightarrow Sn(s)$
oxidation: $Al(s) \rightarrow Al^{3+}(aq) + 3e-$

to balance the overall reaction you need to multiply the first half-reaction by a factor of 3 and the second by a factor of 2.

The oxidization/reduction capabilitites of substances are measured by their standard half-cell potentials E^o. These potentials are relative. The reference was chosen to correspond to the following half-reaction:

$$2\,H^+ \text{ (1 molal)} + 2e^- \rightarrow H_2 \text{ (1 atm) } E^o = 0$$

Standard half-cell potentials for other half-reactions have been tabulated. They are defined for standard conditions, i.e., concentration of all ionic species equal to 1 molal and pressure of all gases involved, if any, equal to 1 atm. The standard temperature is taken as 25 °C. In the case of the Cu^{2+}/Zn reaction the relevant data is tabulated as reduction potentials as follows:

$$Zn^{2+}(aq) + 2e^- \rightarrow Zn(s) \quad E°=-0.76 \text{ volts}$$

$$Cu^{2+}(aq) + 2e^- \rightarrow Cu(s) \quad E°=+0.34 \text{ volts}$$

The more positive the $E°$ value, the more likely the reaction will occur spontaneously as written. The strongest reducing agents have large negative $E°$ values. The strongest oxidizing agents have large positive $E°$ values. Therefore, in our example Cu^{2+} is a stronger oxidizing agent than Zn^{2+}. This conclusion can be expressed in the following practical terms:

(i)   If you put Zn in contact with a solution containing Cu^{2+} ions a spontaneous redox reaction will occur.

(ii)   If you put Cu directly in contact with a solution containing Zn^{2+} ions, no reaction takes place spontaneously.

Thus for the spontaneous reaction:

$$E° = E°_{red} - E°_{ox} = +0.34 - (-0.76) = 1.1 \text{ V}.$$

The positive value confirms the spontaneous nature of the reaction. {A note about terminology: the oxidizing agent is *reduced*; the reducing agent is *oxidized*}

10.2 Galvanic Cells

Batteries are self-contained galvanic cells. A galvanic cell uses a spontaneous redox reaction to produce electricity. For instance, one can design a galvanic cell based on the spontaneous reaction:

$$Zn(s) + CuSO_4(aq) \rightarrow Cu(s) + ZnSO_4(aq)$$

The figure below shows the different parts of such a cell. Note that Zn is not in direct contact with the the Cu^{2+} solution; otherwise electrons will be directly transferred from Zn to Cu^{2+} and no electricity will be produced to an external circuit.

The half-reaction occurring in the left-hand side compartment is the oxidation:

$$Zn(s) \rightarrow Zn^{2+}(aq) + 2e^-$$

The half-reaction occurring in the right-hand side compartment is the reduction:

$$Cu^{2+}(aq) + 2e^- \rightarrow Cu(s)$$

Therefore, electrons flow out of the compartment where the oxidation occurs to the compartment where the reduction takes place.

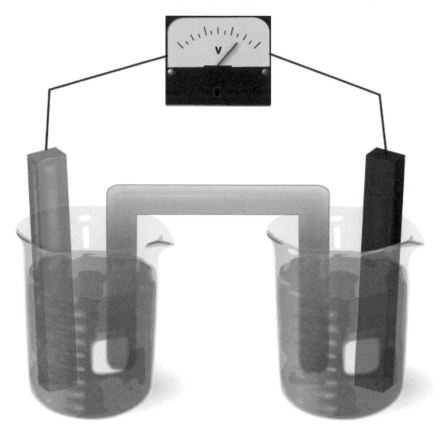

Figure III.A.10.1a: A galvanic (electrochemical) cell.

The metallic parts (Cu(*s*) and Zn(*s*) in our example) of the galvanic cell which allow its connection to an external circuit are called <u>electrodes</u>. The electrode <u>out</u> of which <u>electrons flow</u> is the <u>anode</u>, the electrode <u>receiving</u> these <u>electrons</u> is the <u>cathode</u>. In a galvanic cell the <u>oxidation</u> occurs in the <u>anodic compartment</u> and the <u>reduction</u> in the <u>cathodic compartment</u>. The voltage difference between the two electrodes is called the <u>electromotive force (*emf*)</u> of the cell, if the concentration of all the ions involved is 1 molal, the emf is simply:

$$emf = n \times E^o(\text{reduction}) - m \times E^o(\text{oxidation})$$

Where n and m are the stoichiometric factors by which each half-reaction needs to be multiplied to yield a balanced overall reaction. The stoichiometric factors are *not* used if one is simply calculating the E^o of the cell. The voltage can be measured by the voltmeter. {Mnemonic: LEO is A GERC = <u>L</u>ose <u>E</u>lectrons <u>O</u>xidation is <u>A</u>node, <u>G</u>ain <u>E</u>lectrons <u>R</u>eduction at <u>C</u>athode}

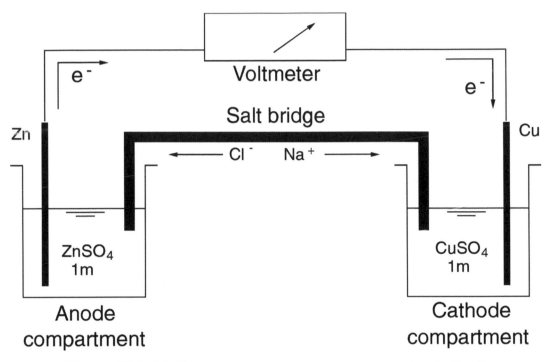

Figure III.A.10.1b: Line diagram of a galvanic (electrochemical) cell.

10.2.1 The Salt Bridge

The salt bridge connects the two compartments chemically (for example, with Na^+ and Cl^-). It has two important functions:

1) Maintenance of Neutrality: As $Zn(s)$ becomes $Zn^{2+}(aq)$, the net charge in the anode compartment becomes positive. To maintain neutrality, Cl^- ions migrate to the anode compartment. The reverse occurs in the cathode compartment: positive ions are lost (Cu^{2+}), therefore positive ions must be gained (Na^+).

2) Completing the Circuit: Imagine the galvanic cell as a circuit. Negative charge leaves the anode compartment via electrons in a wire and then returns via chemicals (i.e. Cl^-) in the salt bridge. Thus the galvanic cell is an electrochemical cell.

As an alternative to a salt bridge, the solutions (i.e. $ZnSO_4$ and $CuSO_4$) can be placed in one container separated by a porous material which allows certain ions to cross (i.e. SO_4^{2-}, Zn^{2-}). Thus it would serve the same functions as the salt bridge.

10.3 Concentration Cell

If the concentration of the ions in one of the compartments of a galvanic cell is not 1 molal, the half-cell potential E is either higher or lower than E^o. Therefore, in principle one could use the same substance in both compartments but with different concentrations to produce electricity. The emf is equal in this case to the difference between the two potentials E. Such a cell is called a concentration cell. To determine the direction of electron flow the same rules as above are used. The cathodic compartment, in which the reduction takes place is the one corresponding to the largest positive (smallest negative) E.

10.4 Electrolytic Cell

There is a fundamental difference between a galvanic cell or a concentration cell and an electrolytic cell: in the first type of electrochemical cell a spontaneous redox reaction is used to produce a current, in the second type a current is actually imposed on the system to drive a non-spontaneous redox reaction. A similarity between the two cells is that the cathode attracts cations, whereas the anode attracts anions.

Remember the following key concepts:

(i)   generally a battery is used to produce a current which is imposed on the electrolytic cell.

(ii)   the battery acts as an electron pump: electrons flow into the electrolytic cell at the cathode and flow out of it at the anode.

(iii)   the half-reaction occurring at the cathode is a reduction since it requires electrons.

(iv)   the half-reaction occurring at the anode is an oxidation since it produces electrons.

10.5 Faraday's Law

Faraday's law relates the amount of elements deposited or gas liberated at an electrode due to current.

We have seen that in a galvanic cell $Cu^{++}(aq)$ can accept electrons to become $Cu(s)$ which will actually plate onto the electrode. Faraday's Law allows us to calculate the amount of $Cu(s)$. In fact, the law states that the weight of product formed at an electrode is proportional to the amount of electricity transferred at the electrode and to the equivalent weight of the material. Thus we can conclude that 1 mole of $Cu^{++}(aq)$ + 2 moles of electrons will leave 1 mole of $Cu(s)$ at the electrode. One mole (= Avogadro's number) of electrons is called a *faraday* ($\mathfrak{F}$). A faraday is equivalent to 96 500 coulombs. As mentioned in Physics 10.1, a coulomb is the amount of electricity that is transferred when a current of one ampere flows for one second ($1C = 1A \cdot S$).

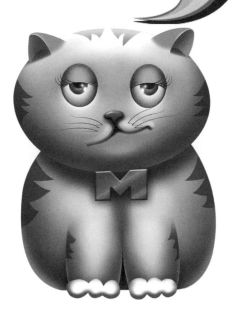

The police stopped a driver who had NaCl and a 9 volt. He was booked for a salt and battery.

10.5.1 Electrolysis Problem

How many grams of copper would be deposited on the cathode of an electrolytic cell if, for a period of 20 minutes, a current of 2.0 amperes is run through a solution of $CuSO_4$?

Calculate the number of coulombs:

$$Q = It = 2.0 \text{ A} \times 20 \text{ min} \times 60 \text{ sec/min} = 2400 \text{ C}$$

Thus

$$\text{Faradays} = 2400 \text{ C} \times 1\mathscr{F}/96\,500 \text{ C} = 0.025 \mathscr{F}$$

Faradays can be related to moles of copper since

$$Cu^{2+} + 2e^- \rightarrow Cu$$

Since 1 mol Cu: 2 mol e^- we can write

$$0.025 \mathscr{F} \times (1 \text{ mol Cu}/2\mathscr{F}) \times (63.5 \text{ g Cu/mol Cu}) = 0.79 \text{ g Cu}$$

Electrolysis would deposit 0.79 g of copper at the cathode.

$= P2 + \rho gh2 + 1/2\ pv22$

$= P2 + \rho gh2 + 1/2\ pv22$

$= P2 + \rho gh2 + 1/2\ pv22$

$v = \sqrt{600} = \sqrt{6(100)} = 10\sqrt{6} = 24 \text{ m/s}$

$Ek = 1/$

$v = \sqrt{600} = \sqrt{6(100)} = 10\sqrt{6} = 24 \text{ m/s}$

$Ek = 1/2\ mv2.$

$P1 + \rho gh1 + 1/2\ pv12$

$P1 + \rho gh1 + 1/2\ pv12$

$Y = \dfrac{(F/A)}{(\Delta l/l)} = \dfrac{F}{A} \cdot \dfrac{l}{\Delta l}$

$ET = Ek + Ep = 1/2mv2 + mgh$

$\overline{00)} = \sqrt{2} = 14 \text{m/s}$

$ET = Ek + Ep = 1/2mv2 + mgh$

$v = \sqrt{2(300) - 2}$

$= P2 + \rho gh2 + 1/2\ pv22$

$v = \sqrt{2(300) - 2(10)20} = \sqrt{2(100)} = \sqrt{2} = 1$

MCAT-Prep.com

PHYSICS

PART III.B: PHYSICAL SCIENCES

Memorize	Understand	Not Required*
* Trigonometric functions: definitions, common values * Pythagorean theorem * Define: displacement, velocity, acceleration * Equations: acceleration, kinematics * Values of standard right angle triangles	* Scalar vs. vector * Add, subtract, resolve vectors * Determine common values of functions * Conversion of the angle to other units * Displacement, velocity, acceleration (avg. and instant.)	* Advanced level college info * Any derivatives with or without vectors * Complex vector systems * Calculus

MCAT-Prep.com

Introduction ▮▮▮▮

Translational motion is the movement of an object (or particle) through space without turning (rotation). Displacement, velocity and acceleration are key vectors – specified by magnitude and direction - often used to describe translational motion. Being able to manipulate and resolve vectors is critical for problem solving in MCAT physics.

Additional Resources

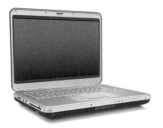

Free Online Q & A

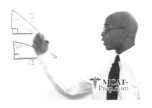

Video: Online or DVD 3

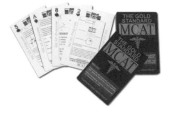

Flashcards

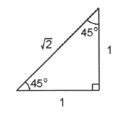

Special Guest

* The real MCAT may have advanced level information presented (ie. in a passage) but previous knowledge of said information is not required to answer the questions that would follow. Practice AAMC and GS practice MCAT CBTs can help you clarify this point.

1.1 Scalars and Vectors

Scalars, such as <u>speed</u>, have magnitude only and are specified by a number with a unit (55 miles/hour). Scalars obey the rules of ordinary algebra. *Vectors,* like <u>velocity</u>, have both magnitude **and** direction (100 km/hour, west). Vectors are represented by arrows where: i) the length of the arrow indicates the magnitude of the vector, and ii) the arrowhead indicates the direction of the vector. Vectors obey the special rules of vector algebra. Thus vectors can be moved in space but their orientation must be kept the same.

<u>Addition of Vectors</u>: Two vectors **a** and **b** can be added geometrically by drawing them to a common scale and placing them head to tail. The vector connecting the tail of **a** to the head of **b** is the sum or <u>resultant</u> vector **r**.

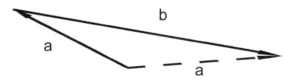

Figure III.B.1.1: The vector sum a + b = r.

<u>Subtraction of Vectors</u>: To subtract the vector **b** from **a**, reverse the direction of **b** then add to **a**.

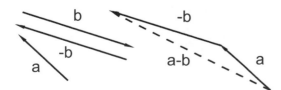

Figure III.B.1.2: The vector difference
a - b = a + (-b).

<u>Resolution of Vectors</u>: Perpendicular projections of a vector can be made on a coordinate axis. Thus the vector **a** can be *resolved* into its x-component (a_x) and its y-component (a_y).

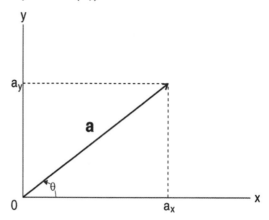

Figure III.B.1.3: The resolution of a vector into its scalar components in a coordinate system.

Analytically, the resolution of vector **a** is as follows:

$$a_x = \mathbf{a}\cos\theta \quad \text{and} \quad a_y = \mathbf{a}\sin\theta$$

Conversely, given the components, we can reconstruct vector **a**:

$$\mathbf{a} = \sqrt{a_x^2 + a_y^2} \quad \text{and} \quad \tan\theta = a_y / a_x$$

Another concept which is sometimes useful is the <u>unit vector</u>. It is a vector of one unit given the special symbols **i**, **j**, and **k** which represent a unit vector in the x-, y- and z-directions, respectively.

Vector **a** can now be written in terms of its components and the unit vectors:

$$\mathbf{a} = \mathbf{i}a_x + \mathbf{j}a_y$$

Thus the vector **a** can be expressed using either scalar components (a_x, a_y) or vector components ($\mathbf{i}a_x$, $\mathbf{j}a_y$).

1.1.1 Trigonometric Functions

The power in trigonometric functions lies in their ability to relate an angle to the ratio of scalar components or *sides* of a triangle. These functions may be defined as follows:

$$sin\ \theta = opp/hyp = y/r$$

$$cos\ \theta = adj/hyp = x/r$$

[*opp* = *the length of the side opposite* angle θ, *adj* = the length of the side *adjacent* to angle θ, *hyp* = the length of the *hypotenuse*]

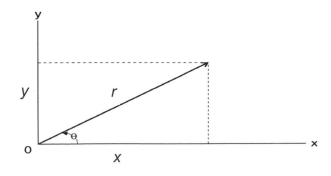

Thus sine ($rsin\ \theta$) gives the *y*-component and cosine ($rcos\ \theta$) gives the x-component of vector r. The tangent function ($tan\ \theta$) and two important trigonometric identities relate sine and cosine:

$$tan\ \theta = sin\ \theta/cos\ \theta = opp/adj = y/x$$

$$sin^2\ \theta + cos^2\ \theta = 1$$

and

$$sin\ 2\theta = 2\ sin\ \theta\ cos\ \theta$$

Other functions of less importance for MCAT physics include: cotangent ($cot\ \theta = x/y$), secant ($sec\ \theta = r/x$) and cosecant ($csc\ \theta = r/y$).

The Pythagorean Theorem relates the sides of the right angle triangle according to the following:

$$r^2 = x^2 + y^2.$$

1.1.2 Common Values of Trigonometric Functions

There are special angles which produce standard values of the trigonometric functions. These values should be memorized. Several of the values are derived from the following triangles:

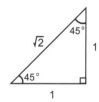
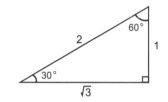

θ	$\sin \theta$	$\cos \theta$	$\tan \theta$
$0°$	0	1	0
$30°$	$1/2$	$\sqrt{3}/2$	$1/\sqrt{3}$
$45°$	$1/\sqrt{2}$	$1/\sqrt{2}$	1
$60°$	$\sqrt{3}/2$	$1/2$	$\sqrt{3}$
$90°$	1	0	∞
$180°$	0	-1	0

Table III.B.1.1:
Common values of trigonometric functions.
The angle θ may be given in radians (R) where $2\pi^R$ = 360°= 1 revolution. Recall $\sqrt{3} \approx 1.7$, $\sqrt{2} \approx 1.4$.

Note that $1° = 60$ arcminutes, 1 arcminute = 60 arcseconds.

Each trigonometric function (i.e. sine) contains an inverse function (i.e. $\sin^{-1}$), where if $\sin \theta = x$, $\theta = \sin^{-1} x$. Thus $\cos 60° = 1/2$, and $60° = \cos^{-1} (1/2)$. Some texts denote the inverse function with "arc" as a prefix. Thus $\operatorname{arcsec} (2) = \sec^{-1} (2)$.

1.2 Distance and Displacement

Distance is the amount of separation between two points in space. It has a magnitude but no direction. It is a scalar quantity and is always positive. Another concept which is sometimes useful is the <u>unit vector</u>.

Displacement of an object between two points is the difference between the final position and the initial position of the object in a given referential system. Thus, a displacement has an origin, a direction and a magnitude. It is a vector.

The sign of the coordinates of the vector displacement depends on the system under study and the chosen referential system. The sign will be positive (+) if the system is moving towards the positive axis of the referential system and negative (-) if not.

The units of distance and displacement are expressed in length units such as *feet (ft), meters (m), miles* and *kilometers (km)*.

Speed is the rate of change of distance with respect to time. It is a scalar quantity, it has a magnitude but no direction, like distance, and it is always positive.

Velocity is the rate of change of displacement with respect to time. It is a vector, and like the displacement, it has a direction and a magnitude. Its value depends on the position of the object. The sign of the coordinates of the vector velocity is the same as that of the displacement.

The <u>instantaneous velocity</u> of a system at a given time is the **slope** of the graph of the displacement of that system vs. time at that time.The magnitude of the velocity decreases if the vector velocity and the vector acceleration have opposite directions.

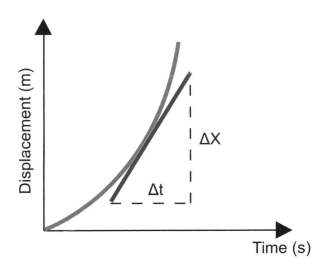

Figure III.B.1.4: Displacement vs. time.

The units of speed and velocity are expressed in length divided by time such as *feet/sec., meters/sec.* and *miles/hour.*

1.4 Acceleration

Acceleration (a) is the rate of change of the velocity (v) with respect to time (t):

$$a = v/t$$

Like the velocity, it is a vector and it has a direction and a magnitude.

The sign of the vector acceleration depends on the net force applied to the system and the chosen referential system. The units of acceleration are expressed as velocity divided by time such as *meters/sec².* The term for negative acceleration is <u>deceleration</u>.

1.4.1 Average and Instantaneous Acceleration

The average acceleration av between two instants t and t' = t + Δt, measures the result of the increase in the speed divided by the time difference,

$$a_v = \frac{v' - v}{\Delta t}$$

The instantaneous acceleration can be determined either by calculating the **slope** (Appendix A.3.1) of a velocity vs. time graph at any time, or by taking the limit when Δt approaches zero of the preceding expression.

$$a_v = \lim_{\Delta t \to 0} \frac{v' - v}{\Delta t}$$

Math involving "limits" does not exist on the MCAT. So let's discuss what this definition is describing in informal terms. The limit is the value of the change in velocity over the change in time as the time approaches 0. It's like saying that the change in velocity is happening in an instant. This allows us to talk about the acceleration in that incredibly fast moment: the instantaneous acceleration which can be determined graphically.

Consider the following events illustrated in the graph (Fig. III.B.1.4): your car starts at rest (0 velocity and time = 0); you steadily accelerate out of the parking lot (the change in velocity increases over time = acceleration); you are driving down the street at constant velocity (change in velocity = 0 and thus acceleration is 0 divided by the change in time which means: a = 0); you see a cat dart across the street safely which made you slow down temporarily (change in velocity is negative thus negative acceleration which, by definition, is deceleration); you now enter the on-ramp for the highway so your velocity is now increasing at a faster and faster rate (increasing acceleration). You can examine the instantaneous acceleration at any one point (or instant) during the period that your acceleration is increasing.

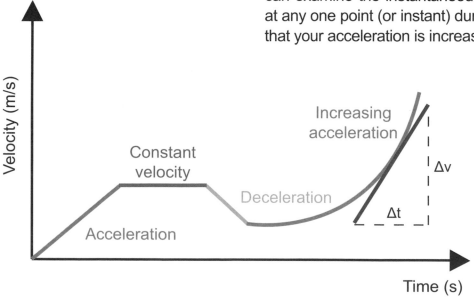

Figure III.B.1.4: Velocity vs. time. Note that at constant velocity, the slope and thus the acceleration are both equal to zero.

The magnitude and direction of the acceleration of a system are solely determined by the exterior forces acting upon the system. If the magnitude of these forces is constant, the magnitude of the acceleration will be constant and the resulting motion is a *uniformly accelerated motion*. The initial displacement, the velocity and the acceleration at any given time contribute to the overall displacement of the system:

$x = x_0$ - displacement due to the initial displacement x_0.

$x = v_0 t$ - displacement due to the initial velocity v at time t.

$x = \frac{1}{2}at^2$ - displacement due the acceleration at time t.

The total displacement of the uniformly-accelerated motion is given by the following formula:

$$x = x_0 + v_0 t + \frac{1}{2}at^2$$

The translational motion is the motion of the center of gravity of a system through space, illustrated by the above equation.

1.6 Equations of Kinematics

Kinematics is the study of objects in motion with respect to space and time. **There are three related equations which must be memorized.** The first is above (PHY 1.5), the others are:

and

$$v = v_0 + at$$

$$v^2 = v_0^2 + 2ax$$

where v is the final velocity; we will put these equations to use in PHY 2.6.

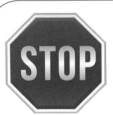

Reminder: Chapter review questions are available online for the owner of this textbook. Doing practice questions will help clarify concepts and ensure that you study in a targeted way. After you login to mcat-prep.com as a Gold Standard Owner*, click on Lessons in the Menu. Your access continues for one full year. Please note that the MCAT is expected to change in 2015 and so access will not continue after the MCAT has changed.

*To become a Gold Standard Owner, you will need to click on FREE MCAT in the top Menu of the mcat-prep.com homepage and then you will find "Click here if you own a Gold Standard textbook". Then follow the directions provided.

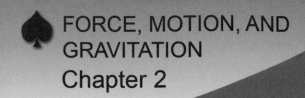

Memorize	Understand	Not Required*
* Define with units: weight, mass * Newton's laws, Law of Gravitation * Values for g including units * Equation for uniformly accelerated motion * Define: drag force, terminal velocity	* Mass, weight, center of gravity * Newton's laws * Law of Gravitation, free fall motion * Projectile motion equations and calculations	* Advanced level college info * Memorizing values for K,G

MCAT-Prep.com

Introduction ▮▮▮

Force is a vector (often a push or pull) that can cause a mass to change velocity thus motion. Forces can be due to gravity, magnetism or anything that causes a mass to accelerate. Nuclear forces (strong) are far greater than electrostatic forces (opposite charges attract), which in turn are far greater than gravitational forces (one of the weakest forces in nature).

Additional Resources

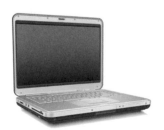

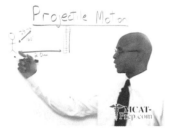

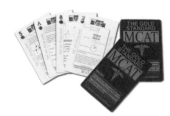

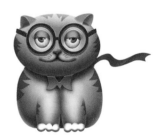

| Free Online Q & A | Video: Online or DVD 1,3 | Flashcards | Special Guest |

2.1 Mass, Center of Mass, Weight

The mass (m) of an object is its measure of inertia. It is the measure of the capacity of that object to remain motionless or to move with a constant velocity if the sum of the forces acting upon it is zero. This definition of inertia is derived from Newton's First Law.

The *center of mass* of an object is a point whose motion can be described like the motion of a particle through space. The center of mass of an object always has the simplest motion of all the points of that object.

The center of gravity (COG) is also the center of mass seen as the center of application of all the gravitational forces acting on the object. For example, for a uniform plank hanging horizontally, the COG is at half the length of the plank.

The COG can be determined experimentally by suspending an object by a string at different points and noting that the direction of the string passes through the COG. The intersection of the projected lines in the different suspensions is the COG.

An object is in *stable equilibrium* if the COG is as low as possible and any change in orientation will lead to an elevation of the COG. An object is in *unstable equilibrium* if the COG is high relative to the support point or surface and any change in orientation will lead to a lowering of the COG.

The *weight* is a force (i.e. newtons, pounds). It is a vector unlike the *mass* which is a scalar (i.e. kilograms, slugs). The weight is proportional to the mass. It is the product of the mass by the vector gravitational acceleration *g*.

$$W = m \times g$$

2.2 Newton's Second Law

Newton's Second Law, also called the fundamental dynamic relation, states that the sum of all the exterior forces acting upon the center of mass of a system is equal to the product of the mass of the system by the acceleration of its center of mass.

Therefore, if there is a net force, the object must accelerate. It is a vectorial equality which asserts that <u>a net force against an object *must* result in acceleration:</u>

$$\Sigma F = m \times a$$

It is important to note that for a system in complex motion, Newton's Second Law can only determine the acceleration of the center of mass. It does not give any indication about the motion of the other parts of the system.

Whereas, for a system in translational motion, Newton's Second Law gives the acceleration of the system.

2.3 Newton's Third Law

For every action there is an equal and opposite reaction. If one object exerts a force, F, on a second object, the second object exerts a force, F', on the first object. F and F' have opposite direction but the same magnitude.

2.4 The Law of Gravitation

The Law of Gravitation states that there is a force of attraction existing between any two bodies of masses m_1 and m_2. The force is proportional to the product of the masses and inversely proportional to the square of the distance between them.

$$F = K_G(m_1 m_2 / r^2)$$

r is the distance between the bodies; K_G is the universal constant of gravitation, and its value depends on the units being used.

2.5 Free Fall Motion

The free fall motion of an object is the upward or downward vertical motion of that object with reference to the earth.

The motion is always uniformly accelerated with the acceleration g: vertical, directed towards the center of the earth and the magnitude is considered constant during the free fall motion.

Also, during the free fall motion, the air resistance is considered negligible. The equation of the motion can easily be derived from Newton's Second Law.

$$\Sigma F = ma$$

Where ΣF represents all the forces acting on the object, m is the mass of the object and a is the acceleration of the center of mass of the object. Hence, a can be replaced by g since $a = g$ by definition. In the free fall motion, the only force acting on the object is the gravitational force, which gives the following equality:

$$K_G m_{object} \frac{M_{earth}}{r^2_{earth}} = m_{object}\, g$$

dividing both sides by m_{object} we get :

$$g = K_G \frac{M_{earth}}{r^2_{earth}}$$

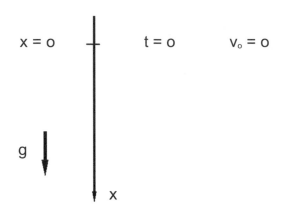

Figure III.B.2.1: Free fall motion.

The values of g which must be committed to memory are: 32 ft/s^2 (Imperial units), 980 cm/s^2 (CGS units), or 9.8 m/s^2 (**SI** units). The equation for uniformly accelerated motion is applicable by replacing a by g:

$$x = x_0 + v_0 t + 1/2 g t^2$$

$$v = gt$$

$$a = g$$

Before doing any calculation, the reference point and a positive direction must be chosen. In the free fall of an actual object, the value of g is modified by the buoyancy of air and resistance of air. This results in a *drag force* which depends on the location on earth, shape and size of the object, and the velocity of the object (as free fall velocity increases, the drag force increases). When the drag force reaches the force of gravity, the object reaches a final velocity called the terminal velocity and continues to fall at that velocity.

The projectile motion is the motion of any object fired or launched at some angle α from the horizontal. The motion defines a parabola (*see Figure III.B.2.2*) in the plane *O-x-y* that contains the initial (*original*) vector velocity v_o.

The motion can be decomposed into two distinct motions: a vertical component, affected by g, and a horizontal component, independent of g.

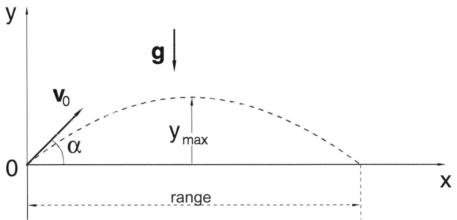

Figure III.B.2.2: Projectile motion.

Vertical component (free fall)
- initial speed : $V_{oy} = V_o \sin \alpha$
- displacement at time t: $y = V_{oy}t + 1/2gt^2$
- speed at any time t: $V_y = V_{oy} + gt$

Horizontal component (linear with constant speed)
- initial speed : $V_{ox} = V_o \cos \alpha$
- displacement at any time t: $x = V_{ox}t$
- speed at any time t: $V_x = V_{ox}$ (speed is constant)

Initial velocity

- magnitude: $|V_o| = \sqrt{V^2_{ox} + V^2_{oy}}$

- direction: *alpha*: $\tan \alpha = V_{oy} / V_{ox}$

- important points to consider:

1)   Neglecting air resistance, there is no acceleration in the horizontal direction: V_x is constant.

2) V_y is zero at Y_{max}, then $V_y = 0 = V_{oy} + gt_{up}$ or $-V_{oy} = gt_{up}$ can be solved for t.

3)   Also, by eliminating the variables y and t in the equations, we can get the following equality :

$$x = \frac{V_o^2 \sin 2\alpha}{g}$$

The horizontal distance from the origin to where the object strikes the ground (= *the range*) is maximum for a given V_o when $\sin 2\alpha = 1$, hence for $2\alpha = (\pi/2)^R$ => $\alpha = (\pi/4)^R$ or $\alpha = 45$ degrees.

2.6.1 Projectile Motion Problem (Imperial units)

In the Superbowl, the punter kicks the football at an angle of 30° from the horizontal with an initial speed of 75 ft/s. Assume that the ball moves in a vertical plane and that air resistance is negligible.

(a) *Find the time at which the ball reaches the highest point of its trajectory.*

{key: height refers to the y-component; we can define gravity as a negative vector since it is directed downwards}

V_y is zero at Y_{max} (= *the highest point*), thus:

$V_y = 0$, $V_o = 75$ ft/s, $\alpha = 30°$, $g = -32$ ft/s²

$V_y = V_o \sin \alpha + g t_{up}$

Isolate t_{up}:

$$t_{up} = \frac{V_y - V_o \sin \alpha}{g} = \frac{-75(\sin 30°)}{-32}$$

$$= 1.2 \text{ seconds}$$

(b) *How high does the ball go?*

$Y_{max} = V_o (\sin \alpha) t_{up} + 1/2 g t_{up}^2$

$Y_{max} = 75(\sin 30°)1.2 + 1/2(-32)(1.2)^2 = 22$ feet

(c) *How long is the ball in the air and what is its range?*

{key: time is the same for x- and y-components, range = x-component}

Once the ball strikes the ground its vertical displacement $y = 0$, thus:

$y = 0 = V_o (\sin \alpha) t + 1/2 g t^2$

Divide through by t then isolate:

$t = 2V_o(\sin \alpha)/g = 2.4$ seconds.

Since $t = 2t_{up}$, we can conclude that the time required for the ball to go up to Y_{max} is the same as the time required to come back down: 1.2 seconds in either direction.

The range $x = V_o(\cos \alpha)t$

$x = 75(\cos 30°)2.4 \approx 150$ feet

or

$x \approx 150$ ft (1 yd/ 3 ft) = 50 yards

{Had the punter kicked the ball at 45° from the horizontal he would have maximized his range. He should be benched for not having done his physics!}

(d) *What is the velocity of the ball as it strikes the ground?*

{*key: velocity* is the resultant vector of V_x and V_y - the final velocities in the *x* and *y* directions}

$$V_x = V_o\cos \alpha = 75(\cos 30°) = 65 \text{ ft/s}$$

$$V_y = V_o\sin \alpha + gt$$

$$= 75(\sin 30°) + (-32)(2.4) = -39 \text{ ft/s}$$

$$V = \sqrt{V^2_x + V^2_y} = \sqrt{(65)^2 + (-39)^2}$$

$$= \sqrt{(13 \times 5)^2 + (13 \times -3)^2}$$

$$V = 13\sqrt{(5)^2 + (-3)^2} = 13\sqrt{34}$$

To estimate $\sqrt{34}$ we must first recognize that the answer must be at least 5 ($5^2 = 25$) but closer to 6 ($6^2 = 36$). Try squaring 5.7, 5.8, 5.9. Squaring 5.8 is the closest estimate (= 33.6), thus

$$V = 13(5.8) = 75 \text{ ft/s.}$$

{*Recall: there are no calculators permitted for the MCAT. You should be able to perform all the preceding calculations with speed and accuracy*}

Dogs have owners.
Cats have staff!

Memorize	Understand	Not Required*
* Equations: f_{max}, μ_s * Centripetal force and acceleration * Circumference and area of a circle	* Static vs. kinetic friction * Resolving vectors, calculate for incline plane * Uniform circular motion * Solve pulley system, free body diagram	* Advanced level college info * Memorizing values of μ

MCAT-Prep.com

Introduction ▪▪▪▪

Particle dynamics is concerned with the physics of motion. Among other topics, particle dynamics includes Newton's laws, frictional forces, and problems dealing with incline planes, uniform circular motion and pulley systems.

Additional Resources

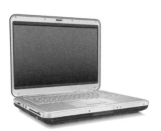

Free Online Q & A

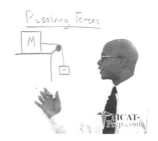

Video: Online or DVD 3,4

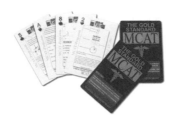

Flashcards

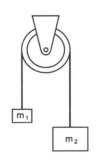

Special Guest

3.1 Overview

For the MCAT, particle dynamics is concerned with the physics of motion. Among other topics, particle dynamics incldes Newton's laws, frictional forces, and problems dealing with incline planes, uniform circular motion and pulley systems.

3.2 Frictional Forces

Frictional forces are nonconservative (mechanical energy is not conserved) and are caused by molecular adhesion between tangential surfaces but are independent of the area of contact of the surfaces. Frictional forces always oppose the motion. The maximal frictional force has the following expression: $f_{max} = \mu N$, where μ is the coefficient of friction and N is the normal force to the surface on which the object rests, it is the reaction of that surface against the weight of the object. Thus N always acts perpendicular to the surface.

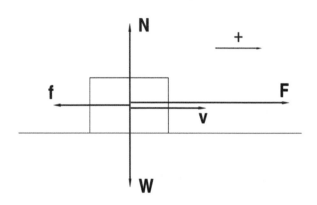

Figure III.B.3.1: Frictional force f and force normal N.

Static friction is when the object is not moving, and it must be overcome for motion to begin. The coefficient of static friction μ_s is given as :

$$\mu_s = \tan \alpha$$

where α is the angle at which the object first begins to move on an inclined plane as the angle is increased from 0 degrees to α degrees (*see Figure III.B.3.2*). There is also a coefficient of kinetic friction, μ_k, which exists when surfaces are in motion; $\mu_k < \mu_s$ always.

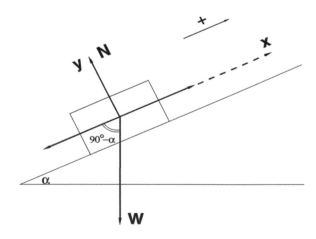

Figure III.B.3.2: Analysis of motion on an incline.

The weight (W) due to gravity (g) may be sufficient to cause motion if friction is overcome. The reference axes are usually chosen as shown such that one (the x) is along the surface of the incline.

Note that W is directed downward and N is directed upward but *perpendicular* to the surface of the incline (i.e. in the positive *y* direction).

3.2.1 Incline Plane Problem with Friction (SI units)

A 50 kilogram block is on an incline of 45°. The coefficient of sliding (= *kinetic*) friction between the block and the plane is 0.10.

Determine the acceleration of the block. {*key: motion* is along the plane, so only the *x*-components of the force is relevant to the acceleration}

Begin with Newton's Second Law:

$$F = m \times a$$

thus

$$F_x = f_k - W\sin\alpha = \mu_k N - W\sin\alpha = m \times a$$

The force normal (*N*) can be determined by summing the forces in the y direction where the acceleration is zero:

$$F_y = N - W\cos\alpha = m \times a = 0$$

Therefore,
$$N = W\cos\alpha$$

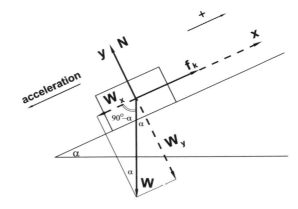

Figure III.B.3.3: Resolving the weight W into its x-component (W sinα) and its y-component (W cosα).

Solving for a and combining our first and last equations we get (*recall: W = mg*):

$$a = (\mu_k W\cos\alpha - W\sin\alpha)/m$$
$$= mg(\mu_k\cos\alpha - \sin\alpha)/m = g(\mu_k\cos\alpha - \sin\alpha)$$

Substituting the values:

$$a = 9.8 \text{ m/s}^2(0.10\cos45° - \sin45°) = -6.2 \text{ m/s}^2$$

• Thus the block accelerates at 6.2 m/s² *down* the plane. Also note that the *mass* of the block is irrelevant.

3.3 Uniform Circular Motion

In Chapter 1 we saw that acceleration is due to a change in velocity (PHY 1.4). For a particle moving in a circle at constant speed (= *uniform circular motion*), the velocity vector changes continuously in <u>direction</u> but the <u>magnitude</u> remains the same.

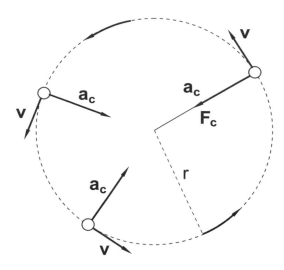

The velocity is always tangent to the circle and since it is always changing (i.e. *direction*) it creates an acceleration directed radially inward called the *centripetal* acceleration (a_c). The magnitude of the acceleration a_c is given by v^2/r where r is the radius of the circle.

Figure III.B.3.4: Uniform Circular Motion.

Every accelerated particle must have a force acting on it according to Newton's Second Law. Thus we can calculate the *centripetal* force,

$$F_c = ma_c = mv^2/r.$$

The centripetal force can be produced in many ways: a taut string which is holding a ball at the end that is spinning in a circle; a radially directed frictional force like when a car drives around a curve on an unbanked road; a contact force exerted by another body like driving around a curve on a banked road or like the wall of an amusement park rotor.

Any particle moving in a circle with *non-uniform* speed will experience both centripetal <u>and</u> tangential forces and accelerations. {Reminder: the circumference of a circle is $2\pi r$ and the area is πr^2}

Consider two unequal masses connected by a string which passes over a frictionless, massless pulley (*see* Figure III.B.3.5). Let us determine the following parameters: i) the tension T in the string which is a force and ii) the acceleration of the masses given that m_2 is greater than m_1.

Always begin by drawing vector or *free-body* diagrams of a problem. The position of each mass will lie at the origin O of their respective axes. Now we assign positivity or negativity to the directions of motion. We can arbitrarily define the upward direction as positive. Thus if the acceleration of m_1 is a then the acceleration of m_2 must be $-a$.

Using Newton's Second Law we can derive the equation of motion for m_1:

$$F = T - m_1 g = m_1 a$$

and for m_2:

$$F = T - m_2 g = -m_2 a$$

Subtracting one equation from the other eliminates T then we can solve for a:

$$a = \frac{m_2 - m_1}{m_2 + m_1} g$$

Solve for a using the equations of motion, equate the formulas, then we can solve for T:

$$T = \frac{2 m_1 m_2}{m_1 + m_2} g$$

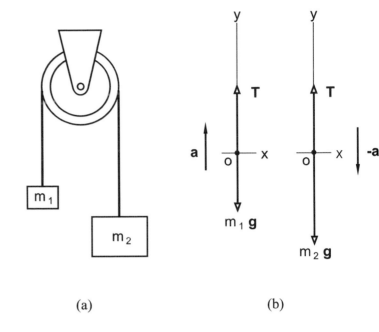

(a)   (b)

Figure III.B.3.5: A Pulley System.
(a) Two unequal masses suspended by a string from a pulley (= Atwood's machine). (b) Free-body diagrams for m_1 and m_2.

Let us solve the problem using Imperial units where m_2 is 3.0 slugs ($W_2 = m_2 g = 96$ pounds - lb) and m_1 is 1.0 slug ($W_1 = m_1 g = 32$ lb):

$$a = \frac{3.0 - 1.0}{3.0 + 1.0} g = g/2 = 16 \text{ ft/s}^2$$

and

$$T = \frac{2 (1.0) (3.0)}{1.0 + 3.0} (32) = 48 \text{ lb.}$$

• Note that T is always between the weight of mass m_1 and that of m_2. The reason is that T must exceed $m_1 g$ to give m_1 an upward acceleration, and $m_2 g$ must exceed T to give m_2 a downward acceleration.

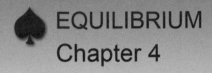
Memorize	Understand	Not Required*
* Definitions and equations to solve torque problems * Newton's First Law, inertia * Equations for momentum, impulse	* Solve torque, collision problems * Choosing an appropriate pivot point * Create vector diagrams * Elastic vs. inelastic vs. conservation of E. * Solve momentum problem, significant figures	* Advanced level college info * Complex torque or collision problems * Torque as a function of time * Machine torque

MCAT-Prep.com

Introduction ▊▊▊▊

Equilibrium exists when a mass is at rest or moves with constant velocity. Translational (straight line) and rotational (turning) equilibria can be resolved using linear forces, torque forces, Newton's first law and inertia. Momentum is a vector that can be used to solve problems involving elastic (bouncy) or inelastic (sticky) collisions.

Additional Resources

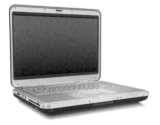

Free Online Q & A

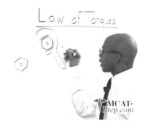

Video: Online or DVD 4

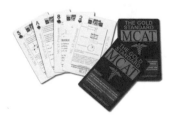

Flashcards

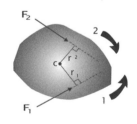

Special Guest

4.1 Translational, Rotational and Complex Motion

When a force acts upon an object, the object will undergo translational, rotational or complex (translational and rotational) motion.

Rotational motion of an object about an axis is the rotation of that object around that axis caused by perpendicular forces to that axis. The effective force causing rotation about an axis is the torque (L).

The torque is like a *turning force*. Consider a hinged door. If you were to apply a force F at the pivot point (*the hinge*), the door would not turn ($L=0$). If you apply the *same* force further and further from the pivot point, the turning force multiplies and the acceleration of the door increases. Thus the torque can be defined as the force applied multiplied by the perpendicular distance from the pivot point (= *lever or moment arm* = r).

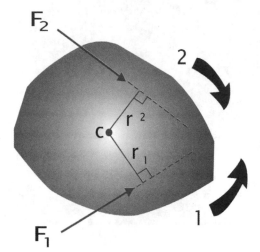

Figure III.B.4.1: Rotational Motion.

$$L = (\text{force}) \times (\text{lever arm})$$

Thus according to Figure III.B.4.1:

$$L_1 = F_1 \times r_1 = \text{counterclockwise torque (1)} = \text{positive}$$

and

$$L_2 = F_2 \times r_2 = \text{clockwise torque (2)} = \text{negative.}$$

Positivity and negativity are arbitrary designations of the two opposite directions of motion. To determine the direction of rotation caused by the torque, imagine the direction the object would rotate if the force is pushing its moment arm at right angles. The net torques acting upon an object is obtained by summing the counterclockwise (+) and the clockwise (-) torques. An object is at equilibrium when the net forces and the net torques acting upon the object is zero. Thus, the object is either motionless or moving at a constant velocity due to its internal inertia.

The conditions of equilibrium are:

For translational equilibrium:

$$\Sigma F_x = 0 \text{ and } \Sigma F_y = 0$$

For rotational equilibrium:

$$\Sigma L = 0$$

If the torques sum to zero about one point in an object, they will sum to zero about any point in the object. If the point chosen as reference (= *pivot point or fulcrum*) includes the line of action of one of the forces, that force need not be included in calculating torques.

4.1.1 Torque Problem (SI units)

A 70 kg person sits 50 cm from the edge of a non-uniform plank which weighs 100 N and is 2.0 m long (*see Figure III.B.4.2*). The weight supported by point *B* is 250 N. Find the center of gravity (COG) of the plank.

{key: draw a vector diagram then choose an unknown value as the pivot point i.e. point A; see section 2.1 for a definition of COG}

(a)

(b)

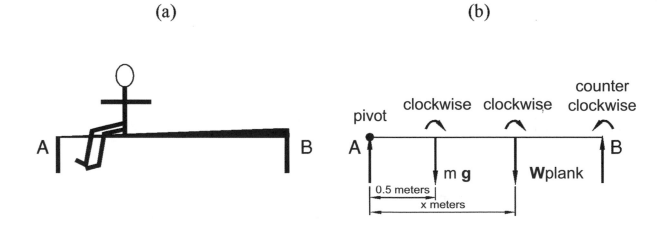

Figure III.B.4.2: Torque Problem.
(a) A person sitting on a non-uniform bench which is composed of a plank with two supports A and B. (b) Vector diagram with point A as the reference point. The torque force at point A is zero since its distance from itself is zero.

The counterclockwise torque (CCW) is given by the force at point B multiplied by its distance from the reference point A:

$$CCW = F_B r_B = 250(2.0) = 500 \text{ Nm}$$

The clockwise torques (CW) are given by the force exerted by the person (= the weight mg) multiplied by the distance from the pivot point (r = 50 cm = 0.5 m) and the force exerted by the plank (= the weight) multiplied by the distance from the pivot point where the weight of the plank acts (= COG):

$$CW = mgr + W(COG)$$
$$= 70(10)0.5 + 100(COG)$$
$$= 350 + 100(COG)$$

Gravity was estimated as 10 m/s². Now we have:

$$\Sigma L = CCW - CW = 500 - 350 - 100(COG) = 0$$

Isolate COG

$$COG = 150/100 = 1.5 \text{ m from point } A.$$

• Note that had the plank been uniform its COG would be at its center which is 1.0 m from either end.

• Had the problem requested the weight supported at point A, it would be easy to determine since $\Sigma F_y = 0$. If we define upward forces as positive, we get:

$$\Sigma F_y = F_A + F_B - mg - W_{plank} = 0$$

Isolate F_A

$$F_A = 70(10) + 100 - 250 = 550 \text{ N.}$$

4.2 Newton's First Law

Newton's First Law states that objects in motion or at rest tend to remain as such unless acted upon by an outside force. That is, objects have inertia (resistance to motion). For translational motion, the mass (m) is a measure of inertia.

For rotational motion, a quantity derived from the mass called the moment of inertia (I) is the measure of inertia. In general $I = \Sigma mr^2$ where r is the distance from the axis of rotation. However, the exact formulation depends on the structure of the object.

The momentum (M) is a vector quantity. The momentum of an object is the product of its mass and its velocity.

$$M = m\,v$$

Linear momentum is a measure of the tendency of an object to maintain motion in a straight line. The greater the momentum (M), the greater the tendency of the object to remain moving along a straight line in the same direction. The momentum (M) is also a measure of the force needed to stop or change the direction of the object.

The impulse I is a measure of the change of the momentum of an object. It is the product of the force applied by the time during which the force was applied to change the momentum.

$$I = F\,\Delta t = \Delta M$$

where F is the acting force and Δt is the elapsed time during which the force was acting. The momentum is also conserved just like energy. The total linear momentum of a system is constant when the resultant external force acting on the system is zero.

4.4 Collisions

During motion, objects can collide. There are two kinds of collisions: elastic and inelastic. During an elastic collision (objects rebound off each other), there is a conservation of momentum and conservation of kinetic energy. Whereas, during an inelastic collision (objects stick together), there is conservation of momentum but not conservation of kinetic energy. Kinetic energy is lost as heat or sound, so total energy is conserved.

Examples of elastic collisions include 2 rubber balls colliding, particle collisions in ideal gases, and the slingshot type gravitational interactions between satellites and planets popularized in science fiction movies. Examples of inelastic collisions include 2 cars colliding at high speed becoming stuck together and a ballistic pendulum

which can be a huge chunk of wood used to measure the speed of a moving object (i.e. bullet) which becomes completely embedded in the wood. If, however, the bullet were to emerge from the wood block, then it would be an elastic collision since the objects did not stick together.

Imagine two spheres with masses m_1 and m_2 and the velocity components before the collision v_{1i} and v_{2i} and after the collision v_{1f} and v_{2f}. If the momentum and the velocity are in the same directions, and we define that direction as positive, from the conservation of momentum we obtain:

$$m_1 v_{1i} + m_2 v_{2i} = m_1 v_{1f} + m_2 v_{2f}\,.$$

If the directions are not the same then each momentum must be resolved into x- and y-components as necessary.

• In the explosion of an object at rest, the total momentum of all the fragments must sum to zero because of the conservation of momentum and because the original momentum was zero.

• If one object collides with a second identical object that is at rest, there is a total transfer of kinetic energy, that is the first object comes to rest and the second object moves off with the momentum of the first one.

4.4.1 Collision Problem (CGS units)

A bullet of mass 10 g and a speed of 5.0×10^4 cm/s strikes a 700 g wooden block at rest on a very smooth surface. The bullet emerges with its speed reduced to 3.5×10^4 cm/s.

Find the resulting speed of the block. {*CGS uses centimeters, grams, and seconds as units; the CGS unit of force is a dyne*}

Let m_1 = the mass of the bullet (10 g), v_{1i} = the speed of the bullet before the collision (5.0×10^4 cm/s), m_2 = the mass of the wooden block (700 g), v_{2i} = the speed of the block before the collision (0 cm/s), v_{1f} = the speed of the bullet after the collision (3.5×10^4 cm/s), and v_{2f} = the speed of the block after the collision (*unknown*), now we have:

$$m_1 v_{1i} + m_2 v_{2i} = m_1 v_{1f} + m_2 v_{2f}$$

Solving for v_{2f}

$$v_{2f} = (m_1 v_{1i} - m_1 v_{1f})/m_2$$
$$= (5.0 \times 10^5 - 3.5 \times 10^5)/(700)$$
$$= 2.1 \times 10^2 \text{ cm/s.}$$

• Note: the least precise figures that we are given in the problem contain at least two digits or significant figures. Thus our answer can not be more precise than two significant figures. The exponent 10^x is not considered when counting significant figures unless you are *told* that the measurement was more precise than is evident {For more on significant figures *see* Appendix A.6 and PHY 8.5.1}.

• Note: you should be comfortable solving physics problems in Imperial, SI or CGS units (Appendix B).

Memorize	Understand	Not Required*
* Define, equation, units: work * Equations and units: potential energy * Equations and units: kinetic energy, power	* Path independence of work done in a g field * Work-Energy Theorem * Conservation of E.; conservative forces * Solving Conservation of E. problems	* Advanced level college info

MCAT-Prep.com

Introduction ▪▪▪▪

Work and energy are used to describe how bodies or masses interact with the environment or other bodies or masses. Conservation of energy, work and power describe the forms of energy and the changes between these forms.

Additional Resources

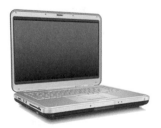

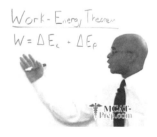

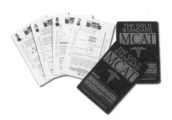

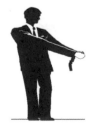

| Free Online Q & A | Video: Online or DVD 1, 3, 4 | Flashcards | Special Guest |

5.1 Work

The work of a force *F* on an object is the product of the force by the distance travelled by the object where the force is in the direction of the displacement.

• *Units*: both work and energy are measured in joules where 1 *joule (J)* = 1 *N* × 1 *m*. {Imperial units: the *foot-pound*, CGS units: the *dyne-centimeter* or *erg*}

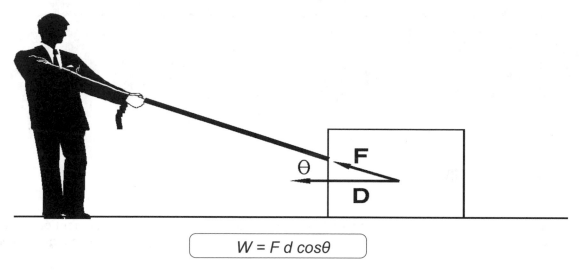

$$W = F\, d\, cos\theta$$

Figure III.B.5.1: Work. The displacement depends on the final and initial positions of the object. The angle θ is necessary to determine the component of a constant force F in the same direction of the displacement. Note that if F acts perpendicular to the displacement then the work $W = F\, d\, cos(90°) = 0$.

5.2 Energy

We usually speak of mechanical, electrical, chemical, potential, kinetic, atomic and nuclear energy, to name a few. In fact, these different kinds of energy are different forms or manifestations of the same energy. Energy is a scalar. It is defined as a physical quantity <u>capable of producing work</u>.

1) *Definition of kinetic energy*

Kinetic energy (E_k) is the energy of motion which can produce work. It is proportional to the mass of the object and its velocity:

$$E_k = 1/2\ mv^2.$$

2) *The Work-Energy Theorem*

A net force is the sum of interior and exterior forces acting upon the system. The variation of the kinetic energy of a system is equal to the work of the net force applied to the system:

$$W \text{ (of the resultant force)} = \Delta E_k .$$

Consequently, if the speed of a particle is constant, $\Delta E_k = 0$, then the work done by the resultant force must be zero. For example, in uniform circular motion the speed of the particle remains constant thus the centripetal force does no work on the particle. A force at right angles to the direction of motion merely changes the direction of the velocity but not its magnitude.

5.4 Potential Energy

Potential energy (E_p) is referred to as potential because it is accumulated by the system that contained it. It varies with the configuration of the system, i.e., when distances between particles of the system vary, the interactions between these particles vary. The variation of the potential energy is equal to the work performed by the interior forces caused by the interaction between the particles of the system. The following are examples of potential energy:

a) potential energy (= electric potential = E_p) derived from the Coulomb force (r is the distance between point charges q_1 and q_2, PHY 9.1.4):

$$E_p = k\,q_1q_2/r$$

b) potential energy derived from the universal attraction force (r is the distance between the COG of masses m_1 and m_2):

$$E_p = G\,m_1m_2/r$$

c) potential energy derived from the gravitational force (h is the height):

$$E_p = mgh$$

d) potential energy derived from the elastic force (i.e. a compressed spring):

$$E_p = kx^2/2 .$$

{k = the spring constant, x = displacement, cf. PHY 7.2.1}

5.5 Conservation of Energy

a) *Definition*

The mechanical energy (E_T) of a system is equal to the sum of its kinetic energy and its potential energy:

$$E_T = E_k + E_p.$$

b) *Theorem of mechanical energy*

The variation of the mechanical energy of a system is equal to the work of exterior forces acting on the system.

c) *Consequence*

An isolated system, i.e., which is not being acted upon by any exterior force, keeps a constant mechanical energy. The kinetic energy and the potential energy may vary separately but their sum remains constant. This makes conservation of energy a very simple way to solve many different types of physics problems.

5.5.1 Conservation of Energy Problem (SI units)

A 6.8×10^3 kg frictionless roller coaster car starts at rest 30 meters above ground level. Determine the speed of the car at (a) 20 m above ground level; (b) at ground level.

$$E_T = E_k + E_p = 1/2mv^2 + mgh$$

Initially v = 0 since the car starts at rest, h = 30 m, and the constant g ≈ 10 m/s2, thus

$$E_T = 0 + m(10)(30) = 300m \text{ joules.}$$

Situation (a) where h = 20 m:

$$E_T = 300m = 1/2mv^2 + mgh$$

m cancels, multiply through by 2, solve for *v*:

$$v = \sqrt{2(300) - 2(10)20} = \sqrt{2(100)} = \sqrt{2}\,(10)$$
$$= 14 \text{ m/s}$$

Situation (b) at ground level h = 0:

$$E_T = 300m = 1/2mv^2 + 0$$

m cancels, multiply through by 2, solve for *v*:

$$v = \sqrt{600} = \sqrt{6(100)} = 10\sqrt{6} = 24 \text{ m/s}$$

• Note: the mass of the roller coaster is irrelevant!

• Note: you must be able to quickly estimate square roots (PHY 1.1.2, 2.6.1).

The three definitions of a conservative force are: i) after a round trip the kinetic energy of a particle on which a force acts must return to its initial value; ii) after a round trip the work done on a particle by a force must be zero; iii) the work done by the force on a particle depends on the initial and final positions of the particle and not on the path taken.

Examples: Friction disobeys all three of the preceding criteria thus it is a non-conservative force. The force $F_s = -kx$ (Hooke's Law, PHY 7.2.1) of an Ideal spring on a frictionless surface is a conservative force. Gravity is a conservative force. If you throw a ball vertically upward, it will return with the same kinetic energy it had when it left your hand (*neglect air resistance*).

5.7 Power

The power P applied during the work W performed by a force F is equal to the work divided by the time necessary to do the work. In other words, power is the rate of doing work:

$$P = \Delta W / \Delta t.$$

• The SI unit for power is the *watt* (W) which equals one *joule per second* (J/s).

Memorize	Understand	Not Required*
* Equations: density, specific gravity * Density of water in 2 different units * Values/units/equations for pressure, pressure change * Pascal's law, Archimedes' principle * Equations: Continuity, hydrostatic pressure	* Buoyancy force, SG and height immersed * Streamline, turbulent flow; continuity/ Bernouilli's equation * Fluid viscosity, Reynolds Number, surface tension * Elastic properties of solids; effect of temperature	* Advanced level college info * Memorizing all the equations for solids

MCAT-Prep.com

Introduction ▮▮▮▮

A fluid is a substance that flows (*deforms*) under sheer stress. This includes all gases and liquids. It is important to understand the properties without movement (hydrostatic pressure, Archimedes' principle) and with movement (continuity, Bernoulli's). On the other hand, a solid *resists* being deformed or submitting to changes in volume. A basic understanding of this *elastic* property of solids is required.

Additional Resources

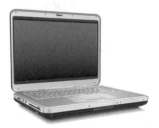

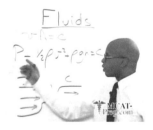

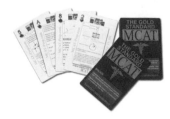

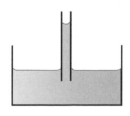

| Free Online Q & A | Video: Online or DVD Disc 4 | Flashcards | Special Guest |

6.1 Fluids

6.1.1 Density, Specific Gravity

The *density* of an object is defined as the ratio of its mass to its volume.

$$density = mass / volume$$

This definition holds for solids, fluids and gases. From the definition, it is easy to see that solids are more dense than liquids which are in turn more dense than gases. This is true because for a given mass, the average distance between molecules of a given substance is bigger in the liquid state than in the solid state. Put simply, the substance occupies a bigger volume in the liquid state than in the solid state and a much bigger volume in gaseous state than in the liquid state.

At a given temperature, the *specific gravity* (SG) is defined as :

$$SG = \frac{density\ of\ a\ substance}{density\ of\ water}$$

The density of water is about 1 g/ml (= 1 g/cm³ = 10^3 kg/m³) over most common temperatures. So in most instances the specific gravity of a substance is the same as its density.

Note that the dimension of density is mass per unit volume, whereas the specific gravity is dimensionless. Density is one of the key properties of fluids (liquids or gases) and the other is pressure.

6.1.2 Hydrostatic Pressure, Buoyancy, Archimedes' Principle

Pressure (P) is defined as the force (F) per unit area (A):

$$P = F/A.$$

The force F is the normal (*perpendicular*) force to the area. The SI unit for pressure is the *pascal* (1 Pa = 1 N/m²). Other units are: 1.00 atm = 1.01×10^5 Pa = 1.01 bar = 760 mmHg = 760 torr = 14.7 lb/in².

Pressure is also formulated as potential energy per unit volume as follows:

$$P = \frac{F}{A} = \frac{mg}{A} = \frac{(mg/a)}{(h/h)} = \frac{mgh}{v} = \rho gh$$

ρ = density and h = depth below surface; if the depth is changing we can write:

$$\Delta P = \rho g \Delta h.$$

Characteristics of force and pressure of incompressible liquid fluids are:

1) Forces exerted by fluids are always perpendicular to the surface of the container.
2) The fluid pressure (*hydrostatic*) is directly proportional to the depth of the fluid and to its density.
3) At any particular depth, the pressure of the fluid is the same in all directions.
4) Fluid pressure is independent of the shape or area of its container.
5) An external pressure applied to an enclosed fluid is transmitted uniformly throughout the volume of the liquid (*Pascal's law*).
6) An object which is completely or partially submerged in a fluid experiences an upward force equal to the weight of the fluid displaced (*Archimedes' principle*).

This buoyant force F_b is :

$$F_b = V\rho g = mg$$

where ρ is the density of the fluid displaced. An object that floats must displace at most its own weight. Archimedes' principle can be used to calculate specific gravity.

And in turn, specific gravity is equivalent to the fraction of the *height* of a buoyant object below the surface of the fluid. Thus if SG = 0.90, then 90% of the height of the object would be immersed in water.

Therefore, less dense objects float. {Note: the constants in PHY 6.1.1 and 6.1.2 should be memorized}

6.1.3 Fluids in Motion, Continuity Equation, Bernoulli's Equation

Fluids in motion are described by two equations, the continuity equation and Bernoulli's equation. Fluids are assumed to have <u>streamline</u> (= *laminar*) flow which means that the motion of every particle in the fluid follows the same path as the particle that preceded it. <u>Turbulent</u> flow occurs when that definition cannot be applied, resulting in molecular collisions, irregularly shaped whirlpools, energy is then dissipated and frictional drag is increased. The rate (R) of streamline flow is given by:

$$R = (volume\ past\ a\ point)/time = Avt\ /\ t = Av$$

volume = (cross-sectional area) (length) = *(A) (vt) = Avt*

length = distance = (velocity) (time) = *vt*

cross-sectional area of a tube = area of a circle = πr^2 where π can be estimated as 3.14 and *r* is the radius of the circle.

• The equation can also be written as the **continuity equation**:

$$A_1v_1 = A_2v_2 = constant$$

where subscripts 1 and 2 refer to different points in the line of flow. The continuity equation can be used for an incompressible fluid flowing in an enclosed tube. For a compressible fluid:

$$\rho_1A_1v_1 = \rho_2A_2v_2 = constant$$

• **Bernoulli's equation** is an application of the law of conservation of energy and is:

$$P + \rho gh + 1/2\, \rho v^2 = constant$$

It follows:

$$P_1 + \rho gh_1 + 1/2\, \rho v_1^2 = P_2 + \rho gh_2 + 1/2\, \rho v_2^2$$

where subscripts 1 and 2 refer to different points in the flow.

A commonly encountered consequence of Bernoulli's equation is that where the height is relatively constant and the velocity of a fluid is high, the pressure is low, and vice versa.

{Various applications of the preceding equations will be explored in GS-1, the first practice test!}

6.1.4 Fluid Viscosity and Determining Turbulence

Viscosity is analogous to friction between moving solids. It may, therefore be viewed as the resistance to flow of layers of fluid (as in streamline or laminar flow) past each other. This also means that viscosity, as in friction, results in dissipation of mechanical energy. As one layer flows over another, its motion is transmitted to the second layer and causes this layer to be set in motion. Since a mass m of the second layer is set in motion and some of the energy of the first layer is lost, there is a transfer of momentum between the layers.

The greater the transfer of this momentum from one layer to another, the more energy that is lost and the slower the layers move.

The viscosity (η) is the measure of the efficiency of transfer of this momentum. Therefore the higher the viscosity coefficient, the greater the transfer of momentum and loss of mechanical energy, and thus loss of velocity. The reverse situation holds for a low viscosity coefficient.

Consequently, a high viscosity coefficient substance flows slowly (e.g. molasses), and a low viscosity coefficient substance flows relatively fast (e.g. water or, especially helium). Note that the transfer of momentum to adjacent layers is in essence, the exertion of a force upon these layers to set them in motion.

Whether flow is streamline or turbulent depends on a combination of factors already discussed. A convenient measure is Reynolds Number (R):

$$R = vd\rho / \eta$$

v = velocity of flow
d = diameter of the tube
ρ = density of the fluid
η = viscosity coefficient

In general, if R < 2000 the flow is streamline; if R > 2000 the flow is turbulent. Note that as v, d or ρ increases or η decreases, the flow becomes more turbulent.

6.1.5 Surface Tension

Molecules of a liquid exert attractive forces toward each other (cohesive forces), and exert attractive forces toward the surface they touch (adhesive forces). If a liquid is in a gravity free space without a surface, it will form a sphere (smallest area relative to volume).

If the liquid is lining an object, the liquid surface will contract (due to cohesive forces) to the lowest possible surface area. The forces between the molecules on this surface will create a membrane-like effect. Due to the contraction, a potential energy (PE) will present in the surface.

This PE is directly proportional to the surface area (A). An exact relation is formed as follows:

$$PE = \gamma A$$

γ = surface tension = PE/A = joules/m^2

An alternative formulation for the surface tension (γ) is:

$$\gamma = F/l$$

F = force of contraction of surface
l = length along surface

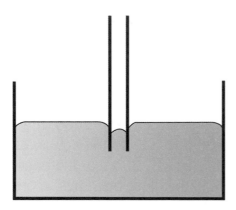

(a) cohesive > adhesive

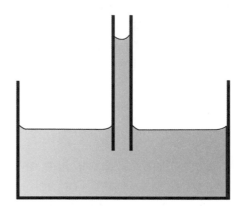

(b) adhesive > cohesive

Figure III.B.6.1: Effects of adhesive and cohesive forces.
The distance the liquid rises or falls in the tube is directly proportional to the surface tension γ and inversely proportional to the liquid density and radius of the tube. Examples of 2 liquids consistent with the illustrations include: (a) mercury; (b) water.

Because of the contraction, a small object which would ordinarily sink in the liquid may float on the surface membrane. For example, a small insect like a "water strider."

The liquid will rise or fall on a wall or in a capillary tube if the adhesive forces are greater than cohesive or vice versa (*see* Figure III.B.6.1).

6.2.1 Elastic Properties of Solids

When a force acts on a solid, the solid is deformed. If the solid returns to its original shape, the solid is elastic. The effect of a force depends on the area over which it acts. Stress is defined as the ratio of the force to the area over which it acts. Strain is defined as the relative change in dimensions or shape of the object caused by the stress. This is embodied in the definition of the modulus of elasticity (ME) as:

$$ME = \frac{stress}{strain}$$

Some different types of stresses are tensile stress (equal and opposite forces directed away from each other), compressive stress (equal and opposite forces directed towards each other), and shearing stress (equal and opposite forces which do not have the same line of action). There are two commonly used moduli of elasticity:

1) Young's Modulus (Y) for compressive or tensile stress:

$$Y = \frac{longitudinal \;\; stress}{longitudinal \;\; strain}$$

$$Y = \frac{(F/A)}{(\Delta l/l)} = \frac{F \times l}{A\Delta l}$$

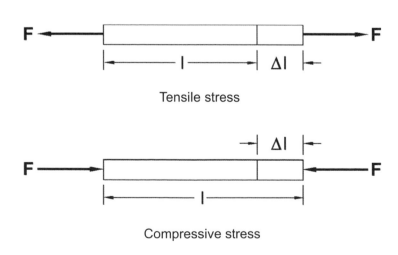

Tensile stress

Compressive stress

Figure III.B.6.2: Compressive and Tensile Stress.

2) Shear modulus (S) or the modulus of rigidity is:

$$S = \text{shearing stress / shearing strain}$$

$$S = (F/A) / \tan\phi$$

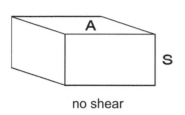

no shear

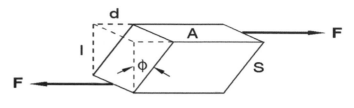

Figure III.B.6.3: Shear Stress. A is the area tangential to the force F.

6.3 The Effect of Temperature on Solids and Liquids

When substances gain or lose heat they usually undergo expansion or contraction.

Expansion or contraction can be by linear dimension, by area or by volume.

Table III.B.6.1: Substance thermal expansion.

Type	Final	Original	Change caused by heat
(1) *Linear*	L $L = L_0 + \alpha\Delta T L_0$ $L = L_0(1 + \alpha\Delta T)$ α = coefficient of linear thermal expansion ΔT = change in temperature	L_0	$\alpha\Delta T L_0$
(2) *Area*	A $A = A_0 + \gamma\Delta T A_0$ $A = A_0(1 + \gamma\Delta T)$ γ = coefficient of area thermal expansion = 2α	A_0	$\gamma\Delta T A_0$
(3) *Volume*	V $V = V_0 + \beta\Delta T V_0$ $V = V_0(1 + \beta\Delta T)$ β = coefficient of volume thermal expansion = 3α	V_0	$\beta\Delta T V_0$

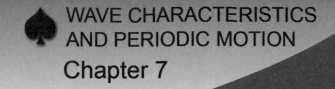
Memorize	Understand	Not Required*
* Define: wavelength, frequency, velocity, amplitude * Define: intensity, constructive/destructive interference, beat freq. * Equation: relating velocity to frequency, wavelength * Equation: Hooke's Law, work (periodic motion)	* SHM, transverse vs. longitudinal waves, phase * Resonance, nodes, antinodes, pipes (standing waves) * Harmonics, overtones * Periodic motion: force, accel., vel., diplace., period * The simple pendulum, theory and calculations	* Advanced level college info * Memorizing displacement/elementar vibration equations * Memorizing equation for harmonics, simple pendulum

MCAT-Prep.com

Introduction

Wave characteristics and periodic motion describe the motion of systems that vibrate. Topics include transverse and longitudinal waves, interference, resonance, Hooke's law and simple harmonic motion (SHM). Some basic equations must be memorized but for most of the material, you must seek a comfortable understanding.

Additional Resources

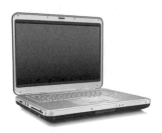

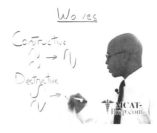

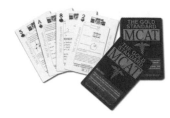

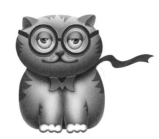

| Free Online Q & A | Video: Online or DVD 2,4 | Flashcards | Special Guest |

7.1 Wave Characteristics

7.1.1 Transverse and Longitudinal Motion

A wave is a disturbance in a medium such that each particle in the medium vibrates about an equilibrium point in a simple harmonic (*periodic*) motion. If the direction of vibration is perpendicular to the direction of propagation of the wave, it is called a <u>transverse wave</u> (e.g. light or an oscillating string under tension).

If the direction of vibration is in the same direction as the propagation of the wave, it is called a <u>longitudinal wave</u> (e.g. sound). Longitudinal waves are characterized by condensations (regions of crowding of particles) and rarefactions (regions where particles are far apart) along the wave in the medium.

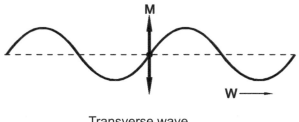

Transverse wave   Longitudinal wave

Figure III.B.7.1: Transverse and longitudinal waves.
W = wave propagation, R = rarefaction, C = condensation, M = motion of particle.

7.1.2 Wavelength, Frequency, Velocity, Amplitude, Intensity

The wavelength (λ) is the distance from crest to crest (or valley to valley) of a transverse wave. It may also be defined as the distance between two particles with the same displacement and direction of displacement. In a longitudinal wave, the wavelength is the distance from one rarefaction (or condensation) to another. The *amplitude* (A) is the maximum displacement of a particle in one direction from its equilibrium point. The *intensity* (I) of a wave is the square of the amplitude.

Frequency (f) is the number of cycles per unit time (per second). *Period (T)* is the duration of one cycle, it is the inverse of the frequency. The *velocity (v)* of a wave is the velocity of the propagation of the disturbance that forms the wave through the medium.

The velocity is inversely proportional to the inertia of the medium. The velocity can be calculated according to the following important equation:

$$v = \lambda f$$

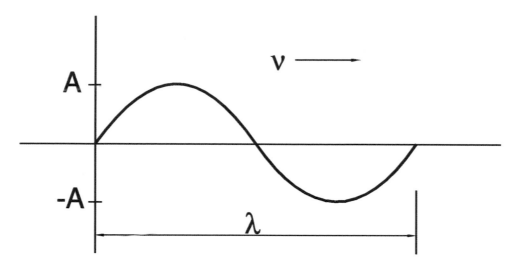

Figure III.B.7.2: Characteristics of waves.

7.1.3 Superposition of Waves, Phase, Interference, Addition

The superposition principle states that the effect of two or more waves on the displacement of a particle is independent. The final displacement of the particle is the resultant effect of all the waves added algebraically, thus the amplitude may increase or decrease. The *phase* of a particle under vibration is its displacement at the time of origin (t=0). The displacement can be calculated as follows:

$$x = A\sin(\omega t + \varphi)$$

where x is the displacement, A is the amplitude, ω is the angular velocity, t is the time, and φ is the phase.

Interference is the summation of the displacements of different waves in a medium. Certain criteria must first be established:

• *synchrony sources*: vibrations emitted by synchrony sources have the same phase.

• *coherent vibrations*: the phases of the vibrations are related, this means that the duration of the light impressions on the retina is much longer than the duration of a wave train between two emissions.

• *parallel vibrations*: the displacements of parallel vibrations keep parallel directions in space.

• *interference conditions*: two or more vibrations can interfere only when the are coherent, parallel and have the same period.

• *beat frequency*: the difference in frequency of two waves creates a new frequency (*see* Beats, PHY 8.4).

Given an elementary vibration $S_i = A_i\sin(w_t + \varphi_i)$ the composition of n vibrations that interfere is given by:

$$S_1 + S_2 + S_3 + ... + S_n = a_1\sin(wt+\varphi_1) + a_2\sin(wt+\varphi_2) + ...+ a_n\sin(wt+\varphi_n) = A\sin(wt+\Phi)$$

where A is the resultant amplitude and Φ the resultant phase. Constructive interference (*see Figure III.B.7.4*) is when the waves add to a larger resultant wave than either original.

This occurs maximally when the phase difference φ is a whole wavelength λ which corresponds to multiples of π.

This occurs at $\varphi = 0, 2\pi, 4\pi$, etc. Since $\varphi = 2\pi\Delta L/\lambda$, where ΔL equals the difference in path to a point of two waves of equal wavelength, these waves interfere constructively when $\Delta L = 0, \lambda, 2\lambda, 3\lambda$, *etc.* See Figure III.B.7.3 for the definition of ΔL.

Destructive interference (*see Figure III.B.7.5*) is when the waves add to a smaller resultant wave than either original wave. This occurs maximally when $\varphi = \pi, 3\pi, 5\pi$, *etc.*, which are multiples of one-half of a wavelength where $180° = \pi$ which corresponds to $\frac{1}{2}\lambda$. This occurs when $\Delta L = \lambda/2, 3\lambda/2, 5\lambda/2$, etc.

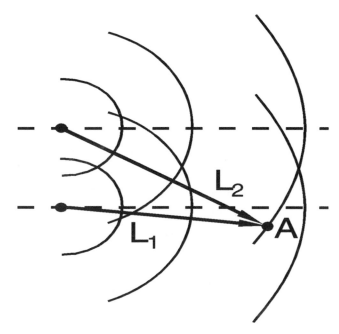

Figure III.B.7.3: Schematic for ΔL.
L_1 and L_2 are distances from the origins of the waves to point A. Thus $\Delta L = |L_2 - L_1|$ (absolute value).

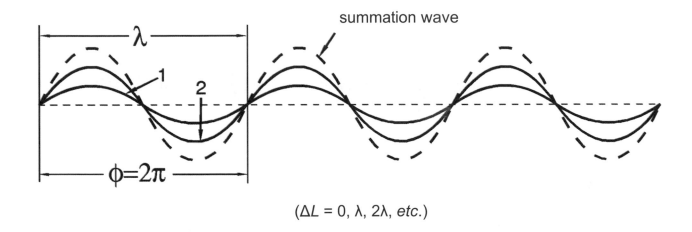

(ΔL = 0, λ, 2λ, *etc.*)

Figure III.B.7.4: Maximal constructive interference.
Waves (1) and (2) begin at the points shown, have the same λ but different amplitudes. The summation wave is maximal (i.e. highest amplitude but same wavelength) since ΔL = λ *in this example.*

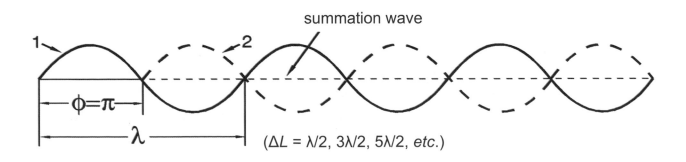

(ΔL = λ/2, 3λ/2, 5λ/2, *etc.*)

Figure III.B.7.5: Maximal destructive interference.

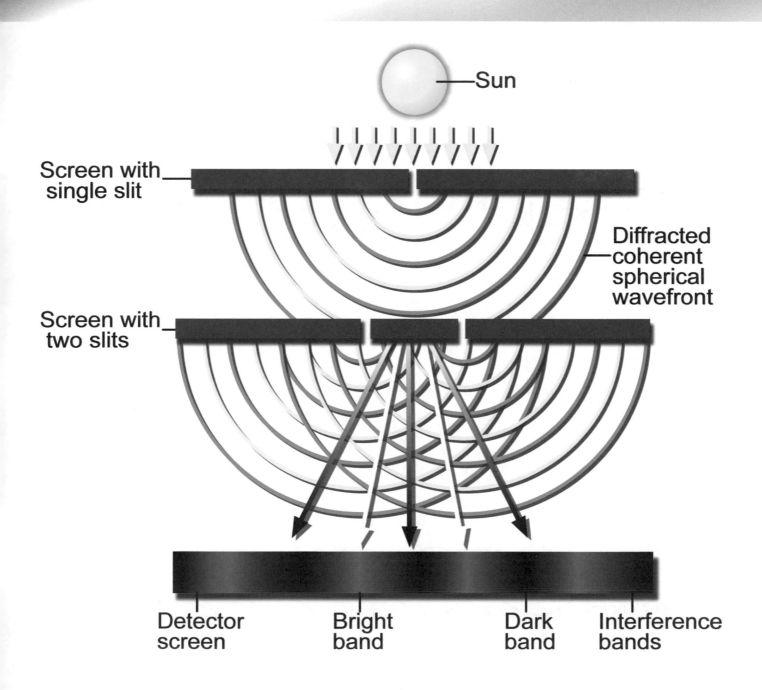

Screen with single slit

Sun

Diffracted coherent spherical wavefront

Screen with two slits

Detector screen

Bright band

Dark band

Interference bands

Figure III.B.7.5.1: Thomas Young's Double Slit Experiment

Young's experiment demonstrates both the wave and particle natures of light. A coherent light source illuminates a thin plate with two parallel slits cut in it, and the light passing through the slits strikes a screen behind them. The wave nature of light causes the light waves passing through both slits to interfere, creating an interference pattern of bright and dark bands on the screen. However, at the screen, the light is always found to be absorbed as though it were made of discrete particles (photons). The double slit experiment can also be performed (using different apparatus) with particles of matter such as electrons with the same results. Again, this provides an additional circumstance demonstrating particle-wave duality.

Forced vibrations occur when a series of waves impinge upon an object and cause it to vibrate. Natural frequencies are the intrinsic frequencies of vibration of a system. If the forced vibration causes the object to vibrate at one of its natural frequencies, the body will vibrate at maximal amplitude. This phenomenon is called *resonance*. Since energy and power are proportional to the amplitude squared, they also are at their maximum.

7.1.5 Standing Waves, Pipes and Strings

Standing waves result when waves are reflected off a stationary object back into the oncoming waves of the medium and super-position results. *Nodes* are points where there is no particle displacement, which are similar to points of maximal destructive inter-ference.

Nodes occur at fixed end points (points that cannot vibrate). Antinodes are points that undergo maximal displacements and are similar to points of maximal constructive interference. Antinodes occur at open or free end points (*see Figure III.B.7.6*).

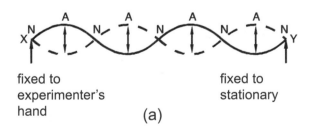

fixed to
experimenter's
hand

fixed to
stationary

(a)

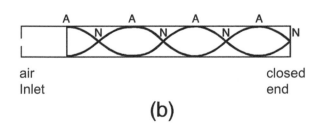

air
Inlet

closed
end

(b)

Figure III.B.7.6: Standing waves.
(a) <u>String</u>: Standing waves produced by an experimenter wiggling a string or rubber tube at point X towards a fixed point Y at the correct frequency. (b) <u>Pipe</u>: Standing wave produced in a pipe with a closed end point i.e. in a closed organ pipe where sound originates in a vibrating air column (A = *antinode* and N = *node*).

7.1.6 Harmonics

Consider a violin. A string is fixed at both ends and is bowed, transverse vibrations travel along the string; these disturbances are reflected at both ends producing a standing wave. The vibrations of the string give rise to longitudinal vibrations in the air which transmits the sound to our ears.

A string of length l, fixed at both ends, can resonate at frequencies f given by:

$$f_n = nv/(2l)$$

where the velocity v is the same for all frequencies and the number of antinodes $n = 1, 2, 3, ...$

The lowest frequency, $f_1 = v/(2l)$, is the *fundamental* frequency, and the others are called *overtones*. The fundamental is the first *harmonic*, the second harmonic $2f_1$ is the first overtone, the third harmonic $3f_1$ is the second overtone, etc. Overtones whose frequencies are integral multiples of the fundamental are called *harmonic series*.

7.2 Periodic Motion

7.2.1 Hooke's Law

The particles that are undergoing displacement when a wave passes through a medium undergo motion called simple harmonic motion (SHM) and are acted upon by a force described by Hooke's Law. SHM is caused by an inconstant force (called a *restoring force*) and as a result has an inconstant acceleration. The force is proportional to the displacement (*distance from the equilibrium point*) but opposite in direction,

$$\boxed{F = -kx \text{ (Hooke's Law)}}$$

where k = the spring constant, x = displacement from the equilibrium. The work W can be determined according to $W = \frac{1}{2}kx^2$.

What do physicists enjoy doing the most at baseball games? The 'wave'.

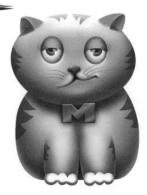

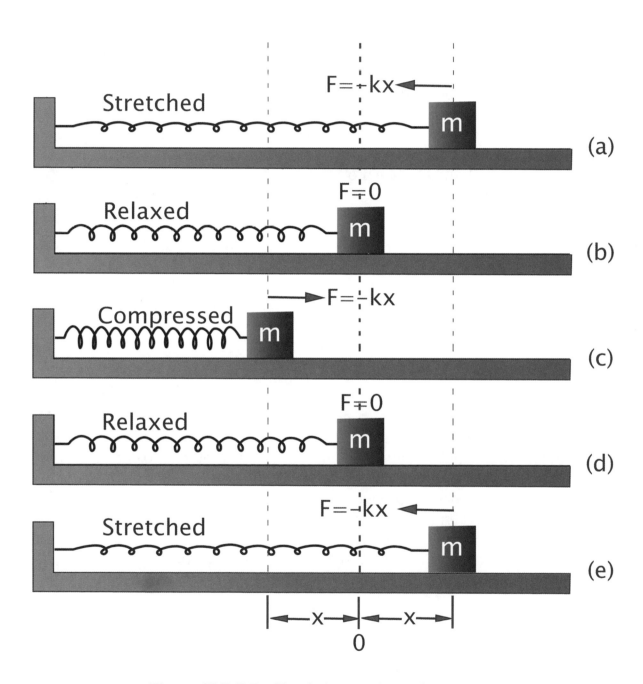

Figure III.B.7.7: Simple harmonic motion.
A block of mass m exhibiting SHM. The force F exerted by the spring on the block is shown in each case.

7.2.2 Features of SHM and Hooke's Law

1) Force and acceleration are always in the same direction.

2) Force and acceleration are always in the opposite direction of the displacement (*this is why there is a negative sign in the equation for force*).

3) Force and acceleration have their maximal value at +A and -A; they are zero at the equilibrium point (*the amplitude A equals the maximum displacement x*).

4) Velocity direction has no constant relation to displacement and acceleration.

5) Velocity is maximum at equilibrium and zero at A and -A.

6) The period T can be calculated from the mass m of an oscillating particle:

$$T = 2\pi\sqrt{m/k}$$

where k is the spring constant. The frequency f is simply $1/T$.

7.2.3 SHM Problem: The Simple Pendulum

A simple pendulum consists of a point mass m suspended by a light inextensible cord of length l. When pulled to one side of its equilibrium position, the pendulum swings under the influence of gravity producing a periodic, oscillatory motion (= *SHM*). Given that the angle θ with the vertical is small, thus $\sin\theta \approx \theta$, determine the general equation for the period T.

The tangential component of mg is the restoring force since it returns the mass to its equilibrium position. Thus the restoring force is:

$$F = -mg\sin\theta.$$

Recall $\sin\theta \approx \theta$, $x = l\theta$, and for SHM $F = -kx$:

$$F = -mg\theta = -mgx/l = -(mg/l)x = -kx.$$

Hence $mg/l = k$, thus the equation for the period T becomes:

$$T = 2\pi\sqrt{\frac{m}{k}} = 2\pi\sqrt{\frac{m}{mg/l}} = 2\pi\sqrt{\frac{l}{g}}$$

The equation for the period in the simple pendulum is therefore independent of the mass of the particle.

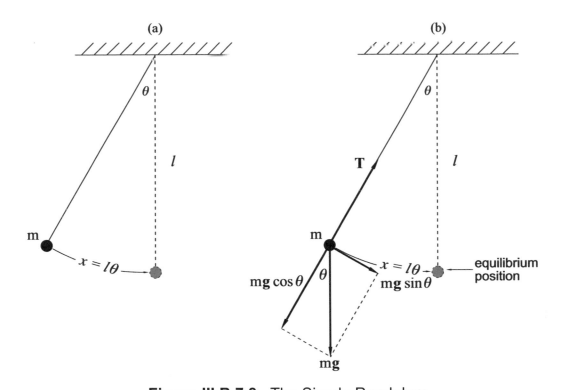

Figure III.B.7.8: The Simple Pendulum.
(a) The problem as it could be presented; the displacement x along the section of the circle (arc) is $l\theta$. (b) The vector components that should be drawn to solve the problem. The forces acting on a simple pendulum are the tension **T** in the string and the weight mg of the mass. The magnitude of the radial component of mg is mgcosθ and the tangential component is mgsinθ.

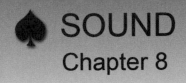

SOUND
Chapter 8

Memorize	Understand	Not Required*
* Sensory vs. physical correspondence of hearing * Equation for beat frequency	* Relative velocity of sound in solids, liquids and gases * The relation of intensity to P, area, f, amplitude * Calculation of the intensity level * Rules of logarithms * Doppler effect and calculations	* Advanced level college info *Memorizing specific frequencies, speed of sound, dB's

MCAT-Prep.com

Introduction ▮▮▮▮

Sound waves are longitudinal waves which can only be transmitted in a material, elastic medium. Speed, intensity, resonance (Chapter 7) and the Doppler effect help to describe the behavior of sound in different media. If the equations for sound intensity or the Doppler effect are required for the MCAT, they are usually provided.

Additional Resources

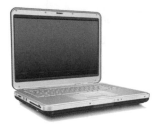

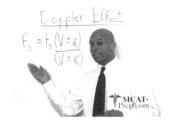

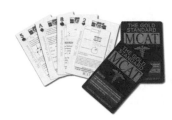

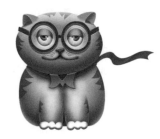

Free Online Q & A	Video: Online or DVD 2, 4	Flashcards	Special Guest

8.1 Production of Sound

Sound is a longitudinal mechanical wave which travels through an elastic medium. Sound is thus produced by vibrating matter. There is no sound in a *vacuum* because it contains no matter.

Compressions (condensations) are regions where particles of matter are close together; they are also high pressure regions. Rarefactions are regions where particles are sparse, they are low pressure regions of sound waves (PHY 7.1.1).

8.2 Relative Velocity of Sound in Solids, Liquids, and Gases

The velocity of sound is proportional to the square root of the elastic restoring force and inversely proportional to the square root of the inertia of the particles (e.g., density is a measure of inertia). Thus as a rule, the velocity of sound is higher in liquids as compared to gases, and highest in solids.

Furthermore, an increase in temperature increases the velocity of sound; conversely, a decrease in temperature decreases the velocity of sound in that medium.

8.3 Intensity, Pitch

Hearing is subjective but its characteristics are closely tied to physical characteristics of sound.

The quality depends on the number and relative intensity of the overtones of the waveform. Frequency, and therefore pitch are perceived by the ear from 20 to 20,000 Hz (hertz = cycles/second = s^{-1}). Frequencies below 20 Hz are called infrasonic. Frequencies above 20,000 Hz are called ultrasonic.

Sensory	Physical
loudness	intensity
pitch	frequency
quality	waveform

Table III.B.8.1:
Sensory and physical correspondence of hearing.

Sound intensity (I) is the rate of energy (power) propagation through space:

$$I = (power/area)$$ which is proportional to $(f^2 A^2)$

where f = frequency, A = amplitude.

The loudness varies with the frequency. The ears are most sensitive (hears sounds of lowest intensity) at approximately 2,000 to 4,000 Hz. I_o is taken to be 10^{-12} watts/cm^2, is barely audible and is assigned a value of 0 dB (zero decibels). Then intensity level (I) of a sound wave in dB is,

$$dB = 10 \log_{10}(I/I_o)$$

where dB = the sound level, I = the intensity at a given level, I_o = the threshold intensity. {To calculate a change in the sound level or volume ΔV in units of dB, given two values for sound intensity, the given equation can be modified thus: $\Delta V = 10\log(I_{new}/I_{old})$}

Examples of some values of dB's are: whisper (20), normal conversation (60), subway car (100), pain threshold (120), and jet engine (160). Continual exposure to sound greater than 90 dB can lead to hearing impairment.

8.3.1 Calculation of the Intensity Level

What is the loudness or intensity level of Mr. Yell Alot's voice when he generates a sound wave ten million times as intense as I_o?

$$I = (10,000,000) I_o = (10^7) I_o$$

Thus

$$\begin{aligned} dB &= 10 \log_{10} (10^7 I_o/I_o) \\ &= 10 \log_{10} 10^7 \\ &= 70 \log_{10} 10 \end{aligned}$$

{See chemistry section 6.5.1 for rules of logarithms}

8.4 Beats

When sound of different frequencies are heard together, they interfere. Constructive interference results in beats. The number of beats per second is the absolute value of the difference of the frequencies ($|f_1 - f_2|$).

Hence, the new frequency heard includes the original frequencies and the absolute difference between them.

THE GOLD STANDARD

8.5 Doppler Effect

The Doppler effect is the effect upon the observed frequency caused by the relative motion of the observer (*o*) and the source (*s*). If the distance is decreasing between them, there is a shift to higher frequencies and shorter wavelengths (to higher pitch for sound and toward blue-violet for light, PHY 8.3 and 9.2.4). If the distance is increasing between them, there is a shift to longer wavelengths and lower frequencies (to lower pitch for sound and toward red for light). The summary equation of the above in terms of frequency (f) is :

$$f_o = f_s(V \pm v_o)/(V \pm v_s)$$

V = speed of the wave, v = speed of the observer (*o*) or the source (*s*).

Choose the sign such that the frequency varies consistently with the relative motion of the source and the observer. In other words, when the distance between the source and observer is *decreasing* use $+v_o$ and $-v_s$; if the distance is *increasing* use $-v_o$ and $+v_s$.

8.5.1 Doppler Effect Problem (SI units)

A car drives towards a bus stop with its car stereo playing opera. The opera singer sings the note middle C (= 262 Hz) loudly; however, the people waiting at the bus stop hear C sharp (= 277 Hz). Given that the speed of sound V in air is 331 m/s, how fast is the car moving?

{Remember the sign convention: since the distance between the source (the car) and the observer (people at the bus stop) is decreasing we use +v$_o$ and -v$_s$}

• the car (the *source* of the frequency) f_s = 262 Hz, v_s = unknown.

• the bus stop (where the *observers* are stationary) f_o = 277 Hz, v_o = 0 m/s.

$$f_o = f_s(V + v_o)/(V - v_s)$$

Thus

$$V - v_s = f_s (V + v_o)/f_o$$

Hence

$$v_s = - f_s (V + v_o)/f_o + V$$

Substitute

$$v_s = - 262(331 + 0)/277 + 331 = 17.9 \text{ m/s}.$$

• Note that the answer contains three significant figures.

The Doppler Effect is when stupid ideas seem smarter when you read them quickly.

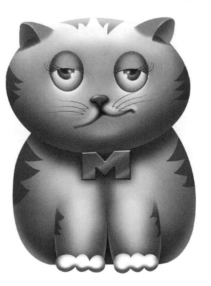

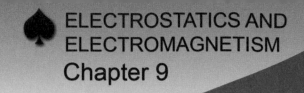

ELECTROSTATICS AND ELECTROMAGNETISM
Chapter 9

Memorize	Understand	Not Required*
* Equations: for charge Q, Coulomb's law, electric field * Equations: potential energy, absolute potential * Equation relating energy, planck's constant, frequency	* Conservation of charge, use of Coulomb's law * Graphs/theory: electric field/potential lines, mag. induction * Potential difference, electric dipoles, mag. induction * Laplace's law, the right hand rule, magnetic field * Direction of F in magn. field; electromagnetism	* Advanced level college info * Memorizing coulomb's, permittivity or planck's constants * Memorizing equation with permittivi constant or dF * Calculus, derivatives, integrals, speed of light

MCAT-Prep.com

Introduction ▌▌▌▌

Electrostatics (statics = usu. at rest) refers to the science of stationary or slowly moving charges. Such charges can interact and behave in ways described by charge, electric force, electric field and potential difference. When a charge is in motion, it creates a magnetic field. Electromagnetism describes the relationship between electricity (moving electrical charge) and magnetism. The electromagnetic spectrum includes light and X-rays.

Additional Resources

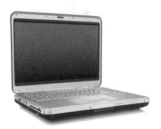

Free Online Q & A

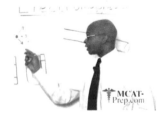

Video: Online or DVD 1, 3, 4

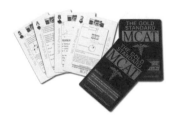

Flashcards

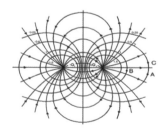

Special Guest

9.1 Electrostatics

9.1.1 Charge, Conductors, Insulators

By friction of matter we create between substances repulsive or attractive electric forces. These forces are due to two kinds of electric charges, distinguished by positive (+) and negative (-) signs. Each has a charge of 1.6×10^{-19} coulombs (C) but differ in sign. The electron is the negative charge carrier, and the proton is the positive charge carrier. Substances with an excess of electrons have a net negative charge. Substances with a deficiency of electrons have a net positive charge. The total amount of charge Q of matter depends on the number of particles n and the charge e on each particle, thus $Q = ne$.

The conservation of charge states that a net charge cannot be created but that charge can be transfered from one object to another. One way of charging substances is by rubbing them (i.e., by contact).

For example, glass rubbed on fur becomes positive and rubber rubbed on fur becomes negative. Objects can also be charged by induction which occurs when one charged object is brought near to another uncharged object causing a charge redistribution in the latter to give net charge regions. Conductors transmit charge readily. Insulators resist the flow of charge.

9.1.2 Coulomb's Law, Electric Force

Charges exert forces upon each other. Like charges repel each other and unlike charges attract. For any two charges q_1 and q_2 the force F is given by Coulomb's Law:

$$\boxed{F = k\,\frac{q_1 q_2}{r^2}} = \frac{1}{4\pi\varepsilon_o}\left(\frac{q_1 q_2}{r^2}\right)$$

where k = coulomb's constant = 9.0×10^9 N-m^2/C^2, ε_o = permittivity constant = 8.85×10^{-12} C^2/N-m^2, and r = the distance between the charges. Note that the relationship of force and distance follows an inverse square law. Thus if the distance r is doubled [$(2r)^2 = 4r^2$], the new force is quartered ($F_{new} = F/4$). {cf. Law of Gravity: PHY 2.4}

9.1.3 Electric Field, Electric Field Lines

A charge generates an electric field (E) in the space around it. Fields (force fields) are vectors. A field is generated by an object and it is that region of space around the object that will exert a force on a second object brought into that field. The field exists independently of that second object and is not altered by its presence. The force exerted on the second object depends upon that object and the field. The electric field E is given by:

$$E = F/q = k\ Q/r^2$$

where E and F are vectors, Q = the charge generating the field, and q = the charge placed in the field.

Charges exert forces upon each other through fields. The direction of a field is the direction <u>a positive charge would move if placed in it</u>. *Electric field lines* are imaginary lines which are in the same direction as E at that point. The direction is away from positive charges and toward negative charges, or put another way, the electric field is directed toward the decreasing potentials.

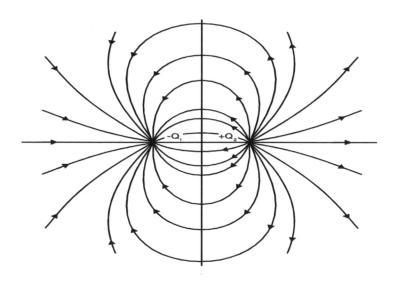

Figure III.B.9.1: Electric field lines.
The electric field is generated by the charges -Q_1 and +Q_2. The arrowheads show the direction of the electric field.

If an electric potential is applied between two plates in a vacuum, and an electron is introduced, the electron will experience an attractive force to the positive plate (*see Figure III.B.9.2*).

The force will cause the electron to accelerate towards the positive plate in a straight line. It suffers no collisions because the area between the plates is *in vacuo*. This effect is used in thermoionic valves.

If the electron is given some motion, and the electric field is applied perpendicular to the motion, interesting things happen (*see Figure III.B.9.3*). For example, a beam of electrons is emitted from a device called an electron gun. These electrons are moving in the *x* direction.

As the electrons pass between the plates they are accelerated in the *y* direction, as explained before, but their velocity in the *x* direction is unaltered. The electron beam is thus deflected as shown.

By varying the potential applied to the plates, the angle of deflection can be controlled. This effect is the basis of the cathode ray oscilloscope.

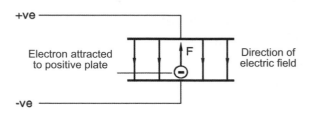

Figure III.B.9.2:
Electric field between parallel plates.

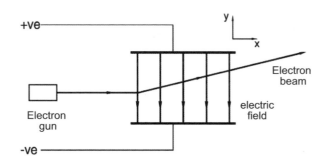

Figure III.B.9.3:
Electrostatic deflection of an electron beam.

9.1.4 Potential Energy, Absolute Potential

The *potential energy* (E_p) of a charged object in a field equals the work done on that object to bring it from infinity to a distance (r) from the charge setting up the electric field,

$$E_p = work = Fr = (qE)r = kQq/r$$

where Q = the charge setting up field, and q = the charge brought in to a distance r.

When a +q moves against E, its E_p increases. When a -q moves against the electric field E, its E_p decreases. If two positive or negative charges were brought together, work would have to be done to the system (and E_p would increase), and vice versa for charges of opposite charges.

The *absolute potential* (V) is a scalar, and it is defined at each distance (r) from a charge (Q) generating an electric field. It represents the negative of the work per unit charge in bringing a +q from infinity to r:

• $V = E_p/q = kQ/r$ in volts where 1 volt = 1 joule/coulomb.

• $V = Ed$ for a parallel plate capacitor where d = distance between the plates (PHY 10.4).

Equipotential lines are lines (and surfaces) of equal V and are *perpendicular* to electric field lines. Work can only be done when moving between surfaces of equal V and is, therefore, independent of the path taken. <u>No work is done</u> when a charge (q) is moved along an <u>equal potential</u> (*equipotential*) surface (or line), because the component of force is zero along it. Potential (V) is defined in terms of positive charges such that V is positive when due to a +Q and negative when due a -Q. Potential (V) is added algebraically at a point (because it is a scalar).

See Figure III.B.9.4:

1) V_1, V_2 are two potentials perpendicular to the electric field E and the force F;
2) $V_2 - V_1$ is the potential difference (*PD*);
3) charge (*q*) moved from A ($V_1 = 0.5$) to B ($V_2 = 1$) has work (*W*) done on it:

$$W = q(V_2 - V_1) = q(PD)$$

4) charge (*q*) moved from A to C has no work done on it because this is along an equipotential surface ($V = 0.5$) and the non-zero component of force (F) is perpendicular to it;
5) the lines of F are along the lines of E.

The *potential difference (PD)* is the difference in V between two points, or it is the work per unit positive charge done by electric forces moving a small test charge from the point of higher potential to the point of lower potential:

$$PD = V_a - V_b = volts = work/charge$$

$$work = q(V_a - V_b) = q(PD).$$

An *electric dipole* consists of two charges separated by some finite distance (d). Usually the charges are equal and opposite. The laws of forces, fields, etc., apply to dipoles. A dipole is characterized by its *dipole moment* which is the product of the charge (q) and d.

Dipoles tend to line up with the electric field (Fig. III.B.9.5). Motion of dipoles against an electric field requires energy as discussed above.

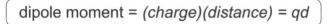

$$\text{dipole moment} = (charge)(distance) = qd$$

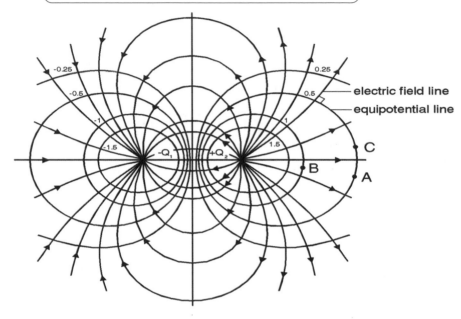

Figure III.B.9.4: Equipotential lines.
The circle-like curves around each charge -Q_1 and +Q_2 are the equipotential lines corresponding to each charge. The numbers represent the electric potential value (i.e. in millivolts) of the respective equipotential lines. Note the electric field lines as in Figure III.B.9.1.

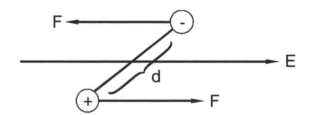

Dipole with equal and opposite charges

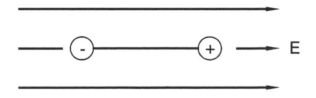

Alignment of dipole with E

Figure III.B.9.5: Dipole and electric field.
E = electric field, F = forces exerted by E on the dipole

9.2.1 Notion of Electromagnetic Induction

Coulomb's Law in electrostatics gives the nature of the forces acting upon electric charges at rest, but when the charges are moving, new forces appear.

They are not of the same nature as the electrostatic forces and they act differently on the electric charges. They are called electromagnetic forces.

9.2.2 Magnetic Induction Vector

Experiments have shown that two straight conductors (e.g. copper wires) traversed by electric currents of intensities I and I′ in the same direction are acted upon by an attractive force proportional to the product of the intensities and inversely proportional to the distance between the two conductors. It can be demonstrated that when the electric current in one of the conductors disappears, the force also disappears.

Therefore, the force is due to the motion of the electric charges in both conductors.

We decompose the phenomenon by introducing a new physical quantity: the magnetic induction vector B, also created by magnets.

The SI unit for B is the tesla where $1\,T = 1\,N/(A\cdot m) = 10^4$ gauss.

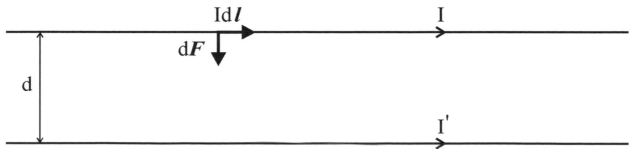

Figure III.B.9.6: Magnetic induction.
Two conductors a distance d apart; the current element *Idl* and the perpendicular force *dF* associated with the magnetic induction vector *B* are both shown. Vector B, which is not shown, has a direction perpendicular to both Idl and dF, pointing out of the page.

Thus, two effects have been shown by the preceding experiment:

1) a moving charge produces a magnetic induction.

2) a magnetic induction exerts a force on any nearby moving charge.

9.2.3 Laplace's Law

A test particle with charge dq moving at a velocity v in a magnetic induction field B is acted upon by a force dF given by the following formula:

$$dF = dq \; v \times B = dq \; v(B\sin \alpha)$$

where α is the angle formed by the direction of v with that of B (= the cross product).

The force dF is perpendicular to the magnetic induction vector and also to the displacement velocity vector of the charge (*see Figure III.B.9.6*).

When many charges are in motion so as to produce an electric current of intensity $I = dq/dt$ the force acting upon an elemental length of conductor dl traversed by that electric current is :

$$dF = I \; dl \times B = I \; dl(B \sin \alpha)$$

where α is the angle formed by the direction of the current element of conductor with that of B (= the cross product).

In order to determine the direction of a cross (= *vector*) product we can use the right-hand rule. If $c = a \times b$ then the right hand is held so that the curled fingers follow the rotation of a to b, the extended right thumb will point in the direction of c (dF in the preceding example). {Student's trick: "Grab the Wire!" Examine Fig. III.B.9.6. Turn the book around such that with your right hand open and thumb extended, the fingers point in the direction of dF and your thumb points in the direction Idl. As you begin to grab the wire, the initial direction of the tips of your fingers move perpendicular to both dF and Idl. Now the tips of your fingers make a circular motion around the wire. Those fingers have just described the direction of the magnetic induction vector B!}

9.2.4 Electromagnetic Spectrum, Radio, Infrared, X Rays

PHYSICS

An electromagnetic field is described as having at every point of the field, two perpendicular vectors: *the electric field* vector E and the magnetic induction field vector B.

Radar (= *radio detection* and ranging) is an example of a radio wave.

Visible light can be broken down into colors remembered by the mnemonic (*from highest to lowest wavelength*), Roy G. BIV: Red, Orange, Yellow, Green, Blue, Indigo, Violet.

The separation of white light into these colors can occur as a result of refraction through a prism (PHY 11.4) or through water (i.e. mist or rain resulting in a rainbow).

Planck developed the relation between energy (E) and the frequency f of the electromagnetic radiation,

$$E = hf$$

where h = planck's constant. Thus high frequency or short wave length corresponds to high energy and vice versa.

{The preceding equation should be memorized in conjunction with the relationship between a wave's velocity, wavelength and frequency; PHY 7.1.2}

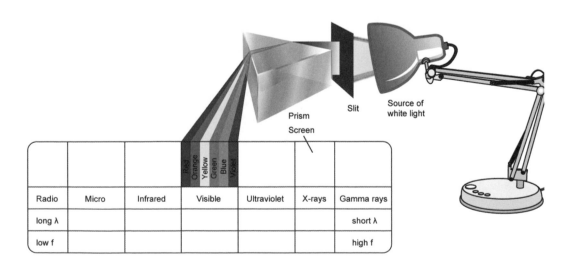

Figure III.B.9.7: The complete electromagnetic spectrum.

THE PHYSICAL SCIENCES   PHY-75

Memorize	Understand	Not Required*
* Definition/equation/units: current, resistance * Ohm's law, resistors in series/parallel * Root-mean-square current, voltage * Capacitance, series, parallel; dielectric * Kirchoff's laws	* Battery, emf, voltage, terminal potential * Internal resistance of the battery, resistivity * Ohm's law, resistors in series/parallel * Parallel plate capacitor, series, parallel * Conductivity, power in circuits, Kirchoff's laws	* Advanced level college info * Complex/discrete/digital circuits * Transistors, FPGAs, microprocessors

MCAT-Prep.com

Introduction

Electric circuits are closed paths which includes electronic components (i.e. resistors, capacitors, power supplies) through which a current can flow. There are 3 basic laws that govern the flow of current in an electrical circuit: Ohm's law and Kirchoff's first and second laws.

Additional Resources

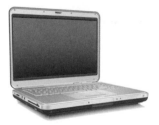

Free Online Q & A

Video: Online or DVD 1, 2, 4

Flashcards

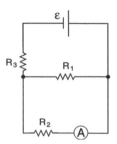

Special Guest

10.1 Current

The current (I) is the amount of charge (Q) that flows past a point in a given amount of time (t),

$$I = Q/t = amperes = coulombs/sec.$$

Current is caused by the movement of electrons between two points of significant potential difference of an electric circuit. Free electrons will accelerate towards the positive connection. As they move they will collide with atoms in the substance, losing energy which we observe as heat. The net effect is a drift of electrons at a roughly constant speed towards the positive connection. The motion of electrons is an *electric current*. As electrons are removed by the electric potential source at the positive connection, electrons are being injected at the negative connection. The potential can be considered as a form of *electron pump*.

This model explains many observed effects.

If the magnitude of the electric potential is increased, the electrons will accelerate faster and their mean velocity will be higher, i.e., the current is increased. The collisions between electrons and atoms transfer energy to the atoms. The collisions manifest themselves as heat. This effect is known as *Joule heating*. Materials such as these are termed ohmic conductors, since they obey the well-known Ohm's Law:

$$V = IR$$

where V is the voltage, I is the current, and R is the resistance.

The potential difference is maintained by a voltage source (emf). The direction of current is taken as the direction of <u>positive charge</u> movement, by convention. It is represented on a circuit diagram by arrows. Ammeters are used to measure the flow of current and are symbolized as in Figure III.B.10.1.

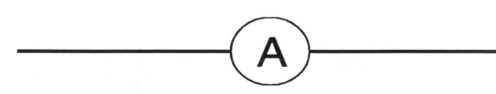

Figure III.B.10.1: Symbol of an ammeter.

Resistance (R) is the measure of opposition to the flow of electrons in a substance. Resistivity (ρ) is an inherent property of a substance. It varies with temperature. For example, the resistivity of metals increases with increasing temperature.

Resistance is directly proportional to resistivity and length *l* but inversely proportional to the cross-sectional area *A*.

$$R = \rho l/A$$

Resistance increases with temperature because the thermal motion of molecules increases with temperature and results in more collisions between electrons which impede their flow.

The units of resistance are ohms, symbolized by Ω (omega). From Ohm's Law, 1 ohm = 1 volt/ampere.

When a positive current flows across a resistor, there is a voltage decrease and an energy loss:

$$energy\ loss = Vq = VIt = joules$$

$$\boxed{power\ loss\ (P) = VIt/t = VI = watts}$$

$$watts = volts \times amperes = joules/sec.$$

The energy loss may be used to perform work. These relations hold for power (P),

$$P = VI = (IR)(I) = I^2R = V(V/R) = V^2/R.$$

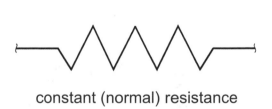

constant (normal) resistance

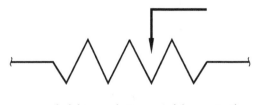

variable resistance (rheostat)

Figure III.B.10.2: Representation of two types of resistors.

Circuit elements are either in series or in parallel. Two components are in series when they have only one point in common; that is, the current travelling from one of them back to the emf source must pass through the other. In a complete series circuit, or for individual series loops of a larger mixed circuit, the current (I) is the same over each component and the total voltage drop in the circuit elements (resistors, capacitors, inductors, internal resistance of emf sources, etc.) is equal to the sum V_t of all the emf sources. The value of the equivalent resistance R_{eq} in a series circuit is:

$$R_{eq} = R_1 + R_2 + R_3 + \ldots$$

Two components are in parallel when they are connected to two common points in the circuit; that is, the current travelling from one such element back to the emf source need not pass through the second element because there is an alternate path.

In a parallel circuit, the total current is the sum of currents for each path and the voltage is the same for all paths in parallel. The equivalent resistance in a parallel circuit is:

$$1/R_{eq} = 1/R_1 + 1/R_2 + 1/R_3 + \ldots$$

10.2.1 Resistance Problem in Series and Parallel

Determine the equivalent resistance between points A and B in Figure III.B.10.3.

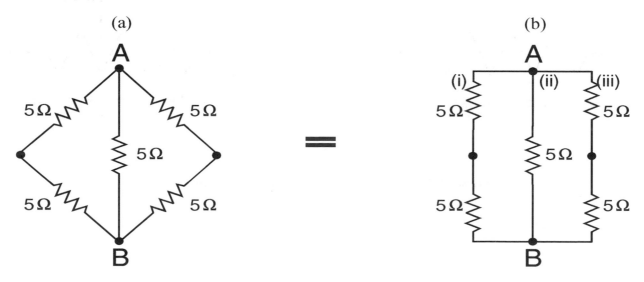

Figure III.B.10.3: Equivalent resistance.
(a) The problem as it could be presented; (b) the way you should interpret the problem.

• Wire (i) has two resistors in a row (*in series*): $R_{(i)} = 5 + 5 = 10\ \Omega$

• Wire (ii) has only one resistor: $R_{(ii)} = 5\ \Omega$

• Wire (iii) has two resistors in series: $R_{(iii)} = 5 + 5 = 10\ \Omega$

Between A and B we have three resistor systems in parallel: (i), (ii) and (iii), thus

$$1/R_{eq} = 1/R_{(i)} + 1/R_{(ii)} + 1/R_{(iii)}$$
$$= 1/10 + 1/5 + 1/10 = 4/10$$

multiply through by $10R_{eq}$ to get: $10 = 4R_{eq}$

thus $R_{eq} = 10/4 = 2.5\ \Omega$.

10.3 Batteries, Electromotive Force, Voltage, Internal Resistance

An *electromotive force (emf)* source maintains between its terminal points, a constant potential difference. The emf source replaces energy lost by moving electrons. Sources of emf are batteries (conversion of chemical energy to electrical energy) and generators (conversion of mechanical energy to electrical energy).

The source of emf does work on each charge to raise it from a lower potential to a higher potential.

Then as the charge flows around the circuit (naturally from higher to lower potential) it loses energy which is replaced by the emf source again.

energy supplied = energy lost

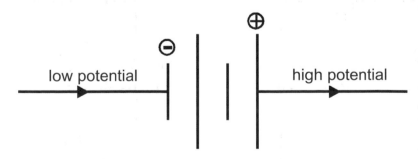

Figure III.B.10.4: Symbol of an emf source.
Arrows show the normal direction of current.

Energy is lost whenever a charge (as current) passes through a resistor. The units of emf are volts. The actual voltage delivered to a circuit is not equal to the value of the source. This is reduced by an internal voltage lost which represents the voltage loss by the *internal resistance (r)* of the source itself. The net voltage is called the terminal voltage or *terminal potential* V_t.

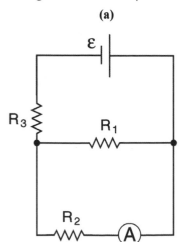

Figure III.B.10.5:
Simplified symbol of an emf source.

$$V_t = V - Ir = IR_t$$

I, R_t = totals for the circuit; V = maximal voltage output of the emf source.

When two emf sources are connected in opposition, (positive pole to positive pole) the charge loses energy when passing in the second emf source.

Therefore, if there is more than one emf source in a circuit, the total emf is the sum of the individual emf sources not in opposition reduced by the sum of individual sources in opposition in a given direction.

10.3.1 Kirchoff's Laws and a Multiloop Circuit Problem

Given that the emf of the battery ε = 12 volts and the resistors R_1 = 12 Ω, R_2 = 4.0 Ω, and R_3 = 6.0 Ω, determine the reading in the ammeter (*see Figure* III.B.10.6).

Ignore the internal resistance of the battery.

{*The ammeter will read the current which flows through it which is i_2*}

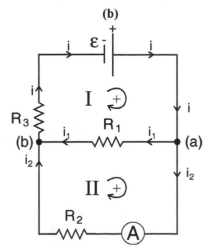

Figure III.B.10.6: A multiloop circuit.
(a) The problem as it could be presented; (b) the way you should label the diagram. Note that the current emanates from the positive terminal and is the same current i which returns to the emf source.

Kirchoff's Law I (*the junctional theorem*): when different currents arrive at a point (= *junction*, as in points (*a*) and (*b*) in the labelled diagram) the sum of current equals zero.

We can arbitrarily define all current *arriving* at the junction as <u>positive</u> and all current *leaving* as <u>negative</u>.

Kirchoff's Law I	$\Sigma i = 0$ at a junction

Thus at junction (a) $i - i_1 - i_2 = 0$

And for junction (b) $i_1 + i_2 - i = 0$

Both (a) and (b) reduce to equation (c):

$$i = i_1 + i_2$$

Kirchoff's Law II (*the loop theorem*): the sum of voltage changes in one continous loop of a circuit is zero. A single loop circuit is simple since the current is the same in all parts of the loop hence the loop theorem is applied only once.

In a multiloop circuit (loops *I* and *II* in the labelled diagram), there is more than one loop thus the current in general will not be the same in all parts of any given loop. We can arbitrarily define all voltage changes around the loop in the *clockwise* direction as <u>positive</u> and in the *counterclockwise* direction as <u>negative</u>.

Thus if by moving in the clockwise direction we can move from the battery's negative terminal (*low potential*) to its positive terminal (*high potential*), the value of the emf ε is negative.

Kirchoff's Law II	$\Sigma \Delta V = 0$ in a loop

Thus in loop *I* (*recall: V=IR*)

$$i_1R_1 + iR_3 - \varepsilon = 0$$
And in loop II
$$i_2R_2 - i_1R_1 = 0$$

We now have simultaneous equations. There are three unknowns (i, i_1, i_2) and three equations (c, loop *I*, and loop *II*). We need only solve for the current i_2 which runs through the ammeter.

Substitute (c) into loop I

$$i_1R_1 + (i_1 + i_2)R_3 - \varepsilon = 0$$
Thus
$$i_1R_1 + i_1R_3 + i_2R_3 - \varepsilon = 0$$

Substitute i_1 from loop *II* where $i_1 = i_2R_2/R_1$, hence
$$i_2R_2 + i_2R_2R_3/R_1 + i_2R_3 = \varepsilon$$
Begin isolating i_2
$$i_2(R_2 + R_2R_3/R_1 + R_3) = \varepsilon$$
Isolate i_2
$$i_2 = \varepsilon(R_2 + R_2R_3/R_1 + R_3)^{-1}$$
Substitute
$$i_2 = 12[4 + (4)(6)/(12) + 6]^{-1} = 12/12 = 1.0$$
ampere.

10.4 Capacitors and Dielectrics

Capacitors can store and separate charge. Capacitors can be filled with dielectrics which are materials which can increase capacitance. The capacitance (C) is an inherent property of a conductor and is formulated as:

$C = charge/electric\ potential = Q/V = farad = coulomb/volt$

The capacitance is the number of coulombs that must be transferred to a conductor to raise its potential by one volt.

The amount of charge that can be stored depends on the shape, size, surroundings and type of the conductor.

The higher the dielectric strength (i.e., the electric field strength at which a substance ceases to be an insulator and becomes a conductor) of the medium, the greater the capacitance of the conductor.

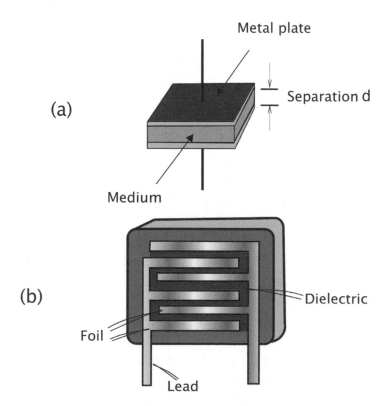

Figure III.B.10.7: (a) Parallel plate capacitor; (b) Ceramic capacitor.

A capacitor is made of two or more conductors with opposite but equal charges placed near each other.

A common example is the parallel plate capacitor. The important formulas for capacitors are:

1) $C = Q/V$ where V = the potential between the plates
2) $V = Ed$ where E = electric field strength, and d = distance between the plates
3) C is directly proportional to the surface area A of the plates and inversely proportional to the distance between the plates

$$C = \varepsilon_o \, A/d$$

for air as a medium between the plates. If the capacitor contains a dielectric, the above equation would by multiplied by the factor κ (= *dielectric constant*) whose value depends on the dielectric being used.

4) The equivalent capacitance C_{eq} for capacitors arranged in series and in parallel is:

$$\text{Series:} \quad 1/C_{eq} = 1/C_1 + 1/C_2 + 1/C_3 \ldots$$

$$\text{Parallel:} \quad C_{eq} = C_1 + C_2 + C_3 \ldots$$

The dielectric substances set up an opposing electric field to that of the capacitor which decreases the net electric field and allows the capacitance of the capacitor to increase ($C = Q/Ed$). The molecules of the dielectric are dipoles which line up in the electric field.

{cf. Fig. III.B.9.5 from PHY 9.1.4 and Fig. III.B.10.8 in this section}

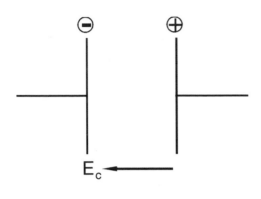

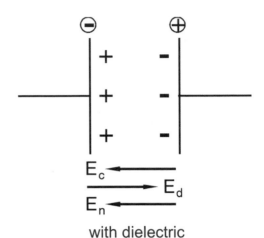

E_c

without dielectric

E_c
E_d
E_n

with dielectric

Figure III.B.10.8: Capacitors and dielectrics.
Note that the capacitor is symbolized by two parallel lines of equal length. The electric fields: E_c generated by the capacitor, E_d generated by the dielectric, and E_n is the resultant electric field.

The energy associated with each charged capacitor is:

Potential Energy $(PE) = W = (1/2V)(Q) = 1/2QV$

also

$$W = 1/2(CV)(V) = 1/2CV^2$$

and

$$W = 1/2Q(Q/C) = 1/2Q^2/C.$$

10.5 Root-Mean-Square Current and Voltage

DC (*direct current*) circuits contain a continuous current. Thus calculating power output is quite simple using $P = I^2R = IV$. However, AC (*alternating current*) circuits pulsate; consequently, we must discuss the average power output P_{av} where

$$P_{av} = (I_{rms})^2R = (I_{rms})(V_{rms})$$

which is true for a purely resistive load where

the root-mean-square (*rms*) values are determined from their maximal (*max*) values:

$$I_{rms} = I_{max}/\sqrt{2} \quad \text{and} \quad V_{rms} = V_{max}/\sqrt{2}.$$

Thus by introducing the *rms* quantities the equations for DC and AC circuits have the same forms. AC circuit voltmeters and ammeters have their scales adjusted to read the *rms* values.

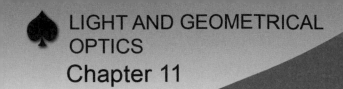

LIGHT AND GEOMETRICAL OPTICS
Chapter 11

Memorize	Understand	Not Required*
* Equations: PHY 11.3, 11.4, 11.5 * Rules for drawing ray diagrams	* Rules/equations: reflection, refraction, Snell's law * Dispersion, total internal reflection * Mirrors, lenses, real/virtual images * Ray diagrams * Lens strength, aberration	* Advanced level college info * Memorization of constants

MCAT-Prep.com

Introduction

Geometrical optics describes the propagation of light in terms of "rays." Rays are then bent at the interface of 2 rather different substances (i.e. air and glass) thus the ray may curve. A basic understanding of the equations and the geometry of light rays is necessary for solving problems in geometrical optics. Discrete questions regarding total internal reflection are frequent.

Additional Resources

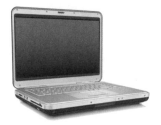

Free Online Q & A

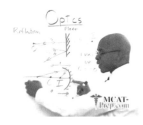

Video: Online or DVD 2, 3

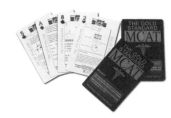

Flashcards

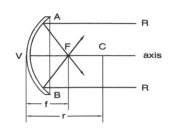

Special Guest

11.1 Visual Spectrum, Color

Geometrical optics is a first approximation of physical optics, which by its wavy nature, is part of the electromagnetic wave theory. The theory of light has a dualistic aspect:

• *particulate*: referring to a packet of energy called a photon when one wants, for example, to explain the photoelectric effect.

• *wavy* : when one wants to explain, for example, light interference and diffraction. Diffraction occurs when waves of light bend at the interface between two different media.

The optics domain of the electromagnetic wave theory corresponds to the following range of wavelengths of the electromagnetic spectrum (expressed in microns $1\mu = 10^{-6}\,m$):

$$0.4\mu < \lambda < 0.8\mu$$

or

$$0.4\mu < visible < 0.8\mu.$$

See PHY 9.2.4 for the colors in the visual spectrum.

11.2 Polarization

An electromagnetic field is described as having at every point of the field two perpendicular vectors: *the electric field vector E and the magnetic induction field vector B.*

The electromagnetic wave front is polarized in a straight line when E and B are fixed at all times. Thus polarized light is light that has waves in only one plane.

11.3 Reflection, Mirrors

Reflection is the process by which light rays (= *imaginary lines drawn perpendicular to the advancing wave fronts*) bounce back into a medium from a surface with another medium (*versus being refracted or absorbed*). The ray that arrives is the *incident* ray while the ray that bounces back is the *reflected* ray. The laws of reflection are:

1) the angle of incidence (I) equals the angle of reflection (R) at the normal (*N*, the line perpendicular to the surface)
2) the I, R, N all lie in the same plane.

After a ray strikes a mirror or a lens it forms an image. A virtual image has no light rays passing through it and cannot be projected upon a screen.

A <u>real image</u> has light rays passing through it and can be projected upon a screen.

Mirrors have a plane surface, like an ordinary household mirror, or a non-plane surface. For a plane mirror, all incident light is reflected in parallel off the mirror and therefore all images seen are virtual, erect, left-right reversed and appear to be just as far (perpendicular distance) behind the mirror as the object is in front of the mirror.

In other words, the object (*o*) and the image (*i*) distances have the same magnitudes but have opposite directions (*i* = -*o*).

Spherical mirrors are non-plane mirrors which may have the reflecting surface convex (*diverges light*) or concave (*converges light*). Note the images formed by a converging mirror (concave) are like those for a converging lens (convex);

and diverging mirrors (convex) and a diverging lens (concave) also form similar images. The terminology for spherical mirrors is :

r = radius of curvature
C = center of curvature
F = focal point

V = vertex (center of the mirror itself)
axis = line through C and V
f = focal length (distance from F to V)

i = image distance (distance from V to image along the axis)
o = object distance (distance from V to object along the axis)
AB = linear aperture (cord connecting the ends of the mirror; the larger the aperture, the better the resolution).

As a rule, capital letters refer to a point (*or position*) and small case letters refer to a distance.

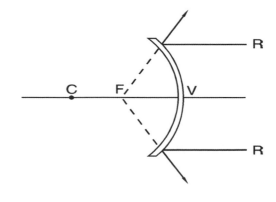

Concave (converging)   Convex (diverging)

Figure III.B.11.1: Reflection by spherical mirrors. R = the light rays.

With concave (spherical) mirrors the incident light is converged toward the axis. The path of light rays is as follows:

1)
if $o < f$, then the image is virtual and erect;
if $o > f$, then the image is real and inverted;
if $o = f$, then no image is formed;
2)
if $o < r$, then the image is enlarged in size;
if $o > r$, then the image is reduced in size;
if $o = r$, then the image is the same.

The relations are similar to those for a converging lens (convex). With convex (spherical) mirrors, the incident light is diverged from the axis after reflection. It is the backward extension (dotted lines in the diagram) that may pass through the focal point F. The path of light rays are as follows:

1) Incident rays parallel to the axis have backward extension of their reflections through F (see Figure III.B.11.1);
2) incident rays along a radius (that would pass C if extended) reflect back along themselves;

3) incident rays that pass through F (if extended) reflect parallel to the axis.

The image formed for a convex mirror is always virtual, erect and smaller than the object. The mirror equation and the derivations from it allow the above relations between object and image to be calculated instead of memorized. The equation is valid for convex and concave mirrors:

$$1/i + 1/o = 1/f$$

$$f = r/2$$

$$M = magnification = -i/o.$$

Convention :
• for i and o, *positive* values mean <u>real</u>, *negative* values mean <u>virtual</u>;
• for r and f, *positive* values mean <u>converging</u>, *negative* values mean <u>diverging</u>;
• for M, a *positive* value means <u>erect</u>, *negative* is <u>inverted</u>;
• for M > 1 the image is <u>enlarged</u>, M < 1 the image is <u>diminished</u>.

11.4 Refraction, Dispersion, Refractive Index, Snell's Law

Refraction is the bending of light as it passes from one transparent medium to another and is caused by the different speeds of light in the two media.

If θ_1 is taken as the angle (to the normal) of the incident light and θ_2 is the angle (to the normal) of the refracted light, where 1 and 2 represent the two different media, the following relations hold (Snell's Law):

If the surface is convex, r is positive (e.g., r_1).
If the surface is concave, r is negative (e.g., r_2).
Subscript 1 refers to the incident side, 2 refers to the refracted side.

C = center of curvature, F = focal point
V = the optical center of the lens or vertex
axis = line through C and V

f = focal length is the distance between V and F
i = image distance (from V to the image)
o = object distance (from V to the object).

The path rays through a lens are:

1) incident rays parallel to the axis refract through F_2 of the converging lens, and appear to come from F_1 of a diverging lens (backward extensions of the refracted ray, see dotted line on diverging diagram);

2) an incident ray through F_1 of a converging lens or through F_2 of a diverging lens (if extended) are refracted parallel to the axis;

3) incident rays through V are deviated (refracted).

For a converging lens (e.g., convex) the image formed depends on the object distance relative to the focal length (f). The relations (note similarity with a converging mirror) are:

1)
if $o < f_1$, then image is virtual and erect;
if $o > f_1$, the image is real and inverted;
if $o = f_1$, then no image is formed;

2)
if $o < 2f_1$, then the image is enlarged is size;
if $o > 2f_1$, then the image is reduced in size;
if $o = 2f_1$, then the image is the same.
remember $2f_1 = r$.

For a diverging lens (e.g., concave), the image is always virtual, erect and reduced in size as for a diverging mirror.

The above relations can be calculated rather than memorized by use of the lens equation (similar to the mirror equation) and derivations from it,

1) $1/o + 1/i = 1/f$ (lens equation, same as mirror equation)

2) $D = 1/f = (n-1)(1/r_1 - 1/r_2)$, (lens maker's equation, n = index of refraction)

3) diopters $(D) = 1/f$ where f is in meters, measures the refractive *power* of the lens; the larger the diopters, the stronger the lens. The diopters has a positive value for a converging lens and a negative value for a diverging lens.

To get the refractive power (D) of lenses in series just add the diopters which can then be converted into focal length:

$$D_T = D_1 + D_2 = 1/f_T \ (T = total).$$

4) Note that you can add only inverses of focal lengths :

$$1/f_T = 1/f_1 + 1/f_2 \ . \ . \ .$$

5) *M = Magnification = -i/o = $M_1 M_2$* for lenses in series.

Convention:
- for i and o, positive values mean real, negative values mean virtual;
- for r and f, positive values mean converging, negative values mean diverging;
- for M, a positive value means erect, negative is inverted.

The lens equation holds only for thin lenses (the thickness is small relative to other dimensions). For combination of lenses not in contact with each other, the image is found for the first lens (nearer the object) and then this image is used as the object of the second lens to find the image formed by it.

It should be noted that since concave lenses are concave on both sides they are sometimes called *biconcave*. Likewise, convex lenses may be called *biconvex*.

11.5.1 Lens Aberrations

In practice, the images formed by various refracting surfaces, as described in the previous section, fall short of theoretical perfection. Imperfections of image formation are due to several mechanisms or *aberrations*.

For example a nick or cut in a convex lens might create a microscopic area of concavity. Thus the light ray which strikes the aberration diverges instead of converging. Therefore the image will be less sharp or clear as the number or sizes of the aberrations increase.

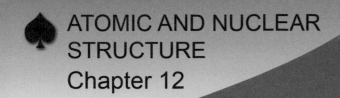
Memorize	Understand	Not Required*
* Equation relating energy and mass; half-life * Alpha, beta, gamma particles * Equation for maximum number of electrons in a shell * Equation relating energy to frequency * Equation for the total energy of the electrons in an atom	* Basic atomic structure, amu * Fission, fusion; the Bohr model of the atom * Problem solving for half-life * Quantized energy levels for electrons * Fluorescence	* Advanced level college info * Memorizing mass: neutrons/protons/elect * Memorizing constants, conversions

MCAT-Prep.com

Introduction ▮▮▮▮

Atomic structure can be summarized as a nucleus orbited by electrons in different energy levels. Transition of electrons between energy levels and nuclear structure (i.e. protons, neutrons) are important characteristics of the atom.

Additional Resources

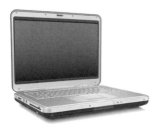

Free Online Q & A

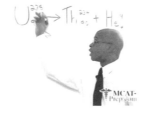

Video: Online or DVD 1

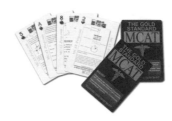

Flashcards

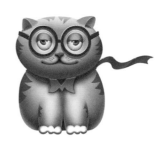

Special Guest

12.1 Protons, Neutrons, Electrons

Only recently, with high resolution electron microscopes, have large atoms been visualized. However, for years their existence and properties have been inferred by experiments. Experimental work on gas discharge effects suggested that an atom is not a single entity but is itself composed of smaller particles. These were termed elementary particles. The atom appears as a small solar system with a heavy nucleus composed of positive particles and neutral particles: *protons* and *neutrons*. Around this nucleus, there are clouds of negatively charged particles, called *electrons*. The mass of a neutron is slightly more than that of a proton (both $\approx 1.7 \times 10^{-24}$ g); the mass of the electron is considerably less (9.1×10^{-28} g).

Since an atom is electrically neutral, the negative charge carried by the electrons must be equal in magnitude (but opposite in sign) to the positive charge carried by the protons.

Experiments with electrostatic charges have shown that opposite charges attract, so it can be considered that electrostatic forces hold an atom together. The difference between various atoms is therefore determined by their *composition*.

A hydrogen atom consists of one proton and one electron; a helium atom of two protons, two neutrons and two electrons. They are shown in diagram form in Figure III.B.12.1.

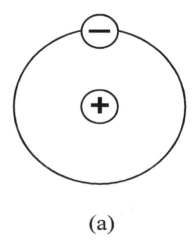

(a)

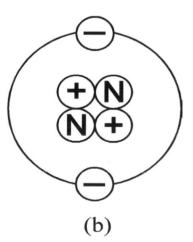

(b)

Figure III.B.12.1: Atomic structure simplified: (a) hydrogen atom; (b) helium atom.

A proton has a mass of 1 a.m.u. (*atomic mass unit*) and a charge of +1, whereas, a neutron has a mass of 1 a.m.u. and no charge. The *atomic number* (*AN*) of an atom is the number of protons in the nucleus.

An *element* is a group of atoms with the same AN. *Isotopes* are elements which have the same AN (= protons) but different numbers of neutrons. It is the number of protons that distinguishes elements from each other.

The *mass number* (*MN*) of an atom is the number of protons and neutrons in an atom. The *atomic weight* (*AW*) is the weighted average of all naturally occurring isotopes of an element.

It is also important to note that as the number of <u>protons</u> distinguishes *elements* from each other, it is their <u>electronic configuration</u> (CHM 2.1, 2.2, 2.3) that determines their *reactivity*.

12.3 Nuclear Forces, Nuclear Binding Energy, Stability, Radioactivity

Coulomb repulsive force (between protons) in the nuclei are overcome by nuclear forces. The nuclear force is a non-electrical type of force that binds nuclei together and is equal for protons and neutrons. The nuclear binding energy (E_b) is a result of the relation between energy and mass changes associated with nuclear reactions,

$$\Delta E = \Delta mc^2$$

in ergs in the CGS system, i.e. m = grams and c = cm/sec; ΔE = energy released or absorbed; Δm = mass lost or gained, respectively; c = velocity of light = 3.0×10^{10} cm/sec.

Conversions:
1 *gram* = 9×10^{20} *ergs*
1 *a.m.u.* = 931.4 *MeV* (*Mev* = 10^6 electron volts)
1 *a.m.u.* = 1/12 the mass of $_6C^{12}$.

The preceding equation is a statement of the law of conservation of mass and energy. The value of E_b depends upon the mass number (MN) as follows, (*see Figure III.B.12.2*):

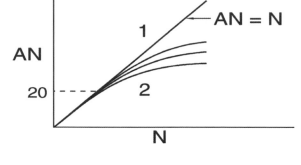

Figure III.B.12.3: Stability of Atoms. AN = atomic number and N = number of neutrons.

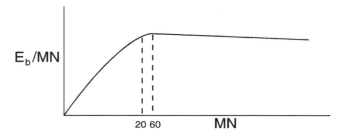

Figure III.B.12.2: Binding Energy per Nucleus. *E_b/MN = binding energy per nucleus; this is the energy released by the formation of a nucleus.*

The peak E_b/MN is at MN=60. Also, E_b/MN is relatively constant after MN=20. <u>Fission</u> is when a nucleus splits into smaller nuclei. <u>Fusion</u> is when smaller nuclei combine to form a larger nucleus. Energy is released from a nuclear reaction when nuclei with MN >> 60 undergo fission or nuclei with MN << 60 undergo fusion.

Not all combinations of protons are stable. The most stable nuclei are those with an even number of protons and an even number of neutrons. The least stable nuclei are those with an odd number of protons and an odd number of neutrons. Also, as the atomic number (AN) increases, there are more neutrons (N) needed for the nuclei to be stable.

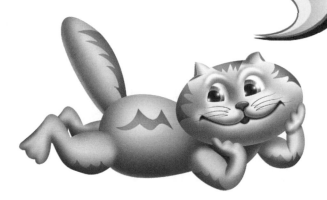

Up to AN = 20 (Calcium) the number of protons is equal to the number of neutrons, after this there are more neutrons. If an atom is in region #1 in Figure III.B.12.3, it has too many protons or too few neutrons and must decrease its protons or increase its neutrons to become stable. The reverse is true for region #2. All nuclei after AN = 84 (Polonium) are unstable.

Unstable nuclei become stable by fission to smaller nuclei or by absorption or emission of small particles. Spontaneous fission is rare. Spontaneous radioactivity (emission of particles) is common. The common particles are:

1) alpha (α) particle = $_2He^4$ (helium nucleus);

2) beta (β) particle = $_{-1}e^0$ (an electron);

3) a positron $_{+1}e^0$ (same mass as an electron but opposite charge);

4) gamma (γ) ray = no mass and no charge, just electromagnetic energy;

5) orbital electron capture - nucleus takes electrons from K shell and converts a proton to a neutron. If there is a flux of particles such as neutrons ($_0n^1$), the nucleus can absorb these also.

12.4 Nuclear Reaction, Radioactive Decay, Half-Life

Nuclear reactions are reactions in which changes in nuclear composition occur. An example of a nuclear reaction which involves uranium and hydrogen:

$$_{92}U^{238} + _1H^2 \longrightarrow _{93}Np^{238} + 2_0n^1$$

for $_{92}U^{238}$: 238 = mass number, 92 = atomic number. The sum of the lower (or higher) numbers on one side of the equation equals the sum of the lower (or higher) numbers on the other side of the equation. Another way of writing the preceding reaction is: $_{92}U^{238}(_1H^2,2_0n^1)_{93}Np^{238}$. {# neutrons (i.e. $_{92}U^{238}$)= superscript (238) - subscript (92) = 146}

Spontaneous radioactive decay is a first order process. This means that the rate of decay is *directly* proportional to the amount of material present:

$$\Delta m/\Delta t = \text{rate of decay}$$

where Δm = change in mass, Δt = change in time.

The preceding relation is equalized by adding a proportionality constant called the decay constant (k) as follows,

$$\Delta m/\Delta t = -km.$$

The minus sign indicates that the mass is decreasing. Also, $k = -(\Delta m/m)/\Delta t$ = fraction of the mass that decays with time.

The *half-life* $(T_{1/2})$ of a radioactive atom is the time required for one half of it to disintegrate. The half-life is related to k as follows,

$$T_{1/2} = 0.693/k.$$

If the number of half-lifes n are known we can calculate the percentage of a pure radioactive sample left after undergoing decay since the fraction remaining = $(1/2)^n$.

For example, given a pure radioactive substance X with $T_{1/2}$ = 9 years, calculating the percentage of substance X after 27 years is quite simple,

$$27 = 3 \times 9 = 3\ T_{1/2}$$

Thus

$$n = 3,\ (1/2)^n = (1/2)^3 = 1/8\ or\ 13\%.$$

After 27 years of disintegration, 13% of pure substance X remains. {Similarly, note that *doubling time* is given by $(2)^n$; *see* BIO 2.2}

12.5 Quantized Energy Levels For Electrons, Emission Spectrum

Work by Bohr and others in the early part of the present century demonstrated that the electron orbits are arranged in shells, and that each shell has a defined maximum number of electrons it can contain.

For example, the first shell can contain two electrons, the second eight electrons (*see* CHM 2.1, 2.2). The maximum number of electrons in each shell is given by:

$$\boxed{N_{electrons} = 2n^2}$$

$N_{electrons}$ designates the number of electrons in shell n.

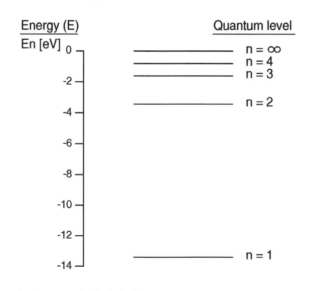

Figure III.B.12.4: Energy levels. The energy E_n in each shell n is measured in electron volts.

The state of each electron is determined by the four quantum numbers:

• *principal quantum number n* determines the number of shells, possible values are: 1 (K), 2 (L), 3 (M), etc...
• *angular momentum quantum number l*, determines the subshell, possible values are: 0 (s), 1 (p), 2 (d), 3 (f), n-1, etc...
• *magnetic momentum quantum number m_l*, possible values are: ±l, ... , 0
• *spin quantum number m_s*, determines the direction of rotation of the electron, possible values are: ±1/2.

Chemical reactions and electrical effects are all concerned with the behavior of electrons in the outer shell of any particular atom. If a shell is full, for example, the atom is unlikely to react with any other atom and is, in fact, one of the noble (inert) gases such as helium.

The energy that an electron contains is not continuous over the entire range of possible energy. Rather, electrons in a atom may contain only discrete energies as they occupy certain orbits or shells. Electrons of each atom are restricted to these discrete energy levels. These levels have an energy below zero.

This means energy is released when an electron moves from infinity into these energy levels.

If there is one electron in an atom, its ground state is n = 1, the lowest energy level available. Any other energy level, n = 2, n = 3, etc., is considered an excited state for that electron. The difference in energy (*E*) between the levels gives the absorbed (or emitted) energy when an electron moves to a higher orbit (or lower orbit, respectively) and therefore, the frequency (*f*) of light necessary to cause excitation.

$$E_2 - E_1 = hf$$

where E_1 = energy level one, E_2 = energy level two, *h* = planck's constant, and *f* = the frequency of light absorbed or emitted.

Therefore, if light is passed through a substance (e.g., gas), certain wavelengths will be absorbed, which correspond to the energy needed for the electron transition. An *absorption* spectrum will result that has <u>dark lines</u> against a <u>light background</u>. Multiple lines result because there are possible transitions from all quantum levels occupied by electrons to any unoccupied levels.

An *emission* spectrum results when an electron is excited to a higher level by another particle or by an electric discharge, for example. Then, as the electron falls from the excited state to lower states, light is emitted that has a wavelength (which is related to frequency) corresponding to the energy difference between the levels since: $E_1 - E_2 = hf$.

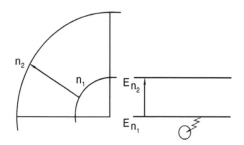

Step 1: light absorption

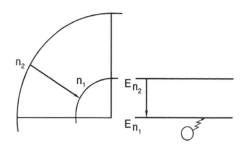

Step 3: light emission

Figure III.B.12.5: The fluorescence process. Represented is an atom with shells n_1, n_2 and their respective energy levels E_n.

The resulting spectrum will have <u>light lines</u> against a <u>dark background</u>. The absorption and emission spectrums should have the same number of lines but often will not. This is because in the absorption spectrum, there is a rapid radiation of the absorbed light in all directions, and transitions are generally from the ground state initially.

These factors result in fewer lines in the absorption than in the emission spectrum.

The total energy of the electrons in an atom can be given by:

$$E_{total} = E_{emission} \ (or \ E_{ionization}) + KE$$

12.6 Fluorescence

Fluorescence is an <u>emission process</u> that occurs after light absorption excites electrons to higher electronic and vibrational levels. The electrons spontaneously lose excited vibrational energy to the electronic states. There are certain molecular types that possess this property, e.g., some amino acids (tryptophan).

The fluorescence process is as follows:
• step 1 - absorption of light;

• step 2 - spontaneous deactivation of vibrational levels to zero vibrational level for electronic state;
• step 3 - fluorescence with light emission (longer wavelength than absorption).

Figure III.B.12.5 shows diagrammatically the steps described above. Step 2 which is not shown in the figure is the intermediate step between light absorption and light emission.

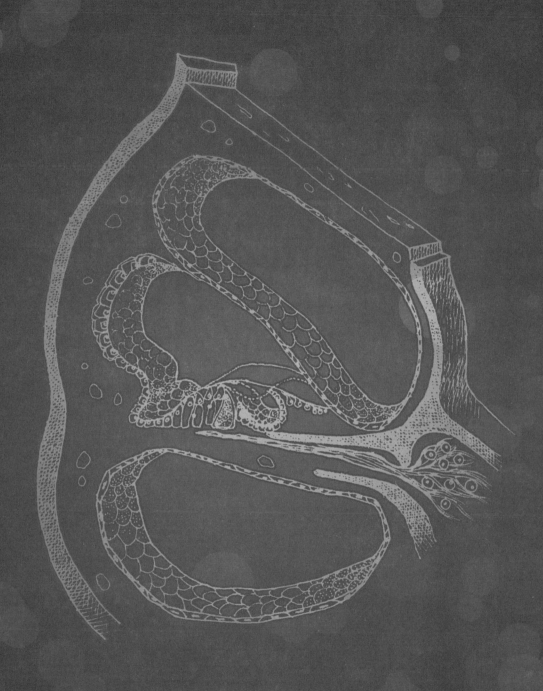

MCAT-Prep.com

BIOLOGY
PART IV.A: BIOLOGICAL SCIENCES

Memorize	Understand	Not Required*
* Structure/function: cell/components * Components and function: cytoskeleton * DNA structure and function * Transmission of genetic information * Mitosis, events of the cell cycle	* Intro level college info * Membrane transport * Hyper/hypotonic solutions * Saturation kinetics: graphs * Unique features of eukaryotes	* Advanced level college info * Molecular bio., detailed mechanisms * Plant cells, chloroplasts * Experiments in genetics * Specify polymerases or such details

MCAT-Prep.com

Introduction

Cells are the basic organizational unit of living organisms. They are contained by a plasma membrane and/or cell wall. Eukaryotic cells (*eu* = true; *karyote* refers to nucleus) are cells with a true nucleus found in all multicellular and nonbacterial unicellular organisms including animal, fungal and plant cells. The nucleus contains genetic information, DNA, which can divide into 2 cells by mitosis.

Additional Resources

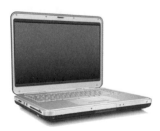

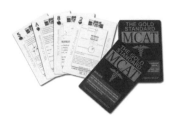

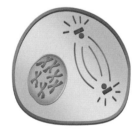

Free Online Q & A   Video: Online or DVD 3   Flashcards   Special Guest

* The real MCAT may have advanced level information presented (ie. in a passage) but previous knowledge of said information is not required to answer the questions that would follow. Practice AAMC and GS practice MCAT CBTs can help you clarify this point.

1.1 Plasma Membrane: Structure and Functions

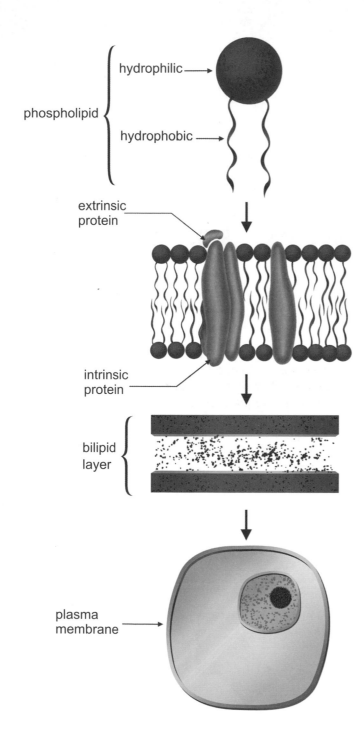

Figure IV.A.1.1: Structure of the plasma membrane.

The plasma membrane is a semipermeable barrier that defines the outer perimeter of the cell. It is composed of lipids (fats) and protein. The membrane is dynamic, selective, active, and fluid. It contains phospholipids which are amphipathic molecules. They are amphipathic because their tail end contains fatty acids which are insoluble in water (hydrophobic), the opposite end contains a charged phosphate head which is soluble in water (hydrophilic). The plasma membrane contains two layers of phospholipids thus it is called a bilipid layer.

The Fluid Mosaic Model tells us that the hydrophilic heads project to the outside and the hydrophobic tails project towards the inside of the membrane. Further, these phospholipids are fluid - thus they move freely from place to place in the membrane. Distributed throughout the membrane is a mosaic of proteins with limited mobility.

Proteins can be found associated with the outside of the membrane (extrinsic or peripheral) or may be found spanning the membrane (intrinsic or integral). Many intrinsic proteins represent channels through which specific molecules and ions can pass, or, receptors which hormones may activate.

The plasma membrane is semipermeable. In other words, it is permeable to small uncharged substances which can freely diffuse across the membrane (i.e. O_2, CO_2, urea). On the other hand, it is relatively impermeable to charged or large substances which may require transport proteins to cross the membrane (i.e. ions, amino acids, sugars) or cannot cross the membrane at all (i.e. protein hormones, intracellular enzymes). Substances which can cross the membrane may do so by simple diffusion, carrier-mediated transport, or by endo/exocytosis.

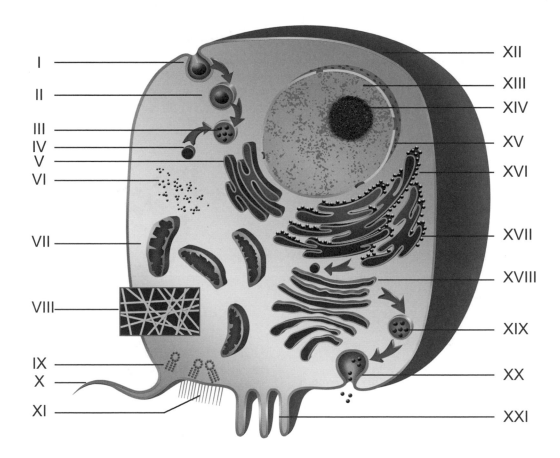

Figure IV.A.1.2: The generalized eukaryotic cell.

I	endocytosis	VIII	cytoskeleton (further magnified)	XV	nuclear envelope
II	endocytotic vesicle	IX	basal body (magnified)	XVI	cytosol
III	secondary lysosome	X	flagellum	XVII	rough endoplasmic reticulum
IV	primary lysosome	XI	cilia	XVIII	Golgi apparatus
V	smooth endoplasmic reticulum	XII	plasma membrane	XIX	exocytotic vesicle
VI	free ribosomes	XIII	nucleus	XX	exocytosis
VII	mitochondrion	XIV	nucleolus	XXI	microvillus

1.1.1 Simple Diffusion

Simple diffusion is the spontaneous spreading of a substance going from an area of higher concentration to an area of lower concentration (i.e. a concentration gradient exists). Gradients can be of a chemical or electrical nature. A chemical gradient arises as a result of an unequal distribution of molecules, and is often called a concentration gradient. In a chemical (or concentration) gradient, there is a higher concentration of molecules in one area than there is in another area, and molecules tend to diffuse from areas of high concentration to areas of lower concentration. An electrical gradient arises as a result of an unequal distribution of charge. In an electrical gradient, there is a higher concentration of charged molecules in one area than in another (this is independent of the concentration of all molecules in the area). Molecules tend to move from areas of higher concentration of charge to areas of lower concentration of charge.

Osmosis is the diffusion of water across a semipermeable membrane moving from an area of higher water concentration (i.e. lower solute concentration = hypotonic) to an area of lower water concentration (i.e. higher solute concentration = hypertonic). The hydrostatic pressure needed to oppose the movement of water is called the osmotic pressure. Thus, an isotonic solution (i.e. the concentration of solute on both sides of the membrane is equal), would have an osmotic pressure of zero.

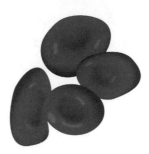

Figure IV.A.1.2.1a: Isotonic Solution.

The fluid bathing the cell (i.e. red blood cell or RBC in this case; see BIO 7.5) contains the same concentration of solute as the cell's inside or cytoplasm. When a cell is placed in an isotonic solution, the water diffuses into and out of the cell at the same rate.

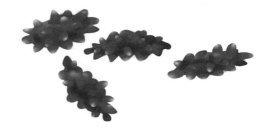

Figure IV.A.1.2.1b: Hypertonic Solution.

Here the fluid bathing the RBC contains a high concentration of solute relative to the cell's cytoplasm. When a cell is placed in a hypertonic solution, the water diffuses out of the cell, causing the cell to shrivel.

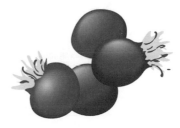

Figure IV.A.1.2.1c: Hypotonic Solution.

Here the surrounding fluid has a low concentration of solute relative to the cell's cytoplasm. When a cell is placed in a hypotonic solution, the water diffuses into the cell, causing the cell to swell and possibly explode.

{Memory guide: notice that the "O" in hyp-Otonic looks like a swollen cell. The O is also a circle which makes you think of the word "around." So IF the environment is hypOtonic

AROUND the cell, then fluid rushes in and the cell swells like the letter O}.

1.1.2 Carrier-Mediated Transport

Amino acids, sugars and other solutes need to reversibly bind to proteins (carriers) in the membrane in order to get across. Because there are a limited amount of carriers, if the concentration of solute is too high, the carriers would be saturated thus the rate of crossing the membrane would level off (= saturation kinetics).

The two carrier-mediated transport systems are:

i) <u>facilitated transport</u> where the carrier

helps a solute diffuse across a membrane it could not otherwise penetrate, and ii) <u>active transport</u> where energy (i.e. ATP) is used to transport solutes <u>against</u> their concentration gradients. The Na^+- K^+ exchange pump uses ATP to actively pump Na^+ to where its concentration is highest (outside the cell) and K^+ is brought within the cell where its concentration is highest (see Neural Cells and Tissues, BIO 5.1.1).

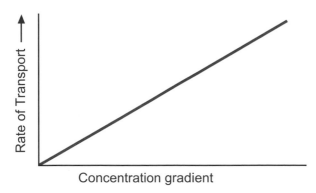

Simple Diffusion: the greater the concentration gradient, the greater the rate of transport across the plasma membrane.

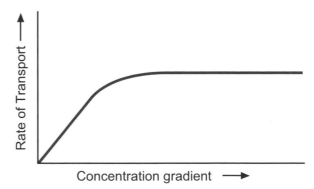

Carrier-Mediated Transport: increasing the concentration gradient increases the rate of transport until a maximum rate at which point all membrane carriers are saturated.

Figure IV.A.1.3: Simple diffusion versus carrier-mediated transport.

1.1.3 Endo/Exocytosis

Endocytosis is the process by which the cell membrane actually invaginates, pinches off and is released intracellularly (endocytotic vesicle). If a solid particle was ingested by the cell (i.e. a bacterium), it is called phagocytosis. If fluid was ingested, it is pinocytosis.

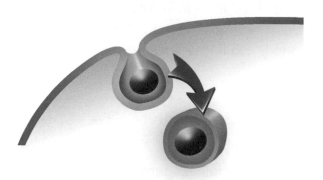

Figure IV.A.1.4: Endocytosis.

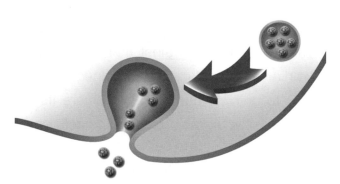

Figure IV.A.1.5: Exocytosis.

Exocytosis is, essentially, the reverse process. The cell directs an intracellular vesicle to fuse with the plasma membrane thus releasing its contents to the exterior (i.e. neurotransmitters, pancreatic enzymes, cell membrane proteins/lipids, etc.).

1.2 The Interior of a Eukaryotic Cell

Cytoplasm is the interior of the cell. It refers to all cell components enclosed by the cell's membrane which includes the cytosol, the cytoskeleton and the membrane bound organelles.

Cytosol is the solution which bathes the organelles and contains numerous solutes like amino acids, sugars, proteins, etc.

Cytoskeleton extends throughout the entire cell and has particular importance in shape and intracellular transportation. The cytoskeleton also makes extracellular complexes with other proteins forming a matrix so that cells can "stick" together. This is called cellular adhesion.

The components of the cytoskeleton in increasing order of size: microfilaments, intermediate filaments, and microtubules. Microfilaments are important for cell movement and contraction (i.e. actin and myosin, see Contractile Cells and Tissues, BIO 5.2).

Intermediate filaments and microtubules extend along axons and dendrites of neurons acting like railroad tracks so organelles or protein particles can shuttle to or from the cell body. Microtubules also form (i) the core of cilia and flagella; (ii) the mitotic spindles which we shall soon discuss; and (iii) centrioles.

A flagellum is a whiplike organelle of locomotion found in sperm and bacteria. Cilia are hair-like vibrating organelles which can be used to move particles along the surface of the cell (i.e. in the fallopian tubes cilia can help the egg move toward the uterus). Centrioles are cylinder-shaped complexes of microtubules associated with the mitotic spindle (MTOC, see later). At the base of flagella and cilia, two centrioles can be found at right angles to each other: this is called a basal body.

Microvilli are regularly arranged finger-like projections with a core of cytoplasm (*see* BIO 9.5). They are commonly found in the small intestine where they help to increase the absorptive and digestive surfaces (= brush border).

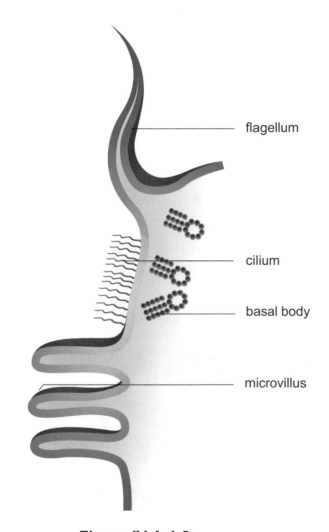

flagellum

cilium

basal body

microvillus

Figure IV.A.1.6:
Cytoskeletal elements and the plasma membrane.

1.2.1 Membrane Bound Organelles

Mitochondrion: The Power House

Mitochondria produce energy (i.e. ATP) for the cell through aerobic respiration. It is a double membraned organelle whose inner membrane has shelf-like folds and are called cristae. The matrix, the fluid within the inner membrane, contains the enzymes for the Kreb's cycle and circular DNA. The latter is the only cellular DNA found outside of the nucleus. There are numerous mitochondria in muscle cells.

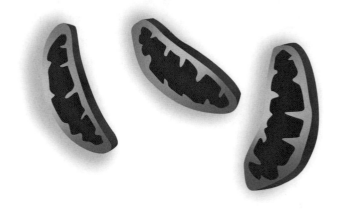

Figure IV.A.1.7: Mitochondria.

Lysosomes: Suicide Sacs

In a diseased cell, lysosomes may release their powerful acid hydrolases to digest away the cell (autolysis). In normal cells, a primary (normal) lysosome can fuse with an endocytotic vesicle to form a secondary lysosome where the phagocytosed particle (i.e. a bacterium) can be digested. This is called heterolysis. There are numerous lysosomes in phagocytic cells of the immune system (i.e. macrophages, neutrophils).

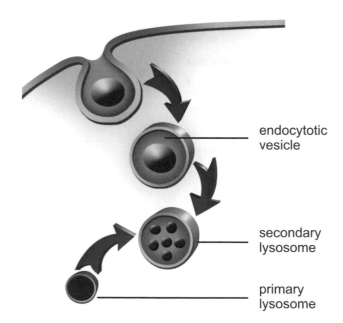

endocytotic vesicle

secondary lysosome

primary lysosome

Figure IV.A.1.8: Heterolysis.

Endoplasmic Reticulum: Synthesis Center

The endoplasmic reticulum (ER) is an interconnected membraned system resembling flattened sacs. There are two kinds: (i) dotted with ribosomes on its surface which is called rough ER and (ii) without ribosomes which is smooth ER.

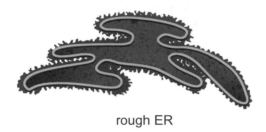

rough ER

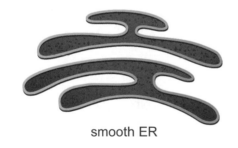

smooth ER

Figure IV.A.1.9: The endoplasmic reticulum.

Rough ER is important in protein synthesis whereas smooth ER is a factor in phospholipid and fatty acid synthesis and metabolism. Smooth ER is also important in the liver to help detoxify many chemicals (i.e. carcinogens, pesticides).

Golgi Apparatus: The Export Department

The Golgi apparatus forms a stack of smooth membranous sacs or *cisternae* that function in protein modification like the addition of polysaccharides (i.e. glycosylation). The Golgi also packages secretory proteins in membrane bound vesicles which can be exocytosed.

An abundant amount of rER and Golgi is found in cells which produce and secrete protein. For example, *B-cells* of the immune system which secrete antibodies, *acinar cells* in the pancreas which secrete digestive enzymes into the intestines, and *goblet cells* of the intestine, which secrete mucus into the lumen.

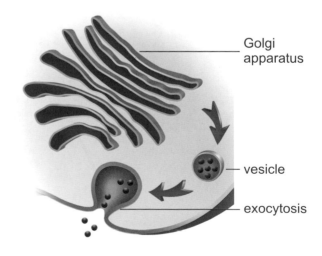

Golgi apparatus

vesicle

exocytosis

Figure IV.A.1.10: Golgi apparatus.

The Nucleus

The nucleus is surrounded by a double membrane called the <u>nuclear envelope</u>. Throughout the membrane are <u>nuclear pores</u> which selectively allow the transportation of large particles to and from the nucleus.

DNA can be found within the nucleus as <u>chromatin</u> (DNA complexed to proteins like *histones*) or as <u>chromosomes</u> which are more clearly visible in a light microscope. The <u>nucleolus</u> is not membrane bound. It contains the DNA necessary to synthesize ribosomal RNA.

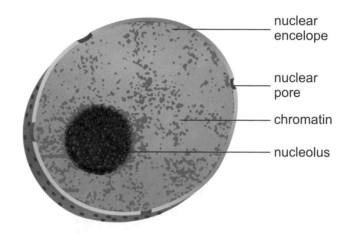

Figure IV.A.1.11: The nucleus.

1.2.2 DNA: The Cell's Architect

Deoxyribonucleic Acid (DNA) and ribonucleic acid (RNA) are essential components in constructing the proteins which act as the cytoskeleton, enzymes, membrane channels, antibodies, etc. It is the DNA which contains the genetic information of the cell.

DNA and RNA are both important nucleic acids. <u>Nucleotides</u> are the subunits which attach in sequence or in other words <u>polymerize</u> via phosphodiester bonds to form nucleic acids. A nucleotide (also called a *nucleoside phosphate*) is composed of a five carbon sugar, a nitrogen base, and an inorganic phosphate.

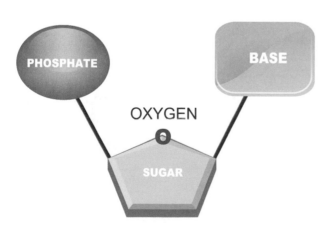

Figure IV.A.1.12: Nucleotide.

The sugar in RNA is ribose but for DNA an oxygen atom is missing in the second position thus it is 2-deoxyribose.

There are two categories of nitrogen bases: *purines* and *pyrimidines*. The purines have two rings and include adenine (A) and guanine (G). The pyrimidines contain one ring and include thymine (T), cytosine (C), and uracil (U).

DNA contains the following four bases: adenine, guanine, thymine, and cytosine. RNA contains the same bases except uracil is substituted for thymine.

Watson and Crick's model of DNA has allowed us to get insight into what takes shape as the nucleotides polymerize to form this special nucleic acid. The result is a double *helical* or *stranded* structure.

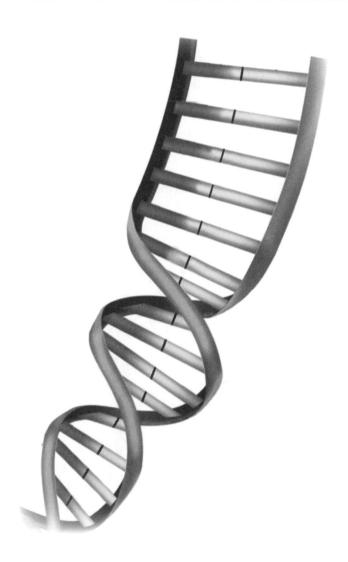

The backbone of each helix is the 2-deoxyribose phosphates. The nitrogen bases project to the center of the double helix in order to hydrogen bond with each other (imagine the double helix as a winding staircase: each stair would represent a pair of bases binding to keep the shape of the double helix intact).

There is specificity in the binding of the bases: one purine binds one pyrimidine. In fact, adenine only binds thymine (through two hydrogen bonds) and guanine only binds cytosine (through three hydrogen bonds). The more the H-bonds (i.e. the more G-C), the more stable the helix will be.

The *replication* (duplication) of DNA is semi-conservative: thus each strand of the double helix can serve as a template to generate a complementary strand. Thus for each double helix there is one parent strand (*old*) and one daughter strand (*new*). The latter is synthesized using one nucleotide at a time, enzymes including DNA polymerase, and the parent strand as a template. The

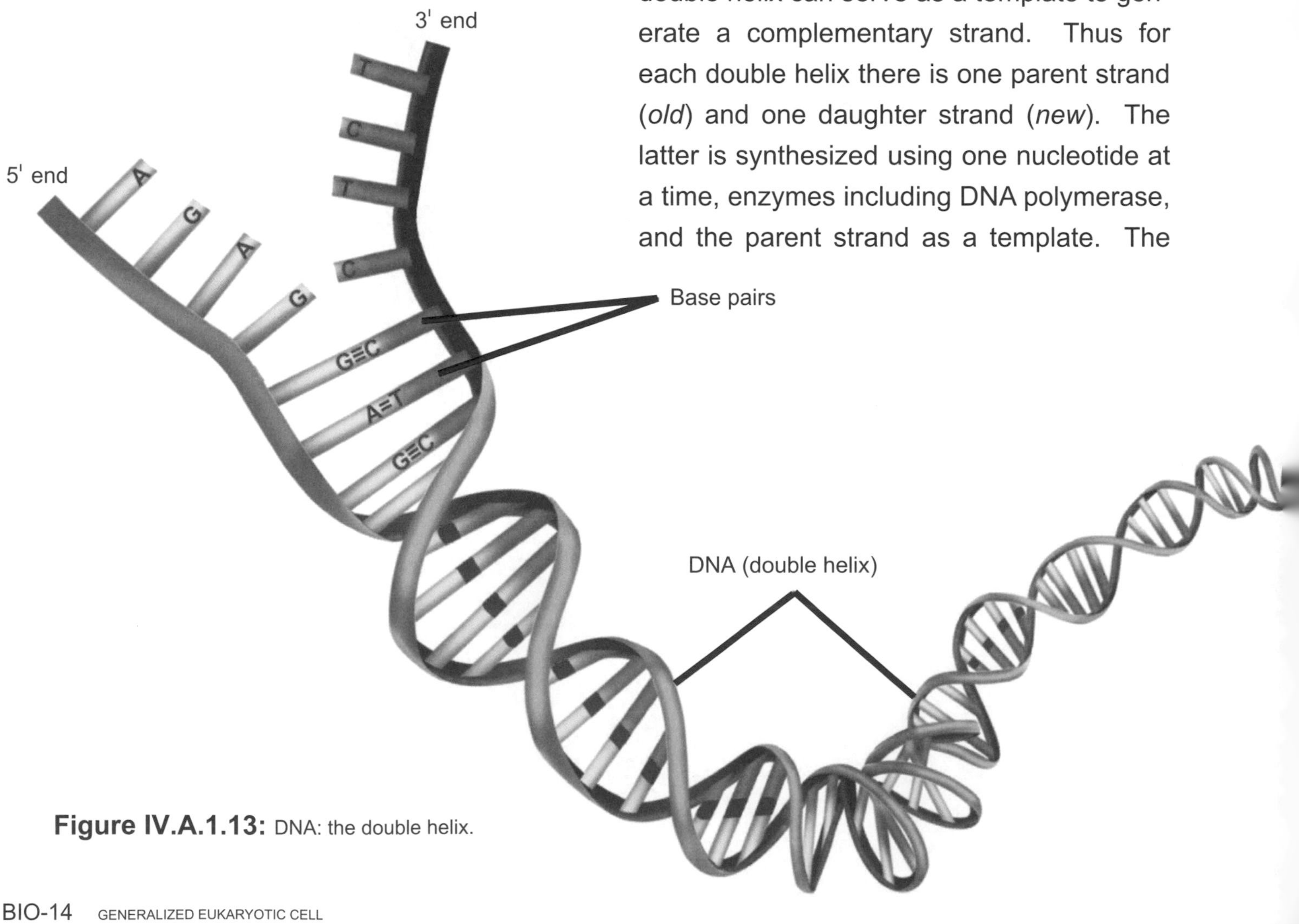

Figure IV.A.1.13: DNA: the double helix.

preceding is termed "DNA Synthesis" and occurs in the S stage of interphase during the cell cycle.

Each nucleotide has a hydroxyl or phosphate group at the 3rd and 5th carbons designated the 3' and 5' positions (see Organic Chemistry 12.3.2 and 12.5). Phosphodiester bonds can be formed between a free 3' hydroxyl group and a free 5' phosphate group. Thus the DNA strand has *polarity* since one end of the molecule will have a free 3' hydroxyl while the other terminal nucleotide will have a free 5' phosphate group. Polymerization of the two strands occurs in opposite directions (= *antiparallel*). In other words, one strand runs in the 5' - 3' direction, while its partner runs in the 3' - 5' direction.

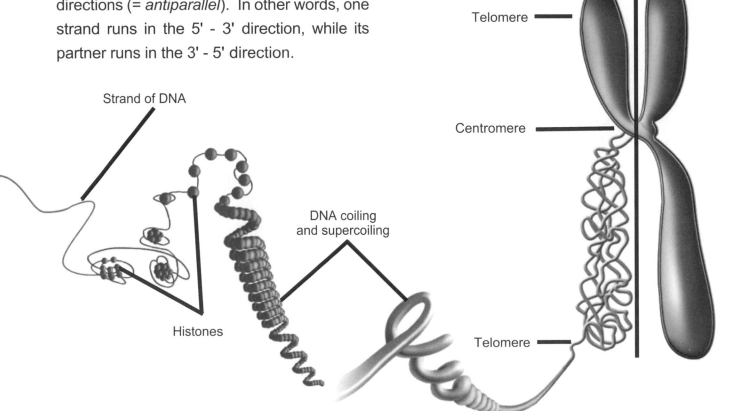

Nucleus

Cell

Chromosome

chromatid   chromatid

Telomere

Centromere

Telomere

Strand of DNA

DNA coiling and supercoiling

Histones

DNA replication is <u>semi-discontinuous</u>. DNA polymerase can only synthesize DNA in the 5' to 3' direction. As a result of the anti-parallel nature of DNA, the 5' - 3' strand is replicated continuously (the *leading strand*), while the 3' - 5' strand is replicated discontinuously (the *lagging strand*) in the <u>reverse direction</u>. In this manner, DNA polymerase synthesizes only from 5' - 3'.

Previous knowledge of recombinant DNA techniques, restriction enzymes, hybridization, DNA repair mechanisms, etc., is not normally required for the new MCAT. If you wish to get a "primer" in these areas, for background information, visit the Forum at www.MCAT-prep.com. The following is an overview regarding DNA repair.

Because of environmental factors including chemicals and UV radiation, any one of the trillions of cells in our bodies may undergo as many as 1 million individual molecular "injuries" per day. Structural damage to DNA may result and could have many effects including inducing mutation. Thus our DNA repair system is constantly active as it responds to damage in DNA structure.

A cell that has accumulated a large amount of DNA damage, or one that no longer effectively repairs damage to its DNA, can: (1) become permanently dormant; (2) exhibit unregulated cell division which could lead to cancer; (3) succumb to cell suicide, also known as *apoptosis* or programmed cell death.

1.3 The Cell Cycle

The cell cycle is a period of approximately 18 - 22 hours during which the cell can synthesize new DNA, partition the DNA equally, thus the cell can divide. These events are divided into a number of phases: interphase (G_1, S, G_2) and mitosis (prophase, metaphase, anaphase and telophase).

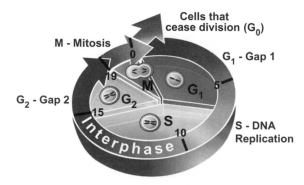

Figure IV.A.1.14: The cell cycle. The numbers represent time in hours. Note how mitosis (M) represents the shortest period of the cycle.

Interphase occupies about 90% of the cell cycle. During interphase, the cell prepares for DNA synthesis (G_1), synthesizes or replicates DNA (S), and ultimately begins preparing for mitosis (G_2). Mitosis begins with prophase.

Prophase: pairs of centrioles migrate away from each other while microtubules appear in between forming a spindle. Other microtubules emanating from the centrioles give a radiating star-like appearance; thus they are called *asters*. Therefore, centrioles form the core of the Microtubule Organizing Centers (MTOC).

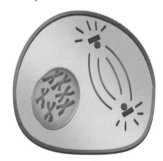

Figure IV.A.1.15: Prophase.

Simultaneously, the diffuse nuclear chromatin condenses into the visible chromosomes which consist of two identical sister chromatids. The area of constriction where the two chromatids are attached is the *centromere*. Just as centromere refers to the center, *telomere* refers to the ends of the chromosome. Ultimately, the nuclear envelope disappears at the end of prophase.

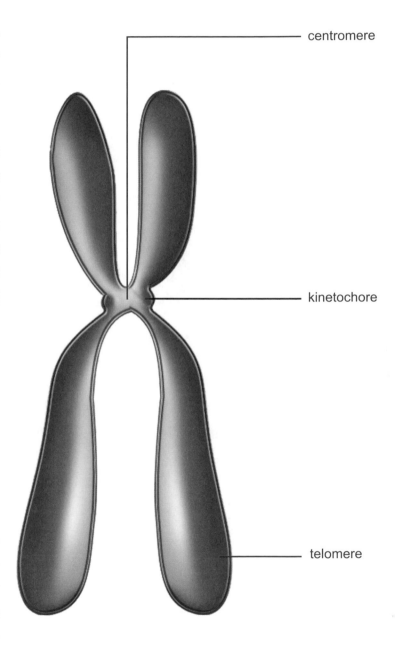

centromere

kinetochore

telomere

Figure IV.A.1.16: Chromosome.

Metaphase: centromeres line up along the equatorial plate. At or near the centromeres are the *kinetochores* which are proteins that face the spindle poles (asters). Microtubules, from the spindle, attach to the kinetochores of each chromosome.

Telophase: new membranes form around the daughter nuclei; nucleoli reappear; the chromosomes uncoil and become less distinct (decondense); and finally, *cytokinesis* (cell separation) occurs.

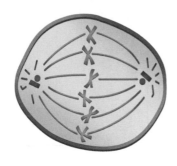

Figure IV.A.1.17: Metaphase.

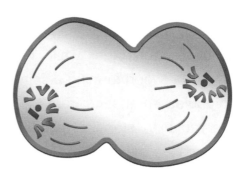

Figure IV.A.1.19: Telophase.

Anaphase: sister chromatids are pulled apart such that each migrates to opposite poles being guided by spindle microtubules.

The cell cycle continues with the next interphase. {Mnemonic for the sequence of phases: P. MATI}

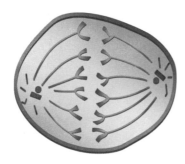

Figure IV.A.1.18: Anaphase.

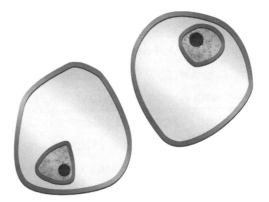

Figure IV.A.1.20: Interphase.

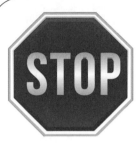

Reminder: Chapter review questions are available online for the owner of this textbook. Doing practice questions will help clarify concepts and ensure that you study in a targeted way. After you login to mcat-prep.com as a Gold Standard Owner*, click on Lessons in the Menu. Your access continues for one full year. Please note that the MCAT is expected to change in 2015 and so access will not continue after the MCAT has changed.

*To become a Gold Standard Owner, you will need to click on FREE MCAT in the top Menu of the mcat-prep.com homepage and then you will find "Click here if you own a Gold Standard textbook". Then follow the directions provided.

Memorize	Understand	Not Required*
* Structures, functions, life cycles * Generalized viral life cycle * Basic categories of bacteria * Equation for bacterial doubling * Differences, similtarities	* Eukaryotes vs. Prokaryotes * General aspects of life cycles * Gen. aspects of genetics/reproduction * Calculation of exponential growth * Scientific method (App. C) and microbiology; the flagellum	* Advanced level college info * Evolutionary history, habitats * Taxonomic (scientific) classification * Role in intfectious diseases * Different viral subtypes, evolution * Prions, viroids

MCAT-Prep.com

Introduction ▦▮▮▮

Microbiology is the study of microscopic organisms including viruses, bacteria and fungi. It is important to be able to focus on the differences and similarities between these microorganisms and the generalized eukaryotic cell you have just studied.

Additional Resources

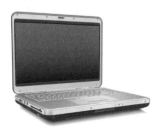

Free Online Q & A

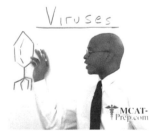

Video: Online or DVD 2

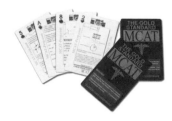

Flashcards

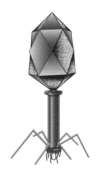

Special Guest

2.1 Viruses

Unlike cells, viruses are too small to be vvseen directly with a light microscope. Viruses infect all types of organisms, from animals and plants to bacteria and archaea (BIO 2.2). Only a very basic and general understanding of viruses is required for the MCAT.

Viruses are obligate intracellular para-sites; in other words, in order to replicate their genetic material and thus multiply, they must gain access to the inside of a cell. Viruses are often considered non-living for several reasons:

(i) they do not grow by increasing in size
(ii) they cannot carry out independent metabolism
(iii) they do not respond to external stimuli
(iv) they have no cellular structure.

The genetic material for viruses may be either DNA <u>or</u> RNA, never both. The nucleic acid core is encapsulated by <u>a</u> protein coat (capsid) which together forms the <u>head</u> region in some viruses. The tail region helps to anchor the virus to a cell. An extracellular viral particle is called a *virion*.

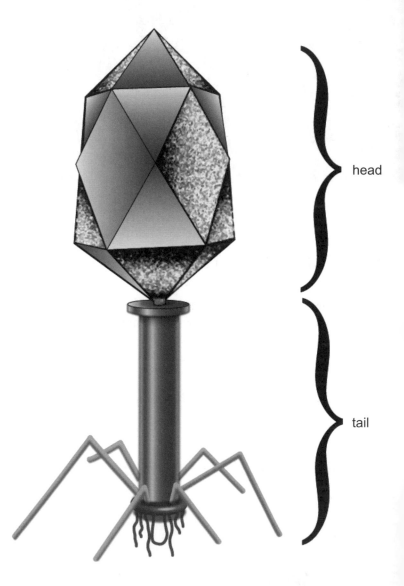

head

tail

Figure IV.A.2.1: A virus.

Viruses are much smaller than prokaryotic cells (i.e. bacteria) which, in turn, are much smaller than oukaryotes (i.e. animal cells, fungi). A virus which infects bacteria is called a bacteriophage or simply a phage.

The life cycle of viruses has many variants; the following represents the main themes for MCAT purposes. A virus attaches to a specific receptor on a cell. Some viruses may now enter the cell; others, as in the diagram, will simply inject their nucleic acid. Either way, viral molecules induce the metabolic machinery of the host cell to produce more viruses.

The new viral particles may now exit the cell by lysing (bursting). The preceding is deemed lytic or virulent. Some viruses lie latent for long periods of time without lysing the host cell. These are called lysogenic or temperate viruses.

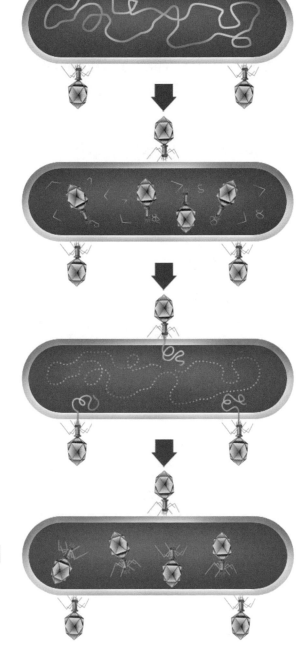

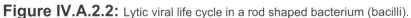

Figure IV.A.2.2: Lytic viral life cycle in a rod shaped bacterium (bacilli).

2.1.1 Retroviruses

A retrovirus uses RNA as its genetic material. It is called a retrovirus because of an enzyme (reverse transcriptase) that gives these viruses the unique ability of transcribing RNA (their RNA) into DNA (see Biology Chapter 3 for the central dogma regarding protein synthesis). The retroviral DNA can then integrate into the chromosomal DNA of the host cell to be expressed there. The human immunodeficiency virus (HIV), the cause of AIDS, is a retrovirus.

Retroviruses are used, in genetics, to deliver DNA to a cell (= a vector); in medicine, they are used for gene therapy.

2.2 Prokaryotes

Prokaryotes (= pre-nucleus) are organisms without a membrane bound nucleus which includes 2 types of organisms: bacteria (= Eubacteria) and archaea (= bacteria-like organisms that live in extreme environments). For the purposes of the MCAT, we will focus on bacteria. They are haploid and have a long circular strand of DNA in a region called the nucleoid. Bacteria also have smaller circular DNA called plasmids which help to confer resistance to antibiotics.

Bacteria do not have mitochondria, Golgi apparatus, lysosomes, nor endoplasmic reticulum. Instead, metabolic processes can be carried out in the cytoplasm or associated with bacterial membranes. Bacteria have ribosomes (smaller than eukaryotes), plasma membrane, and a cell wall. The cell wall, made of peptidoglycans, helps to

Typical eukaryotic cell

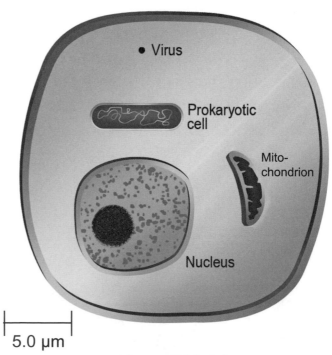

5.0 µm

Figure IV.A.2.3

Comparing the size of a typical eukaryote, prokaryote and virus. Note that both the prokaryote and mitochondrion are similar in size and both contain circular DNA suggesting an evolutionary link.

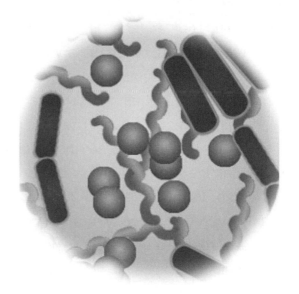

prevent the hypertonic bacterium from bursting. Some bacteria have a slimy polysaccharide mucoid-like capsule on the outer surface for protection.

Bacteria can achieve movement with their whiplike flagella. The form and rotary engine of flagella are maintained by proteins (i.e. flagellin) which interact with the plasma

Figure IV.A.2.5
Schematic representation of bacteria colored for the purpose of identification: cocci (spherical, green), bacilli (cylindrical, purple) and spirilli (helical, orange).

membrane and the basal body (BIO 1.2). Power is generated by a proton motive force similar to the proton pump in metabolism (Biology, Chapter 4).

Bacteria are partially classified according to their shapes: <u>cocci</u> which are spherical or sometimes elliptical; <u>bacilli</u> which are rod shaped or cylindrical (Fig. IV.A.2.2 in BIO 2.1 showed phages attacking a bacillus bacterium); <u>spirilli</u> which are helical or spiral. They are also classified according to whether or not their cell wall reacts to a special dye called a Gram stain; thus they are gram-positive if they retain the stain and gram-negative if they do not.

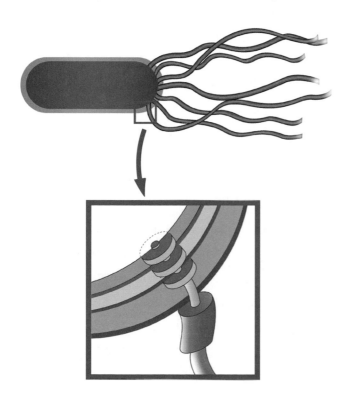

Figure IV.A.2.4
Schematic representation of the basis for flagellar propulsion. The flagellum, similar to a flexible hook, is anchored to the membrane and cell wall by a series of protein rings forming a motor. Powered by the flow of protons, the motor can rotate the flagellum more than 100 revolutions per second.

Most bacteria engage in a form of asexual reproduction called binary fission. Two identical DNA molecules migrate to opposite ends of a cell as a transverse wall forms, dividing the cell in two. The cells can now separate and enlarge to the original size. Under ideal conditions, a bacterium can undergo fission every 10-20 minutes producing over 10^{30} progeny in a day and a half. If resources are unlimited, exponential growth would be expected. The doubling time of bacterial populations can be calculated as follows:

$$b = B \times 2^n$$

where b is the number of bacteria at the end of the time interval, B is the number of bacteria at the beginning of the time interval and n is the number of generations. Thus if we start with 2 bacteria and follow for 3 generations then we get:

$$b = B \times 2^n = 2 \times 2^3 = 2 \times 8 = 16$$
bacteria after 3 generations.

{Note: bacterial doubling time is a relatively popular question type.}

Bacteria do not produce gametes nor zygotes, nor do they undergo meiosis; however, three forms of genetic recombination do occur: transduction, transformation, and conjugation. In transduction, phages act as a vector transferring DNA between bacteria. In transformation, bacteria incorporate free DNA from its immediate environment (i.e. from a dead cell which has released its DNA). In conjugation, part of the DNA strand may be passed from one mating type to another through a hollow tube (i.e. a pilus) while the two cells are in contact.

Most bacteria cannot synthesize their own food and thus depend on other organisms for it; such a bacterium is heterotrophic. Most heterotrophic bacteria obtain their food from dead organic matter; this is called saprophytic. Some bacteria are autotrophic meaning they can synthesize organic compounds from simple inorganic substances. Thus some are photosynthetic producing carbohydrate and releasing oxygen, while others are chemoautotrophic obtaining energy via chemical reactions including the oxidation of iron, sulfur, nitrogen, or hydrogen gas.

Bacteria can be either aerobic or anaerobic. The former refers to metabolism in the presence of oxygen and the latter in the absence of oxygen (i.e. fermentation). An obligate anaerobe would die in the presence of oxygen while a facultative anaerobe would survive.

Symbiosis generally refers to close and often long term interactions between different biological species. Bacteria have various symbiotic relationships with, for example, humans. These include mutualism (both benefit: GI tract bacteria, BIO 9.5), parasitism (parasite benefits over the host: tuberculosis, appendicitis) and commensalism (one benefits and the other is not significantly harmed or benefited: some skin bacteria).

2.3 Fungi

Fungi are eukaryotic (= true nucleus) organisms which absorb their food through their chitinous cell walls. They may either be unicellular (i.e. yeast) or filamentous (i.e. mushrooms, molds) with individual filaments called hyphae which collectively form a mycelium.

Fungi often reproduce asexually. Spores (i.e. conidia) can be produced and then liberated from outside of a sporangium; or, as in yeast, a simple asexual budding process may be used. Sexual reproduction can involve the fusion of opposite mating types to produce asci (singular: ascus), basidia (singular: basidium), or zygotes. All of the three preceding diploid structures must undergo meiosis to produce haploid spores. If resources are unlimited, exponential growth would be expected.

Fungi are relatively important for humans as a source of disease and a decomposer of both food and dead organic matter. On the lighter side, they also serve as food (mushrooms, truffles), for alcohol and food production (cheese molds, bread yeast) and they have given us the breakthrough antibiotic, penicillin (from penicillium molds).

GOLD NOTES

PROTEIN SYNTHESIS
Chapter 3

Memorize	Understand	Not Required*
* The genetic code (triplet) * Central Dogma: DNA RNA protein * Definitions: mRNA, tRNA, rRNA * Codon-anticodon relationship * Initiation, elongation and termination	* Mechanism of transcription * Mechanism of translation * Roles of mRNA, tRNA, rRNA * Role and structure of ribosomes	* Advanced level college info * Splicosomes, heterphil nuclear RNA * Inhibitory, signal peptides * Specific post translation changes * Memorizing the ribosomal subunits in Svedberg units * Memorizing stop or start codons

MCAT-Prep.com

Introduction

Protein synthesis is the creation of proteins using DNA and RNA. Individual amino acids are connected to each other in peptide linkages in a specific order given by the sequence of nucleotides in DNA. Thus the process occurs through a precise interplay directed by the genetic code and involving mRNA, tRNA and amino acids - all in an environment provided by a ribosome.

Additional Resources

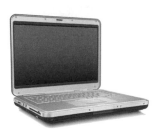

Free Online Q & A

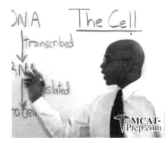

Video: DVD Disc 1

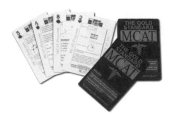

Flashcards

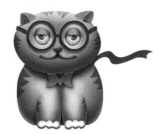

Special Guest

Proteins (which comprise many hormones, all enzymes, antibodies, etc.) are long chains formed by peptide bonds between combinations of twenty amino acid subunits. Each amino acid is encoded in a sequence of three nucleotides (a triplet code = the genetic code). A gene is a conglomeration of such codes and thus is a section of DNA which encodes for a protein (or a polypeptide which is exactly like a protein but much smaller).

The information in DNA is rewritten (transcribed) into a messenger composed of RNA (= mRNA); the reaction is catalyzed by the enzyme RNA polymerase. The newly synthesized mRNA (the primary transcript) contains regions called introns that are not expressed in the synthesized protein. The introns are removed and the regions that are expressed (exons) are spliced together to form the final functional mRNA molecule. {EXons EXpressed; INtrons IN the garbage!} The messenger then leaves the nucleus with the information necessary to make a protein. It attaches to a small subunit of a ribosome which will then attach to a larger ribosomal subunit thus creating a full ribosome. A ribosome is composed of a complex of protein and ribosomal RNA (= rRNA).

Floating in the cytoplasm is yet another form of RNA; this RNA specializes in taking amino acids and transfering them onto other amino acids when contained within the environment of the ribosome. More specifically, this transfer RNA (tRNA) molecule can attach itself to a specific amino acid, enter

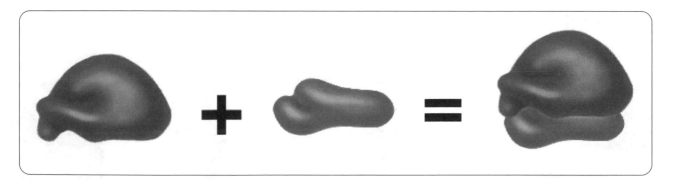

Figure IV.A.3.1: A ribosome provides the environment for protein synthesis. Ribosomes are composed of a large and a small subunit.

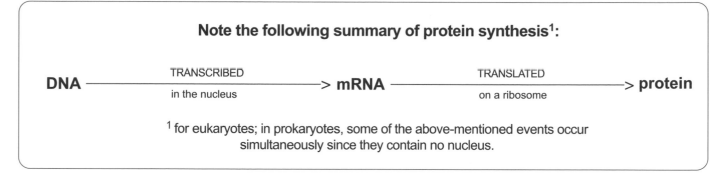

Note the following summary of protein synthesis[1]:

DNA ———————TRANSCRIBED——————> mRNA ———————TRANSLATED——————> protein
in the nucleus   on a ribosome

[1] for eukaryotes; in prokaryotes, some of the above-mentioned events occur
simultaneously since they contain no nucleus.

the environment of the ribosome, recognize the triplet code (= codon) on mRNA which codes for the amino acid tRNA is carrying (tRNA can do this since it has its own triplet code - an anticodon); and finally, tRNA can transfer its amino acid onto the preceding one thus elongating the polypeptide chain. In a way, tRNA translates the code that mRNA carries into a sequence of amino acids which can produce a protein. According to the base pair matching already discussed, if the codon on mRNA is AUG then the anticodon to match on tRNA would be UAC.

A nonsense mutation is a point mutation in a sequence of DNA that results in a premature stop codon (there are 3: UAA, UAG, UGA), or a nonsense codon in the transcribed mRNA. Either way, an incomplete, and usually nonfunctional protein is the result. A missense mutation is a point mutation where a single nucleotide is changed to cause substitution of a different

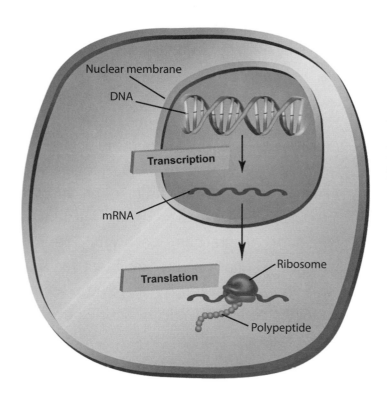

Figure IV.A.3.2: The central dogma of protein synthesis.

amino acid. Some genetic disorders (i.e. thalassemia) result from nonsense mutations.

Protein made on free ribosomes in the cytoplasm may be used for intracellular purposes (i.e. enzymes for glycolysis, etc.). Whereas proteins made on rER ribosomes are usually modified by both rER and the Golgi apparatus en route to the plasma membrane or exocytosis (i.e. antibodies, intestinal enzymes, etc.).

Note the following: i) the various kinds of RNA are single stranded molecules which are produced using DNA as a template; ii) hormones can have a potent regulatory effect on protein synthesis (esp. enzymes); iii) allosteric enzymes (= proteins with two different configurations - each with different biological properties) are important regulators of transcription; iv) there are many protein factors which trigger specific events in the <u>initiation</u> (using a start codon, AUG),

<u>elongation</u> and <u>termination</u> (using a stop codon) of the synthesis of a protein; v) one end of the protein has an amino group ($-NH_2$, which projects from the first amino acid), while the other end has a carboxylic acid group (-COOH, which projects from the last amino acid). {Amino acids and protein structure will be explored in ORG 12.1 and 12.2}

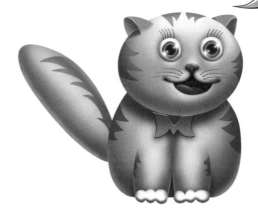

Peptide: the result of the moon pulling on the Pepsi.

Memorize	Understand	Not Required*
* Define: catabolism, anabolism, activation energy * Define: metabolism, active/allosteric sites * Substrates/products, especially: Acetyl CoA, pyruvate * Enzymes: kinase, phosphatase	* Feedback, competitive, non-competitive inhibition * Krebs cycle, electron transport chain: main features * Oxidative phosphorylation, substrates and products, general features * Metabolism: carbohydrates (glucose), fats and proteins	* Advanced level college info * Photosynthesis, gluconeogenesis, fatty acid oxidation * Knowing the deficiencies in the theoretical yield (36 ATP) calculation

MCAT-Prep.com

Introduction ▌▌▌▌

Cells require energy to grow, reproduce, maintain structure, respond to the environment, etc. Biochemical reactions and other energy producing processes that occur in cells, including cellular metabolism, are regulated in part by enzymes.

Additional Resources

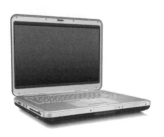

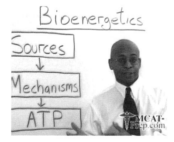

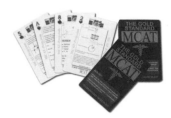

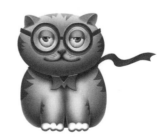

Free Online Q & A   Video: Online or DVD 2   Flashcards   Special Guest

4.1 Overview

In an organism or an individual many biochemical reactions take place. All these biochemical reactions are collectively termed metabolism. In general, metabolism can be broadly divided into two main categories. They are:

(a) Catabolism which is the breakdown of macromolecules (larger molecules) such as glycogen to micromolecules (smaller molecules) such as glucose.

(b) Anabolism which is the building up of macromolecules such as protein using micromolecules such as amino acids.

As we all know, chemical reactions in general involve great energy exchanges when they occur. Similarly both catabolic and anabolic reactions would involve massive amounts of energy if they were to occur in vitro (outside the cell). However, all these reactions could be carried out within a lower temperature range using substances called enzymes.

What is an enzyme?

An enzyme is a protein catalyst. A protein is a large polypeptide made up of amino acid subunits. A catalyst is a substance that alters the rate of a chemical reaction without itself being permanently changed into another compound. A catalyst accelerates a reaction by decreasing the free energy of activation

(see Chemistry 9.7).

Enzymes fall into two general categories:

(a) Simple proteins which contain only amino acids like the digestive enzymes ribonuclease, trypsin and chymotrypsin.

(b) Complex proteins which contain amino acids and a non-amino acid cofactor. Thus the complete enzyme is called a holoenzyme and it is made up of a protein portion (apoenzyme) and a cofactor.

> Holoenzyme = Apoenzyme + Cofactor.

A metal may serve as a cofactor. Zinc, for example, is a cofactor for the enzymes carbonic anhydrase and carboxypeptidase. An organic molecule such as pyridoxal phosphate or biotin may serve as a cofactor. Cofactors such as biotin, which are covalently linked to the enzyme are called prosthetic groups or ligands.

In addition to their enormous catalytic power which accelerates reaction rates, enzymes exhibit exquisite specificity in the types of reactions that each catalyzes as well as specificity for the substrates upon which they act. Their specificity is linked to the concept of an active site. An active site is a cluster of amino acids within the tertiary (i.e. 3-dimensional) configuration of the enzyme where the actual catalytic event occurs. The active site is often similar to a pocket or groove with properties (chemical or structural) that accommodate the intended substrate with high specificity.

Examples of such specificity are as follows: Phosphofructokinase catalyzes a reaction between ATP and fructose-6-phosphate. The enzyme does not catalyze a reaction between other nucleoside triphosphates. It is worth mentioning the specificity of trypsin and chymotrypsin though both of them are proteolytic (i.e. they degrade or *hydrolyse* proteins). Trypsin catalyzes the

hydrolysis of peptides and proteins only on the carboxyl side of polypeptidic amino acids lysine and arginine. Chymotrypsin catalyzes the hydrolysis of peptides and proteins on the carboxyl side of polypeptidic amino acids phenylalanine, tyrosine and tryptophan. The degree of specificity described in the previous examples originally led to the **Lock and Key Model** which has been generally replaced by the **Induced Fit Hypothesis.** While the former suggests that the molecular interaction is rigid, the latter describes a greater flexibility at the active site.

4.2 Enzyme Kinetics and Inhibition

There is an increase in reaction velocity with an increase in the concentration of substrate. At increasingly higher substrate concentrations the increase in activity is progressively smaller. From this, it could be inferred that enzymes exhibit saturation kinetics. The mechanism of the preceding lies largely with <u>feedback inhibition</u>. Feedback inhibition is when the product of the enzyme catalysed reaction returns (*feeds*

back) to prevent or *inhibit* further reactions between the enzyme and its substrate.

Enzyme inhibitors are classified as reversible and irreversible. Irreversible inhibitors usually react covalently to render the enzyme inactive. Reversible inhibitors generally interact non-covalently and virtually instantaneously with an enzyme.

4.3 Regulation of Enzyme Activity

The activity of enzymes in the cell is subject to a variety of regulatory mechanisms. The amount of enzyme can be altered by increasing or decreasing its synthesis or

degradation. Enzyme induction refers to an enhancement of its synthesis. Repression refers to a decrease in its biosynthesis.

Enzyme activity can also be altered by covalent modification. Phosphorylation of specific serine residues by protein kinases increases or decreases catalytic activity depending upon the enzyme. Proteolytic cleavage of proenzymes (e.g., chymotrypsinogen, trypsinogen, protease and clotting factors) converts an inactive form to an active form (e.g., chymotrypsin, trypsin, etc.).

Enzyme activity can be greatly influenced by its environment (esp. pH and temperature). For example, most enzymes exhibit optimal activity at a pH in the range 6.5 to 7.5. However, pepsin (an enzyme found in the stomach) has an optimum pH of ~ 2.0. Thus it cannot function adequately at a higher pH (i.e. in the small intestine). Likewise, enzymes function at an optimal temperature. When the temperature is lowered, kinetic energy decreases and thus the rate of reaction decreases. If the temperature is raised too much then the enzyme may become denatured and thus non-functional.

Enzyme activity can also be modified by non - covalent or allosteric mechanisms. Isocitrate dehydrogenase is an enzyme in the Kreb's Tricarboxylic Acid Cycle, which is activated by ADP. ADP is not a substrate or substrate analogue. It is postulated to bind a site *distinct* from the active site called the *allosteric site*.

Some enzymes fail to behave by simple saturation kinetics. In such cases a phenomenon called <u>positive co-operativity</u> is explained in which binding of one substrate or ligand makes it easier for the second to bind.

4.4 Bioenergetics

Biological species must transform energy into readily available sources in order to survive. ATP (adenosine triphosphate) is the body's most important short term energy storage molecule. It can be produced by the breakdown or oxidation of protein, lipids (i.e. fat) or carbohydrates (esp. glucose). If the body is no longer ingesting sources of energy it can access its own stores: glucose is stored in the liver as glycogen, lipids are stored throughout the body as fat, and ultimately, muscle can be catabolized to release protein (esp. amino acids).

We will be examining four key processes that can lead to the production of ATP: glycolysis, Krebs Citric Acid Cycle, the electron transport chain (ETC), and oxidative phosphorylation. Figure IV.A.4.1 is a schematic summary.

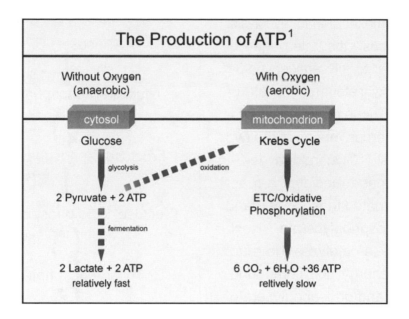

[1]from 1 molecule of glucose

Figure IV.A.4.1: Summary of ATP production.

4.5 Glycolysis

The initial steps in the catabolism or *lysis* of D-glucose constitute the Embden - Meyerhof glyco*lytic* pathway. This pathway can occur in the absence of oxygen (anaerobic). The enzymes for glycolysis are present in all human cells and are located in the cytosol. The overall reaction can be depicted as follows (ADP: adenosine diphosphate, NAD: nicotinamide adenine dinucleotide, Pi: inorganic phosphate):

$$\text{Glucose} + 2\text{ADP} + 2\,\text{NAD}^+ + 2\text{P}_i \longrightarrow 2\text{Pyruvate} + 2\text{ATP} + 2\text{NADH} + 2\text{H}^+$$

The first step in glycolysis involves the phosphorylation of glucose by ATP. The enzyme that catalyzes this irreversible reaction is either hexokinase or glucokinase. Phosphohexose isomerase then catalyzes the conversion of glucose-6-phosphate to fructose-6-phosphate. Phosphofructokinase (PFK) catalyzes the second phosphorylation. It is an irreversible reaction. This step, which produces fructose-1,6-diphosphate, is said to be the rate limiting or pacemaker step in glycolysis. Aldolase then catalyzes the cleavage of fructose-1,6-diphosphate to glyceraldehyde-3-phosphate and dihydroxyacetone phosphate (= 2 triose phosphates). Triose phosphate isomerase catalyzes the interconversion of the two preceding compounds. Glyceraldehyde-3-phosphate dehydrogenase mediates a reaction between the designated triose, NAD^+ and P_i to yield 1,3-diphosphoglycerate. Next, phosphoglycerate kinase catalyzes the reaction of the latter, an energy rich compound, with ADP to yield ATP and phosphoglycerate. Phosphoglycerate mutase catalyzes the transfer of the phosphoryl group from carbon two to yield 2-phosphoglycerate. Enolase catalyzes an isogonic dehydration to yield phosphoenolpyruvate. The enzyme enolase is inhibited by fluoride at high, non-physiological concentrations. This is why blood samples that are drawn for estimation of glucose are added to fluoride to inhibit glycolysis. Phosphoenolpyruvate is then acted upon by pyruvate kinase to yield pyruvate which is a three carbon compound.

Under **aerobic** conditions (i.e. in the presence of oxygen) pyruvate is converted to Acetyl CoA which will enter the Kreb's Cycle followed by oxidative phosphorylation producing a total of 38 ATP per molecule of glucose (i.e. 2 pyruvate). Under **anaerobic** conditions (i.e. absence of oxygen),

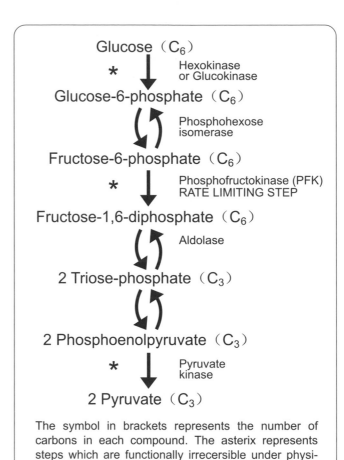

The symbol in brackets represents the number of carbons in each compound. The asterix represents steps which are functionally irrecersible under physiologic conditions. PFK is involved in the rate limiting step which is activated by ADP and inhibited by ATP.

Figure IV.A.4.2: Summary of glycolysis.

pyruvate is quickly reduced by NADH to lactic acid using the enzyme lactate dehydrogenase. A net of only 2 ATP is produced per molecule of glucose (this process is called *fermentation*).

Oxygen Debt: after running a 100m dash you may find yourself gasping for air even if you have completely ceased activity. This is because during the race you could not get an adequate amount of oxygen to your muscles and your muscles needed energy quickly; thus the anaerobic pathway was used. The lactic acid which built up during the race will require you to *pay back* a certain amount of oxygen in order to oxidize lactate to pyruvate and continue along the more energy efficient aerobic pathway.

4.6 Glycolysis: A Negative Perspective

An interesting way to summarize the main events of glycolysis is to follow the fate of the phosphate group which contains a negative charge. Note that *kinases* and *phosphorylases* are enzymes that can add or subtract phosphate groups.

The first event in glycolysis is the phosphorylation of glucose. Thus glucose becomes negatively charged which prevents it from leaking out of the cell. Then glucose-6-phosphate becomes its isomer (= *same molecular formula, different structure*) fructose-6-phosphate which is further phosphorylated to fructose-1,6-diphosphate. Imagine that this six carbon sugar (fructose) now contains two large negatively charged ligands which repel each other! The six carbon sugar (*hexose*) sensibly breaks into two three-carbon compounds (*triose phosphates*).

A triose phosphate is ultimately converted to 1,3-diphosphoglycerate which is clearly an unstable compound (i.e. *two negative phosphate groups*). Thus it transfers a high energy phosphate group onto ADP to produce ATP. When ATP is produced from a substrate (i.e. 1,3-diphosphoglycerate), the reaction is called *substrate level phosphorylation*.

4.7 Krebs Citric Acid Cycle

Aerobic conditions: for further breakdown of pyruvate it has to enter the mitochondria where a series of reactions will cleave the molecule to water and carbon dioxide. All these reactions (which were discovered by Hans. A. Krebs) are collectively known as the Tricarboxylic Acid Cycle (TCA) or Krebs Citric Acid Cycle. Not only carbohydrates but also lipids and proteins use the TCA for channelling their metabolic pathways. This is why TCA is often called the final common pathway of metabolism.

The glycolysis of glucose (C_6) produces 2 pyruvate (C_3) which in turn produces 2 CO_2 and 2 acetyl CoA (C_2). The catabolism of both glucose and fatty acids yield acetyl CoA. Metabolism of amino acids yields acetyl CoA or actual intermediates of the TCA Cycle. The Citric Acid Cycle provides a pathway for the oxidation of acetyl CoA. The pathway includes eight discrete steps. Seven of the enzyme activities are found in the mitochondrial matrix; the eighth (succinate dehydrogenase) is associated with the Electron Transport Chain (ETC) within the inner mitochondrial membrane.

The following includes key points to remember about the TCA Cycle: i) glucose → 2 acetyl CoA → 2 turns around the TCA Cycle; ii) 2 CO_2 per turn is generated as a waste product which will eventually be blown off in the lungs; iii) one GTP (guanosine triphosphate) per turn is produced by substrate level phosphorylation; one GTP is equivalent to one ATP ($GTP + ADP \rightarrow GDP + ATP$); iv) *reducing equivalents* are <u>hydrogens</u> which are carried by NAD^+ ($\rightarrow$ NADH + H^+) three times per turn and FAD ($\rightarrow$ $FADH_2$) once per turn; these reducing equivalents will eventually be oxidized to produce ATP (*oxidative phosphorylation*) and eventually produce H_2O as a waste product (the last step in the ETC); v) the hydrogens (*H*) which are reducing equivalents are not protons (*H^+*) - quite the contrary! Often the reducing equivalents are simply called electrons.

4.8 Oxidative Phosphorylation

The term oxidative phosphorylation refers to reactions associated with oxygen consumption and the phosphorylation of ADP to yield ATP. Oxidative phosphorylation is associated with an Electron Transport Chain or Respiratory Chain which is found in the inner mitochondrial membrane of eukaryotes. A similar process occurs within the plasma membrane of prokaryotes such as *E.coli.*

The importance of oxidative phosphorylation is that it accounts for the reoxidation of reducing equivalents generated in the reactions of the Krebs Cycle as well as in glycolysis. This process accounts for the preponderance of ATP production in humans. The ETC transfers electrons from reductants (hydrogens) to oxygen in a series of exergonic (exothermic) reactions thus producing H_2O. A schematic summary is in Figure IV.A.4.3.

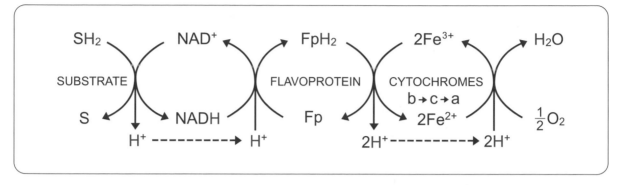

Figure IV.A.4.3: Transport of reducing equivalents through the respiratory chain. Examples of substrates (S) which provide reductants are isocitrate, malate, etc. Cytochromes contain iron (Fe).

4.9 Electron Transport Chain (ETC)

The following are the components of the ETC: iron - sulphur proteins, cytochromes c, b, a and coenzyme Q or *ubiquinone*. The respiratory chain proceeds from NAD-specific dehydrogenases through flavoprotein, ubiquinone, then cytochromes and ultimately molecular oxygen. Reducing equivalents can enter the chain at two locations. Electrons from NADH are transferred to NADH dehydrogenase. In reactions involving iron - sulphur proteins electrons are transferred to coenzyme Q; protons are translocated from the mitochondrial matrix to the exterior of the inner membrane during this process. This creates a proton gradient which is coupled to the production of ATP.

Electrons entering from succinate dehydrogenase ($FADH_2$) are donated directly to coenzyme Q. Electrons are transported from reduced coenzyme Q to cytochrome b and then cytochrome c. Electrons are then carried by cytochrome c to cytochrome a. Cytochrome a is also known as *cytochrome oxidase*. It catalyzes the reaction of electrons and protons with molecular oxygen to produce water. Cyanide is a powerful inhibitor of cytochrome oxidase.

4.10 Summary of Energy Production

Process of reaction	ATP yield
1. Glycolysis (Glucose → 2 Pyruvate)	2
2. Glycolysis (2NADH from glyceraldehyde-3-phosphate dehydrogenase)	6
3. Pyruvate dehydrogenase (2NADH)	6
4. Isocitrate dehydrogenase (2NADH)	6
5. Alpha-ketoglutarate dehydrogenase (2NADH)	6
6. Succinate thiokinase	2
7. Succinate dehydrogenase (2FADH$_2$)	4
8. Malate dehydrogenase (2NADH)	6
TOTAL	38 ATP yield per hexose.

Note the following: i) 1 NADH produces 3 ATP molecules while 1 FADH$_2$ produces only 2 ATP; ii) there is a *cost* of 2 ATP to get the two molecules of NADH generated in the cytoplasm (see the preceding point # 2.) to enter the mitochondrion, thus the *net yield for eukaryotes is 36 ATP*.

The efficiency of ATP production is far from 100%. Energy is lost from the system primarily in the form of heat. Under standard conditions, less than 40% of the energy generated from the complete oxidation of glucose is converted to the production of ATP. As a comparison, a gasoline engine fairs much worse with an efficiency rating generally less than 20%. Further inefficien-

cies reduce the net theoretical yield in the (non-MCAT!) real world.

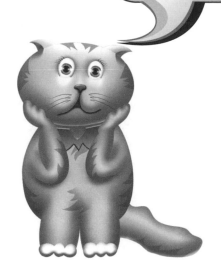

I'm low on energy. What do you mean I can't have a CAT scan and a PET scan ?!!?

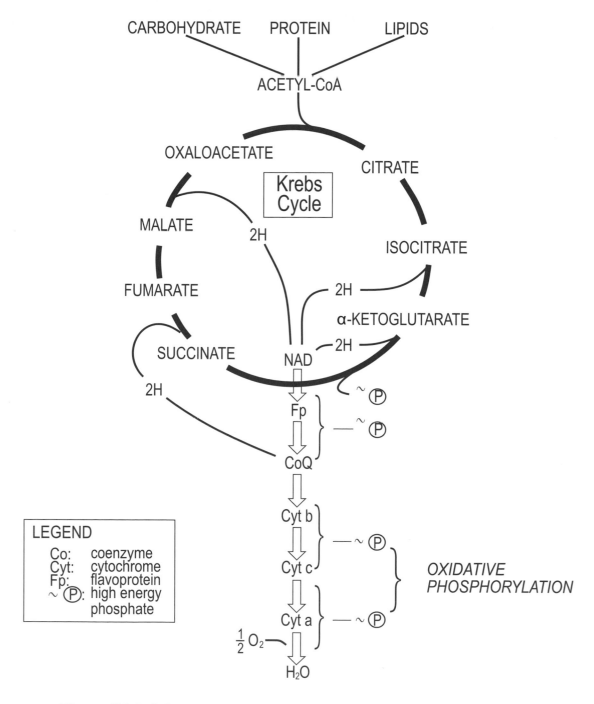

Figure IV.A.4.4: Summary of the Krebs Cycle and the Electron Transport Chain.
Note: Acetyl CoA can be the product of carbohydrate, protein, or lipid metabolism. Thick black arrows represent the Krebs Cycle while white arrows represent the Electron Transport Chain. High energy phosphate groups are transferred from ADP to produce ATP. Ultimately, oxygen accepts electrons and hydrogen from Cyt a to produce water.

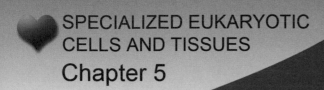
Memorize	Understand	Not Required*
* Neuron: basic structure and function * Reasons for the membrane potential * Structural characteristics of striated, smooth, and cardiac muscle * Sarcomeres: "I" and "A" bands, "M" and "Z" lines, "H" zone * Basic structure/function: epithelial cells, connective tissue cells	* Resting potential: electrochemical gradient/action potential, graph * Excitatory and inhibitory nerve fibers: summation, frequency of firing * Organization of contractile elements: actin and myosin filaments * Cross bridges, sliding filament model; calcium regulation of contraction	* Advanced level college info * Memorizing details about epithelial cells, connective tissue

MCAT-Prep.com

Introduction

To build a living organism, with all the various tissues and organs, cells must specialize. Communication among cells and organs, movement, protection and support are achieved to a great degree by neurons, muscle cells, epithelial cells and the cells of connective tissue, respectively.

Additional Resources

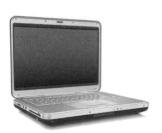

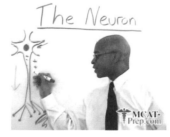

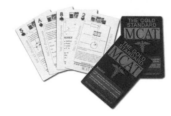

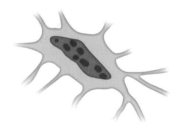

| Free Online Q & A | Video: Online or DVD 2 | Flashcards | Special Guest |

5.1 Neural Cells and Tissues

The brain, spinal cord and peripheral nervous system are composed of nerve tissue. The basic cell types of nerve tissue is the *neuron* and the *glial cell*. Glial cells support and protect neurons and participate in neural activity, nutrition and defense processes. Neurons, which we will examine in detail, conduct and transmit nerve impulses.

Each neuron consists of a nerve cell body (*perikaryon or soma*), and one or more nerve processes (*fibers*). The cell body of a typical neuron contains a nucleus, *Nissl* material which is rough endoplasmic reticulum, free ribosomes, Golgi apparatus, mitochondria, many neurotubules, neurofilaments and pigment inclusions. The cell processes of neurons occur as *axons* and *dendrites*. Dendrites contain most of the components of the cell body except the nucleus and Golgi apparatus whereas axons contain major structures found in dendrites except for the Nissl material. As a rule, dendrites conduct impulses *to* the cell body and ultimately through to the axon. At the synaptic (terminal) ends of axons the presynaptic process contains vesicles from which are elaborated excitatory or inhibitory substances.

The functional dendrites of some neurons, such as the sensory pseudounipolar neurons of spinal nerves, are structurally the

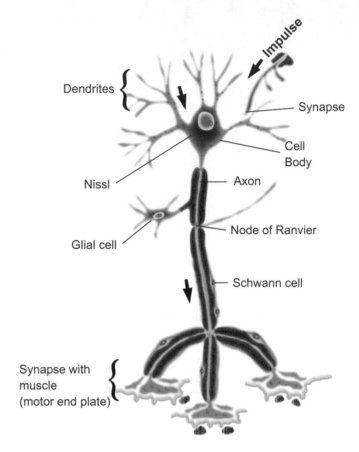

Figure IV.A.5.1: A neuron and other cells of nerve tissue, showing the neuromuscular junction, or motor end plate.

same as axons. **Unmyelinated** fibers in peripheral nerves lie in grooves on the surface of the neurolemma (= plasma membrane) of a type of glial cell (*Schwann cell*). **Myelinated** peripheral neurons are invested by numerous layers of Schwann cell plasma membrane that constitute a *myelin sheath*. There are many Schwann cells along each myelinated fiber. In junctional areas between adjacent Schwann cells there is a lack of myelin. These junctional areas along the myelinated process constitute the nodes of Ranvier.

The neurons of the nervous system are arranged so that each neuron stimulates or inhibits other neurons and these in turn may stimulate or inhibit others until the functions of the nervous system are performed. The area between a neuron and the successive cell (i.e. another neuron, muscle fiber or gland) is called a *synapse*. When a neuron makes a synapse with muscle, it is called a *motor end plate* (*see* Fig. IV.A.5.1). The terminal endings of the nerve filament that synapse with the next cell are called presynaptic terminals, synaptic knobs, or more commonly - synaptic boutons.

At the synapse there is no physical contact between the two cells. The space between the dendrite of one neuron and the axon of another neuron is called the synaptic cleft and it measures about 200 - 300 angstroms (1 angstrom = 10^{-10} m). The chemical mediators which are housed in vesicles at the presynaptic terminal are exocytosed in response to an increase in intracellular calcium (Ca^{2+}) concentration. The mediators or *transmitters* diffuse through the synaptic cleft when an impulse reaches the terminal. This transmitter substance may either excite the *postsynaptic* neuron or inhibit it. They are therefore called either excitatory or inhibitory transmitters (examples include *acetylcholine* and *GABA*, respectively).

5.1.1 The Membrane Potential

A membrane or resting potential (V_m) occurs across the plasma membranes of all cells. In large nerve and muscle cells this potential amounts to about 90 millivolts with positivity outside the cell membrane and negativity inside (V_m = -90 mV). The development of this potential occurs as follows: every cell membrane contains a Na^+ - K^+ ATPase that pumps each ion to where its concentration is highest: Na^+ to the outside of the cell and K^+ to the inside. However, more Na^+ is pumped outward than K^+ inward ($3Na^+$ per $2K^+$). Also, the membrane is relatively permeable to K^+ so that it can leak out of the cell with relative ease. Therefore, the net effect is a loss of positive charges from inside the membrane and a gain of positive charges on the outside. The resulting

membrane potential is the basis of all conduction of impulses by nerve and muscle

fibers.

5.1.2 Action Potential

The action potential is a sequence of changes in the electric potential that occurs within a small fraction of a second when a nerve or muscle membrane impulse spreads over the surface of the cell. Any factor which makes the membrane suddenly permeable over and above a threshold potential (i.e. pinching a nerve fiber) will cause the membrane to become very permeable to sodium ions. As a result, the positive sodium ions on the outside of the membrane now flow rapidly to the more negative interior. Therefore, the membrane potential suddenly becomes reversed with positivity on the inside and negativity on the outside. This state is called *depolarization*.

Once a portion of a nerve fiber is depolarized the mechanisms in the nerve or muscle fiber function to achieve the previous polarity. This is called *repolarization*. The depolarized nerve goes on depolarizing the adjacent nerve membrane in a wavy manner which is called an impulse. In other words, an impulse is a wave of depolarization. The impulse is

fastest in myelinated fibers since the wave of depolarization "jumps" from node to node of Ranvier: this is called *saltatory* conduction.

After depolarization the neuron will pass through three stages in the following order: a) it can no longer depolarize = *absolute refractory period*; b) it can depolarize but with difficulty = *relative refractory period*; c) it returns to its original resting potential and thus can depolarize as easily as it originally did.

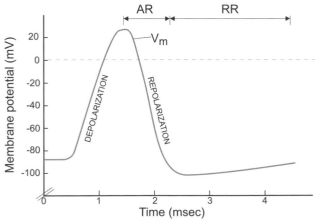

Action Potential: V_m is the membrane voltage or potential, AR is the absolute refractory period, RR is the relative refractory period.

Figure IV.A.5.2: Action potential.

The action potential is an all-or-none event. The magnitude or strength of the action potential is not graded according to the strength of the stimulus. It occurs with the same magnitude each time it occurs, or it does not occur at all.

5.1.3 Action Potential: A Positive Perspective

To better understand the action potential it is useful to take a closer look at what occurs to the positive ions Na^+ and K^+. To begin with, there are protein channels in the plasma membrane that act like gates which guard the passage of specific ions. Some gates open or close in response to V_m and are thus called *voltage gated channels*.

Once a threshold potential is reached, the voltage gated Na^+ channels open allowing the permeability or *conductance* of Na^+ to increase. The Na^+ ions can now diffuse across their chemical gradient: from an area of high concentration (*outside the membrane*) to an area of low concentration (*inside the membrane*). The Na^+ ions will also diffuse across their electrical gradient: from an area of relative positivity (*outside the membrane*) to an area of relative negativity (*inside the membrane*). Thus the inside becomes positive and the membrane is depolarized. Repolarization occurs as the Na^+ channels close and the voltage gated K^+ channels open. As K^+ conductance increases to the outside (where K^+ concentration is lowest), the membrane repolarizes to once again become relatively negative on the inside.

5.2 Contractile Cells and Tissues

There are three types of muscle tissue: smooth, skeletal and cardiac. All three types are composed of muscle cells (fibers) that contain myofibrils possessing contractile filaments of actin and myosin.

Smooth muscle:- Smooth muscle cells are spindle shaped and are organized chiefly into sheets or bands of smooth muscle tissue. This tissue is found in blood vessels and other tubular visceral structures (i.e. intestines). Smooth muscles contain both actin and myosin filaments but actin predominates. The filaments are not organized into patterns that give cross striations as in cardiac and skeletal muscle. Filaments course obliquely in the cells and attach to the plasma membrane.

Skeletal muscle:- Skeletal muscle fibers are characterised by their peripherally located multiple nuclei and striated myofibrils. The cross striations are due to the organization and distribution of actin and myosin filaments. These striations are organized within each muscle fiber into fundamental contractile units called sarcomeres which are joined end to end at the Z-lines. The striations in a sarcomere consists of an A-band (dark) bordered towards the Z-lines by I-bands (light). The mid-region of the A-band contains a variable light H-band that is bisected by an M-line. The light I-band contains actin filaments that insert into the Z-line. The filaments interdigitate and are cross-bridged in the A-band with myosin filaments forming a hexagonal pattern of one myosin filament surrounded by six actin filaments. In the contraction of a muscle fiber a chemical reaction takes place in the region of the cross bridges causing the actin filaments of the I-bands to move deeper into the A-band thus resulting in a shortening of the I-bands.

Each skeletal muscle fiber is invested with a sarcolemma (= plasmalemma = plasma membrane) that extends into the fiber as numerous small transverse tubes called T-tubules. These tubules ring the myofibrils at the A-I junction and are bounded on each side by terminal cisternae of the endoplasmic (*sarcoplasmic*) reticulum. The sarcoplasmic reticulum is involved in catalysing the chemical reaction between the actin and myosin filaments in the region of the cross bridges.

The thin filaments within a myofibril are composed of actin and to a lesser degree two smaller proteins: *troponin and tropomyosin*. In muscle contraction, calcium is elaborated by the sarcoplasmic reticulum and attaches to a subunit of troponin resulting in the movement of tropomyosin and the uncovering of the active sites for the attachment of actin to the cross bridging heads of myosin. Due to this attachment, ATP in the

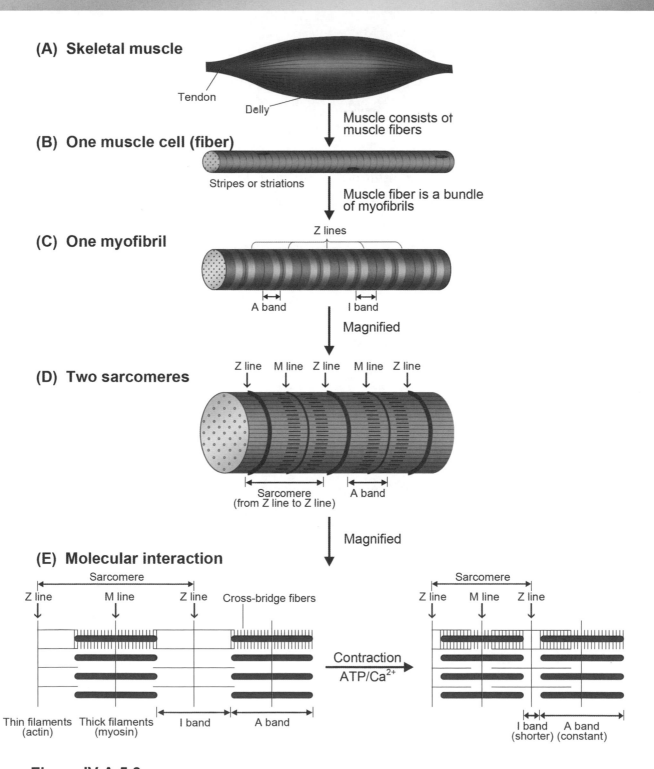

(A) Skeletal muscle

Tendon

Delly

Muscle consists of muscle fibers

(B) One muscle cell (fiber)

Stripes or striations

Muscle fiber is a bundle of myofibrils

(C) One myofibril

Z lines

A band   I band

Magnified

(D) Two sarcomeres

Z line   M line   Z line   M line   Z line

Sarcomere (from Z line to Z line)   A band

Magnified

(E) Molecular interaction

Sarcomere

Z line   M line   Z line   Cross-bridge fibers

Contraction
ATP/Ca^{2+}

Sarcomere

Z line   M line   Z line

Thin filaments (actin)   Thick filaments (myosin)   I band   A band

I band (shorter)   A band (constant)

Figure IV.A.5.3: A schematic view of the molecular basis for muscle contraction. Note: the "H zone" is the central portion of an A band and is characterized by the presence of myosin filaments.

myosin head hydrolyses, producing energy, P_i and ADP which results in a bending of the myosin head and a pulling of the actin filament into the A-band. These actin - myosin bridges detach when myosin binds a new ATP molecule and when calcium returns to the terminal cisternae at the conclusion of neural stimulation.

There are three interesting consequences to the preceding:

i) neither actin nor myosin change length during muscle contraction; rather, shortening of the muscle fiber occurs as the filaments slide over each other increasing the area of overlap.

ii) initially a dead person is very stiff (*rigor mortis*) since they can no longer produce the ATP necessary to detach the actin-myosin bridges thus their muscles remain locked in position.

iii) Ca^{2+} is a critical ion both for muscle contraction and for transmitter release from presynaptic neurons.

Cardiac muscle:- Cardiac muscle contains striations and myofibrils that are similar to those of skeletal muscle. It differs from skeletal muscle in several major ways. Cardiac muscle fibers branch and contain centrally located nuclei (characteristically, one nucleus per cell) and large numbers of mitochondria. Individual cardiac muscle cells are attached to each other at their ends by *intercalated disks*. These disks contain several types of membrane junctional complexes, the most important of which is the *gap junction*.

The gap junction electrically couples one cell to its neighbor (= *syncytium*) so that electric depolarization is propagated throughout the heart by cell-to-cell contact rather than by nerve innervation to each cell. The sarcoplasmic reticulum - T-tubule system is arranged differently in cardiac muscle than in skeletal muscle. In cardiac muscle each T-tubule enters at the Z-line and forms a diad with only one terminal cisterna of sarcoplasmic reticulum.

5.3 Epithelial Cells and Tissues

Epithelia have the following characteristics:

1) they cover all body surfaces (i.e. skin, organs, etc.)

2) they are the principal tissues of glands

3) their cells are anchored by a non-living layer (= the *basement membrane*)

4) they lack blood vessels and are thus nourished by diffusion.

Epithelial tissues are classified according to the characteristics of their cells. Tissues with elongated cells are called *colum-nar*, those with thin flattened cells are *squamous*, and those with cube-like cells are *cuboidal*. They are further classified as **simple** if they have a single layer of cells and **stratified** if they have multiple layers of cells. As examples of the classification, skin is composed of a stratified squamous epithelium while various glands (i.e. thyroid, salivary, etc.) contain a simple cuboidal epithelium. The former epithelium serves to protect against microorganisms, loss of water or heat, while the latter epithelium functions to secrete glandular products.

5.4 Connective Cells and Tissues

Connective tissue connects and joins other body tissue and parts. It also carries substances for processing, nutrition, and waste release. Connective tissue is characterized by the presence of relatively few cells surrounded by an extensive network of material which is intercellular (*between cells*).

The adult connective tissues are: connective tissue proper, cartilage, bone and blood (see *The Circulatory System*, section 7.5). Connective tissue proper is further classified into loose irregular connective tissue and dense irregular connective tissue. These tissues contain cells and a preponderance of intercellular fibers and ground substance.

5.4.1 Loose Irregular Connective Tissue

Loose connective tissue is found in the superficial and deep *fascia*. It is generally considered as the *packaging material* of the body. Fascia helps to bind skin to underlying organs, to fill spaces between muscles, etc. Loose connective tissue contains most of the cell types and all the fiber types found in the other connective tissues. The most common cell types are the fibroblast, macrophage, adipose cell, mast cell, plasma cell and wandering cells from the blood (which include several types of white blood cells).

Fibroblasts contain the organelles that permit them to produce all of the fiber types and the intercellular material.

Macrophages are part of the *reticuloendothelial system* (tissue which predominately destroys foreign particles). They possess large lysosomes containing digestive enzymes which are necessary for the digestion of phagocytosed materials. Mast cells occur mostly along blood vessels and contain granules which contain *heparin* and *histamine*.

Heparin is a compound which prevents blood clotting while histamine is associated with allergic reactions. Plasma cells are part of the immune system in that they produce circulatory antibodies. They contain extensive amounts of rough endoplasmic reticulum (rER). Adipose cells are found in varying quantities, when they predominate, the tissue is called adipose (fat) tissue.

Collagenous reticular and elastic fibers are irregularly distributed in loose connective tissue. **Collagenous fibers** are usually found in bundles and provide **strength** to the tissue. Many different types of collagen are identified on the basis of their molecular structure.

Of the five most common types, collagen type I is the most abundant, being found in dermis, bone, dentine, tendons, organ capsules, fascia and sclera. Type II is located in hyaline and elastic cartilage. Type III is probably the collagenous component of reticular fibers. Type IV is found in a specific part (*the basal lamina*) of basement membranes. Type V is a component of placental basement membranes. **Reticular fibers** are smaller, more delicate fibers that form the basic framework of reticular connective tissue. **Elastic fibers** branch and provide elasticity and support to connective tissue.

Ground substance is the gelatinous material that fills most of the space between the cells and the fibers. It is composed of acid mucopolysaccharides and structural glycoproteins and its properties are important in determining the permeability and consistency of the connective tissue.

5.4.2 Dense Connective Tissue

Dense irregular connective tissue is found in the dermis, periosteum, perichondrium and capsules of some organs. All of the fiber types are present, but collagenous fibers predominate. Dense irregular connective tissue occurs as aponeuroses, ligaments and tendons. In most ligaments and tendons collagenous fibers are most prevalent and are oriented parallel to each other. Fibroblasts are practically the only cell type present.

5.4.3 Cartilage

Cartilage is composed of chondrocytes (= cartilage cells) embedded in an intercellular (= extracellular) matrix, consisting of fibers and an amorphous firm ground substance. In cases of injury, cartilage repairs slowly since it has no direct blood supply. Three types of cartilage are distinguished on the basis of the amount of ground substance and the relative abundance of collagenous and elastic fibers. They are hyaline, elastic and fibrous cartilage.

Hyaline Cartilage is found as costal (rib) cartilage, articular cartilage and cartilage of the nose, larynx, trachea and bronchi. The extracellular matrix consists primarily of collagenous fibers and a ground substance rich in chondromucoprotein, a copolymer of a protein and chondroitin sulphates.

Elastic Cartilage is found in the pinna of the ear, auditory tube and cartilage of the larynx. Elastic fibers predominate and thus provide greater flexibility. Calcification of this type of cartilage is rare.

Fibrous Cartilage occurs in the anchorage of tendons and ligaments, in intervertebral disks, in the symphysis pubis, and in some interarticular disks and in some ligaments. Chondrocytes occur singly or in rows between large bundles of collagenous fibers. Compared with hyaline cartilage, only small amounts of hyaline matrix surround the chondrocytes of fibrous cartilage.

5.4.4 Bone

Bone tissue consists of three **cell types** and an **extracellular matrix** that contains organic and inorganic components. The three cell types are: *osteocytes* which are embedded in cavities (lacunae) within the matrix; *osteoblasts* which synthesize the organic components of the matrix; and *osteoclasts* which help to resorb and remodel bone.

The organic matrix consists of dense collagenous fibers and an osteomucoid substance containing chondroitin sulphate which is important in providing flexibility and tensile strength to bone. The inorganic component is responsible for the *rigidity* of the bone and is composed chiefly of calcium phosphate and calcium carbonate with small amounts of magnesium, fluoride, hydroxide, sulphate and hydroxyapatite.

Compact bone contains haversian systems (osteons), interstitial lamellae and circumferential lamellae. Lamellae are usually a concentric deposit (*circumferential*) of bone matrix around tiny tubes called Haversian canals. Haversian systems are the structural units for bone. Haversian systems consist of extensively branching haversian canals that are oriented chiefly longitudinally in long bones. Each canal contains blood vessels and is surrounded by 8 to 15 concentric lamellae and osteocytes.

Nutrients from blood vessels in the haversian canals pass through canaliculi and lacunae to reach all osteocytes in the system. Volkmann's canals traverse the bone transversely and interconnect the haversian systems. They enter through the outer circumferential lamellae and carry blood vessels and nerves which are continuous with those of the haversian canals and the periosteum. The periosteum is the connective tissue layer which envelopes bone.

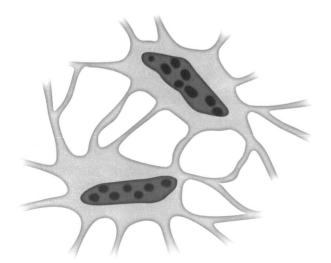

Figure IV.A.5.4: Osteocytes.

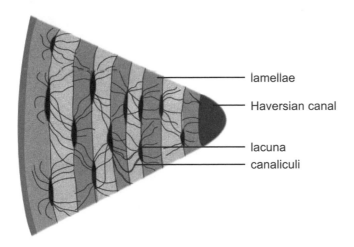

Figure IV.A.5.5: Schematic drawing of part of a haversian system.

Bones are supplied by a loop of blood vessels that enter from the periosteal region, penetrate the cortical bone, and enter the medulla before returning to the periphery of the bone. Long bones are specifically supplied by arteries which pass to the marrow through diaphyseal, metaphyseal and epiphyseal arteries.

Bone undergoes extensive remodelling, and harvesian systems may break down or be resorbed in order that calcium can be made available to other parts of the body. Bone resorption occurs by osteocytes engaging in osteolysis or by osteoclastic activity.

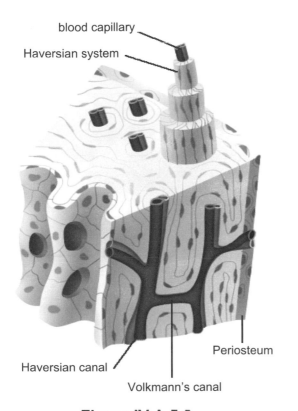

Figure IV.A.5.6
Schematic drawing of the wall of a long bone.

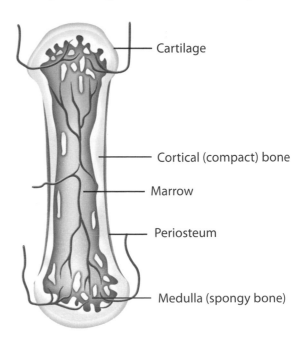

Figure IV.A.5.7
Schematic drawing of adult bone structure.

Memorize	Understand	Not Required*
* Nervous system: basic structure, major functions * Basic sensory reception and processing * Basic ear, eye: structure and function * Define: endocrine gland, hormone * Major endocrine glands: names, locations, major hormones	* Organization of the nervous system; sensor and effector neurons * Feedback loop, reflex arc: role of spinal cord, brain * Endocrine system: specific chemical control at cell, tissue, and organ level * Cellular mechanisms of hormone action, transport of hormones * Integration with nervous system: feedback control	* Advanced level college info * Memorizing all cranial nerves (just memorize vagus) * Details regarding ear, eye: structure and function * Details regarding endocrine glands: names

MCAT-Prep.com

Introduction

The nervous and endocrine systems are composed of a network of highly specialized cells that can communicate information about an organism's surroundings and itself. Thus together, these two systems can process incoming information and then regulate and coordinate responses in other parts of the body.

Additional Resources

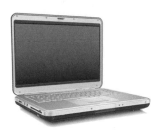

Free Online Q & A

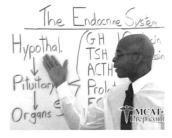

Video: Online or DVD 2

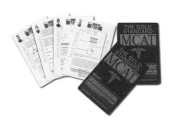

Flashcards

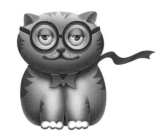

Special Guest

* The real MCAT may have advanced level information presented (ie. in a passage) but previous knowledge of said information is not required to answer the questions that would follow. Practice AAMC and GS practice MCAT CBTs can help you clarify this point.

6.1 Organisation of the Vertebrate Nervous System

The role of the nervous system is to control and coordinate body activities in a rapid and precise mode of action. The nervous system is composed of central and peripheral nervous systems.

The **central nervous system** (CNS) is enclosed within the cranium (skull) and vertebral (spinal) canal and consists respectively of the brain and spinal cord. The **peripheral nervous system** (PNS) is outside the bony encasement and is composed of peripheral nerves, which are branches or continuations of the spinal or cranial nerves. The PNS can be divided into the **somatic nervous system** and the **autonomic nervous system** which are *anatomically* a portion of both the central and peripheral nervous systems. As a rule, a collection of nerve cell bodies in the CNS is called a *nucleus* and outside the CNS it is called a *ganglion*.

The spinal cord is a long cylindrical structure whose hollow core is called the *central canal*. The central canal is surrounded by a gray matter which is in turn surrounded by a white matter (the reverse is true for the brain: outer gray matter and inner white matter). Basically, the gray matter consists of the cell bodies of neurons whereas the white matter consists of the nerve fibers (axons and dendrites). There are 31 pairs of spinal nerves each leaving the spinal cord at various levels: 8 cervical (neck), 12 thoracic (chest), 5 lumbar (abdomen), 5 sacral and 1 coccygeal (these latter 6 are from the pelvic region). The lower end of the spinal cord is cone shaped and is called the *conus medullaris*.

The brain can be divided into three main regions: the forebrain which contains the telencephalon and the diencephalon; the midbrain; and the hindbrain which contains the cerebellum, the pons and the medulla. The **brain stem** includes the latter two structures and the midbrain.

The telencephalon is the **cerebral hemispheres** (cerebrum) which contain an outer surface (cortex) of gray matter. Its function is in higher order processes (i.e. learning, memory, emotions, voluntary motor activity, processing sensory input, etc.). For most people, the *left* hemisphere specializes in *language*, while the right hemisphere specializes in patterns and spatial relationships. Each hemisphere is subdivided into four lobes: *occipital* which receives input from the optic nerve for vision; *temporal* which receives auditory signals for hearing; *parietal* which receives somatosensory information from the opposite side of the body (= heat, cold, touch, pain, and the sense of body movement); and *frontal* which is involved in problem solving and controls voluntary movements for the opposite side of the body.

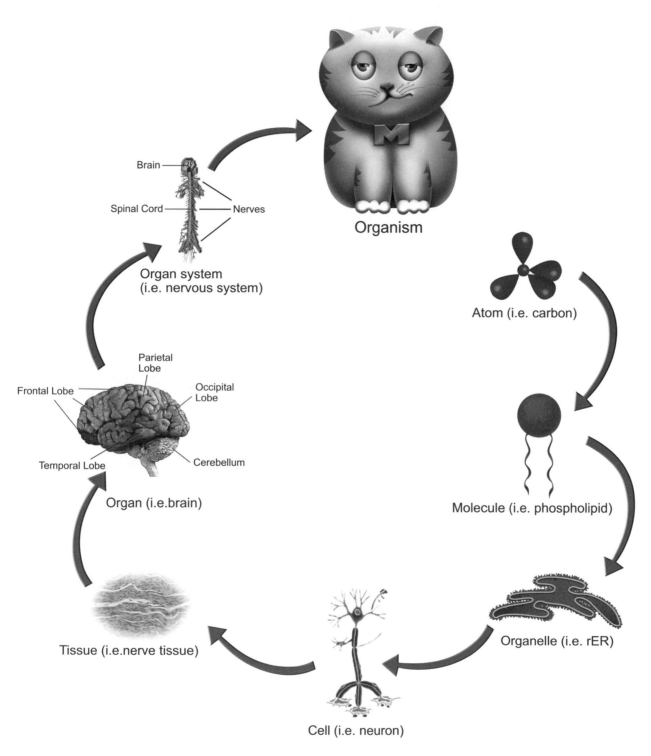

Figure IV.A.6.0: Levels of organization.

The diencephalon contains the **thalamus** which is a relay center for sensory input, and the **hypothalamus** which is crucial for homeostatic controls (heart rate, body temperature, thirst, sex drive, hunger, etc.). Protruding from its base and greatly influenced by the hypothalamus is the **pituitary** which is an endocrine gland. The limbic system, which functions to produce emotions, is composed of the diencephalon and deep structures of the cerebrum (esp. basal ganglia). The **cerebellum** plays an important role in coordination and the control of muscle tone. The **medulla** contains many vital centers (i.e. for breathing, heart rate, arteriole blood pressure, etc.).

There are 12 pairs of cranial nerves which emerge from the base of the brain (esp. the brain stem): *olfactory* (I) for smell; *optic* (II) for vision; *oculomotor* (III), *trochlear* (IV) and *abducens* (VI) for eye movements; *trigeminal* (V) for motor (i.e. *mastication*

which is chewing) and sensory activities (i.e. pain, temperature, and pressure for the head and face); *facial* (VII) for taste (sensory) and facial expression (motor); *vestibulo-cochlear* (VIII) for the senses of equilibrium (vestibular branch) and hearing (cochlear branch); *glosso-pharyngeal* (IX) for taste and swallowing; *vagus (X)* for speech, swallowing, slowing the heart rate, and many sensory and motor innervations to smooth muscles of the viscera (internal organs) of the thorax and abdomen; *accessory* (XI) for head rotation and shoulder movement; and *hypoglossal* (XII) for tongue movement.

Both the brain and the spinal cord are surrounded by three membranes (= meninges). The outermost covering is called the dura mater, the innermost is called the pia mater (which is in direct contact with nervous tissue), while the middle layer is called the arachnoid mater. {DAP = **d**ura - **a**rachnoid - **p**ia, repectively, from out to in}

6.1.1 The Sensory Receptors

The sensory receptors include any type of nerve ending in the body that can be stimulated by some physical or chemical stimulus either outside or within the body. These receptors include the rods and cones of the eye, the cochlear nerve endings of the ear, the taste endings of the mouth, the olfactory endings in the nose, sensory nerve endings in the skin, etc. Afferent neurons carry sense signals to the central nervous system.

6.1.2 The Effector Receptors

These include every organ that can be stimulated by nerve impulses. An important effetor system is skeletal muscle. Smooth muscles of the body and the glandular cells are among the important effector organs. Efferent neurons carry motor signals from the CNS to effector receptors.

6.1.3 Reflex Arc

One basic means by which the nervous system controls the functions in the body is the reflex arc, in which a stimulus excites a receptor, appropriate impulses are transmitted into the CNS where various nervous reactions take place, and then appropriate effector impulses are transmitted to an effector organ to cause a reflex effect (i.e. removal of one's hand from a hot object, the knee jerk reflex, etc.). The preceding can be processed at the level of the spinal cord.

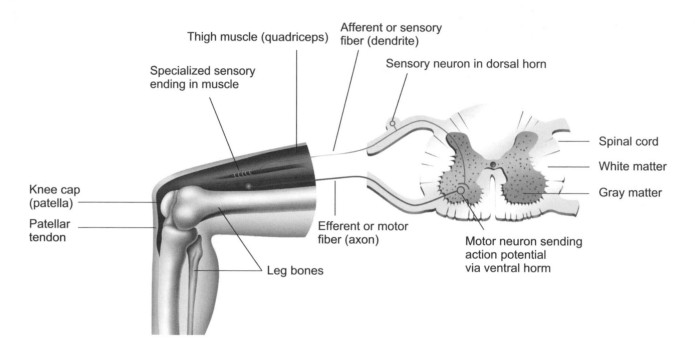

Figure IV.A.6.1: Schematic representation of the basis of the knee jerk reflex.

6.1.4 Autonomic Nervous System

While the Somatic Nervous System controls voluntary activities (i.e. innervates skeletal muscle), the Autonomic Nervous System (ANS) controls involuntary activities. The ANS consists of two components which often antagonize each other: the sympathetic and parasympathetic nervous systems.

The **Sympathetic Nervous System** originates in neurons located in the lateral horns of the gray matter of the spinal cord. Nerve fibers pass by way of anterior (ventral)

nerve roots first into the spinal nerves and then immediately into the sympathetic chain. From here fiber pathways are transmitted to all portions of the body, especially to the different visceral organs and to the blood vessels.

This division of the nervous system is crucial in the "fight, fright, or flight" responses (i.e. pupillary dilation, increase in breathing and heart rates, increase of blood flow to skeletal muscle, etc.).

Parasympathetic Nervous System: The parasympathetic fibers pass mainly through the *vagus nerves*, though a few fibers pass through several of the other cranial nerves and through the anterior roots of the sacral segments of the spinal cord. Parasympathetic fibers do not spread as extensively through the body as do sympathetic fibers, but they do innervate some of the thoracic and abdominal organs, as well as the pupillary sphincter and ciliary muscles of the eye and the salivary glands.

This division of the nervous system is crucial for "vegetative" responses (i.e. pupillary constriction, decrease in breathing and heart rates, increase in blood flow to the gastro-intestinal tract, etc.).

6.1.5 Autonomic Nerve Fibers

The nerve fibers from the ANS are primarily motor fibers. Unlike the motor pathways of the somatic nervous system, which usually include a single neuron between the CNS and an effector, those of the ANS involve *two* neurons. The first neuron has its cell body in the brain or spinal cord but its axon (= *preganglionic fiber*) extends outside of the CNS. The axon synapses with the cell body of a second neuron in an autonomic ganglion (*recall: a ganglion is a collection of nerve cell bodies outside the CNS*). The axon of the second neuron (= *postganglionic fiber*) extends to a visceral effector.

The sympathetic ganglia form chains which, for example, may extend longitudinally along each side of the vertebral column. Conversely, the parasympathetic ganglia are located *near* or *within* various visceral organs (i.e. bladder, intestine, etc.) thus requiring relatively short postganglionic fibers.

Both divisions of the ANS secrete *acetylcholine* from their preganglionic fibers. Most sympathetic postganglionic fibers secrete *norepinephrine* (= nor*adren*alin), and for this reason they are called **adren**ergic fibers. The parasympathetic postganglionic fibers secrete acetyl**choline** and are called ***cholinergic fibers.***

6.2 Sensory Reception and Processing

Each modality of sensation is detected by a particular nerve ending. The most common nerve ending is the free nerve ending. Different types of free nerve endings result in different types of sensations such as pain, warmth, pressure, touch, etc. In addition to free nerve endings, skin contains a number of specialized endings that are adapted to respond to some specific type of physical stimulus.

Sensory endings deep in the body are capable of detecting *proprioceptive sensations* such as joint receptors, which detect the degree of angulation of a joint, Golgi tendon organs which detect the degree of tension in the tendons, and muscle spindles which detect the degree of stretch of a muscle fiber.

6.2.1 Olfaction

Olfaction (the sense of smell) is perceived by the brain following the stimulation of the olfactory epithelium located in the nostrils. The olfactory epithelium contain large numbers of neurons with chemoreceptors called *olfactory cells* which are responsible for the detection of different types of smell. It is believed that there might be seven or more primary sensations of smell which combine to give various types of smell that we perceive in life.

6.2.2 Taste

Taste buds in combination with olfaction give humans the taste sensation. Taste buds are primarily located on the surface of the tongue with smaller numbers found in the roof of the mouth and the walls of the pharynx (throat). Taste buds contain chemoreceptors which are activated once the chemical is dissolved in saliva which is secreted by the salivary glands.

Four different types of taste buds are known to exist, each of these responding principally to saltiness, sweetness, sourness and bitterness.

When a stimulus is received by either a taste bud or an olfactory cell for the second time, the intensity of the response is diminished. This is called *sensory adaptation*.

6.2.3 Ears: Structure and Function

Ears function in both hearing and balance. The external ear is composed of the external cartilaginous portion, the pinna or *auricle*, and the external auditory meatus or canal. The external auditory meatus connects the auricle and the middle ear or *tympanic cavity*. The tympanic cavity is bordered on the outside by the tympanic membrane, and inside the air-filled cavity are the <u>auditory ossicles</u> - the *malleus* (hammer), *incus* (anvil), and *stapes* (stirrup). The stapes is held by ligaments to a part of inner ear called the *oval window*.

The inner ear or *labyrinth* consists of an osseous labyrinth containing a membranous labyrinth. Three semicircular canals, which are oriented at right angles to each other, and the cochlea are the important structures of the inner ear. The semicircular canals function in providing a sense of equilibrium (balance).

The eustachian tube connects the middle ear to the pharynx. This tube is important in maintaining equal pressure on both sides of the tympanic membrane.

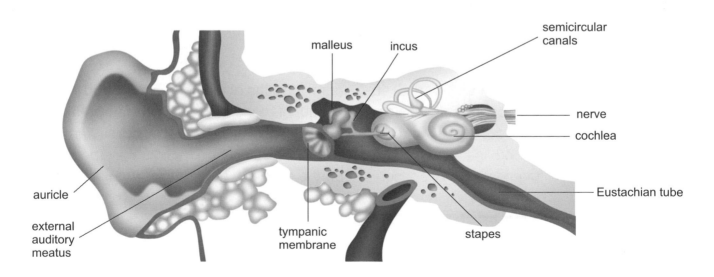

Figure IV.A.6.2: Structure of the external, middle and inner ear.

Mechanism of hearing: Sound is caused by compression of waves that travel through the air. Each compression wave is funneled by the external ear to strike the tympanic membrane (ear drum). Thus the sound vibrations are transmitted through the osseous system which consists of three tiny bones (the malleus, incus, and stapes) into the cochlea at the oval window. The sound waves then travel through the lymph of the cochlea and stimulate the hairy cells found in the **basilar membrane** which is called the *organ of Corti*. From here the auditory nerves carry the impulses to the auditory area of the brain (*temporal lobe*) where it is interpreted as sound.

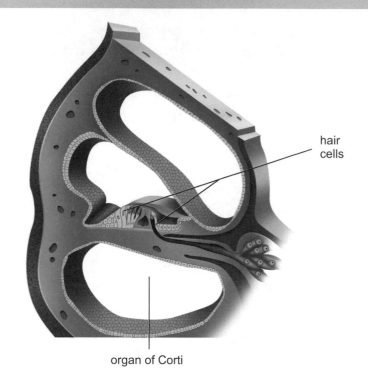

hair cells

organ of Corti

Figure IV.A.6.3: Cross-section of the cochlea.

6.2.4 Vision: Eye Structure and Function

The eyeball consists of three layers: i) an outer fibrous tunic composed of the sclera and cornea; ii) a vascular coat (*uvea*) of choroid, the ciliary body and iris; and iii) the retina formed of pigment and sensory (nervous) layers. The anterior chamber lies between the cornea anteriorly (in front) and the iris and pupil posteriorly (behind); the posterior chamber lies between the iris anteriorly and the ciliary processes and the lens posteriorly.

The cornea constitutes the anterior one sixth of the eye. The sclera forms the posterior five sixths of the fibrous tunic and is composed of dense fibrous connective tissue. The choroid layer consists of vascular loose connective tissue. The lens can focus light on the retina by the contraction or relaxation of muscles in the ciliary body which transmit tension along *suspensory ligaments* to the lens. The iris helps to control the intensity of light impinging on the retina by alternating the diameter of the pupil.

The retina is divisible into ten layers. Layers two to five contain the rod and cone receptors of the light pathway.

Rods and Cones: The light sensitive receptors (*photoreceptors*) of the retina are millions of minute cells called rods and cones. The rods ("*night vision*") distinguish only the black and white aspects of an image while the cones ("*day vision*") are capable of distinguishing three colors: red, green and blue. From different combinations of these three colors, all colors can be seen.

Photoreceptors contain photosensitive pigments. For example, rods contain the membrane protein *rhodopsin* which is covalently linked to a form of vitamin A. Light causes an isomerization of the pigment which can affect Na^+ channels in a manner as to start an action potential.

The central portion of the retina which is called the *fovea centralis* has only cones, which allows this portion to have very sharp vision, while the peripheral areas, which contain progressively more and more rods, have progressively more diffuse vision.

Each point of the retina connects with a discrete point in the visual cortex which is in the back of the brain (i.e. the *occipital lobe*). The image that is formed on the retina is upside down and reversed from left to right. This information leaves the eye via the optic nerve en route to the visual cortex which corrects the image.

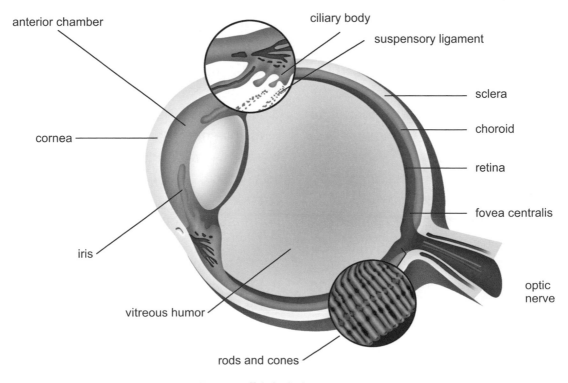

Figure IV.A.6.4: Structure of the eye.

Defects of vision

1. **Myopia** (short-sighted or nearsighted): In this condition, an image is formed in front of the retina because the lens converges light too much since the eyeballs are long. A diverging (concave) lens helps focus the image on the retina and it is used for the correction of myopia.

2. **Hyperopia** (long-sighted or farsighted): In this condition, an image is formed behind the retina since the eyeballs are too short. A converging (convex) lens helps focus the image on the retina.

3. **Astigmatism**: In this condition, the curvatures of either the cornea or the lens are different at different angles. A cylindrical lens helps to improve this condition.

4. **Presbyopia**: This condition is characterized by the inability to focus (especially objects which are closer). This condition, which is often seen in the elderly, is corrected by using a converging lens.

6.3 Endocrine Systems

The endocrine system is the set of glands, tissues and cells that secrete hormones directly into bodily fluids (usu. blood). The hormones are transported by the blood system, sometimes bound to plasma proteins, en route to having an effect on the cells of a target organ. Hormones control many of the body's functions. Hormones function in three major ways:

1. By controlling transport of substances through cell membranes

2. By controlling the activity of some of the specific genes, which in turn determine the formation of specific enzymes

3. By controlling directly some metabolic systems of cells.

Steroid hormones can diffuse across the plasma membrane thus they tend to have a direct intracellular effect (i.e. on DNA; ORG 12.4.1). Non-steroid hormones do not diffuse across the membrane. They tend to bind plasma membrane receptors which increase intracellular *cyclic AMP* concentration which, in turn, brings about cellular changes which are recognized as the hormone's actions.

Of the following hormones, if there is no mention as to its chemical nature, then it is a non-steroidal hormone (i.e. protein, polypeptide, etc.).

6.3.1 Pituitary Hormones

The **pituitary gland** secretes hormones that regulate a wide variety of functions in the body. This gland is divided into two major divisions: the *anterior* and the *posterior* pituitary gland. Six hormones are secreted by the anterior pituitary gland whereas two hormones are secreted by the posterior gland. The **hypothalamus** influences the secretion of hormones from both parts of the pituitary in different ways: i) it secretes specific *releasing factors* into special blood vessels (*a portal system*) which carries these factors (hormones) which affect the cells in the anterior pituitary; ii) the hypothalamus contains neurosecretory cells that secrete their products (esp. the two hormones oxytocin and vasopressin) directly <u>into</u> the posterior pituitary where they can be released.

The hormones secreted by the anterior pituitary gland are as follows:

1. Growth hormone (GH)
2. Thyroid Stimulating Hormone (TSH)
3. Adrenocorticotropic hormone (ACTH)
4. Prolactin
5. Follicle Stimulating Hormone (FSH) or Interstitial Cell Stimulating Hormone (ICSH)

6. Luteinizing Hormone (LH)

[N.B. these latter two hormones will be discussed in the section on "Reproduction"]

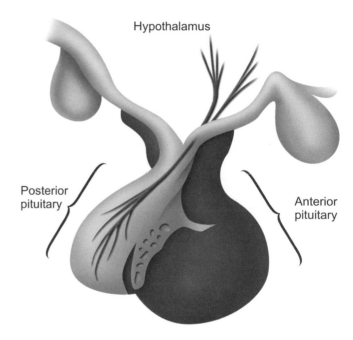

Figure IV.A.6.5: The pituitary gland.

The hormones secreted by the posterior pituitary are:

1. Vasopressin or Anti-diuretic Hormone (ADH)
2. Oxytocin

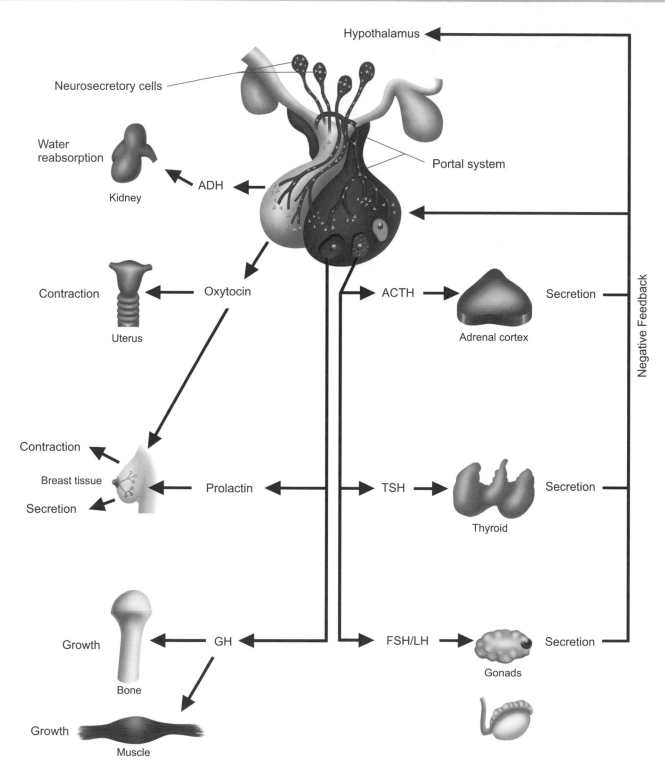

Figure IV.A.6.6: Pituitary hormones and their target organs.

The Adrenal Medulla

The **adrenal medulla** synthesizes epinephrine (= *adrenal*ine) and norepineph-rine which: i) are non-steroidal stimulants of the sympathetic nervous system and ii) raise blood glucose concentrations.

6.3.3 Thyroid Hormones

The thyroid gland is located anteriorly in the neck and is composed of follicles lined with thyroid glandular cells. These cells secrete a glycoprotein called *thyroglobulin*. Thyroxine, which is a thyroid hormone, is formed within the thyroglobulin molecule. The rate of synthesis of thyroid hormone is influenced by TSH from the pituitary.

Once thyroid hormones have been released into the blood stream they combine with several different plasma proteins. Then they are released into the cells from the blood stream. They increase the rate of synthesis of proteins in most cells. They also increase the size and numbers of mitochondria and these in turn increase the rate of production of ATP, which is a factor that promotes cellular metabolism.

Hyperthyroidism is an excess of thyroid hormone secretion above that needed for normal function. Basically, an increased rate of metabolism throughout the body is observed.

Hypothyroidism is an inadequate amount of thyroid hormone secreted into the blood stream. Generally it slows down the metabolic rate and enhances the collection of mucinous fluid in the tissue spaces, creating an edematous (fluid filled) state called myxedema.

The thyroid and parathyroid glands affect blood calcium concentration in different ways. The thyroid produces *calcitonin* which inhibits osteoclast activity and stimulates osteoblasts to form bone tissue; thus blood $[Ca^{2+}]$ decreases. The parathyroid glands produce parathormone (= parathyroid hormone = PTH), which stimulates osteoclasts to break down bone, thus raising $[Ca^{2+}]$ and $[PO_4^{3-}]$ in the blood.

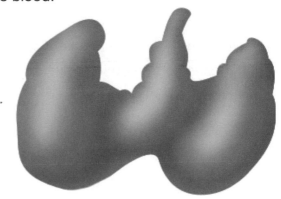

Figure IV.A.6.8: The thyroid gland.

6.3.4 Pancreatic Hormones

The pancreas contains clusters of cells (= *islets of Langerhans*) closely associated with blood vessels. The islets of Langerhans contain alpha cells which secrete *glucagon* and beta cells which secrete *insulin*. Glucagon increases blood glucose concentration by promoting the following events in the liver: the conversion of glycogen to glucose (*glycogenolysis*) and the production of glucose from amino acids (*gluconeogenesis*). Insulin decreases blood glucose by increasing cellular uptake of glucose. A deficiency in insulin results in *diabetes mellitus*.

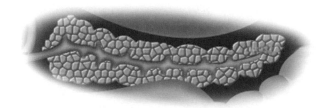

Figure IV.A.6.9: The pancreas.

6.3.5 Kidney Hormones

The kidney produces and secretes *renin, erythropoietin* and it helps in the activation of vitamin D. Renin increases water resorption and blood pressure through the activation of the **Renin-Angiotensin System** which produces angiotensin II from angiotensin I. Angiotensin II acts on the adrenal cortex to increase the synthesis and release of aldosterone <u>and</u> it constricts blood vessels. Erythropoietin increases the production of *erythro-* cytes by acting on red bone marrow. Vitamin D is a steroid which is critical for the proper absorption of calcium from the small intestine; thus it is essential for the normal growth and development of bone and teeth. Vitamin D can either be ingested or produced from a precursor by the activity of ultraviolet light on skin cells. It must be further activated in the liver and kidney by hydroxylation.

6.3.6 A Negative Feedback Loop

In order to maintain the internal environment of the body in equilibrium (= *homeostasis*), our hormones engage in various negative feedback loops.

For example, if the body is exposed to extreme cold, the hypothalamus will activate systems to conserve heat (see *Skin as an Organ System*, BIO 13.1) and to produce heat. Heat production can be attained by increasing the basal metabolic rate. To achieve this, the hypothalamus secretes a releasing factor (thyrotropin releasing factor - TRF) which stimulates the anterior pituitary to secrete TSH. Thus the thyroid gland is stimulated to secrete the thyroid hormones.

Body temperature begins to return to normal. The high levels of circulating thyroid hormones begin to *inhibit* the production of TRF and TSH (= *negative feedback*) which in turn ensures the reduction in the levels of the thyroid hormones. Thus homeostasis is maintained.

Memorize	Understand	Not Required*
* Circ. and lymphatic systems: basic structures and functions * Composition of blood, lymph, purpose of lymph nodes * RBC production and destruction; spleen, bone marrow * Basics: coagulation, clotting mechanisms	* Circ: structure/function; 4 chambered heart: systolic/diastolic pressure * Oxygen transport; hemoglobin, oxygen content/affinity * Substances transported by blood, lymph * Source of lymph: diffusion from capillaries by differential pressure	* Advanced level college info * Memorizing names of small to medium arteries, veins * Circulatory systems in other vertebrates * Memorizing Starling's equation

MCAT-Prep.com

Introduction

The circulatory system is concerned with the movement of nutrients, gases and wastes to and from cells. The circulatory or cardiovascular system (closed) distributes blood while the lymphatic system (open) distributes lymph.

Additional Resources

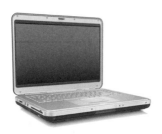

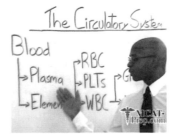

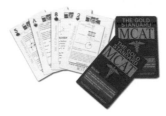

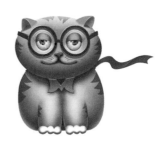

| Free Online Q & A | Video: Online or DVD 3 | Flashcards | Special Guest |

7.1 Generalities

The circulatory system is composed of the heart, blood, and blood vessels. The heart (which acts like a pump) and its blood vessels (which act like a closed system of ducts) are called the *cardiovascular system* which moves the blood throughout the body. The following represents some important functions of blood within the circulatory system.

* It transports:
- hormones from endocrine glands to target tissues
- molecules and cells which are components of the immune system

- nutrients from the digestive tract (usu. to the liver)
- oxygen from the respiratory system to body cells
- waste from the body cells to the respiratory and excretory systems.

* It aids in temperature control (*thermoregulation*) by:
- distributing heat from skeletal muscle and other active organs to the rest of the body
- being directed to or away from the skin depending on whether or not the body wants to release or conserve heat, respectively.

7.2 The Heart

The heart is a muscular, cone-shaped organ about the size of a fist. The heart contains four chambers: two thick muscular walled *ventricles* and two thinner walled *atria*. An inner wall or *septum* separates the heart (and therefore the preceding chambers) into left and right sides. The atria contract or *pump* blood more or less simultaneously and so do the ventricles.

Deoxygenated blood returning to the heart from all body tissues except the lungs (= *systemic circulation*) enters the right atrium through large veins (= *venae cavae*). The blood is then pumped into the right ventricle through the tricuspid valve (which is one of

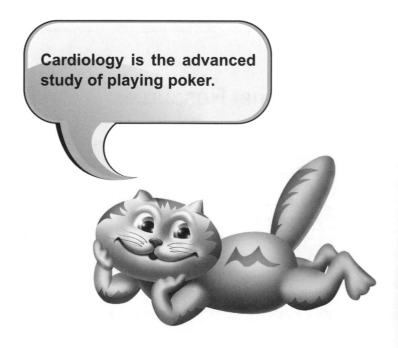

Cardiology is the advanced study of playing poker.

many one-way valves in the cardiovascular system). Next the blood is pumped to the lungs (= *pulmonary circulation*) through semilunar valves and pulmonary arteries {remember: blood in <u>ar</u>teries goes <u>a</u>way from the heart}.

The blood loses CO_2 and is **oxygenated** in the lungs and returns through pulmonary veins to the left atrium. Now the blood is pumped through the mitral (= bicuspid) valve into the largest chamber of the heart: the left

ventricle. This ventricle's task is to return blood into the systemic circulation by pumping into a huge artery: the *aorta* (its valve is the aortic valve).

The mitral (= <u>bi</u>cuspid = <u>2</u> leaflets) and tricuspid (<u>tri</u> = <u>3</u> leaflets) valves are prevented from everting into the atria by strong fibrous cords (*chordae tendineae*) which are attached to small mounds of muscle (*papillary muscles*) in their respective ventricles. A major cause of heart murmurs is the inadequate functioning of these valves.

7.3 Blood Vessels

Blood vessels include arteries, arterioles, capillaries, venules and veins. Whereas arteries tend to have smooth muscular walls and contain blood at high pressure, veins have thinner walls and lower blood pressures. The wall of a blood vessel is composed of an outer <u>adventitia</u>, an inner <u>intima</u> and a *m*iddle *m*uscle layer, the <u>media</u>.

Oxygenated blood entering the systemic circulation must get to all the body's tissues. The aorta must divide into smaller and smaller arteries (small artery = **arteriole**) in order to get to the level of the capillary

which i) is the smallest blood vessel; ii) often forms branching networks called *capillary beds*; and iii) is the level at which the exchange of wastes and gases (i.e. O_2 and CO_2) occurs by diffusion. Next the newly deoxygenated blood enters very small veins (= **venules**) and then into larger and larger veins until the blood enters the venae cavae and then the right atrium. There are two venae cavae: one drains blood from the upper body while the other drains blood from the lower body (*superior* and *inferior* venae cavae, respectively). <u>Coronary arteries</u> branch off the aorta to supply the heart muscle.

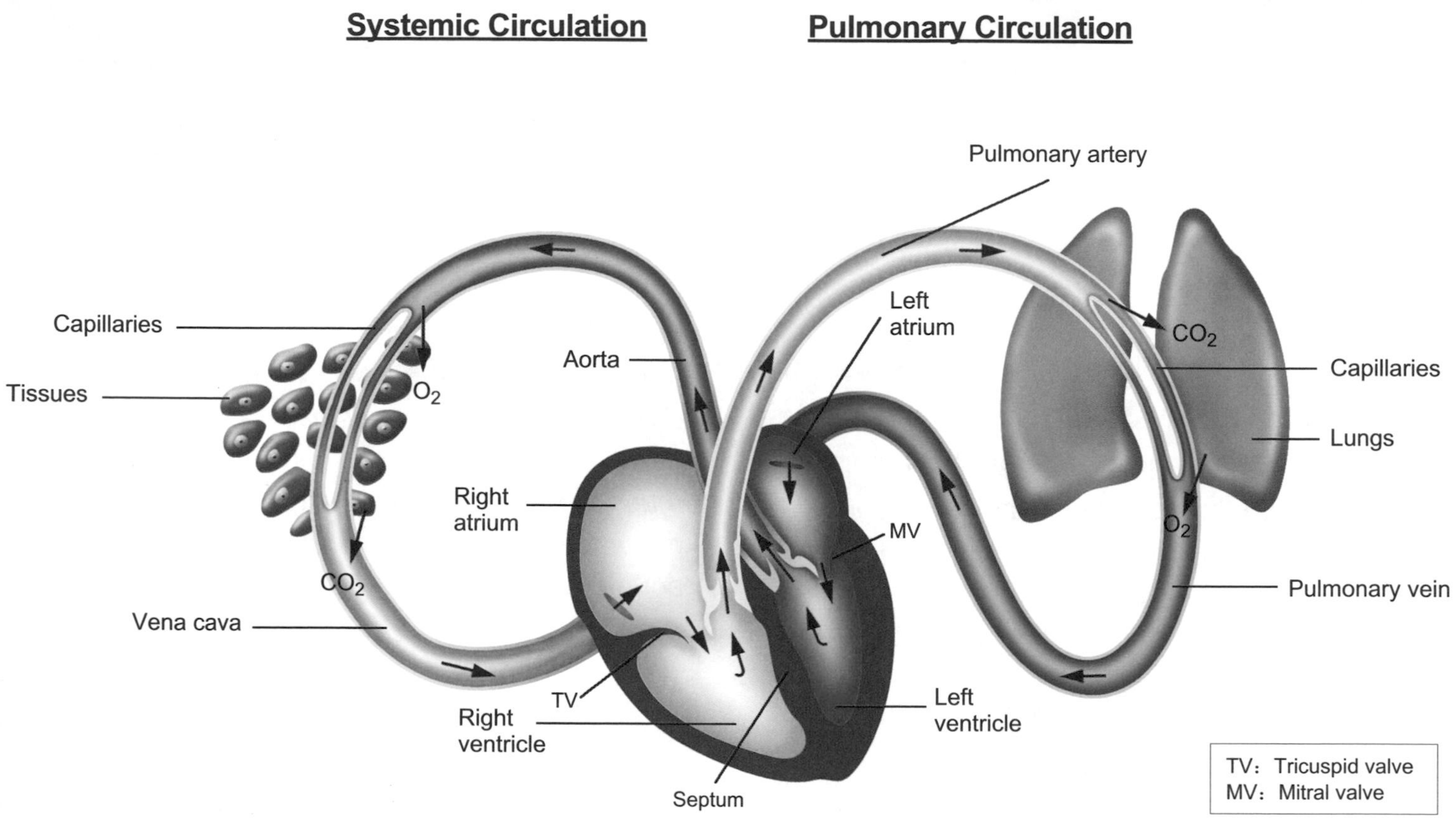

Systemic Circulation   Pulmonary Circulation

Figure IV.A.7.1: Schematic representation of the circulatory system.

7.4 Blood Pressure

Blood pressure is the force exerted by the blood against the inner walls of blood vessels (esp. arteries). Maximum arterial pressure is when the ventricles contract (= *systolic pressure*). Minimal pressure is when the ventricles relax (= *diastolic pressure*). Blood pressure is usually measured in the brachial artery in the arm. A pressure of 120/80 signifies a systolic pressure of 120 mmHg and a diastolic pressure of 80 mmHg. The *pulse pressure* is the difference (i.e. 40 mmHg).

Peripheral resistance is essentially the result of arterioles and capillaries which resist the flow of blood from arteries to veins (the narrower the vessel, the higher the resistance). An increase in peripheral resistance causes a rise in blood pressure.

7.5 Blood Composition

Blood contains *plasma* (55%) and *formed elements* (45%). Plasma is a straw colored liquid which is mostly composed of water (92%), electrolytes, and the following plasma proteins:

  * **Albumin** which is important in maintaining the osmotic pressure and helps to transport many substances in the blood

  * **Globulins** which include both transport proteins and the proteins which form antibodies

  * **Fibrinogen** which polymerizes to form the insoluble protein *fibrin* which is essential for normal blood clotting. If you take away fibrinogen and some other clotting factors from plasma you will be left with a fluid called *serum*.

The formed elements of the blood originate from precursors in the bone marrow which produce the following for the circulatory system: 99% red blood cells (= *erythrocytes*), then there are platelets (= *thrombocytes*), and white blood cells (= *leukocytes*). **Red blood cells** are biconcave cells without nuclei whose primary function is the transport of O_2 and CO_2.

Platelets are cytoplasmic fragments of large bone marrow cells (*megakaryocytes*) which are involved in blood clotting by adhering to the collagen of injured vessels, releasing mediators which cause blood vessels to constrict (= *vasoconstriction*), etc.

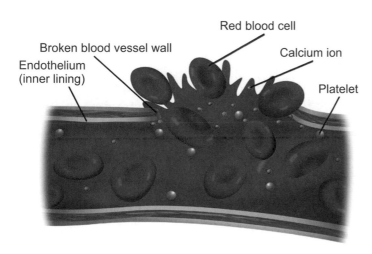 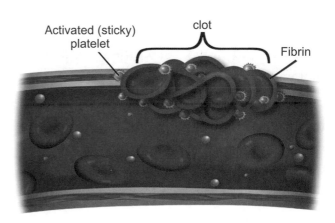

Figure IV.A.7.1.1: Schematic representation of blood clotting.

Calcium ions (Ca²⁺) are also important in blood clotting because they help in signaling platelets to aggregate.

White blood cells help in the defense against infection; they are divided into *granulocytes* and *agranulocytes* depending on whether or not the cell does or does not contain granules, respectively.

Granulocytes (= *polymorphonuclear leukocytes*) are divided into: i) neutrophils which are the first white blood cells to respond to injury, they destroy microorganisms (i.e. bacteria, viruses) by phagocytosis and are the main cellular constituent of pus; ii) eosinophils which, like neutrophils, are phagocytic and have a variety of inflammatory and immune responses; iii) basophils which can release both anticoagulants (heparin) and substances important in hypersensitivity reactions (histamine).

Agranulocytes (= *mononuclear leukocytes*) are divided into: i) lymphocytes which are vital to the immune system (*see Immune System*, chapter 8); and monocytes (often called *phagocytes* or *macrophages* when they are outside of the circulatory system) which can phagocytose large particles. {*See* BIO 15.2 *for ABO Blood Types*}

The hematocrit measures how much space (volume) in the blood is occupied by red blood cells. Normal hematocrit in adults is about 45%.

7.5.1 Hemoglobin

Each red blood cell carries hundreds of molecules of a substance which is responsible for their red color: **hemoglobin**. Hemoglobin (Hb) is a complex of *heme*, which contains iron, and *globin*, which is a protein. In the lungs, oxygen concentration or *partial pressure* is high, thus O_2 dissolves in the blood; oxygen can then quickly combine with the iron in Hb forming bright red *oxyhemoglobin*. The binding of oxygen to hemoglobin is cooperative. In other words, each oxygen that binds to Hb facilitates the binding of the next

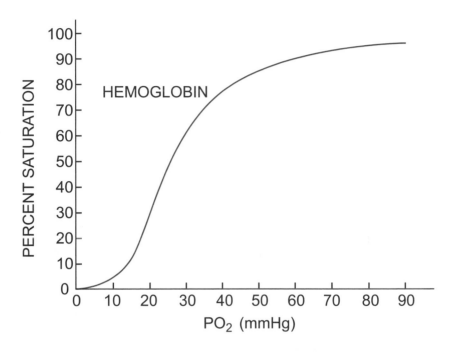

Figure IV.A.7.2: Oxygen dissociation curve: percent O_2 saturation versus O_2 partial pressure.

oxygen. Consequently, the dissociation curve for oxyhemoglobin is sigmoidal.

Examine Figure IV.A.7.2 carefully. Notice that P_{50}, which is the partial pressure of oxygen (PO_2) when the per cent saturation is 50, is approximately 27 mmHg. The curve can: (i) <u>shift to the left</u> which means that for a given PO_2 in the tissue capillary there is *decreased* unloading (release) of oxygen; or (ii) <u>shift to the right</u> which means that for a given PO_2 in the tissue capillary there is increased unloading of oxygen. The latter occurs when the tissue (i.e. muscle) is very active and thus requires more oxygen. Thus

a rightward shift occurs when the muscle is hot ($\uparrow$ temperature), acid ($\downarrow$ pH due to lactic acid, *see* BIO 4.4 and 4.5), hypercarbic ($\uparrow CO_2$ means $\downarrow$ pH, *see* BIO 4.4 and 12.4.1), or contains high levels of organic phosphates (esp. 2,3 DPG in red blood cells).

In the body tissues where the partial pressure of O_2 is low and CO_2 is high, O_2 is released and CO_2 combines with the protein component of Hb forming the darker colored *carbaminohemoglobin* (also called: deoxyhemoglobin). The red color of muscle is due to a different form of hemoglobin concentrated in muscle called *myoglobin*.

7.5.2 Capillaries: A Closer Look

Capillary fluid movement can occur as a result of two processes: diffusion (dominant role) and filtration (secondary role but critical for the proper function of organs, especially the kidney; BIO 10.3). Osmotic pressure (CHM 5.1.3) due to proteins in blood plasma is sometimes called colloid osmotic pressure or oncotic pressure. The Starling equation is an equation that describes the role of hydrostatic and oncotic forces (= Starling forces) in the movement of fluid across capillary membranes as a result of filtration.

When blood enters the arteriole end of a capillary, it is still under pressure produced by the contraction of the ventricle. As a result of this pressure, a substantial amount of water (hydrostatic) and some plasma proteins filter through the walls of the capillaries into the tissue space. This fluid, called interstitial fluid (BIO 7.6), is simply blood plasma minus most of the proteins.

Interstitial fluid bathes the cells in the tissue space and substances in it can enter the cells by diffusion (mostly) or active transport. Substances, like carbon dioxide, can diffuse out of cells and into the interstitial fluid.

Near the venous end of a capillary, the blood pressure is greatly reduced. Here

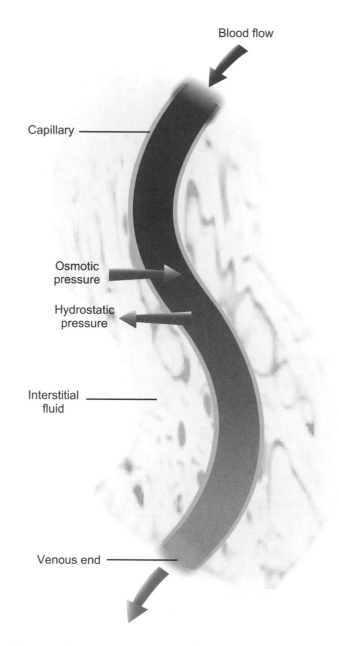

Figure IV.A.7.2b: Circulation at the level of the capillary. The exchange of water, oxygen, carbon dioxide, and many other nutrient and waste chemical substances between blood and surrounding tissues occurs at the level of the capillary

another force comes into play. Although the composition of interstitial fluid is similar to that of blood plasma, it contains a smaller concentration of proteins than plasma and thus a somewhat greater concentration of water. This difference sets up an osmotic pressure. Although the osmotic pressure is small, it is greater than the blood pressure at the venous end of the capillary. Thus the fluid reenters the capillary here.

To summarize: when the blood pressure is greater than the osmotic pressure, filtration of interstitial fluid occurs; when the blood pressure is less than the osmotic pressure, reabsorption of interstitial fluid occurs.

7.6 The Lymphatic System

Body fluids can exist in blood vessels (intravascular), in cells (intracellular) or in a *3rd space* which is intercellular (between cells) or extracellular (outside cells). Such fluids are called interstitial fluids. The **lymphatic system** is a network of vessels which can circulate fluid from the 3rd space to the cardiovascular system.

Aided by osmotic pressure, interstitial fluids enter the lymphatic system via small closed-ended tubes called *lymphatic capillaries* (in the small intestine they are called *lacteals*). Once the fluid enters it is called **lymph**. The lymph continues to flow into larger and larger vessels propelled by muscular contraction (esp. skeletal) and one-way valves. Then the lymph will usually pass through *lymph nodes* and then into a large vessel (esp. *the thoracic duct*) which drains into one of the large veins which eventually leads to the right atrium.

Lymph functions in important ways. Most protein molecules which leak out of blood capillaries are returned to the bloodstream by lymph. Also, microorganisms which invade tissue fluids are carried to lymph nodes by lymph. Lymph nodes contain *lymph*ocytes and macrophages which are components of the immune system.

Memorize	Understand	Not Required*
* Roles in immunity: T-lymphocytes; * B-lymphocytes * Tissues in the immune system including bone marrow * Spleen, thymus, lymph nodes	* Concepts of antigen, antibody, interaction * Structure of antibody molecule * Mechanism of stimulation by antigen	* Advanced level college info * The 5 antibody isotypes * Life cycle of pathogens * Anatomy of lymph nodes * Class switching

MCAT-Prep.com

Introduction

The immune system protects against disease. Many processes are used in order to identify and kill various microbes (see Microbiology, Chapter 2, for examples) as well as tumor cells (more detail when you get into medical school!). There are 2 acquired responses of the immune system: cell-mediated and humoral.

Additional Resources

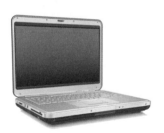

Free Online Q & A

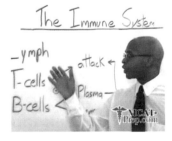

Video: Online or DVD 3

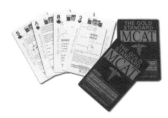

Flashcards

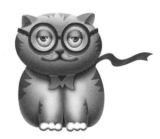

Special Guest

8.1 Overview

The immune system is composed of various cells and organs which defend the body against pathogens, toxins or any other foreign agents. Substances (usu. proteins) on the foreign agent causing an immune response are called **antigens**. There are two acquired responses to an antigen: the **cell-mediated response** where T-lymphocytes are the dominant force and the **humoral response** where B-lymphocytes are the dominant force.

8.2 Cells of the Immune System

B-lymphocytes originate in the bone marrow. Though T-lymphocytes also originate in the bone marrow, they go on to mature in the thymus gland. T-lymphocytes learn with the help of macrophages to recognize and attack only *foreign* substances (i.e. antigens) in a direct cell to cell manner (= *cell-mediated* or *cellular immunity*). Some T-cells (T_4, T_H or T *helper*) mediate the cellular response by secreting substances to activate macrophages, other T-cells and even B-cells. {T_H-cells are specifically targeted and killed by the HIV virus in AIDS patients}

B-lymphocytes act indirectly against the foreign agent by producing and secreting antigen-specific proteins called **antibodies**, which are sometimes called immunoglobulins (= *humoral immunity*). Antibodies are "designer" proteins which can specifically attack the antigen for which it was designed.

The antibodies along with other proteins (i.e. *complement proteins*) can attack the antigen-bearing particle in many ways:

* **Lysis** by digesting the plasma membrane of the foreign cell

* **Opsonization** which is the altering of cell membranes so the foreign particle is more susceptible to phagocytosis by neutrophils and macrophages

* **Agglutination** which is the clumping of antigen-bearing cells

* **Chemotaxis** which is the attracting of other cells (i.e. phagocytes) to the area

* **Inflammation** which includes migration of cells, release of fluids and dilatation of blood vessels.

The activated antibody secreting B-lymphocyte is called a *plasma cell.* After the first or *primary* response to an antigen, both T- and B-cells produce *memory cells* which will make the next or *secondary* response much faster. {Note: though lymphocytes are vital to the immune system, it is the neutrophil which responds to injury first; BIO 7.5}

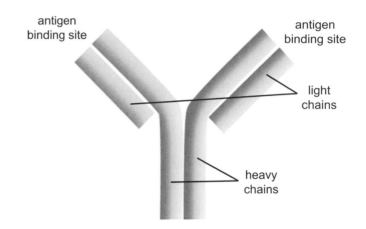

Figure IV.A.8.1: Schematic representation of an antibody.

8.3 Tissues of the Immune System

The important tissues of the immune system are the bone marrow, and the lymphatic organs which include the thymus, the lymph nodes and the spleen. The roles of the bone marrow and the thymus have already been discussed. It is of value to add that the thymus secretes a hormone (= *thymosin*) which appears to help stimulate the activity of T-lymphocytes.

Lymph nodes are often the size of a pea and are found in groups or chains along the paths of the larger lymphatic vessels. Their functions can be broken down into two general categories: i) a non-specific filtration of bacteria and other particles from the lymph using the phagocytic activity of macrophages; ii) the storage and proliferation of T-cells, B-cells and antibody production.

The **spleen** is the largest lymphatic organ and is situated in the upper left part of the abdominal cavity. Within its lobules it has tissue called red and white pulp. In the white pulp there are white blood cells which help to filter: i) damaged red blood cells; ii) cellular debris, and iii) foreign particles from the blood. The spleen is sometimes considered a blood storage organ (the red pulp has a high concentration of red blood cells).

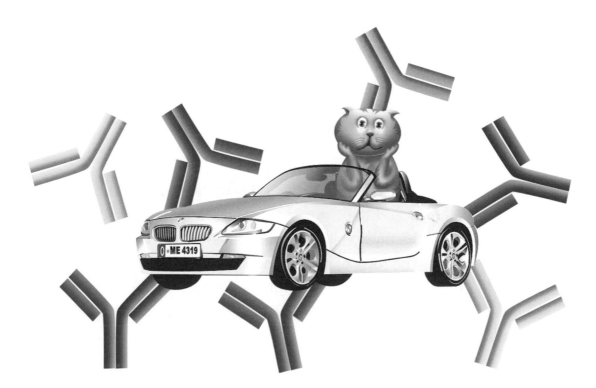

Autoimmunity!

Figure IV.A.8.1: Actually "autoimmunity" refers to a disease process where the immune system attacks one's own cells and tissues as opposed to one's own car.

Memorize	Understand	Not Required*
* Basic anatomy of the upper GI and lower GI tracts * Saliva as lubrication and enzyme source * Stomach low pH, gastric juice, mucal protection against self-destruction * Sites for production of digestive enzymes, sites of digestion * Liver: nutrient metabolism, vitamin storage; blood glucose regulation, detoxification	* Basic function of the upper GI and lower GI tracts * Bile: storage in gallbladder, function * Pancreas: production of enzymes; transport of enzymes to small intestine * Small intestine: production of enzymes, site of digestion, neutralize stomach acid * Peristalsis; structure and function of villi	* Advanced level college info

MCAT-Prep.com

Introduction

The digestive system is involved in the mechanical and chemical break down of food into smaller components with the aim of absorption into, for example, blood or lymph. Thus digestion is a form of catabolism.

Additional Resources

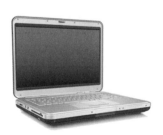

Free Online Q & A

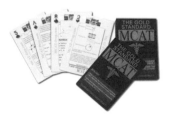

Video: Online or DVD 3

Flashcards

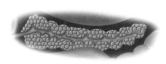

Special Guest

9.1 Overview

The digestive or *gastrointestinal* (= GI) system is principally concerned with the intake and reduction of food into subunits for absorption. These events occur in five main phases which are located in specific parts of the GI system: i) **ingestion** which is the taking of food or liquid into the mouth; ii) **fragmentation** which is when larger pieces of food are *mechanically* broken down; iii) **digestion** where macromolecules are *chemically* broken down into subunits which can be absorbed; iv) **absorption** through cell membranes; and v) **elimination** of the waste products.

The GI tract or *alimentary canal* is a muscular tract about 9 meters long covered by a layer of mucosa which has definable characteristics in each area along the tract. The GI tract includes the oral cavity (mouth), pharynx, esophagus, stomach, small intestine, large intestine, and anus. The GI system includes the accessory organs which release secretions into the tract: the salivary glands, gallbladder, liver, and pancreas (*see Figure IV.A.9.1*).

9.2 The Oral Cavity and Esophagus

Ingestion, fragmentation and digestion begin in the oral cavity. Children have twenty teeth (= *deciduous*) and adults have thirty-two (= *permanent*). From front to back, each quadrant (= quarter) of the mouth contains: two incisors for cutting, one cuspid (= *canine*) for tearing, two bicuspids (= *premolars*) for crushing, and three molars for grinding. Chewing fragments the food as three pairs of salivary glands (*parotid, sublingual,* and *submaxillary*) secrete their products - esp. salivary amylase and mucous. Amylase is an enzyme which splits starch and glycogen into disaccharide subunits. The mucous helps to bind food particles together and lubricate it as it is swallowed. Swallowing (= *deglutition*) occurs by the action of the tongue and pharyngeal muscles which role the bolus of food into the esophagus. The epiglottis is a small flap of tissue which covers the opening to the airway (= *glottis*) while swallowing. Gravity and peristalsis help bring the food through the esophagus to the stomach.

Peristalsis, which is largely the result of two muscle layers in the GI tract (i.e. the inner circular and outer longitudinal layers), is the sequential wave-like muscular contractions which propell food along the tract. The rate, strength and velocity of muscular contractions

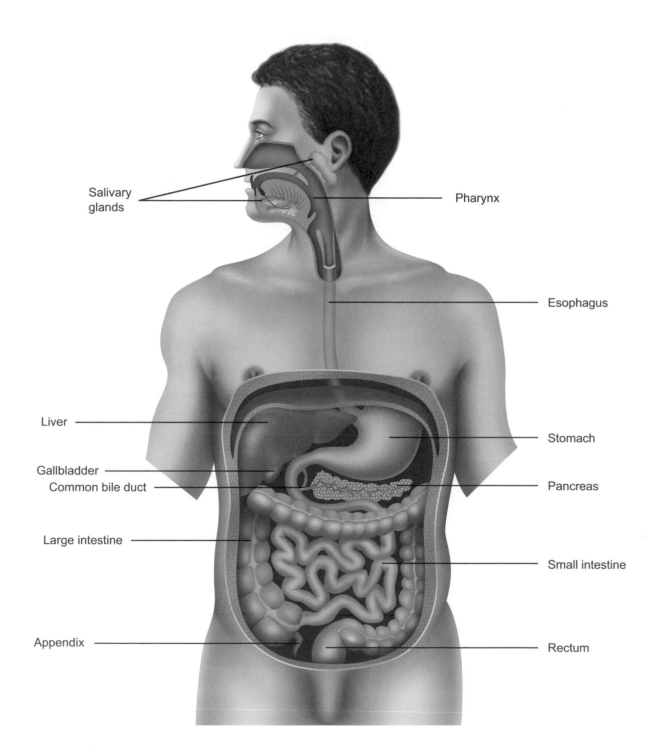

Salivary glands

Pharynx

Esophagus

Liver

Stomach

Gallbladder

Common bile duct

Pancreas

Large intestine

Small intestine

Appendix

Rectum

Figure IV.A.9.1: Schematic drawing of the major components of the digestive system.

are modulated by the ANS. Parasympathetic impulses tend to activate the GI system while sympathetic impulses tend to do the opposite.

9.3 The Stomach

The stomach continues in fragmenting the food with its strong muscular activity and it more completely aids in digestion due to the secretion of gastric juice. Goblet cells of the G.I. tract protect the lumen from the acidic gastric juice by secreting mucous. Both the hormone *gastrin*, which is produced in the stomach, and parasympathetic impulses can increase the production of gastric juice. The important components of gastric juice are: i) HCl which keeps the pH low (approx. = 2) to kill microorganisms, to aid in hydrolysis, and to provide the environment for ii) *pepsinogen* which is an inactive enzyme (= *zymogen*) which is converted to its active form *pepsin* in the presence of a low pH. Pepsin digests proteins.

The preceding events turns food into a semi-digested fluid called chyme. Chyme is squirted through a muscular sphincter in the stomach, the *pylorus*, into the first part of the small intestine, the *duodenum*. Many secretions are produced by exocrine glands in the liver and pancreas and enter the duodenum via the *common bile duct*. Exocrine secretions eventually exit the body through ducts which includes any gland or cell which secretes its product to the skin or into the intestine. For example, *goblet cells*, which are found in the stomach and throughout the intestine, are exocrine secretory cells which produce mucus which lines the epithelium of the gastrointestinal tract.

9.4 The Exocrine Roles of the Liver and Pancreas

9.4.1 The Liver

The liver occupies the upper right part of the abdominal cavity. It has many roles including: the conversion of glucose to glycogen; the synthesis of glucose from non-carbohydrates; the production of plasma proteins; the destruction of red blood cells; the deamination of amino acids and the formation of urea; the storage of iron and certain vitamins; the alteration of toxic substances (*detoxification*); and its exocrine role - the production of **bile** by liver cells (= *hepatocyles*).

Bile is a yellowish-green fluid mainly composed of water, cholesterol, pigments (from the destruction of red blood cells) and salts. It is the **bile salts** which have a digestive function by the emulsification of fats. Emulsification is the dissolving of fat globules into tiny droplets called *micelles* which have hydrophobic interiors and hydrophilic exteriors (cf. Plasma Membrane, BIO 1.1). Emulsification also helps in the absorption of the fat-soluble vitamins A, D, E, and K.

Thus bile is produced by the liver, stored and concentrated in a small muscular sac, the **gallbladder**, and then secreted into the duodenum via the common bile duct.

9.4.2 The Pancreas

The pancreas is close to the duodenum and extends behind the stomach. The pancreas has both endocrine (*see Endocrine Systems*; BIO 6.3.4) and exocrine functions. It secretes pancreatic juice into the pancreatic duct which joins the common bile duct. Pancreatic juice is secreted both due to parasympathetic and hormonal stimuli. The hormones *secretin* and *CCK* are produced and released by the duodenum in response to the presence of chyme. They make the pancreas secrete alkaline bicarbonate ions (to neutralize the acidic chyme) and digestive enzymes, respectively. The **digestive enzymes** can break down molecules of carbohydrates (*pancreatic amylase*), fat (*pancreatic lipase*), nucleic acids (*nucleases*), and proteins in a very specific manner (*trypsin, chymotrypsin, carboxypeptidase*).

9.5 The Intestines

The **small intestine** is divided into the duodenum, the jejunum, and the ileum, in that order. It is this part of the GI system that completes the digestion of chyme, absorbs the nutrients (i.e. monosaccharides, amino acids, nucleic acids, etc.), and passes the rest onto the large intestine. Peristalsis is the primary mode of transport.

Absorption is aided by the great surface area involved including the finger-like projections **villi** (which contain blood capillaries and lacteals) and **microvilli** (*see the Generalized Eukaryotic Cell,* BIO 1.1F and 1.2). They both project into the passageway or lumen of the small intestines. The lacteals absorb most fat products into the lymphatic system while the blood capillaries absorb the rest taking these nutrients to the liver for processing via a special vein - the *hepatic portal vein* [A portal vein carries blood from one capillary bed to another]. Goblet cells secrete a copious amount of mucus in order to lubricate the passage of material through the intestine and to protect the epithelium from abrasive chemicals (i.e. acids, enzymes, etc.).

The **large intestine** is divided into: the cecum which connects to the ileum and projects a closed-ended tube - the *appendix*; the colon which is subdivided into ascending, transverse, descending, and sigmoid portions; the rectum which can store feces; and the anal canal which can expel feces (*defecation*) through the anus with the relaxation of the anal sphincter and the increase in abdominal pressure. The large intestine has little or no digestive functions. It absorbs water and electrolytes from the residual chyme and it forms feces. Feces is mostly water, undigested material, bacteria, mucous, bile pigments (responsible for the characteristic color) and bacteria (= gut flora = 60% of the dry weight of feces). The average human body consists of about 10 trillion (10,000,000,000,000) cells but about ten times that number of bacteria are in the lower GI tract (mostly colon).

Essentially, it is a mutualistic, symbiotic relationship (BIO 2.2). Though people can survive with no bacterial flora, these microorganisms perform a host of useful functions, such as fermenting unused energy substrates, training the immune system, preventing growth of harmful species, producing vitamins for the host (i.e. vitamin K), etc. and bile pigments.

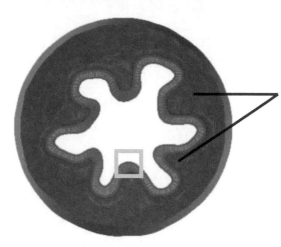

Cross-section of the small intestine.

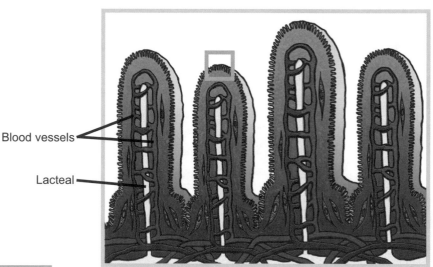

4 intestinal villi.

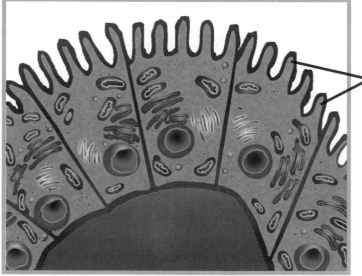

Columnar cells (i.e. intestinal cells arranged in columns) with microvilli facing the lumen (brush border).

Figure IV.A.9.2: Levels of organization of the small intestine.

Memorize	Understand	Not Required*
* Kidney structure: cortex, medulla * Nephron structure: glomerulus, Bowman's capsule, proximal tubule, etc. * Loop of Henle, distal tubule, collecting duct * Storage and elimination: ureter, bladder, urethra	* Roles of the excretory system in homeostasis * Blood pressure, osmoregulation, acid-base balance, N waste removal * Formation of urine: glomerular filtration, secretion and reabsorption of solutes * Concentration of urine; counter-current multiplier mechanism	*Advanced level college info

MCAT-Prep.com

Introduction

The excretory system excretes waste. The focus of this chapter, in keeping with the goals of the MCAT, is to examine the kidney's role in excretion. This includes eliminating nitrogen waste products of metabolism such as urea.

Additional Resources

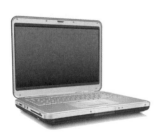

Free Online Q & A

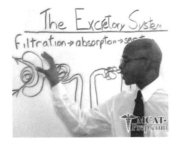

Video: Online or DVD 4

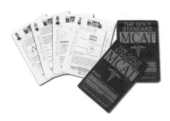

Flashcards

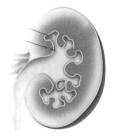

Special Guest

* The real MCAT may have advanced level information presented (ie. in a passage) but previous knowledge of said information is not required to answer the questions that would follow. Practice AAMC and GS practice MCAT CBTs can help you clarify this point.

10.1 Overview

Excretion is the elimination of substances (usu. wastes) from the body. It begins at the level of the cell. Broken down red blood cells are excreted as bile pigments into the GI tract; CO_2, an end product of cellular aerobic respiration, is blown away in the lungs; urea and ammonia (NH_3), breakdown products of amino acid metabolism, creatinine, a product of muscle metabolism, and H_2O, a breakdown product of aerobic metabolism, are eliminated by the urinary system. In fact, the urinary system eliminates such a great quantity of waste it is often called the excretory system.

The composition of body fluids remains within a fairly narrow range. The urinary system is the dominant organ system involved in electrolyte and water homeostasis (*osmoregulation*). It is also responsible for the excretion of toxic nitrogenous compounds (i.e. urea, uric acid, creatinine) and many drugs into the urine. The urine is produced in the kidneys (mostly by the filtration of blood) and is transported, with the help of peristaltic waves, down the tubular ureters to the muscular sack which can store urine, the bladder. Through the process of urination (= *micturition*), urine is expelled from the bladder to the outside via a tubular urethra.

The amount of volume within blood vessels (= *intravascular* or blood volume) and blood pressure are proportional to the rate the kidneys filter blood. Hormones act on the kidney to affect urine formation (*see Endocrine Systems*, BIO 6.3).

10.2 Kidney Structure

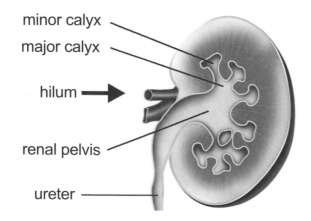

minor calyx
major calyx
hilum
renal pelvis
ureter

Figure IV.A.10.1: Kidney structure.

The kidney resembles a bean with a concave border (= *the hilum*) where the ureter, nerves, and vessels (blood and lymph) attach. The upper end of the ureter expands into the *renal pelvis* which can be divided into two or three *major calyces*. Each major calyx can be divided into *minor calyces*. The kidney can be grossly divided into an outer granular-looking **cortex** and an inner dark striated **medulla**.

The kidney is a *filtration-reabsorption-secretion* (excretion) organ. These events are clearly demonstrated at the level of the nephron.

10.3 The Nephron

The nephron is the functional unit of the kidney and consists of the **renal corpuscle** and the **renal tubule**. A renal corpuscle is responsible for the filtration of blood and is composed of a tangled ball of blood capillaries (= *the glomerulus*) and a sac-like structure which surrounds the glomerulus (= *Bowman's capsule*). *Afferent* and *efferent* arterioles lead towards and away from the glomerulus, respectively. The renal tubule is divided into *proximal* and *distal convoluted tubules* with a *loop of Henle* in between. The tube ends in a *collecting duct*.

Blood plasma is **filtered** by the glomerulus through three layers before entering Bowman's capsule. The first layer is formed by the *endothelial cells* of the capillary; the second layer is the *glomerular basement membrane*; and the third layer is formed by the negatively charged cells (= *podocytes*) in Bowman's capsule which help repel proteins (most proteins are negatively charged). The rate of filtration is proportional to the *hydrostatic* (or blood) pressure and osmotic pressure.

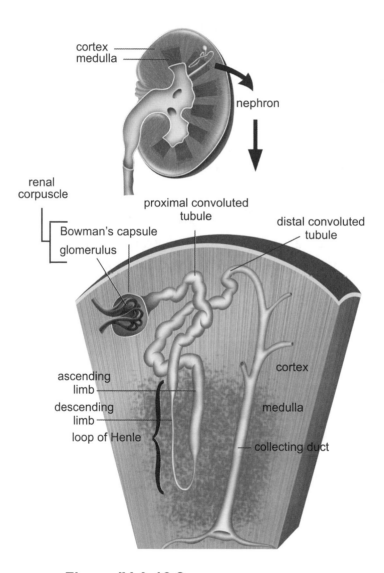

Figure IV.A.10.2: The kidney and its functional unit, the nephron.

The filtrate, which is similar to plasma but with minimal proteins, now passes into the proximal convoluted tubule (PCT). It is here that the body actively **reabsorbs** compounds that it needs (i.e. proteins, amino acids, and especially glucose); and over 75% of all ions and water are reabsorbed by *obligate* (= required) reabsorption from the PCT. To increase the surface area for absorption, the cells of the PCT have a lot of microvilli (= *brush border*; cf. BIO 1.2). Some substances like H^+, urea and penicillin are **secreted** into the PCT.

From the PCT the filtrate goes through the descending and ascending limbs of the loop of Henle which extend into the renal medulla. The purpose of the loop of Henle is to concentrate the filtrate by the transport of ions (Na^+ and Cl^-) into the medulla which produces an osmotic gradient (= *a countercurrent mechanism*). As a consequence of this system, the medulla of the kidney becomes concentrated with ions and tends to "pull" water out of the renal tubule by osmosis.

The filtrate now passes on to the distal convoluted tubule (DCT) which reabsorbs ions actively and water passively and secretes various ions (i.e. H^+). Hormones can modulate the reabsorption of substances from the DCT (= *facultative* reabsorption). Aldosterone acts at the DCT to absorb Na^+ which is coupled to the secretion of K^+ and the passive retention of H_2O.

Finally the filtrate, now called urine, passes into the collecting duct which drains into larger and larger ducts which lead to renal papillae, calyces, the renal pelvis, and then the ureter. ADH concentrates urine by increasing the permeability of the DCT and the collecting ducts allowing the medulla to draw water out by osmosis. Water returns to the circulation via a system of vessels called the *vasa recta*.

Renin is a hormone (BIO 6.3.5) which is secreted by cells that are "near the glomerulus" (= *juxtaglomerular* cells). At the beginning of the DCT is a region of modified tubular cells which can influence the secretion of renin (= *macula densa*). The juxtaglomerular cells and the macula densa are collectively known as the juxtaglomerular apparatus.

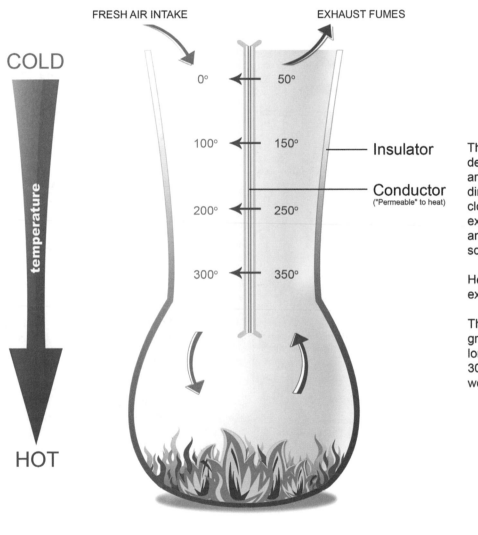

COLD

temperature

HOT

FRESH AIR INTAKE

EXHAUST FUMES

0°   50°

100°   150°   Insulator

Conductor
("Permeable" to heat)

200°   250°

300°   350°

Furnace

The countercurrent principle depends on a parallel flow arrangement moving in 2 different directions (countercurrent) in close proximity to each other. Our example is that of the air intake and exhaust pipe in this simplified schematic of a furnace.

Heat is transferred from the exhaust fumes to the incoming air.

The small horizontal temperature gradient of only 50° is multiplied longitudinally to a gradient of 300°. This conserves heat that would otherwise be lost.

Figure IV.A.10.3: The countercurrent principle (= counter-current mechanism) using a simplified furnace as an example.

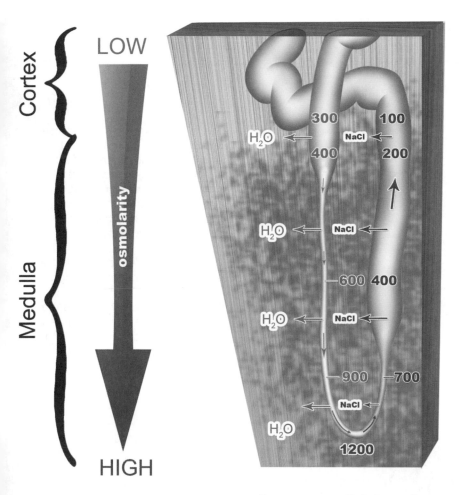

The descending limb of the loop of Henle is highly permeable to water and relatively impermeable to NaCl. The ascending limb is impermeable to water but relatively (through active transport) permeable to NaCl.

Due to the increased osmolarity of the interstitial fluid, water moves out of the descending limb into the interstitial fluid by osmosis. Volume of the filtrate decreases as water leaves. Osmotic concentration of the filtrate increases (1200) as it rounds the hairpin turn of the loop of Henle.

Some of the NaCl leaving the ascending limb moves by diffusion into the descending limb from the interstitial fluid thus increasing the solute concentration in the descending limb. Also, new NaCl in the filtrate continuously enters the tubule inflow to be transported out of the ascending limb into the interstitial fluid. Thus this recycling multiplies NaCl concentration.

Loop of Henle

Figure IV.A.10.4: The countercurrent principle (= counter-current mechanism) in the loop of Henle.

Memorize	Understand	Not Required*
* Structure of three basic muscle types: striated, smooth, cardiac * Voluntary/involuntary muscles; sympathetic/parasympathetic innervation * Basics: cartilage, ligaments, tendons * Bone basics: structure, calcium/protein matrix, growth	* Muscle system, important functions * Support, mobility, peripheral circulatory assistance, thermoregulation (shivering reflex) * Control: motor neurons, neuromuscular junctions, motor end plates * Skeletal system: structural rigidity/support, calcium storage, physical protection * Skeletal structure: specialization of bone types, basic joint, endo/exoskeleton	* Advanced level college info

MCAT-Prep.com

Introduction ▮▮▮▮

The musculoskeletal system (= locomotor system) permits the movement of organisms with the use of muscle and bone. Other uses include providing form and stability for the organism; protection of vital organs (i.e. skull, rib cage); storage for calcium and phosphorous as well as containing a critical component to the production of blood cells (skeletal system).

Additional Resources

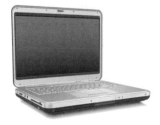

Free Online Q & A

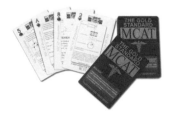

Flashcards

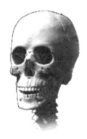

Special Guest

11.1 Overview

The musculoskeletal system supports, protects and enables body parts to move. Muscles convert chemical energy (i.e. ATP, creatine phosphate) into mechanical energy (→ contraction). Thus body heat is produced, body fluids are moved (i.e. lymph), and body parts can move in accordance with lever systems of muscle and bone.

11.2 Muscle

There are many general features of muscle. A latent period is the lag between the stimulation of a muscle and its response. A twitch is a single contraction which lasts for a fraction of a second. Muscles can either *contract* or *relax* but they can not actively expand. Tetany is a sustained contraction (a summation of multiple contractions) that lacks even partial relaxation. Muscle tone (*tonus*) occurs because even when a muscle appears to be at rest, some degree of sustained contraction is occurring.

The cellular characteristics of muscle have already been described (*see Contractile Cells and Tissues,* BIO 5.2). We will now examine the gross features of the three basic muscle types.

Cardiac muscle forms the walls of the heart and is responsible for the pumping action. Its contractions are continuous and are initiated by inherent mechanisms and modulated by the autonomic nervous system. Its activity is decreased by the parasympathetic nervous system and increased by the sympathetic nervous system. The sinoatrial node (SA node) or *pacemaker* contains specialized cells in the right atrium which initiate the contraction of the heart.

Smooth Muscle has two forms. One type occurs as separate fibers and can contract in response to motor nerve stimuli. These are found in the iris (*pupillary dilation or constriction*) and the walls of blood vessels (*vasodilation or constriction*). The second and more dominant form occurs as sheets of muscle fibers and is sometimes called *visceral muscle*. It forms the walls of many hollow visceral organs like the stomach, intestines, uterus, and the urinary bladder. Like cardiac muscle, its contractions are inherent, involuntary, and rhythmic. Visceral muscle is responsible for peristalsis. Its contractility is usually slow and can be modulated by the autonomic nervous system, hormones, and local metabolites. The activity of visceral muscle is increased by the parasympathetic nervous system and decreased by the sympathetic nervous system.

Skeletal muscle is responsible for voluntary movements. This includes the skeleton and organs such as the tongue and the globe of the eye. Its cells can form a syncytium which is a mass of cells which merge and can function together. Thus skeletal muscle can contract and relax relatively rapidly (*see the Reflex Arc*, BIO 6.1.3). Control of skeletal muscle originates in the cerebral cortex. Most skeletal muscles act across joints. Each muscle has a movable end (= *the insertion*) and an immovable end (= *the origin*). When a muscle contracts its insertion is moved towards its origin. When the angle of the joint decreases it is called flexion, when it increases it is called extension. Abduction is movement away from the midline of the body and adduction is movement toward the midline. {Adduction is addicted to the middle (= midline)}

Muscles which assist each other are synergistic (for example: while the deltoid muscle abducts the arm, other muscles hold the shoulder steady). Muscles that can move a joint in opposite directions are antagonistic (for example: at the elbow the biceps can flex while the triceps can extend).

Skeletal muscle is innervated by the somatic nervous system. Motor (*efferent*) neurons carry nerve impulses from the CNS to synapse with muscle fibers at the *neuromuscular junction*. The terminal end of the motor neuron (motor end plate) can secrete acetylcholine which can depolarize the muscle fiber. One motor neuron can depolarize many muscle fibers (= a *motor unit*).

The autonomic nervous system can supply skeletal muscle with more oxygenated blood in emergencies (sympathetic response) or redirect the blood to the viscera during relaxed states (parasympathetic response).

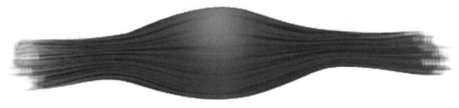

Skeletal muscle

11.3 The Skeletal System

The microscopic features of bone and cartilage have already been described (*see Connective Cells and Tissues*, BIO 5.4.3/4). We will now examine the relevant gross features of the skeletal system.

The bones of the skeleton have many functions: i) acting like levers that aid in **body movement**; ii) the **storage** of inorganic salts like calcium and phosphorus (and to a lesser extent sodium and magnesium); iii) the production of blood cells (= **hematopoiesis**) in the metabolically active red marrow of the spongy parts of many bones. Bone also has a yellow marrow which contains fat storage cells.

11.3.1 Bone Structure and Development

Bone structure can be classified as follows: i) long bones which have a long longitudinal axis and expanded ends, like arm and leg bones; ii) short bones which are shaped like long bones but are smaller and have less prominent ends; iii) flat bones which have broad surfaces like the skull, ribs, and the scapula; iv) irregular bones like the vertebrae and many facial bones.

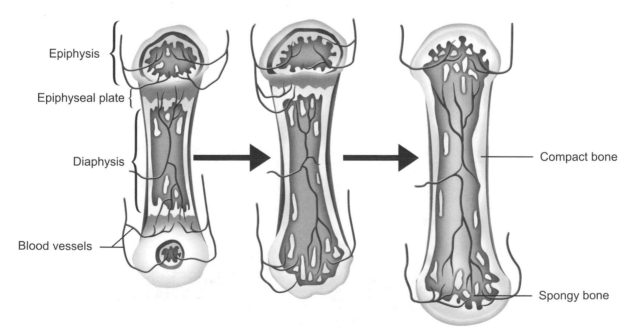

Epiphysis

Epiphyseal plate

Diaphysis

Blood vessels

Compact bone

Spongy bone

Figure IV.A.11.1: Bone structure and development.

The rounded expanded end of a long bone is called the *epiphysis* which contains spongy bone. The epiphysis is covered by fibrous tissue (*the periosteum*) and it forms a joint with another bone. Spongy bone contains bony plates called *trabeculae*. The shaft of the bone which connects the expanded ends is called the *diaphysis*. It is predominately composed of compact bone. This kind of bone is very strong and resistant to bending. Animals that fly have less dense, more light bones (spongy bone) in order to facilitate flying. Animals that swim do not need to have as strong bones as land animals as the buoyant force of the water takes away from the everyday stress on the

bones. In the adult, yellow marrow is likely to be found in the diaphysis while red marrow is likely to be found in the epiphysis.

Bone growth occurs in two ways: i) the bone first appears as layers of membranous connective tissue and is thus called membranous bone; ii) cartilage appears first and is replaced by bone which is then called cartilaginous or endochondral bone. In children one can detect an **epiphyseal growth plate** on X-ray. This plate is a disk of cartilage between the epiphysis and diaphysis where bone is being actively deposited (= *ossification*).

11.3.2 Joint Structure

Articulations or joints are junctions between bones. They can be **immovable** like the dense connective tissue sutures which hold the flat bones of the skull together; **partly movable** like the hyaline and fibrocartilage joints on disks of the vertebrae; or **freely movable** like the synovial joints which are the most prominent joints in the skeletal system. Synovial joints contain a joint capsule composed of outer ligaments

and an inner layer (= *the synovial membrane*) which secretes a lubricant (= *synovial fluid*).

Freely movable joints can be of many types. For example, ball and socket joints have a wide range of motion, like the shoulder and hip joints. On the other hand, hinge joints allow motion in only one plane like a hinged door (i.e. the knee, elbow, and interphalangeal joints).

11.3.3 Cartilage

The microscopic aspects of cartilage have already been discussed (*see Dense Connective Tissue,* BIO 5.4.2/3). Opposing and mobile surfaces of bone are covered by various forms of cartilage. As already mentioned, joints with hyaline or fibrocartilage allow little movement.

Ligaments attach bone to bone. They are formed by dense bands of fibrous connective tissue which reinforce the joint capsule and help to maintain bones in the proper anatomical arrangement.

Tendons connect muscle to bone. They are formed by the densest kind of fibrous connective tissue. Tendons allow muscular forces to be exerted even when the body (*or belly*) of the muscle is at some distance from the action.

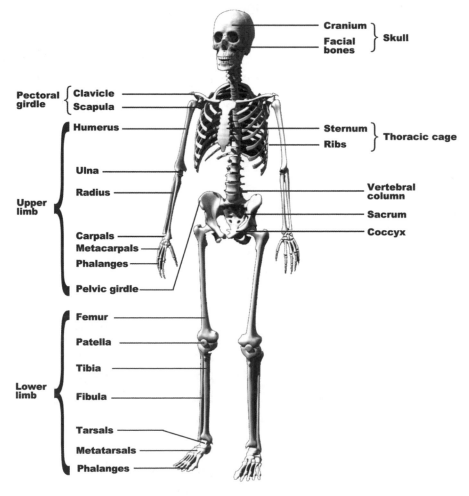

Figure IV.A.11.2: Skeletal structure. Note: in brackets some common relations - scapula (shoulder blade), clavicle (collarbone), carpals (wrist), metacarpals (palm), phalanges (fingers), tibia (shin), patella (kneecap), tarsals (ankle), metatarsals (foot), phalanges (toes), vertebral column (backbone).

Memorize	Understand	Not Required*
* Basic anatomy and order	* Basic functions: gas exchange, thermoregulation, . . . * Protection against disease, particulate matter * Breathing mechanisms: diaphragm, rib cage, differential pressure * Resiliency and surface tension effects	* Advanced level college info

MCAT-Prep.com

Introduction

The respiratory system permits the exchange of gases with the organism's environment. This critical process occurs in the microscopic space between alveoli and capillaries. It is here where molecules of oxygen and carbon dioxide passively diffuse between the gaseous external environment and the blood.

Additional Resources

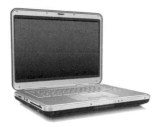

Free Online Q & A

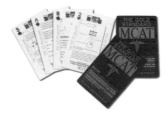

Flashcards

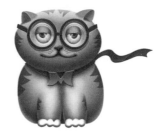

Special Guest

12.1 Overview

There are two forms of respiration: <u>cellular respiration</u> which refers to the oxidation of organic molecules (*see* BIO 4.4 - 4.10) and <u>mechanical respiration</u> where the gases related to cellular respiration are exchanged between the atmosphere and the circulatory system (O_2 in and CO_2 out).

The respiratory system, which is concerned with mechanical respiration, has the following principal functions:

* providing a <u>conducting system</u> for the exchange of gases
* the <u>filtration</u> of incoming particles
* to help control the <u>water content and temperature</u> (= *thermoregulation*) of the incoming air
* to assist in <u>speech production</u>, the <u>sense of smell</u>, and the <u>regulation of pH</u>.

12.2 The Upper Respiratory Tract

The <u>respiratory system</u> can be divided into an *upper* and *lower respiratory tract* which are separated by the pharynx. The **upper respiratory tract** is composed of <u>the nose</u>, <u>the nasal cavity</u>, <u>the sinuses</u>, and <u>the nasopharynx</u>. The nose (*nares*) has receptors for the sense of smell. It is guarded by hair to entrap coarse particles. The nasal cavity, the hollow space behind the nose, contains a ciliated mucous membrane (= a form of *respiratory epithelium*) to entrap smaller particles and prevent infection (this arrangement is common throughout the respiratory tract; for cilia *see the Generalized Eukaryotic Cell*, BIO 1.2). The nasal cavity adjusts the humidity and temperature of incoming air. The nasopharynx helps to equilibrate pressure between the environment and the middle ear via the eustachian tube.

12.3 The Lower Respiratory Tract

The **lower respiratory tract** is composed of <u>the larynx</u> which contains the vocal cords, <u>the trachea</u> which divides into left and right <u>main bronchi</u> which continue to divide into smaller airways ($\rightarrow 2°$ bronchi $\rightarrow 3°$ bronchi $\rightarrow$ bronchioles $\rightarrow$ terminal bronchioles $\rightarrow$ respiratory bronchioles $\rightarrow$ alveolar ducts $\rightarrow$ alveolar sacs) until the level of <u>the alveolus</u>.

It is in these microscopic air sacs called *alveoli* that O_2 diffuses through the alveolar walls and enters the blood in nearby capillaries (where the concentration or *partial pressure* of O_2 is lowest and CO_2 is highest) and CO_2 diffuses from the blood through the walls to enter the alveoli (where the partial pressure of CO_2 is lowest and O_2 is highest). *Alveolar macrophages* are phagocytes which help to engulf particles which reach the alveolus. A *surfactant* is secreted into alveoli by special lung cells (*pneumocytes type II*). The surfactant reduces surface tension and prevents the fragile alveoli from collapsing.

Sneezing and coughing, which are reflexes mediated by the medulla, can expel particles from the upper and lower respiratory tract, respectively.

The **lungs** are separated into left and right and are enclosed by the diaphragm and the thoracic cage. It is covered by a membrane (= *pleura*) which secretes a lubricant to reduce friction while breathing. The lungs contain the air passages, nerves, alveoli, blood and lymphatic vessels of the lower respiratory tract.

12.4 Breathing: Structures and Mechanisms

Inspiration is <u>active</u> and occurs according to the following main events: i) nerve impulses from the <u>phrenic nerve</u> cause the muscular <u>diaphragm</u> to contract; as the dome shaped diaphragm moves downward, the thoracic cavity increases; ii) simultaneously, the intercostal (= *between ribs*) muscles and/or certain neck muscles may contract further increasing the thoracic cavity (the muscles mentioned here are called *accessory respiratory muscles* and under normal circumstances the action of the diaphragm is much more important); iii) as the size of the thoracic cavity increases, its <u>internal pressure</u>

decreases leaving it relatively negative; iv) the relatively positive <u>atmospheric pressure</u> forces air into the respiratory tract thus inflating the lungs.

Expiration is <u>passive</u> and occurs according to the following main events: i) the diaphragm and the accessory respiratory muscles relax; ii) the elastic tissues of the lung, thoracic cage, and abdominal organs suddenly recoil; iii) this recoil increases the pressure within the lungs (making the pressure relatively positive) thus forcing air out of the lungs and passageways.

12.4.1 Control of Breathing

Though voluntary breathing is possible (!), normally breathing is involuntary, rhythmic, and controlled by the *respiratory center* in the medulla of the brain stem. <u>Low</u> blood O_2 but more importantly <u>high</u> blood CO_2 or <u>low</u> pH increase the breathing rate. The latter two events are interrelated since CO_2 can be picked up by hemoglobin forming carbamino-hemoglobin (about 20%, BIO 7.5.1), but it can also be <u>converted into carbonic acid</u> by dissolving in blood plasma (about 5%) or by conversion in red blood cells by the enzyme *carbonic anhydrase* (about 75%). The reaction is summarized as follows:

$$CO_2 + H_2O \leftrightarrow \underset{\substack{\text{carbonic} \\ \text{acid}}}{H_2CO_3} \leftrightarrow \underset{\text{bicarbonate}}{HCO_3^-} + H^+$$

According to Henry's Law, the concentration of a gas dissolved in solution is directly proportional to its partial pressure. From the preceding you can see why the respiratory system, through the regulation of the partial pressure of CO_2 in blood, also helps in maintaining pH homeostasis.

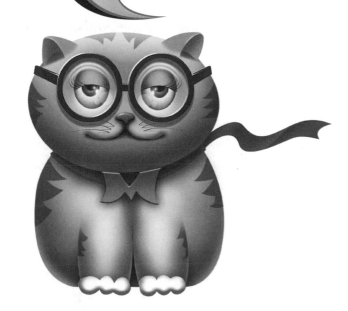

So the anesthetist said: "Breathe in, breathe out"; to which I replied: "Is there any other way?!?"

Memorize

* Structure and function of skin, layer differentiation
* Sweat glands, location in dermis

Understand

* Skin system: homeostasis and osmoregulation
* Functions in thermoregulation: hair, erectile musculature, fat layer for insulation
* Vasoconstriction and vasodilation in surface capillaries
* Physical protection: nails, calluses, hair; protection against abrasion, disease organisms
* Relative impermeability to water

Not Required*

* Advanced level college info

MCAT-Prep.com

Introduction

Skin is composed of layers of epithelial tissues which protects underlying muscle, bone, ligaments and internal organs. Thus skin has many roles including protecting the body from microbes, insulation, temperature regulation, sensation and synthesis of vitamin D.

Additional Resources

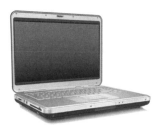

Free Online Q & A

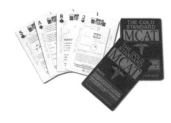

Flashcards

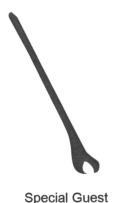

Special Guest

* The real MCAT may have advanced level information presented (ie. in a passage) but previous knowledge of said information is not required to answer the questions that would follow. Practice AAMC and GS practice MCAT CBTs can help you clarify this point.

13.1 Overview

The skin, or *integument*, is the body's largest organ. The following represents its major functions:

* **Physical protection**: The skin protects against the onslaught of the environment including uv light, chemical, thermal or even mechanical agents. It also serves as a barrier to the invasion of microorganisms.

* **Sensation**: The skin, being the body's largest sensory organ, contains a wide range of sensory receptors including those for pain, temperature, light touch, and pressure.

* **Metabolism**: Vitamin D synthesis can occur in the epidermis of skin (*see Endocrine Systems*, BIO 6.3). Also, energy is stored as fat in subcutaneous adipose tissue.

* **Thermoregulation and osmoregulation**: Skin is vital for the homeostatic mechanism of thermoregulation and to a lesser degree osmoregulation. Hair (*piloerection*, which can trap a layer of warm air against the skin's surface) and especially subcutaneous fat (*adipose tissue*) insulate the body against heat loss. Shivering, which allows muscle to generate heat, and decreasing blood flow to the skin (= *vasoconstriction*) are important in emergencies. On the other hand, heat and water loss can be increased by increasing blood flow to the multitude of blood vessels (= *vasodilation*) in the dermis (cooling by radiation), the production of sweat, and the evaporation of sweat due to the heat at the surface of the skin; thus the skin cools. {Remember: the **hypothalamus** also regulates body temperature (*see The Nervous System*, BIO 6.1); it is like a thermostat which uses other organs as tools to maintain our body temperatures at about 37 °C (98.6 °F)}.

13.2 The Structure of Skin

Skin is divided into three layers: i) the outer **epidermis** which contains a stratified squamous epithelium; ii) the inner **dermis** which contains vessels, nerves, muscle, and connective tissues; iii) the innermost **subcutaneous layer** which contains adipose and a loose connective tissue; this layer binds to any underlying organs.

The epidermis is divided into several different layers or *strata*. The deepest layer, *stratum basale*, contains actively dividing cells which are nourished by the vessels in the dermis. As these cells continue to divide, older epidermal cells are pushed towards the surface of the skin - *away from the nutrient providing dermal layer*, thus in time they die. Simultaneously, these cells are actively producing strands of a tough, fibrous, water-proof protein called keratin. This process is called *keratinization*. The two preceding events lead to the formation of an outermost layer (= the *stratum corneum*) of keratin-filled dead cells which are devoid of organelles and can be easily shed (= *desquamation*).

Melanin is a dark pigment produced by

cells (= *melanocytes*) whose cell bodies are usually found in the stratum basale. Melanin absorbs light thus protects against uv light induced cell damage (i.e. sunburns, skin cancer). Individuals have about the same number of melanocytes - regardless of race. Melanin production depends on genetic factors (i.e. race) and it can be stimulated by exposure to sunlight (i.e. tanning).

The dermis contains the blood vessels which nourish the various cells in the skin. It also contains motor and many sensory nerve fibers.

13.3 Skin Appendages

The **appendages** of the skin include hair, sebaceous glands and sweat glands. Hair is a modified keratinized structure produced by a cylindrical downgrowth of epithelium (= *hair follicle*). The follicle extends into the dermis (sometimes the subcutaneous tissue as well). When the bundle of smooth muscle which is attached to the connective tissue of the follicle contracts (= *piloerection*), 'goose bumps' are produced.

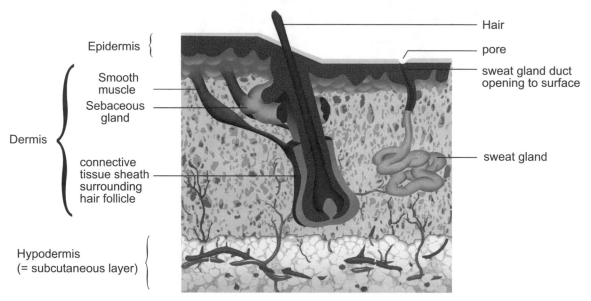

Epidermis {

Smooth
muscle

Sebaceous
gland

Dermis {

connective
tissue sheath
surrounding
hair follicle

Hypodermis
(= subcutaneous layer) {

Hair

pore

sweat gland duct
opening to surface

sweat gland

Figure IV.A.13.1: Skin structure with appendages.

13.3.1 Nails, Calluses

Nails are flat, translucent, keratinized coverings near the tip of fingers and toes. They are useful for scratching and fine manipulation (including picking up dimes!).

A callus is a toughened, thickened area of skin. It is usually created in response to repeated friction or pressure thus they are normally found on the hands or feet.

Memorize	Understand	Not Required*
* Male and female reproductive structures, functions * Ovum, sperm: differences in formation, relative contribution to next generation * Reproductive sequence: fertilization; implantation; development * Major structures arising out of primary germ layers	* Gametogenesis by meiosis * Formation of primary germ layers: endoderm, mesoderm, ectoderm * Embryogenesis: stages of early development: order and general features of each * Cell specialization, communication in development, gene regulation in development * Programmed cell death; basic: the menstrual cycle	* Advanced level college info

MCAT-Prep.com

Introduction

Reproduction refers to the process by which new organisms are produced. The process of development follows as the single celled zygote grows into a fully formed adult. These two processes are fundamental to life as we know it.

Additional Resources

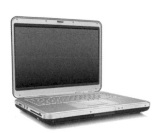

Free Online Q & A

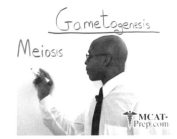

Video: Online or DVD 3, 4

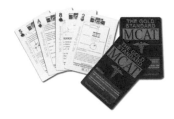

Flashcards

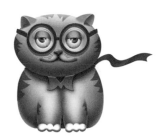

Special Guest

* The real MCAT may have advanced level information presented (ie. in a passage) but previous knowledge of said information is not required to answer the questions that would follow. Practice AAMC and GS practice MCAT CBTs can help you clarify this point.

14.1 Organs of the Reproductive System

The female gonads are the two ovaries which lie in the pelvic cavity. Opening around the ovaries and connecting to the uterus are the Fallopian tubes (= *oviducts*) which conduct the egg (= *ovum*) from the ovary to the uterus. The uterus is a muscular organ. Part of the uterus (= the cervix) protrudes into the vagina or *birth canal*. The vagina leads to the external genitalia. The vulva includes the openings of the vagina, various glands, and folds of skin which are large (= labia majora) and small (= labia minora). The clitoris is found between the labia minora at the anterior end of the vulva. Like the glans penis, it is very sensitive as it is richly innervated.

The male gonads are the two testicles (= *testes*) which are suspended by spermatic cords in a sac-like scrotum outside the body cavity (this is because the optimal temperature for spermatogenesis is less than body temperature). Sperm (= *spermatozoa*) are produced in the seminiferous tubules in the testes and then continue along a system of

ducts including: the epididymis where sperm complete their maturation and are collected and stored; the vas deferens which leads to the ejaculatory duct which in turn leads to the penile urethra which conducts to the exterior. The accessory organs include the seminal vesicles, the bulbourethral and prostate glands. They are exocrine glands whose secretions contribute greatly to the volume of the *ejaculate* (= semen = seminal fluid). The penis is composed of a body or shaft, which contains an erectile tissue which can be engorged by blood; a penile urethra which can conduct either urine or sperm; and a very sensitive head or glans penis which may be covered by foreskin (= *prepuce*, which is removed by circumcision).

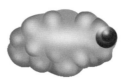
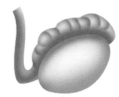

Figure IV.A.14.0: An ovulating ovary and a testicle with spermatic cord.

14.2 Gametogenesis

Gametogenesis refers to the production of gametes (eggs and sperm) which occurs by meiosis (*see Mitosis, BIO 1.3, for comparison*). Meiosis involves two succes-

sive divisions which can produce four cells from one parent cell. The first division, the reduction division, reduces the number of chromosomes from 2N (= *diploid*) to N (= *hap-

loid) where N = 23 for humans. This reduction division occurs as follows: i) in **prophase I** the chromosomes appear (= *condense*), the nuclear membrane and nucleoli disappear, the spindle fibers become organized, homologous chromosomes pair[1] (= *synapsis*) and exchange genetic information by crossing over at particular sites (= *chiasmata formation*); ii) in **metaphase I** the synaptic pairs of chromosomes line up midway between the poles of the developing spindle (= *the equatorial plate*). Thus each pair consists of 2 chromosomes (= 4 chromatids), each attached to a spindle fiber; iii) in **anaphase I** the homologous chromosomes migrate to opposite poles of the spindle. Consequently, the centromeres do *not* divide; iv) in **telophase I** the parent cell divides into two daughter cells (= *cytokinesis*), the nuclear membranes and nucleoli reappear, and the spindle fibers are no longer visible.

The first meiotic division is followed by a short interphase I and then the second meiotic division which proceeds essentially the same as mitosis. Thus prophase II, metaphase II, anaphase II, and telophase II proceed like the corresponding mitotic phases.

Gametogenesis in males (= *spermatogenesis*) proceeds as follows: before the age of sexual maturity only a small number of primordial germ cells (= *spermatogonia*) are present in the testes. After sexual maturation these cells prolifically multiply throughout a male's life. In the seminiferous tubules, the spermatogonia (2N) differentiate by mitosis into primary spermatocytes (2N) which undergo meiotic divisions producing secondary spermatocytes (1N) followed by spermatids (1N). Each primary spermatocyte results in the production of **four** spermatids which are transformed into **four** motile sperm by *spermiogenesis.*

Sperm can be divided into: i) a *head* which is oval and contains the nucleus with its 23 chromosomes {since the nucleus carries either an X or Y sex chromosome, sperm determine the sex of the offspring}. The head is partly surrounded by the *acrosome* which contains enzymes (esp. *hyaluronidase*) which help the sperm penetrate the egg; ii) the *body* of the sperm contains a central core surrounded by a large number of mitochondria for power; and iii) the *tail* constitutes a flagellum which is critical for the cell's locomotion. Also in the seminiferous tubules are Sertoli cells which support and nourish developing sperm and Leydig cells which produce and secrete testosterone. While LH stimulates the latter, FSH stimulates primary spermatocytes to undergo meiosis. {Remember:

---

[1]synapsing homologous chromosomes are often called *tetrads* or *bivalents*.

Spermatogenesis   Oogenesis

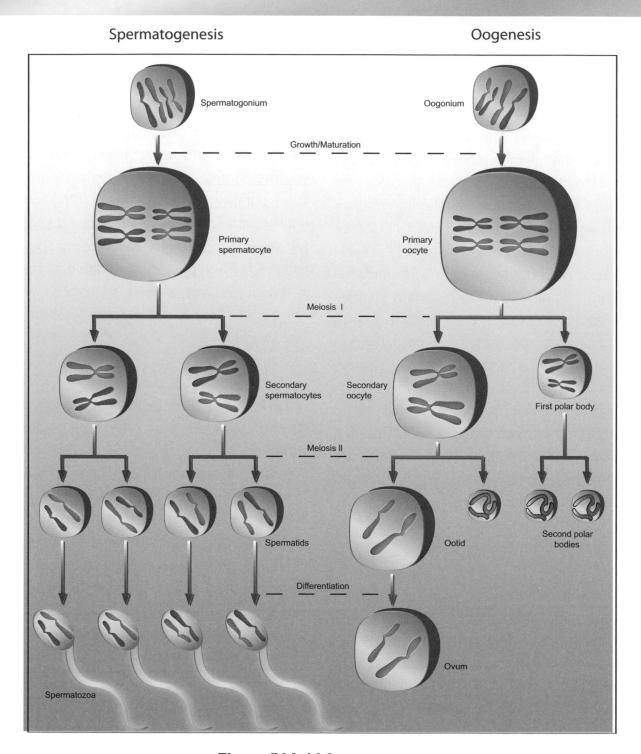

Figure IV.A.14.0a: Gametogenesis.

LH = Leydig, FSH = spermatogenesis}

Gametogenesis in females (= *oogenesis*) proceeds as follows: in fetal develop ment, groups of cells (= *ovarian* or *primordial follicles*) develop from the germinal epithelium of the ovary. Oogonia (2N) produce primary oocytes (2N) which are surrounded by epithelia (= *follicular cells*) in the primordial follicle. The oocytes remain arrested in prophase I of meiosis until ovulation which occurs between the ages of about 13 (sexual maturity) and 50 (menopause). Thus, unlike males, all female germ cells are present at birth. Some follicles degenerate and are called *atretic*. During puberty, when the ovarian cycle begins, up to 20 primordial follicles may begin to differenti ate to Graafian follicles. During this develop ment meiosis continues as the primary oocyte (2N) produces a secondary oocyte (1N) by a reduction division. The latter is surrounded by (from the inside out): a thick, tough mem brane (= *the zona pellucida*), follicular cells (= the corona radiata), and estrogen-secreting *thecal* cells.

Of the twenty or so maturing follicles, all will degenerate (= *atresia*) except one which is expelled from the ovary in the process called ovulation. This ovum, along with its zona pellucida and corona radiata, migrate to and through the Fallopian tubes where a sperm may penetrate the ovum (= *fertilization*). If fertilization occurs then the second meiotic division proceeds; if fertilization does not occur, then the ovum degenerates. Unlike in males, each primary germ cell (oocyte) produces one gamete and not four. This is a consequence of the production of *polar bodies* which are degenerated nuclear mate rial. Up to three polar bodies can be formed: one from the division of the primary oocyte, one from the division of the secondary oocyte, and sometimes the first polar body divides.

14.3 The Menstrual Cycle

The "period" or menstrual cycle occurs in about 28 days and can be divided as follows: i) **Menses**: the first five days of the cycle are notable for the menstrual blood flow. This occurs as a result of an estrogen and proges- terone withdrawal which leads to vasocon striction in the uterus causing the uterine lining (= *endometrium*) to disintegrate and slough away; ii) **Follicular** (ovary) or **Pro liferative Phase** (uterus): FSH stimulates the maturation of the <u>follicle</u> which in turn produces and secretes estrogen. Estrogen causes the uterine lining to thicken (= <u>proliferate</u>); iii) **Ovulation**: a very high concentration of estrogen is followed by an LH surge at about day 14 (midcycle) which stimulates ovulation; iv) **Luteal** (ovary) or **Secretory Phase** (uterus): the follicular cells degenerate into the <u>corpus luteum</u> which secretes estrogen *and* progesterone. Progesterone is responsible for a transient body temperature rise immediately after ovulation and it stimulates the uterine lining to become more vascular and glandular. Estrogen continues to stimulate uterine wall development and, along with progesterone, inhibits the secretion of LH and FSH (= <u>negative feedback</u>).

If the ovum <u>is fertilized</u>, the implanted embryo would produce the hormone *human chorionic gonadotropin* (= hCG) which would stimulate the corpus luteum to continue the secretion of estrogen and progesterone {hCG is the basis for most pregnancy tests}. If there is <u>no fertilization</u>, the corpus luteum degenerates causing a withdrawal of estrogen and progesterone thus the cycle continues [*see* i) *above*].

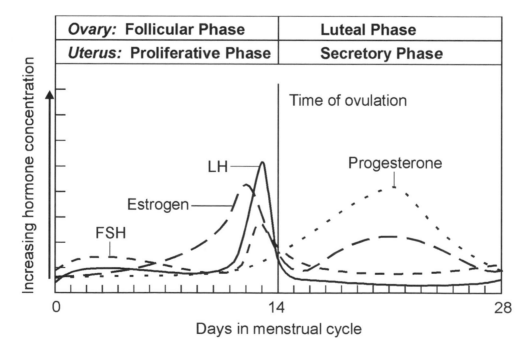

Figure IV.A.14.1: Changing hormoneconcentration during the menstrual cycle.

During sexual stimulation parasympathetic impulses in the male lead to the dilatation of penile arteries combined with restricted flow in the veins resulting in the engorgement of the penis with blood (= *an erection*). In the female, the preceding occurs in a similar manner to the clitoris, along with the expansion and increase in secretions in the vagina. Intercourse or copulation may lead to orgasm which includes many responses from the sympathetic nervous system. In the male, the ejaculation of semen accompanies orgasm. In the female, orgasm is accompanied by many reflexes including an increase in muscular activity of the uterus and the Fallopian tubes. The latter may help in the transport of the already motile sperm to reach the tubes where the egg might be.

14.5 Embryogenesis

The formation of the embryo or *embryogenesis* occurs in a number of steps within two weeks of fertilization. Many parts of the developing embryo take shape during this period (= *morphogenesis*).

Fertilization is a sequence of events which include: the sperm penetrating the corona radiata and the zona pellucidum due to the release of lytic enzymes from the acrosome; the fusion of the plasma membranes of the sperm and egg; the egg, which is really a secondary oocyte, becomes a mature ovum by completing the second meiotic division; the nuclei of the ovum and sperm are now called *pronuclei*; the male and female pronuclei fuse forming a zygote (2N). Fertilization, which normally occurs in the Fallopian tubes, is completed within 24 hours of ovulation.

Cleavage consists of rapid, repeated mitotic divisions beginning with the zygote. Because the resultant daughter cells or blastomeres are still contained within the zona pellucidum, the cytoplasmic mass remains constant. Thus the increasing number of cells requires that each daughter cell be smaller than its parent cell. A morula is a solid ball of about 16 blastomeres which enters the uterus.

Blastulation is the process by which the morula develops a fluid filled cavity (= *blastocoel*) thus converting it to a blastocyst (= *blastula*). Since the zona pellucidum degenerates at this point, the blastocyst is free to implant in the uterine lining or endometrium. The blastocyst contains some centrally located cells (= *the inner cell mass*) which develops into the embryo.

Gastrulation is the process by which the blastula invaginates, and the inner cell mass is converted into a three layered (= *trilaminar*) disk. The trilaminar disk includes the **three primary germ layers**: an outer ectoderm, a middle mesoderm, and an inner endoderm. The ectoderm will develop into the epidermis and the nervous system; the mesoderm will become muscle, connective tissue (incl. blood, bone), and circulatory, reproductive and excretory organs; the endoderm will become the epithelial linings of the respiratory tract, and digestive tract, including the glands of the accessory organs (i.e. the liver and pancreas). During this stage the embryo may be called a gastrula.

Neurulation is the process by which the neural plate and neural folds form and close to produce the neural tube. The neural plate is formed by the thickening of ectoderm which is induced by the developing *notochord*. The notochord is a cellular rod that defines the axis of the embryo and provides some rigidity. Days later, the neural plate invaginates along its central axis producing a central neural groove with neural folds on each side. The neural folds come together and fuse thus converting the neural plate into a neural tube which separates from the surface ectoderm. Special cells on the crest of the neural folds (= *neural crest cells*) migrate to either side of the developing neural tube to a region called the neural crest.

As a consequence, we are left with **three** regions: the surface ectoderm which will become the epidermis; the neural tube which will become the central nervous system (CNS); and the neural crest which will become cranial and spinal ganglia and nerves and the medulla of the adrenal gland. During this stage the embryo may be called a *neurula*.

Though this is a subject which is still poorly understood, it seems clear that morphogenesis relies on the coordinated interaction of genetic and environmental factors. When the zygote passes through its first few divisions, the blastomeres remain indeterminate or uncommitted to a specific fate. As development proceeds the cells become increasingly committed to a specific outcome (i.e. neural tube cells → CNS). This is called **determination**.

In order for a cell to specialize it must differentiate into a committed or determined cell. Since essentially all cells in a person's body have the same amount of genetic information, differentiation relies on the *difference* in the way these genes are *activated*. For example, though brain cells (neurons) have the same genes as osteoblasts, neurons do not activate such genes (otherwise we would have bone forming in our brains!). The general mechanism by which cells differentiate is called **induction**.

Induction can occur by many means. If two cells divide unevenly, the cell with more cytoplasm might have the necessary amount of a substance which could *induce* its chromosomes to activate cell-specific genes. Furthermore, sometimes a cell, through contact (i.e. *contact inhibition*) or the release of a chemical mediator, can influence the development of nearby cells (*recall that the notochord induces the development of the neural plate*). The physical environment (pH, temperature, etc.) may also influence the development of certain cells. Irrespective of what form of induction is used, the signal must be translated into an intracellular message which influences the genetic activity of the responding cells.

Programmed cell-death (PCD = apoptosis) is death of a cell in any form, which is controlled by an intracellular program. PCD is carried out in a regulated process directed by DNA which normally confers advantage during an organism's life-cycle. PCD serves fundamental functions during tissue development. For example, the development of the spaces between your fingers requires cells to undergo PCD.

Thus cells specialize and develop into organ systems (morphogenesis). The embryo develops from the second to the ninth week, followed by the fetus which develops from the ninth week to birth (*parturition*).

14.6 The Placenta

The **placenta** is a complex vascular structure formed by part of the maternal endometrium (= *the decidua basalis*) and cells of embryonic origin (= *the chorion*). The placenta begins to form when the blastocyst implants in the endometrium. A cell layer from the embryo invades the endometrium with fingerlike bumps (= *chorionic villi*) which project into intervillous spaces which contain maternal blood. Maternal spiral arteries enter the intervillous spaces allowing blood to circulate.

The placenta has three main functions: i) the **transfer** of substances necessary for the development of the embryo or fetus from the mother (O_2, H_2O, carbohydrates, amino acids, certain antibodies, vitamins, etc.) and the **transfer** of wastes from the embryo or fetus to the mother (CO_2, urea, uric acid, etc.); ii) the placenta can synthesize substances (i.e. glycogen, fatty acids) to use as an energy source for itself and the embryo or fetus; iii) the placenta produces and secretes a number of hormones including hCG, estrogen and progesterone.

14.7 Fetal Circulation

Consider the following: the fetus has lungs but does not breathe O_2. In fact, the placenta is, metaphorically, the "fetal lung." Oxygenated blood from the placenta carried via umbilical veins is largely directed to the inferior vena cava by the ductus venosus. Most of this oxygenated blood is diverted from pulmonary circulation to the left atrium via a hole in the atrial septum: the patent foramen ovale (for adult circulation and anatomy, see chapter 7).

Deoxygenated blood from the superior vena cava enters the right heart then pulmonary artery as in an adult. However, resistance in the collapsed lung is high. Thus pulmonary artery pressure is higher than it is in the aorta. Consequently, most of the blood bypasses the lung via the ductus arteriosus to the aorta. Blood from the aorta now enters systemic circulation. Umbilical arteries divert some aortal blood to the placenta for oxygenation. In normal infants, the foramen ovale and the ductus arteriosus both fuse shut. {Consider what would happen if they remained open}

The normal sexual development of the fetus depends on the genotype (XX female, XY male), the morphology of the internal organs and gonads, and the phenotype or external genitalia. Later, these many factors combine to influence the individual's self-perception along with the development of secondary sexual characteristics (i.e. breast development in females, hair growth and lower pitched voice in males).

Every fetus, regardless of genotype, has the capacity to become a normally formed individual of either sex. Development naturally proceeds towards "female" unless there is a Y chromosome factor present. Thus the XX genotype leads to the maturation of the Müllerian ducts into the uterus, fallopian tubes, and part of the vagina. The primitive gonad will develop into a testis only if the Y chromosome is present and encodes the appropriate factor and eventually the secretion of testosterone. Thus the XY genotype leads to the involution of the Müllerian ducts and the maturation of the Wolffian ducts into

the vas deferens, seminiferous tubules and prostate.

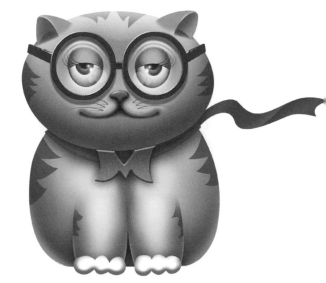

Reproductive biology is the only science where multiplication and division mean the same thing.

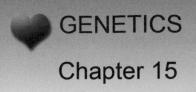

Memorize	Understand	Not Required*
* Define: phenotype, genotype, gene, locus, allele: single and multiple * Homo/heterozygosity, wild type, recessiveness, complete/co-dominance * Incomplete dominance, leakage, penetrance, expressivity, gene pool * Sex-linked characteristics, sex determination, cytoplasmic inheritance * Types of mutations: random, translation error, transcription error, base subs., etc.	*Importance of meiosis; compare/contrast with mitosis *Segregation of genes, assortment, linkage, recombination *Single/double crossovers; relationship of mutagens to carcinogens *Hardy-Weinberg Principle, inborn errors of metabolism *Test cross: back cross, concepts of parental, F1 and F2 generations	* Advanced level college info

MCAT-Prep.com

Introduction

Genetics is the study of heredity and variation in organisms. The observations of Gregor Mendel in the mid-nineteenth century gave birth to the science which would reveal the physical basis for his conclusions, DNA, about 100 years later.

Additional Resources

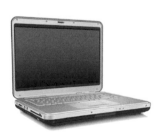

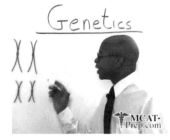

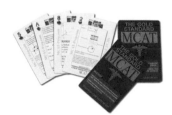

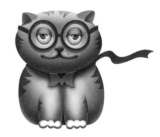

| Free Online Q & A | Video: Online or DVD 4 | Flashcards | Special Guest |

* The real MCAT may have advanced level information presented (ie. in a passage) but previous knowledge of said information is not required to answer the questions that would follow. Practice AAMC and GS practice MCAT CBTs can help you clarify this point.

15.1 Background Information

Genetics is a branch of biology which deals with the principles and mechanics of heredity; in other words, the *means* by which *traits* are passed from parents to offspring. To begin, we will first examine some relevant definitions - a few of which we have already discussed.

Chromosomes are a complex of DNA and proteins (incl. histones). A gene is that sequence of DNA that codes for a protein or polypeptide. A locus is the *position* of the gene on the DNA molecule. Recall that humans inherit 46 chromosomes - 23 from maternal origin and 23 from paternal origin (BIO 14.2). A given chromosome from maternal origin has a counterpart from paternal origin which codes for the same products. This is called a **homologous pair** of chromosomes. Any homologous pair of chromosomes have a pair of genes which codes for the same product (i.e. hair color). Such pairs of genes are called **alleles**. Thus for one gene product, a nucleus contains one allele from maternal origin and one allele from paternal origin. If both alleles are identical (i.e. they code for the same hair color), then the individual is called **homozygous** for that trait. If the two alleles differ (i.e. one codes for dark hair while the other codes for light hair), then the individual is called **heterozygous** for that trait.

The set of genes possessed by a particular organism is its genotype. The appearance or phenotype of an individual is expressed as a consequence of the genotype and the environment. Consider a heterozygote that expressed one gene (dark hair) but not the other (light hair). The expressed gene would be called dominant while its allele is recessive. The individual would have dark hair as their phenotype, yet their genotype would be heterozygous for that trait.

It is common to symbolize dominant genes with capital letters (A) and recessive genes with small letters (a). From the preceding paragraphs, we can conclude that with two alleles, three genotypes are possible: homozygous dominant (AA), heterozygous (Aa), and homozygous recessive (aa). Note that this only results in two phenotypes since both AA and Aa express the dominant gene, while only aa expresses the recessive gene.

Each individual carries **two** alleles while populations may have many or **multiple alleles**. Sometimes these genes are not strictly dominant or recessive. There may be degrees of blending (= *incomplete dominance*) or sometimes two alleles may be equally dominant (= *codominance*). ABO blood types are an important example of multiple alleles with codominance.

15.2 ABO Blood Types

Red blood cells can have various antigens or *agglutinogens* on their plasma membranes which aid in blood typing. The important two are antigens A and B. If the red blood cells have only antigen A, the blood type is A; if they have only antigen B, then the blood type is B; if they have both antigens, the blood type is AB; if neither antigen is present, the blood type is O. There are three allelic genes in the population (I^A, I^B, i^O). Two are codominant (I^A, I^B) and one is recessive (i^O). Thus in a given population, there are six possible genotypes which result in four possible phenotypes:

Genotype	Phenotype
$I^A I^A$, $I^A i^O$	blood type A
$I^B I^B$, $I^B i^O$	blood type B
$I^A I^B$	blood type AB
$i^O i^O$	blood type O

Blood typing is critical before doing a blood transfusion. This is because people with blood type A have anti-B antibodies, those with type B have anti-A, those with type AB have neither antibody, while type O has both anti-A and anti-B antibodies. If a person with type O blood is given types A, B, or AB, the clumping of the red blood cells will occur (= *agglutination*). Though type O can only receive from type O, it can give to the other blood types since its red blood cells have **no** antigens {type O = universal donor}. Type AB has neither antibody so it can receive blood from all blood types. The only other antigens which have some importance are the Rh factors which are coded by different genes at different loci from the A and B antigens. Rh factors are either there (Rh+) or they are not there (Rh-). 85% of the population are Rh+. The problem occurs when a woman is Rh- and has been exposed to Rh+ blood and then forms anti-Rh+ antibodies (note: unlike the previous case, exposure is necessary to produce these antibodies). If this woman is pregnant with an Rh+ fetus her antibodies may cross the placenta and cause the fetus' red blood cells to agglutinate (*erythroblastosis fetalis*). This condition is fatal if left untreated.

15.3 Mendelian Genetics

Recall that in gametogenesis homologous chromosomes separate during the first meiotic division. Thus alleles that code for the same trait are segregated: this is **Mendel's First Law of Segregation. Mendel's Second Law of Independent Assortment** states that different chromosomes (*or factors which carry different traits*) separate independently of each other. For example, consider a primary spermatocyte (2N) undergoing its first meiotic division. It is not the case that all 23 chromosomes of paternal origin will end up in one secondary spermatocyte while the other 23 chromosomes of maternal origin ends up in the other. Rather, each chromosome in a homologous pair separates *independently* of any other chromosome in other homologous pairs.

However, it has been noted experimentally that sometimes traits on the same chromosome assort independently! This non-Mendelian concept is a result of *crossing over* (recall that this is when homologous chromosomes exchange parts, BIO 14.2). In fact, it has been shown that two traits located far apart on a chromosome are more likely to cross over and thus assort independently, as compared to two traits that are close. The propensity for some traits to refrain from assorting independently is called linkage. Double crossovers occur when two cross-overs happen in a chromosomal region being studied.

Another exception to Mendel's laws involves **sex linkage**. Mendel's laws would predict that the results of a genetic cross should be the same regardless of which parent introduces the allele. However, it can be shown that some traits follow the inheritance of the sex chromosomes. Humans have one pair of sex chromosomes (XX = female, XY = male), and the remaining 22 pairs of homologous chromosomes are called **autosomes**. Since females have two X chromosomes and a male only has one, a *single* recessive allele on an X chromosome could be expressed in a male! {the preceding occurs only when the Y chromosome has no homologous counterpart to the X chromosome - which is commonly the case} In fact, a typical pattern of sex linkage is when a mother passes her phenotype to **all** her sons but **none** of her daughters. Her daughters become *carriers* for the recessive allele. Certain forms of hemophilia, colorblindness, and one kind of muscular dystrophy are well-known recessive sex-linked traits.{*in what was once known as Lyon's Hypothesis, it has been shown that every female has a condensed, inactivated X chromosome in her body or somatic cells called a Barr body*}

Let us examine the predictions of Mendel's First Law. Consider two parents, one homozygous dominant (AA) and the other homozygous recessive (aa). Each parent can only form one type of gamete with respect to that trait (*either* A *or* a, *respectively*). The next generation (*called first filial or* F_1) must then be uniformly heterozygotes or *hybrids* (Aa). Now the F_1 hybrids can produce gametes that can be either A *half the time* or a *half the time*. With this information we can predict the outcome in the next generation (F_2) using a Punnett square:

	1/2 A	1/2 a
1/2 A	1/4 AA	1/4 Aa
1/2 a	1/4 Aa	1/4 aa

Here is an example as to how you derive the information within the square: when you cross A with A you get AA (i.e. 1/2 A × 1/2 A = 1/4 AA). Thus by doing a simple *mono*hybrid cross (Aa × Aa) with random mating, the Punnett square indicates that in the F_2 generation,

1/4 of the population would be AA, 1/2 would be Aa (1/4 + 1/4), and 1/4 would be aa. In other words the *genotypic* ratio of homozygous dominant to heterozygous to homozygous recessive is 1:2:1. However, since AA and Aa demonstrate the same *phenotype* (i.e. dominant) the ratio of dominant to recessive is 3:1.

Now we will consider the predictions of Mendel's Second Law. To examine independent assortment, we will have to consider a case with two traits (usu. on different chromosomes) or a *di*hybrid cross. Imagine a parent which is homozygous dominant for two traits (AABB) while the other is homozygous recessive (aabb). Each parent can only form one type of gamete with respect to those traits (*either* AB *or* ab, *respectively*). The F_1 generation will be uniform for the dominant trait (i.e. *the genotypes would all be* AaBb). In the gametes of the F_1 generation, the alleles will assort independently. Consequently, an equal amount of all the possible gametes will form: 1/4 AB, 1/4 Ab, 1/4 aB, and 1/4 ab. With this information we can predict the outcome in the F_2 generation using the Punnett square:

	1/4 AB	1/4 Ab	1/4 aB	1/4 ab
1/4 AB	1/16 AABB	1/16 AABb	1/16 AaBB	1/16 AaBb
1/4 Ab	1/16 AABb	1/16 AAbb	1/16 AaBb	1/16 Aabb
1/4 aB	1/16 AaBB	1/16 AaBb	1/16 aaBB	1/16 aaBb
1/4 ab	1/16 AaBb	1/16 Aabb	1/16 aaBb	1/16 aabb

Thus by doing a dihybrid cross with random mating, the Punnett square indicates that there are nine possible genotypes (*the frequency is given in brackets*): AABB (1), AABb (2), AaBb (4), AaBB (2), Aabb (2), aaBb (2), AAbb (1), aaBB (1), and aabb (1). Since A and B are dominant, there are only four phenotypic classes in the ratio 9:3:3:1 which are: the expression of <u>both</u> traits (AABB + AABb + AaBb + AaBB = 9), the expression of only the <u>first</u> trait (AAbb + Aabb = 3), the expression of only the <u>second</u> trait (aaBB + aaBb = 3), and the expression of <u>neither</u> trait (aabb = 1). Now we know, for example, that 9/16 represents that fraction of the population which will have the phenotype of both dominant traits.

15.3.1 A Word about Probability

If you were to flip a quarter, the probability of getting "heads" is 50% (p = 0.5). If you flipped the quarter ten times and each time it came up heads, the probability of getting heads on the next trial is still 50%. After all, previous trials have no effect on the next trial.

Since chance events, such as fertilization of a particular kind of egg by a particular kind of sperm, occur independently, the genotype of one child has no effect on the genotypes of other children produced by a set of parents. Thus in the previous example of the dihybrid cross, the chance of producing the genotype AaBb is 4/16 (25%) irrespective of the genotypes which have already been produced.

15.4 The Hardy-Weinberg Law

The Hardy-Weinberg Law deals with population genetics. A **population** includes all the members of a species which occupy a more or less well defined geographical area and have demonstrated the ability to reproduce from generation to generation. A **gene pool** is the sum of all the genes in a population. A central component to evolution is the changing of alleles in a gene pool from one generation to the next. The Hardy-Weinberg Law or *equilibrium* predicts the outcome of a randomly mating population of sexually reproducing diploid organisms who are not undergoing evolution.

For the Hardy-Weinberg Law to be applied, the idealized population must meet the following conditions: i) **random mating**: the members of the population must have no mating preferences; ii) **no mutations**: there must be no errors in replication nor similar event resulting in a change in the genome; iii) **isolation**: there must be no exchange of genes between the population being considered and any other population; iv) **large population**: since the law is based on statistical probabilities, to avoid sampling errors, the population cannot be small; v) **no selection pressures**: there must be no reproductive advantage of one allele over the other.

To illustrate a use of the law, consider an idealized population that abides by the preceding conditions and have a gene locus occupied by either A or a. Let p = the frequency of allele A in the population and let q = the frequency of allele a. Since they are the only alleles, p + q = 1. Squaring both sides we get:

$$(p + q)^2 = (1)^2$$

OR

$$p^2 + 2pq + q^2 = 1$$

The preceding equation (= *the Hardy-Weinberg equation*) can be used to calculate genotype frequencies once the allelic frequencies are given. This can be summarized by the following:

	pA	qa
pA	p^2AA	pqAa
qa	pqAa	q^2aa

The Punnett square illustrates the expected frequencies of the three genotypes in the next generation: AA = p^2, Aa = 2pq, and aa = q^2.

For example, let us calculate the percentage of heterozygous individuals in a population where the recessive allele q has a frequency of 0.2. Since p + q = 1, then p = 0.8. Using the Hardy-Weinberg equation and squaring p and q we get:

$$0.64 + 2pq + 0.04 = 1$$
$$2pq = 1 - 0.68 = 0.32$$

Thus the percentage of heterozygous (2pq) individuals is 32%.

A practical application of the Hardy-Weinberg equation is the prediction of how many people in a generation are carriers for a particular recessive allele. The values would have to be recalculated for every generation since humans do not abide by all the conditions of the Hardy-Weinberg Law (i.e. *humans continually evolve*).

15.4.1 Back Cross, Test Cross

A back cross is the cross of an individual (F_1) with one of its parents (P) or an organism with the same genotype as a parent. Back crosses can be used to help identify the genotypes of the individual in a specific type of back cross called a test cross. A test cross is a cross between an organism whose genotype for a certain trait is unknown and an organism that is homozygous recessive for that trait so the unknown genotype can be determined from that of the offspring. For example, for P: AA x aa and F1: Aa, we get:

Backcross #1: Aa x AA
Progeny #1: 1/2 Aa and 1/2 AA

Backcross #2: Aa x aa
Progeny #2: 1/2 Aa and 1/2 aa

15.5 Genetic Variability

Meiosis and mutations are sources of genetic variability. During the first division of meiosis, crossing over occurs which leads to a **recombination** of parental genes in a new way. Thus recombination can result in alleles of linked traits separating into different gametes. However, the closer two traits are on a chromosome, the more likely they will be linked and thus remain together, and vice versa.

Further recombination occurs during the random fusion of gametes during fertilization. Consequently, taking Mendel's two laws and recombination together, we can predict that parents can give their offspring combinations of alleles which the parents never had. This leads to **genetic variability**.

Mutations are rare, inheritable, random changes in the genetic material (DNA) of a cell. Mutations are much more likely to be either neutral (esp. *silent mutations*) or negative (i.e. cancer) than positive for an organism's survival. Nonetheless, such a change in the genome increases genetic variability. Only mutations of gametes, and not somatic cells, are passed on to offspring.

The following are some forms of mutations:

* **Point mutation** is a change affecting a single base pair in a gene

* **Deletion** is the removal of a sequence of DNA, the regions on either side being joined together

* **Inversion** is the reversal of a segment of DNA

* **Translocation** is when one chromosome breaks and attaches to another

* **Duplication** is when a sequence of DNA is repeated.

* **Frame shift mutations** occur when bases are added or deleted in numbers other than multiples of three. Such deletions or additions cause the rest of the sequence to be shifted such that each triplet reading frame is altered.

A mutagen is any substance or agent that can cause a mutation. A mutagen is not the same as a carcinogen. Carcinogens are agents that cause cancer. While many mutagens are carcinogens as well, many others are not. The Ames test is a widely used test to screen chemicals used in foods or medications for mutagenic potential.

Mutations can produce many types of genetic diseases including inborn errors of metabolism. These disorders in normal metabolism are usually due to defects of a single gene that codes for one enzyme.

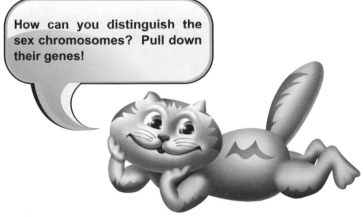

How can you distinguish the sex chromosomes? Pull down their genes!

EVOLUTION
Chapter 16

Memorize	Understand	Not Required*
* Define: species, genetic drift *Basics: chordates, vertebrates	*Natural selection, speciation *Genetic drift *Basics: origin of life *Basics: comparative anatomy	* Advanced level college info

MCAT-Prep.com

Introduction

Evolution is, quite simply, the change in the inherited traits of a population of organisms from one generation to another. This change over time can be traced to 3 main processes: variation, reproduction and selection. The major mechanisms that drive evolution are natural selection and genetic drift.

Additional Resources

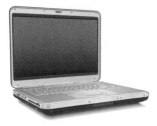

Free Online Q & A

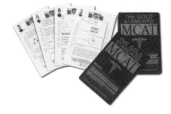

Flashcards

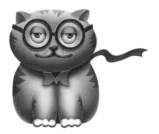

Special Guest

16.1 Overview

Evolution is the change in frequency of one or more alleles in a population's gene pool from one generation to the next. The evidence for evolution lies in the fossil record, biogeography, embryology, comparative anatomy, and experiments from artificial selection. The most important mechanism of evolution is the **selection** of certain phenotypes provided by the **genetic variability** of a population.

16.2 Natural Selection

Natural selection is the non-random differential survival and reproduction from one generation to the next. Natural selection contains the following premises: i) genetic and phenotypic variability exist in populations; ii) more individuals are produced than live to grow up and reproduce; iii) individuals with some genes are more likely to survive (*greater fitness*) than those with other genes.

It is not necessarily true that natural selection leads to the "survival of the fittest"; rather it is the genes, and not necessarily the individual, which are likely to survive.

Evolution goes against the foundations of the Hardy-Weinberg Law. For example, natural selection leads to non-random mating due to phenotypic differences. Evolution occurs when those phenotypic changes depend on an underlying genotype; thus non-random mating can lead to changes in allelic frequencies. Consider an example: if female pea-cocks decide to only mate with a male with long feathers, then there will be a selection pressure against any male with a genotype which is expressed as short feathers. Because of this differential reproduction, the alleles which are expressed as short feathers will be eliminated from the population. Thus this population evolves.

The two common forms of natural selection are : i) **stabilizing selection** in which average phenotypes have a selective advantage over extremes (*phenotypes have a 'bell curve' distribution*); ii) **directional selection** when one extreme has a selective advantage over the average phenotype (*thus the curve can become squewed to the left or right*). A derivative of directional selection is disruptive selection where both extremes are selected over the average phenotype; this would produce a split down the middle of the 'bell curve' such that two new and separate 'bell curves' would result. For example, if a bird only ate medium sized seeds and left the large and small ones alone, two new populations or groups of seeds would have a reproductive advantage. Thus by selecting against one group of seeds, two new groups of seeds with, possibly, different allelic frequencies for seed size will result. This is an example of *group selection* causing *disruptive selection*.

16.3 Species and Speciation

Species can be defined as the members of populations that interbreed or can interbreed under natural conditions. There are great variations within species. A **cline** is a gradient of variation in a species across a geographical area. **Speciation** is the evolution of new species by the isolation of gene pools of related populations. The isolation of gene pools is typically geographic. An ocean, a glacier, a river or any other physical barrier can isolate a population and prevent it from mating with other populations of the same species. The two populations may begin to differ because their mutations may be different, or, there may be different selection pressures from the two different environments, or, genetic drift may play a role.

Genetic drift is the random change in frequencies of alleles or genotypes in a population (recall that this is antagonistic to the Hardy-Weinberg Law). Genetic drift normally occurs when a small population is isolated from a large population. Since the allelic frequencies in the small population may be different from the large population (*sampling error*), the two populations may evolve in different directions.

Populations or species can be sympatric (= live together), or allopatric (= live apart). Mechanisms involved in allopatric speciation are represented in the two preceding paragraphs. The following represents some isolating mechanisms that prevent sympatric populations of different species from breeding together: i) habitat differences; ii) different breeding times or seasons; iii) mechanical differences (i.e. different anatomy of the genitalia); iv) behavioral specificity (i.e. different courtship behavior); v) gametic isolation (= fertilization cannot occur); vi) hybrid inviability (i.e. the hybrid zygote dies before reaching the age of sexual maturity); vii) hybrid sterility; viii) hybrid breakdown: the hybrid offspring is fertile but produces a next generation (F_2) which is infertile or inviable.

16.4 Origin of Life

Evidence suggests that the primitive earth had a reducing atmosphere with gases such as H_2 and the reduced compounds H_2O (vapor), $NH_{3(g)}$ (ammonia) and $CH_{4(g)}$ (methane). Such an atmosphere has been shown (i.e. Miller, Fox) to be conducive to the formation and stabilization of organic compounds. Such compounds can sometimes polymerize (*possibly due to autocatalysis*) and evolve into living systems with metabolism, reproduction, digestion, excretion, etc...

Critical in the early history of the earth was the evolution of: photosynthesis which releases O_2 and thus converted the atmosphere into an oxidizing one; respiration, which could use the O_2 to efficiently produce ATP; and the development of membrane bound organelles (*a subset of prokaryotes which evolved into eukaryotes*) which allowed eukaryotes to develop meiosis, sexual reproduction, and fertilization.

It is important to recognize that throughout the evolution of the earth, organisms and the environment have and will continue to shape each other.

16.5 Comparative Anatomy

Anatomical features of organisms can be compared in order to derive information about their evolutionary histories. Structures which originate from the same part of the embryo are called homologous. **Homologous** structures may have different functions in different species. **Analogous** structures have similar functions but arise from different embryological structures. **Vestigial** structures represent further evidence for evolution since they are organs which are useless in their present owners, but are homologous with organs which are important in other species.

Taxonomy is the branch of biology which deals with the classification of organisms. Humans are classified as follows:

Kingdom	Animalia
Phylum (= Division)	Chordata
Class	Mammalia
Order	Primates
Family	Hominidae
Genus	*Homo*
Species	*Homo sapiens*

{Mnemonic for remembering the taxonomic categories: King Philip came over for great soup}

The subphyla Vertebrata and Invertebrata are subdivisions of the phylum Chordata. Acorn worms, tunicates, sea squirts and amphioxus are invertebrates. Humans, birds, frogs, fish, and crocodiles are vertebrates. We will examine features of both the chordates and the vertebrates.

Chordates have the following characteristics at some stage of their development: i) a notochord; ii) pharyngeal gill slits which lead from the pharynx to the exterior; iii) a hollow dorsal nerve cord. Other features which are less defining but are nonetheless present in chordates are: i) a more or less segmented anatomy; ii) an internal skeleton (= *endoskeleton*); iii) a tail at some point in their development.

Vertebrates have all the characteristics of chordates. In addition, vertebrates have: i) a vertebral column; ii) well developed sensory and nervous systems; iii) a ventral heart with a closed vascular system; iv) some sort of a liver, endocrine organs, and kidneys; and v) cephalization which is the concentration of sense organs and nerves to the front end of the body producing an obvious head.

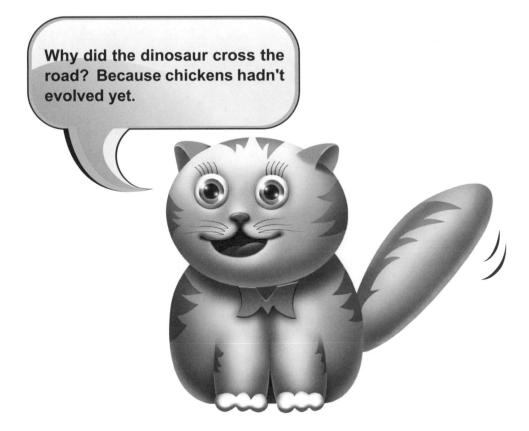

Why did the dinosaur cross the road? Because chickens hadn't evolved yet.

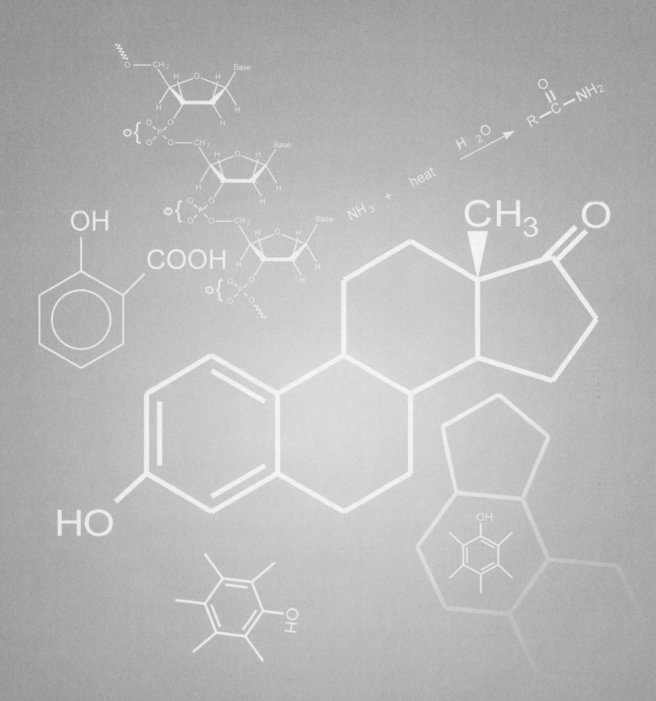

**ORGANIC
CHEMISTRY**

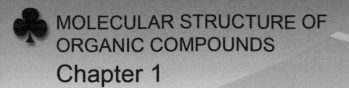

MOLECULAR STRUCTURE OF ORGANIC COMPOUNDS
Chapter 1

Memorize	Understand	Not Required*
* Hybrid orbitals and geometries * Periodic table trends * Define: Lewis, dipole moments * Ground rules for reaction mechanisms * Spectator, nucleophile, leaving group	* Delocalized electrons and resonance * Multiple bonds, length, energies * Basic stereochemistry * Principles for reaction mechanisms	* Advanced level college info * Alkenes and alkynes: NOT required * Hybrids involving d, f, etc.

MCAT-Prep.com

Introduction ▮▮▮▮

Organic chemistry is the study of the structure, properties, composition, reactions, and preparation (i.e. synthesis) of chemical compounds containing carbon. Such compounds may contain hydrogen, nitrogen, oxygen, the halogens as well as phosphorus, silicon and sulfur. If you master the basic rules in this chapter, you will be able to conquer MCAT mechanisms with little or no further memorization.

Additional Resources

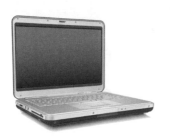

Free Online Q & A

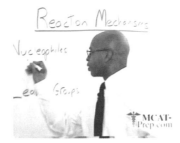

Video: DVD Disc 1

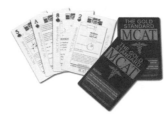

Flashcards

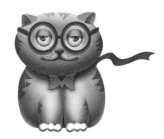

Special Guest

Organic chemistry may be defined as the chemistry of the compounds of carbon. Organic chemistry is very important, as living systems are composed mainly of water and organic compounds. Other important organic molecules form essential components of fuels, plastics and other petroleum derivatives.

Carbon (C), hydrogen (H), oxygen (O), nitrogen (N) and the halides (i.e. fluorine - F, chlorine - Cl, bromine - Br, etc.) are the most common atoms found in organic compounds. The atoms in most organic compounds are held together by covalent bonds (*the sharing of an electron pair between two atoms*). Some ionic bonding (*the transfer of electrons from one atom to another*) does exist. Common to both types of chemical bonds is the fact that the atoms bond such that they can achieve the electron configuration of the nearest noble gas, usually eight electrons. This is known as the *octet rule*.

A **carbon** atom has one s and three p orbitals in its outermost shell, allowing it to form 4 single bonds. As well, a carbon atom may be involved in a double bond, where two electron pairs are shared, or a triple bond, where three electron pairs are shared. An **oxygen** atom may form 2 single bonds, or one double bond. It has 2 unshared (lone) electron pairs. A **hydrogen** atom will form only one single bond. A **nitrogen** atom may form 3 single bonds. As well, it is capable of double and triple bonds. It has one unshared electron pair. The **halides** are all able to form only one (single) bond. Halides all have three unshared electron pairs.

Throughout the following chapters we will be examining the structural formulas of molecules involving H, C, N, O, halides and phosphorus (P). However it should be noted that less common atoms often have similar structural formulas within molecules as compared to common atoms. For example, silicon (Si) is found in the same group as carbon in the periodic table; thus they have similar properties. In fact, Si can also form 4 single bonds leading to a tetrahedral structure (i.e. SiH_4, SiO_4). Likewise sulfur (S) is found in the same group as oxygen. Though it can be found as a solid (S_8), it still has many properties similar to those of oxygen. For example, like O in H_2O, sulfur can form a bent, polar molecule which can hydrogen bond (H_2S). We will later see that sulfur is an important component in the amino acid cysteine. {*To learn more about molecular structure, hybrid orbitals, polarity and bonding, review General Chemistry chapters 2 and 3* }

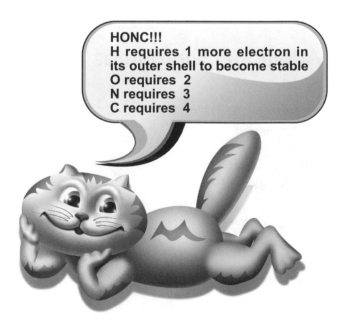

HONC!!!
H requires 1 more electron in its outer shell to become stable
O requires 2
N requires 3
C requires 4

1.2 Hybrid Orbitals

In organic molecules, the orbitals of the atoms are combined to form **hybrid orbitals**, consisting of a mixture of the s and p orbitals. In a carbon atom, if the one s and three p orbitals are mixed, the result is four hybrid sp^3 orbitals. Three hybridized sp^2 orbitals result from the mixing of one s and two p orbitals, and two hybridized sp orbitals result from the mixing of one s and one p. The geometry of the hybridized orbitals is shown in Figure IV.B.1.1.

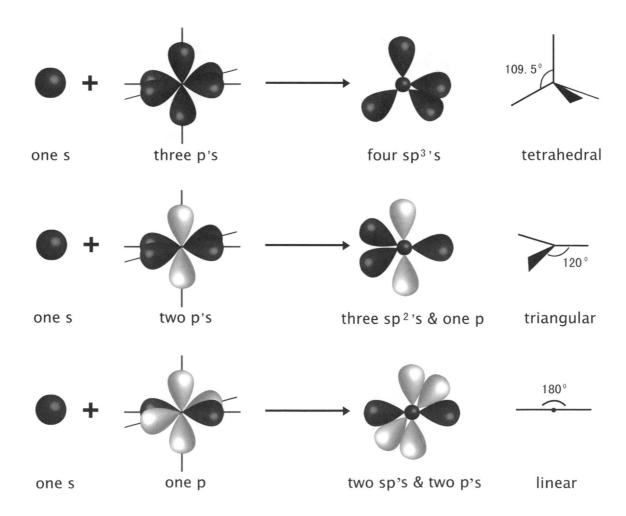

Figure IV.B.1.1: Hybrid orbital geometry

1.3 Bonding

Sigma (or single) bonds are those in which the electron density is between the nuclei. They are symmetric about the axis, can freely rotate, and are formed when orbitals (regular or hybridized) overlap directly. They are characterized by the fact that they are circular when a cross section is taken and the bond is viewed along the bond axis. The electron density in pi bonds overlaps both above and below the plane of the atoms. A single bond is a sigma bond; a double bond is one sigma and one pi bond; a triple bond is one sigma (σ) and two pi (π) bonds.

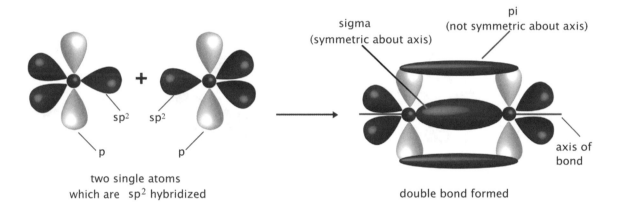

Figure IV.B.1.2: Sigma and pi bonds. The sp^2 hybrids overlap between the nuclei to form a σ bond; the p orbitals overlap above and below the axis between the nuclei to form a π bond.

1.3.1 The Effects of Multiple Bonds

The pi bonds in doubly and triply bonded molecules create a barrier to free rotation about the axis of the bond. Thus multiple bonds create molecules which are much more rigid than a molecule with only a single bond which can freely rotate about its axis.

As a rule, the length of a bond decreases with multiple bonds. For example, the carbon-carbon triple bond is shorter than the carbon-carbon double bond which is shorter than the carbon-carbon single bond.

Bond strength and thus the amount of energy required to break a bond (= *BE, the bond dissociation energy*) varies with the number of bonds. One σ bond has a BE $\approx$ 110 kcal/mole and one π bond has a BE $\approx$ 60 kcal/mole. Thus a single bond (one σ) has a BE $\approx$ 110 kcal/mole while a double bond (one σ + one π) has a BE $\approx$ 170 kcal/mole. Hence multiple bonds have greater bond strength than single bonds.

1.4 Delocalized Electrons and Resonance

Delocalization of charges in the pi bonds is possible when there are hybridized orbitals in adjacent atoms. This delocalization may be represented in two different ways, the molecular orbital (MO) approach or the resonance (*valence bond*) approach. The differences are found in Figure IV.B.1.3.

The MO approach takes a linear combination of atomic orbitals to form molecular orbitals, in which electrons form the bonds. These molecular orbitals cover the whole molecule, and thus the delocalization of electrons is depicted. In the resonance approach, there is a linear combination of different structures with localized pi bonds and electrons, which together depict the true molecule, or **resonance hybrid**. There is no single structure that represents the molecule.

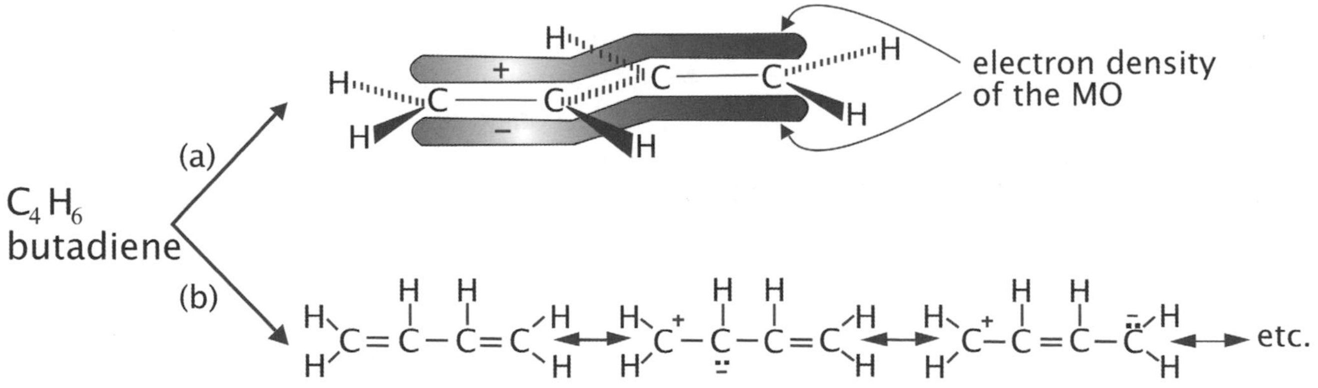

C_4H_6
butadiene

Figure IV.B.1.3: A comparison of MO and resonance approaches. (a) The electron density of the MO covers the entire molecule such that π bonds and p orbitals are not distinguishable. (b) No singular resonance structure accurately portrays butadiene; rather, the true molecule is a composite of all of its resonance structures.

1.5 Lewis Structures, Charge Separation and Dipole Moments

The outer shell (or **valence**) electrons are those that form chemical bonds. **Lewis dot structures** are a method of showing the valence electrons and how they form bonds. These electrons, along with the octet rule (*which states that a maximum of eight electrons are allowed in the outermost shell of an atom*) holds only for the elements in the second row of the periodic table (C,N,O,F). The elements of the third row (Si, P, S, Cl) use d orbitals, and thus can have more than eight electrons in their outer shell.

Let us use CO_2 as an example. Carbon has four valence electrons and oxygen has six. By covalently bonding, electrons are shared and the octet rule is followed,

$$\cdot \overset{\displaystyle \cdot}{\underset{\displaystyle \cdot}{C}} \cdot \quad + \quad 2 \; \vdots \overset{\displaystyle \cdot \cdot}{\underset{\displaystyle \cdot \cdot}{O}} \vdots \quad \longrightarrow$$

$$\vdots \overset{\displaystyle \cdot \cdot}{\underset{\displaystyle \cdot \cdot}{O}} :: C :: \overset{\displaystyle \cdot \cdot}{\underset{\displaystyle \cdot \cdot}{O}} \vdots \quad \text{or} \quad \vdots \overset{\displaystyle \cdot \cdot}{\underset{\displaystyle \cdot \cdot}{O}} = C = \overset{\displaystyle \cdot \cdot}{\underset{\displaystyle \cdot \cdot}{O}} \vdots$$

Carbon and oxygen can form resonance structures in the molecule CO_3^{-2}. The -2 denotes two extra electrons to place in the molecule. Once again the octet rule is followed,

In the final structure, each element counts one half of the electrons in a bond as its own, and any unpaired electrons are counted as its own. The sum of these two quantities should equal the number of valence electrons that were originally around the atom.

If the chemical bond is made up of atoms of different electronegativity, there is a **charge separation:**

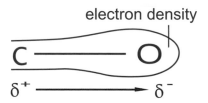

electron density

$$\delta^+ \xrightarrow{\hspace{2cm}} \delta^-$$

There is a slight pulling of electron density by the more electronegative atom (oxygen in the preceding example) from the less electronegative atom (carbon in the preceding example). This results in the C-O bond having **partial ionic character** (i.e. *a polar bond; see* CHM 3.3). The charge separation also causes an <u>electrical dipole</u> to be set up in the direction of the arrow. A dipole has a positive end (carbon) and a negative end (oxygen). A dipole will line up in an electric field.

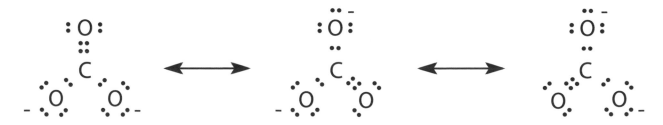

The most electronegative elements (in order, with electronegativities in brackets) are fluorine (4.0), oxygen (3.5), nitrogen (3.0), and chlorine (3.0) [To examine trends, see the periodic table in CHM 2.3]. These elements will often be paired with hydrogen (2.1) and carbon (2.5), resulting in bonds with partial ionic character. The **dipole moment** is a measure of the charge separation and thus, the electronegativities of the elements that make up the bond; the larger the dipole moment, the larger the charge separation.

No dipole moment is found in molecules with no charge separation between atoms (i.e. Cl_2, Br_2), or, when the charge separation is <u>symmetric</u> resulting in a cancellation of bond polarity like vector addition in physics (i.e. CH_4, CO_2).

A molecule where the charge separation between atoms is <u>not symmetric</u> will have a non-zero dipole moment (i.e. CH_3F, H_2O, NH_3 - *see* ORG 11.1.2).

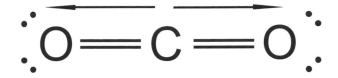

Figure IV.B.1.4: CO_2 - polar bonds but overall it is a non-polar molecule; therefore, CO_2 has a zero dipole moment.

1.5.1 Strength of Polar vs. Non-Polar Bonds

Non-polar bonds are generally stronger than polar covalent and ionic bonds, with ionic bonds being the weakest. However, in compounds with ionic bonding, there is generally a large number of bonds between molecules and this makes the compound as a whole very strong. For instance, although the ionic bonds in one compound are weaker than the non-polar covalent bonds in another compound, the ionic compound's melting point will be higher than the melting point of the covalent compound. Polar covalent bonds have a partially ionic character, and thus the bond strength is usually intermediate between that of ionic and that of non-polar covalent bonds. The strength of bonds generally decreases with increasing ionic character.

Opposites attract. Like charges repel. Such simple statements are fundamental in solving over 90% of mechanisms in organic chemistry. Once you are comfortable with the basics - electronegativity, polarity and resonance - you will not need to memorize the grand majority of outcomes of given reactions. You will be capable of quickly deducing the answer even when new scenarios are presented.

A substance which has a formal positive charge ($^+$) or a partial positive charge ("delta$^+$" or δ^+) is attracted to a substance with a formal negative charge ($^-$) or a partial negative charge (δ^-). In general, a substance with a formal charge would have a greater force of attraction than one with a partial charge when faced with an oppositely charged species. There is an important exception: spectator ions. Ions formed by elements in the first two groups of the periodic table (i.e. Na^+, K^+, Ca^{++}) do not actively engage in reactions in organic chemistry. They simply watch the reaction occur then at the very end they associate with the negatively charged product.

In most carbon-based compounds the carbon atom is bonded to a more electronegative atom. For example, in a carbon-oxygen bond the oxygen is δ^- resulting in a δ^+ carbon (see ORG 1.5). Because opposites attract, a δ^- carbon (which is unusual) could create a carbon-carbon bond with a δ^+ carbon (which is common). There are two important categories of compounds which can create a carbon-carbon bond; a) alkyl lithiums

(RLi) and b) Grignard reagents (RMgBr), because they each have a δ^- carbon. Note that the carbon is δ^- since lithium is to the left of carbon on the periodic table (for electronegativity trends see CHM 2.3).

For nucleophiles, the general trend is that the stronger the nucleophile, the stronger the base it is. For example:

$$RO^- > HO^- >> RCOO^- > ROH > H_2O$$

For information on the quality of leaving groups, see ORG 6.2.4.

Memorize	Understand	Not Required*
* Categories of stereoisomers * Define enantiomers, diastereomers, meso * Convention: R, S and E, Z forms * Define ligand, chiral, racemic mixture	* Basic stereochemistry only	* Advanced level college info * Assign R/S/E/Z to complex molecul * Memorize specific rotation equatio

MCAT-Prep.com

Introduction ▪▪▪▪

Stereochemistry is the study of the relative spatial (3 D) arrangement of atoms within molecules. An important branch of stereochemistry, and most relevant to the new MCAT, is the study of chiral molecules.

Additional Resources

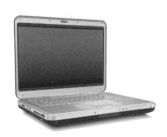

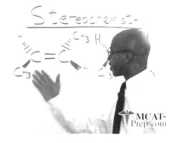

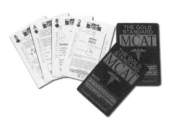

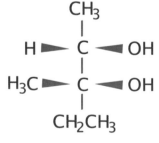

Free Online Q & A   Video: DVD Disc 1   Flashcards   Special Guest

2.1 Isomers

Stereochemistry is the study of the arrangement of atoms in a molecule, in three dimensions. Two *different molecules* with the same number and type of atoms (= *the same molecular formula*) are called isomers. There are several different types of isomers:

Structural isomers have different atoms and/or bonding patterns in relation to each other:

$$H_3C-\overset{\overset{\displaystyle CH_3}{|}}{\underset{\underset{\displaystyle H}{|}}{C}}-CH_2CH_2CH_3$$

and $H_3C-\overset{\overset{\displaystyle H}{|}}{\underset{\underset{\underset{\displaystyle CH_3}{|}}{\underset{\displaystyle CH_2}{|}}}{C}}-CH_2CH_3$

Conformational isomers are isomers which differ only by the rotation about multiple single bonds or just one single bond (= *rotamer*). As a result, substituents (= *ligands = attached atoms or groups*) can be maximally close (*eclipsed conformation*), maximally apart (*anti or staggered conformation*) or anywhere in between (i.e. *gauche conformation*). Though all conformations occur at room temperature, anti is most stable since it minimizes electron shell repulsion.

Geometric isomers occur because carbons that are in a ring or double bond structure are *unable* to freely rotate. Geometric isomers occur only as alkenes and cyclic compounds. This results in *cis* and *trans* compounds. When the substituents (i.e. Br) are on the same side of the ring or double bond, it is designated cis. When they are on opposite sides, it is designated trans. The trans isomer is more stable since the substituents are further apart, thus electron shell repulsion is minimized.

$$\underset{Br}{\overset{H}{\diagdown}}C=C\underset{Br}{\overset{H}{\diagup}}$$

cis-dibromoethene

and

$$\underset{Br}{\overset{H}{\diagdown}}C=C\underset{H}{\overset{Br}{\diagup}}$$

trans-dibromoethene

In general, structural and geometric isomers have different reactivity, spectra and physical properties (i.e. boiling points, melting points, etc.).

Stereoisomers are different compounds with the same structure, differing only in the spatial orientation of the atoms (= *configuration*). Stereoisomers may be further divided into enantiomers and diastereomers.

2.2 Enantiomers and Diastereomers

Enantiomers come in pairs. They are two non-superimposable molecules, which are mirror images of each other. In order to have an enantiomer, a molecule must be chiral. Chiral molecules contain a carbon atom that has four different substituents attached to it.

Enantiomers have the same chemical and physical properties. The only difference is with their interactions with other chiral molecules, and their rotation of plane polarized light.

Conversely, diastereomers are any pair of stereoisomers that are not enantiomers. Diastereomers are both chemically and physically different from each other.

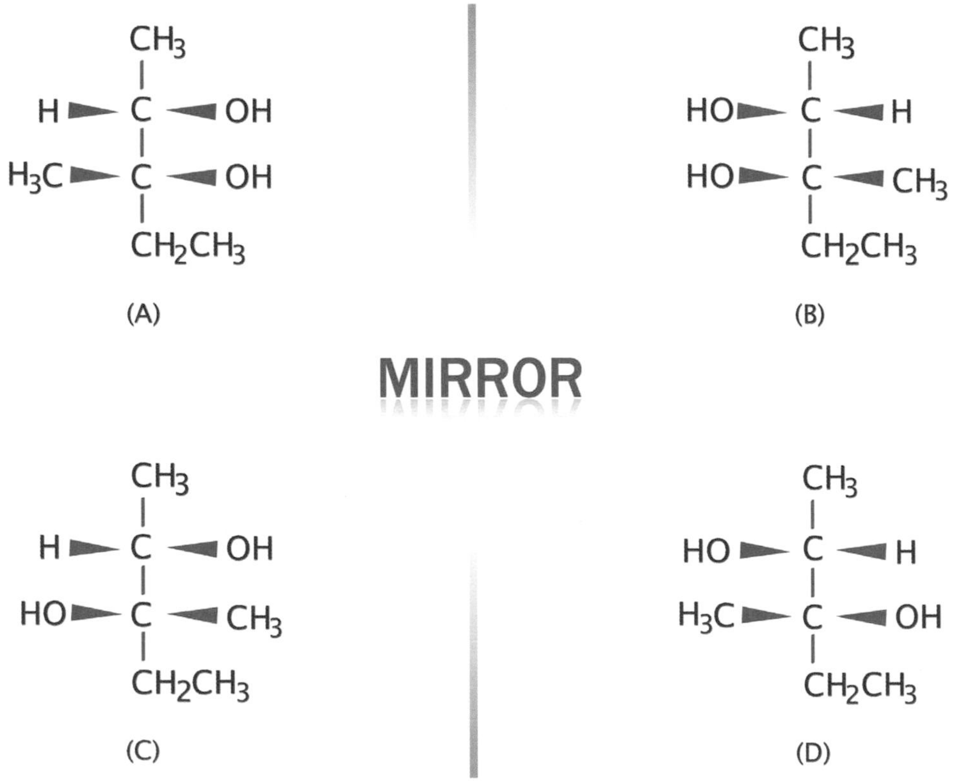

MIRROR

Figure IV.B.2.1: Enantiomers and diastereomers. The enantiomers are A & B, C & D. The diastereomers are A & C, A & D, B & D, B & C.

2.3 Absolute and Relative Configuration

Before 1951, the absolute three dimensional arrangement or <u>configuration</u> of chiral molecules was not known. Instead chiral molecules were compared to an arbitrary standard (*glyceraldehyde*). Thus the *relative* configuration could be determined. Once the actual spatial arrangements of groups in molecules were finally determined, the *absolute* configuration could be known.

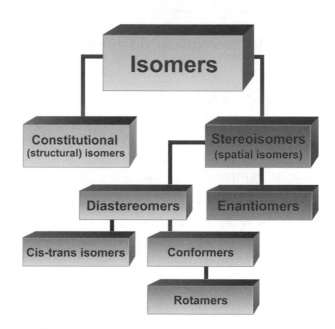

Figure IV.B.2.1.1: Categories of isomers.

2.3.1 The R, S System

One consequence of the existence of enantiomers, is a special system of nomenclature: the <u>R, S system</u>. This system provides information about the absolute configuration of a molecule. This is done by assigning a stereochemical configuration at each asymmetric (*chiral*) carbon in the molecule by using the following steps:

1. Identify an asymmetric carbon, and the four attached groups.

2. Assign priorities to the four groups, using the following rules:

i. Atoms of higher atomic number have higher priority.

ii. An isotope of higher atomic mass receives higher priority.

iii. The higher priority is assigned to the group with the atom of higher atomic number or mass at the first point of difference.

iv. If the difference between the two groups is due to the number of otherwise identical atoms, the higher priority is assigned to the group with the greater number of atoms of higher atomic number or mass.

v. To assign priority of double and triple bonded groups, these atoms are replicated:

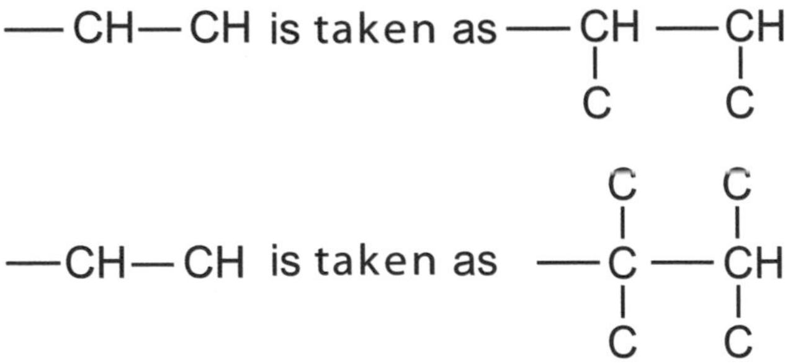

—CH—CH is taken as —CH—CH
C C
—CH—CH is taken as —C—CH
C C C C

3. View the molecule along the bond from the asymmetric carbon to the group of lowest priority (i.e. the asymmetric carbon is near, and the low priority group is far away).

4. Consider the clockwise or counterclockwise order of the priorities of the remaining groups. If they increase in a clockwise direction, the asymmetric carbon is said to have the R configuration. If they decrease in a clockwise direction, the asymmetric carbon is said to have the S configuration.

A stereoisomer is named by indicating the configurations of each of the asymmetric carbons.

3
CH3
C
4 H
CH=CH2
1
C2H5
2
clockwise

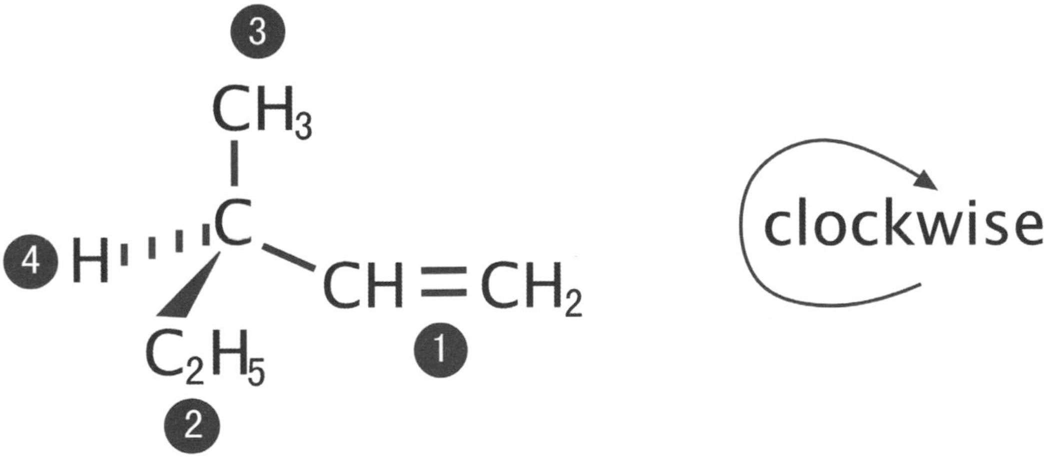

(R) - 3 - methyl - 1 - pentene

Figure IV.B.2.2: Assigning Absolute Configuration. In organic chemistry, the directions of the bonds are symbolized as follows: a broken line extends away from the viewer (i.e. INTO the page), a solid triangle projects towards the viewer, and a straight line extends in the plane of the paper. According to rule #3, we must imagine that the lowest priority group (H) points away from the viewer.

2.3.2 Optical Isomers and the D, L System

Optical Isomers are stereoisomers that differ by different spatial orientations about a chiral carbon atom. Light is an electromagnetic wave that contains oscillating fields. In ordinary light, the electric field oscillates in all directions. However, it is possible to obtain light with an electric field that oscillates in only one plane. This type of light is known as **plane polarized light**. When plane polarized light is passed through a sample of a chiral substance, it will emerge vibrating in a different plane than it started. Optical isomers differ only in this rotation. If the light is rotated in a clockwise direction, the compound is dextrorotary, and is designated by a D or (+). If the light is rotated in a counterclockwise direction, the compound is levrorotary, and is designated by an L or (-). All L compounds have the same relative configuration as L-glyceraldehyde.

A racemic mixture will show no rotation of plane polarized light. This is a consequence of the fact that a racemate is a mixture with equal amounts of the D and L forms of a substance.

Specific rotation (α) is an inherent physical property of a molecule. It is defined as follows:

$$\alpha = \frac{\text{Observed rotation in degrees}}{(\text{ tube length in dm}) (\text{concentration in g/ml})}$$

The observed rotation is the rotation of the light passed through the substance. The tube length is the length of the tube that contains the sample in question. The specific rotation is dependent on the solvent used, the temperature of the sample, and the wavelength of the light.

It should be noted that there is no clear correlation between the absolute configuration (i.e. R, S) and the direction of rotation of plane polarized light.

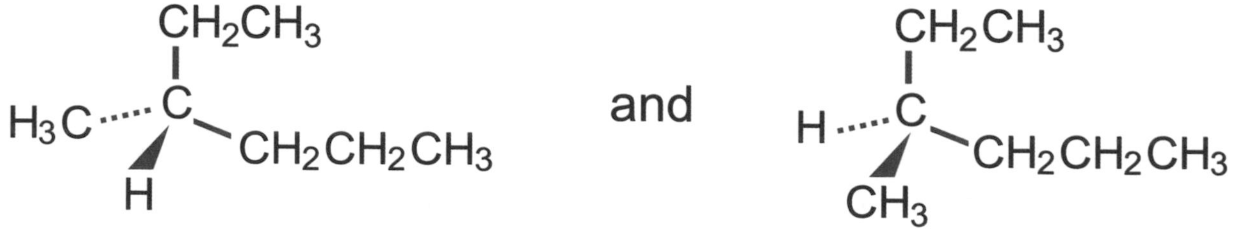

Figure IV.B.2.3: Optical isomers.

2.3.3 Meso Compounds

Tartari acid(= 2,3-dihydroxybutanedioic acid which, for MCAT purposes, please feel free to forget its IUPAC name!) has two chiral centers that have the same four substituents and are equivalent. As a result, two of the four possible stereoisomers of this compound are identical due to a plane of symmetry. Thus there are only three stereoisomeric tartaric acids. Two of these stereoisomers are enantiomers and the third is an achiral diastereomer, called a *meso* compound. Meso compounds are achiral (optically inactive) diastereomers of chiral stereoisomers {**MeS**o = **M**irror of **S**ymmetry}.

(+)-tartaric acid   (-)-tartaric acid

MIRROR

meso-tartaric acid   *meso*-tartaric acid

2.3.4 E, Z Designation

The E, Z notation is the IUPAC preferred method for designating the stereochemistry of double bonds (yes, we are aware of the irony that the AAMC lists this topic as one of your responsibilities for the MCAT despite the fact that alkene chemistry is no longer part of the new MCAT!). Anyways (!!), ORG 2.1 reviewed how to use cis/trans. The E, Z notation is quite similar but more precise.

To begin with, each substituent at the double bond is assigned a priority (*see* ORG 2.3.1 for rules). If the two groups of higher priority are on opposite sides of the double bond, the bond is assigned the configuration E, (from *entgegen*, the German word for "opposite"). If the two groups of higher priority are on the same side of the double bond, the bond is assigned the configuration Z, (from *zusammen*, the German word for "together"). {Learning German is NOT required for the MCAT!}

GOLD NOTES

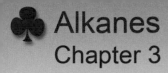

Memorize	Understand	Not Required*
* IUPAC nomenclature * Physical properties " Steps: free radical substitution	* Trends based on length, branching * Ring strain, ESR * Complete combustion	* Advanced level college info * Reactions involving alkenes, alkyne * Technical categorization of "cyclic alkanes"

MCAT-Prep.com

Introduction ▪▪▪▪

Alkanes (a.k.a. paraffins) are compounds that consist only of the elements carbon (C) and hydrogen (H) (i.e. hydrocarbons). In addition, C and H are linked together exclusively by single bonds (i.e. they are saturated compounds). Methane is the simplest possible alkane while saturated oils and fats are much larger.

Additional Resources

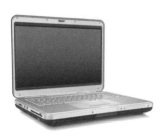

Free Online Q & A

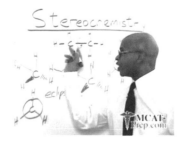

Video: DVD Discs 1,3

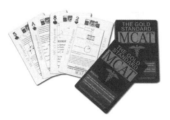

Flashcards

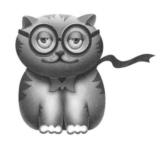

Special Guest

Alkanes are hydrocarbon molecules containing only sp3 hybridized carbon atoms (single bonds). They may be unbranched, branched or cyclic. Their general formula is C_nH_{2n+2} for a straight chain molecule; 2 hydrogen (H) atoms are subtracted for each ring. They contain no functional groups and are fully saturated molecules (= *no double or triple bonds*). As a result, they are chemically unreactive except when exposed to heat or light.

Systematic naming of compounds (= *nomenclature*) has evolved from the International Union of Pure and Applied Chemistry (IUPAC). **The nomenclature of alkanes is the basis of that for many other organic molecules.** The root of the compound is named according to the number of carbons in the longest carbon chain:

C_1 = meth	C_5 = pent	C_8 = oct
C_2 = eth	C_6 = hex	C_9 = non
C_3 = prop	C_7 = hept	C_{10} = dec
C_4 = but		

When naming these as fragments, (alkyl fragments: *the alkane minus one H atom*, symbol: R), the suffix '-yl' is used. If naming the alkane, the suffix '-ane' is used. Some prefixes result from the fact that a carbon with *one* R group attached is a *primary* (normal or n -) carbon, *two* R groups is *secondary* (sec) and with *three* R groups it is a *tertiary* (tert or t -) carbon. Some alkyl groups have special names:

C—C—C— n - propyl

C—C—C—C— n - butyl

H_3C CH— isopropyl

H_3C-C- tert - butyl

CH_3CH_2CH— sec - butyl

$H_3C-C-CH_2$— neopentyl

Cyclic alkanes are named in the same way (according to the number of carbons), but the prefix 'cyclo' is added. The shorthand for organic compounds is a geometric figure where each corner represents a carbon; hydrogens need not be written, though it should be remembered that the number of hydrogens would exist such that the number of bonds at each carbon is four.

cyclobutane

cyclohexane

The nomenclature for branched-chain alkanes begins by determining the longest straight chain (i.e. *the highest number of carbons attached in a row*). The groups attached to the straight or *main* chain are numbered so as to achieve the lowest set of numbers. Groups are cited in alphabetical order. If a group appears more than once, the prefixes di-(2), tri-(3), tetra-(4) are used. If two chains of equal length compete for selection as the main chain, choose the chain with the most substituents. For example:

4,6-Diethyl-2,5,5,6,7-pentamethyl octane (7 substituents) or 3,5-Diethyl-2,3,4,4,7-pentamethyl octane (a bit better for keeners! i.e. not MCAT level) NOT 2,5,5,6-Tetramethyl-4-ethyl-6-isopropyl octane (6 substituents)

3.1.1 Physical Properties of Alkanes

At room temperature and one atmosphere of pressure straight chain alkanes with 1 to 4 carbons are gases (i.e. CH_4 - methane, CH_3CH_3 - ethane, etc.), 5 to 17 carbons are liquids, and more than 17 carbons are solid. Boiling points of straight chain alkanes (= *aliphatic*) show a regular increase with increasing number of carbons. This is because they are nonpolar molecules, and have weak intermolecular forces. Branching of alkanes leads to a dramatic decrease in the boiling point. As a rule, as the number of carbons increase the melting points also increase.

Alkanes are soluble in nonpolar solvents (i.e. benzene, CCl_4 - carbon tetrachloride, etc.), and not in aqueous solvents (= *hydrophobic*). They are insoluble in water because of their low polarity and their inability to hydrogen bond. Alkanes are the least dense of all classes of organic compounds (<< ρ_{water}, 1 g/ml). Thus petroleum, a mixture of hydrocarbons rich in alkanes, floats on water.

3.2 Important Reactions of Alkanes

3.2.1 Combustion

Combustion may be either complete or incomplete. In complete combustion, the hydrocarbon is converted to carbon dioxide (CO_2) and water (H_2O). If there is insufficient oxygen for complete combustion, the reaction gives other products, such as carbon monoxide (CO) and soot (molecular C). This strongly exothermic reaction may be summarized:

$$C_nH_{2n+2} + \text{excess } O_2 \rightarrow nCO_2 + (n+1)H_2O.$$

3.2.2 Radical Substitution Reactions

Radical substitution reactions with halogens may be summarized:

$$RH + X_2 + \text{uv light}(hf) \text{ or heat} \rightarrow RX + HX$$

The halogen X_2, may be F_2, Cl_2, or Br_2. I_2 does not react. The mechanism of *halogenation* may be explained and summarized by example:

i. Initiation: This step involves the formation of *free radicals* (highly reactive substances which contain an unpaired electron, which is symbolized by a single dot):

$$Cl{:}Cl + \text{uv light or heat} \rightarrow 2Cl\cdot$$

ii. Propagation: In this step, the chlorine free radical begins a series of reactions that form new free radicals:

$$CH_4 + Cl\cdot \rightarrow \cdot CH_3 + HCl$$
$$\cdot CH_3 + Cl_2 \rightarrow CH_3Cl + Cl\cdot$$

iii. Termination: These reactions end the radical propagation steps. Termination reactions destroy the free radicals (coupling).

$$Cl\cdot + \cdot CH_3 \rightarrow CH_3Cl$$
$$\cdot CH_3 + \cdot CH_3 \rightarrow CH_3CH_3$$
$$Cl\cdot + Cl\cdot \rightarrow Cl_2$$

Radical substitution reactions can also occur with halide acids (i.e. HCl, HBr) and peroxides (i.e. HOOH - hydrogen peroxide). Chain propagation (step ii) can destroy many organic compounds fairly quick. This step can be inhibited by using a resonance stabilized free radical to "mop up" (*termination*) other destructive free radicals in the medium. For example, BHT is a resonance stabilized free radical added to packaging of many breakfast cereals in order to inhibit free radical destruction of the cereal (= *spoiling*).

The stability of a free radical depends on the ability of the compound to stabilize the unpaired electron. This is analogous to stabilizing a positively charged carbon (= *carbocation*). Thus, in both cases, a tertiary compound is more stable than secondary which, in turn, is more stable than a primary compound.

3.3 Ring Strain in Cyclic Alkanes

Cyclic alkanes are strained compounds. This **ring strain** results from the bending of the bond angles in greater amounts than normal. This strain causes cyclic compounds of 3 and 4 carbons to be unstable, and thus not often found in nature. The usual angle between bonds in an sp^3 hybridized carbon is $109.5°$ (= *the normal tetrahedral angle*).

The expected angles in some cyclic compounds can be determined geometrically: $60°$ in cyclopropane; $90°$ in cyclobutane and $108°$ in cyclopentane. Cyclohexane, in the chair conformation, has normal bond angles of $109.5°$. The closer the angle is to the normal tetrahedral angle of $109.5°$, the more stable the compound. In fact, cyclohexane can be found in a chair or boat conformation or any conformation in between; however, at any given moment, 99% of the cyclohexane molecules would be found in the chair conformation because it is the most stable (lower energy).

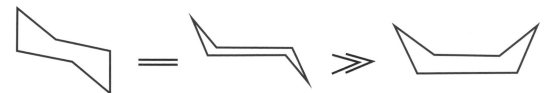

Figure IV.B.3.1: The chair and boat conformations of cyclohexane.

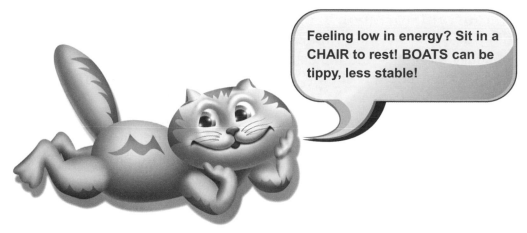

Feeling low in energy? Sit in a CHAIR to rest! BOATS can be tippy, less stable!

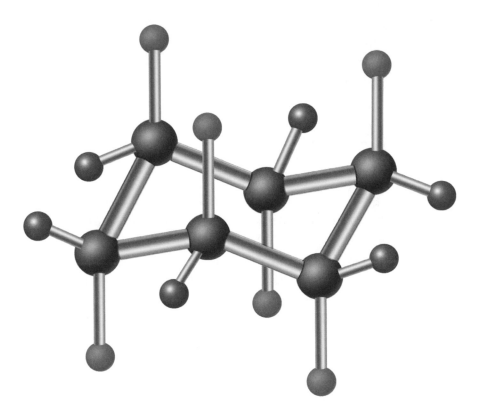

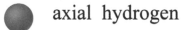 axial hydrogen

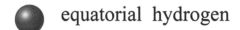 equatorial hydrogen

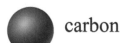 carbon

Figure IV.B.3.2: The chair conformation of cyclohexane. The hydrogens which are generally in the same plane as the ring are <u>equatorial</u>. The hydrogens which are generally perpendicular to the ring are <u>axial</u>. The hydrogen atoms are maximally separated and staggered to minimize electron shell repulsion.

It is important to have a clear understanding of electron shell repulsion (ESR). Essentially all atoms and molecules are surrounded by an electron shell (CHM 2.1, ORG 1.2) which is more like a cloud of electrons. Because like charges repel, when there are options, atoms and molecules assume the conformation which minimizes ESR.

For example, when substituents are added to a cyclic compound (i.e. Fig. IV.B.3.2), the most stable position is equatorial (equivalent to the anti conformation, ORG 2.1) which minimizes ESR. This conformation is most pronounced when the substituent is bulky (i.e. isopropyl, t-butyl, phenyl, etc.). In other words, a large substituent takes up more space thus ESR has a more prominent effect.

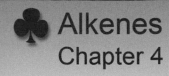

Alkenes
Chapter 4

Memorize	Understand	Not Required*
* Nothing	* Nothing	* Alkenes!

MCAT-Prep.com

Introduction ▊▊▊

An alkene (a.k.a. olefin) is an unsaturated chemical compound containing at least one carbon-to-carbon double bond. Alkene chemistry, including electrophilic addition, is no longer required for the new MCAT.

Additional Resources

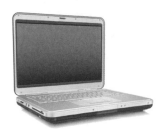

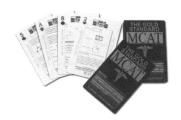

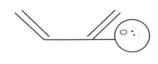

| Free Online Q & A | Video: DVD Discs 1,3,4 | Flashcards | Special Guest |

4.0 MCAT Changes

In 2003, the MCAT changed to no longer require previous knowledge of Alkenes, Benzene, Phenols and Ethers. Some questions on the *new* MCAT may, however, refer to these subjects but relevant information would be provided. It is therefore not necessary for you to memorize chapters containing such information. The following is presented only for completeness and to provide background information for questions that you may be asked but it is not required reading.

4.1 Description and Nomenclature

Alkenes are unsaturated hydrocarbon molecules containing carbon-carbon double bonds. Their general formula is C_nH_{2n} for a straight chain molecule; 2 hydrogen (H) atoms are subtracted for each ring. The *functional group* in these molecules is the double bond which determines the chemical properties of alkenes. Double bonds are sp^2 hybridized (*see* ORG 1.2, 1.3). The nomenclature is the same as that for alkanes, except that i) the suffix 'ene' replaces 'ane' and ii) the double bond is (are) numbered in the molecule, trying to get the smallest number for the double bond(s). For cycloalkenes, the carbons of the double bond are given the 1- and 2- positions.

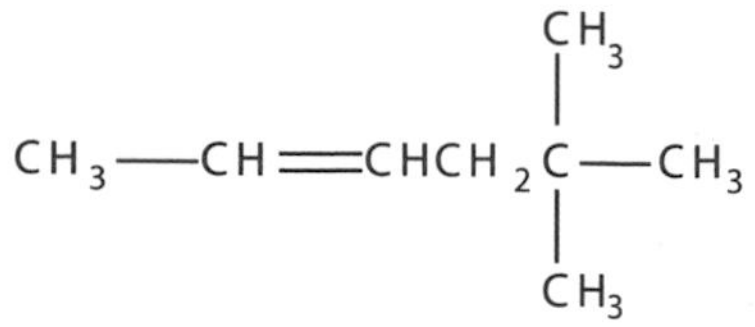

Two frequently encountered groups are sometimes named as if they were substituents.

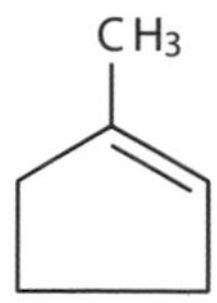

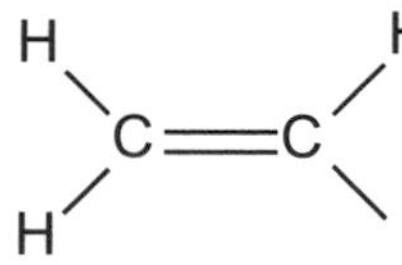

or $CH_2 \!=\! CH \!-\!$

the vinyl group

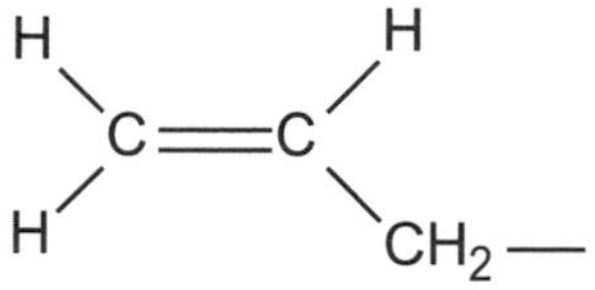

or $CH_2 \!=\! CHCH_2 \!-\!$

the allyl group

5,5-Dimethyl-2-hexene   1-methylcyclopentene

Alkenes have similar physical properties to alkanes. Trans compounds tend to have higher melting points (due to better symmetry), and lower boiling points (due to less polarity) than its corresponding cis isomer. Alkenes, however, due to the nature of the double bond may be polar:

has a small
dipole moment

has no dipole
moment

(cis)
small dipole
moment

(trans)
no dipole
moment

The greater the number of attached alkyl groups (i.e. *the more highly substituted the double bond*), the greater is the alkene's stability. The reason is that <u>alkyl</u> groups are somewhat electron donating, thus they stabilize the double bond.

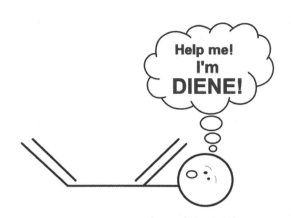

Help me!
I'm
DIENE!

4.2 Important Chemical Reactions

4.2.1 Electrophilic Addition

The chemistry of alkenes may be understood in terms of their functional group, the double bond. When <u>electrophiles</u> (*substances which seek electrons*) add to alkenes, carbocations (= *carbonium ions*) are formed. An important electrophile is H^+ (i.e. in HBr, H_2O, etc.). A <u>nucleophile</u> is a molecule with a free pair of electrons, and sometimes a negative charge, that seeks out partially or completely positively charged species (i.e. a carbon nucleus). Some important nucleophiles are OH^- and CN^-.

E = electrophile

carbocation
(intermediate)

Nu = nucleophile

Another important property of the double bond is its ability to stabilize carbocations, carbanions or radicals attached to adjacent carbons (*allylic carbons*). Note that all the following are resonance stabilized:

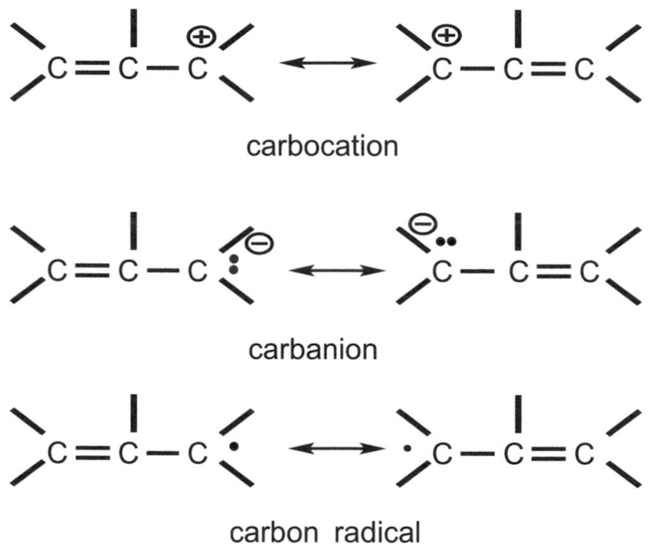

carbocation

carbanion

carbon radical

The stability of the intermediate carbocation depends on the groups attached to it, which can either stabilize or destabilize it. In general, groups which can share electrons by pi orbital overlap (resonance) stabilize the carbocation. As well, groups which place a partial or total positive charge adjacent to the carbocation withdraw electrons inductively, by sigma bonds, to destabilize it.

These points are useful in predicting which carbon will become the carbocation, and to which carbon the electrophile and nucleophile will bond. The intermediate carbocation formed must be the most stable. **Markovnikoff's rule** is a result of this, and it states: *the nucleophile will be bonded to the most substituted carbon* (fewest hydrogens attached) *in the product. Equivalently, the electrophile will be bonded to the least substituted carbon* (most hydrogens attached) *in the product.* An example of this is:

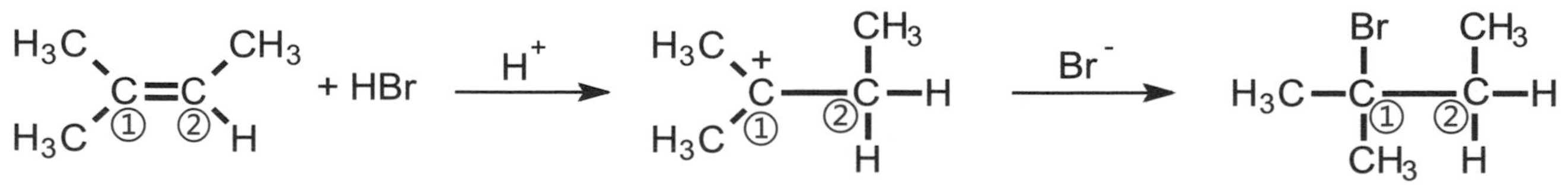

H^+ = electrophile
Br^- = nucleophile

① most substituted carbon
② least substituted carbon

① forms the most stable carbonium ion.

The product, 2-bromo-2-methyl butane, is the more likely or major product (*the Markovnikoff product*). Had the H$^+$ added to the most substituted carbon (which has a much lower probability of occurrence) the less likely or minor product would be formed (*the anti-Markovnikoff product*).

Markovnikoff's rule is true for the ionic conditions presented in the preceding reaction. However, for radical conditions the reverse occurs. Thus *anti-Markovnikoff* products are the major products under free radical conditions.

4.2.2 Oxidation

Alkenes can undergo a variety of reactions in which the carbon-carbon double bond is oxidized. Using potassium permanganate (KMnO$_4$) under mild conditions (*no heat*), or osmium tetroxide (OsO$_4$), a glycol (= *a dialcohol*) can be produced:

$$CH_2 = CH_2 + KMnO_4$$

$$\xrightarrow[OH^-]{Cold}$$

CH$_2$——CH$_2$
|OH |OH
Ethylene glycol

Using KMnO$_4$ under more abrasive conditions leads to an oxidative cleavage of the double bond:

$$CH_3 CH = CHCH_3 \xrightarrow[heat]{KMnO_4 , OH^-}$$

$$2CH_3C \overset{O}{\underset{O^-}{\diagdown}} \xrightarrow{H^+} 2CH_3C \overset{O}{\underset{OH}{\diagdown}}$$

Acetate ion   Acetic acid

Ozone (O$_3$) reacts vigorously with alkenes. The reaction (= *ozonolysis*) leads to an oxidative cleavage of the double bond which can produce a ketone and an aldehyde:

$$CH_3C = CHCH_3 \xrightarrow[\text{(2) Zn, H}_2\text{O}]{\text{(1) O}_3} CH_3C = O + CH_3CH$$

(with CH_3 substituent above the central carbons and O above the carbonyl)

2 - Methyl - 2 - butene   Acetone   Acetaldehyde

4.2.3 Hydrogenation

Alkenes react with hydrogen in the presence of a variety of metal catalysts (i.e. Ni - nickel, Pd - palladium, Pt - platinum). The reaction that occurs is an *addition* reaction since one atom of hydrogen adds to each carbon of the double bond (= *hydrogenation*). Since there are two phases present in the process of hydrogenation (the hydrogen and the metal catalyst), the process is referred to as a heterogenous catalysis.

A carbon with multiple bonds is not bonded to the maximum number of atoms that potentially that carbon could possess. Thus it is *unsaturated*. Alkanes, which can be formed by hydrogenation, are *saturated* since each carbon is bonded to the maximum number of atoms it could possess (= *four*). Thus hydrogenation is sometimes called the process of saturation.

$$CH_3CH = CH_2 + H_2 \longrightarrow CH_3CH_2 - CH_3$$

4.3 Alkynes

Alkynes are unsaturated hydrocarbon molecules containing carbon-carbon triple bonds. The nomenclature is the same as that for alkenes, except that the suffix 'yne' replaces 'ene'. Alkynes have similar physical properties and chemical reactions (i.e. electrophilic addition, oxidation) to alkenes. The current MCAT exam does not require any knowledge specific to alkyne chemistry.

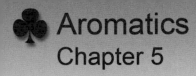

Aromatics
Chapter 5

Memorize	Understand	Not Required*
* Nothing	* Nothing	* Aromatics!

MCAT-Prep.com

Introduction ▊▊▊▊

Aromatics are cyclic compounds with unusual stability due to cyclic delocalization and resonance. Aromatic chemistry, including electrophilic aromatic substitution, is no longer required for the new MCAT.

Additional Resources

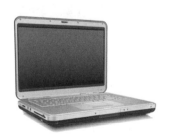

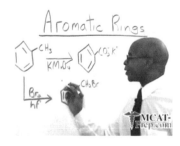

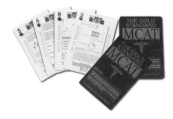

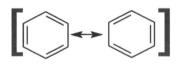

Free Online Q & A   Video: DVD Disc 4   Flashcards   Special Guest

* The real MCAT may have advanced level information presented (ie. in a passage) but previous knowledge of said information is not required to answer the questions that would follow. Practice AAMC and GS practice MCAT CBTs can help you clarify this point.

NB: Please do not read this chapter until you have read ORG 4.0

5.1 Description and Nomenclature

Aromatic compounds are cyclic and have their π electrons delocalized over the entire ring and are thus stabilized by π-electron delocalization. Benzene is the simplest of all the aromatic hydrocarbons. The term *aromatic* has historical significance in that many well known fragrant compounds were found to be derivatives of benzene. Although at present, it is known that not all benzene derivatives have fragrance, the term remains in use today to describe benzene derivatives and related compounds.

Benzene is known to have only one type of carbon-carbon bond, with a bond length of ≈ 1.4 Å (angstroms, 10^{-10}m) somewhere between that of a single and double bond. The benzene molecule may thus be represented by two different resonance structures, showing it to be the average of the two:

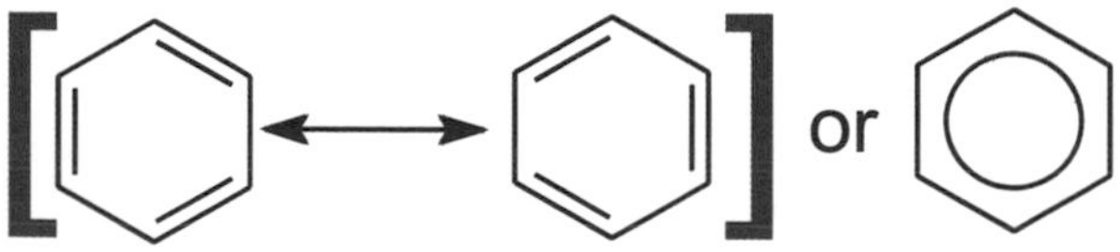

Many monosubstituted benzenes have common names by which they are known. Others are named by substituents attached to the aromatic ring. Some of these are:

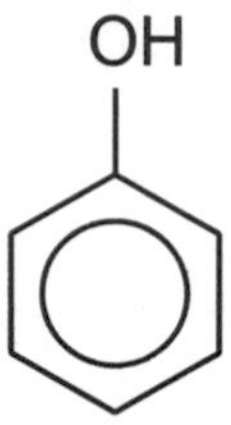

phenol 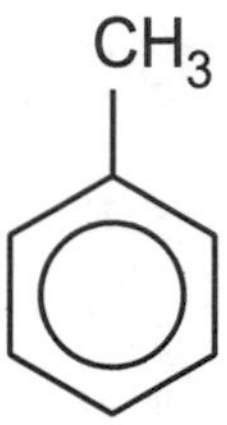   toluene 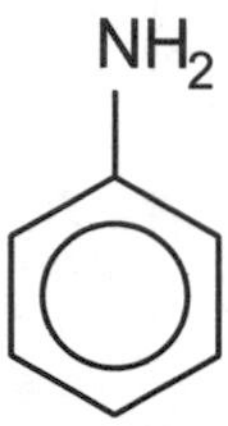   aniline

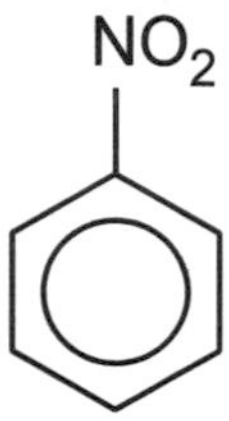

nitrobenzene 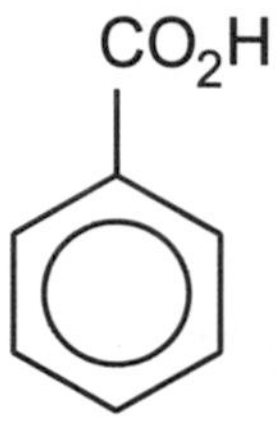   benzoic acid

Disubstituted benzenes are named as derivatives of their primary substituents. In this case, either the usual numbering or the ortho-meta-para system may be used. Ortho (*o*) substituents are at the 2nd position from the primary substituent; meta (*m*) substituents are at the 3rd position; para (*p*) substituents are at the 4th position. If there are more than two substituents on the aromatic ring, the numbering system is used. Some examples are:

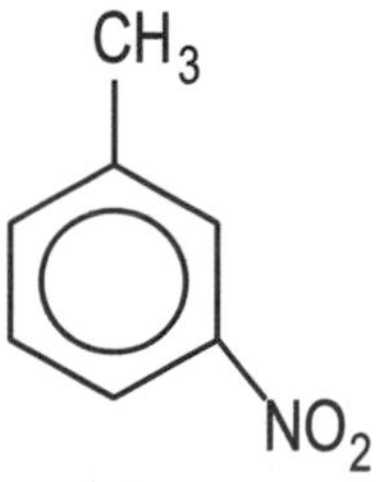

m - Nitrotoluene 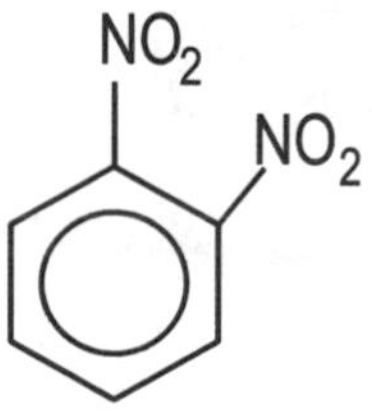   o - Dinitrobenzene

o - Methylaniline
o - Aminotoluene

3 - nitro - 4 -
hydroxybenzoic acid

When benzene is a substituent, it is called a *phenyl or aryl group*. The shorthand for phenyl is Ph. Toluene without a hydrogen on the methyl substituent is called a *benzyl group.*

5.2 Electrophilic Aromatic Substitution

One important reaction of aromatic compounds is known <u>as electrophilic aromatic substitution</u>, which occurs with electrophilic reagents. The reaction is similar to a S_N1 mechanism in that an addition leads to a rearrangement which produces a substitution. However, in this case it is the electrophile (*not a nucleophile*) which substitutes for an atom in the original molecule. The reaction may be summarized:

Note that the intermediate positive charge is stabilized by resonance.

It is important to understand that the electrophile used in electrophilic aromatic substitution must always be a powerful electrophile. After all, the resonance stabilized aromatic ring is resistant to many types of routine chemical reactions (i.e. oxidation with $KMnO_4$ - ORG 4.2.2, electrophilic addition with acid - ORG 4.2.1, and hydrogenation - ORG 4.2.3). Remembering that Br, a halide, is already very electronegative (CHM 2.3), Br^+ is an example of a powerful electrophile. In a reaction called bromination, $Br_2/FeBr_3$ is used to generate the Br^+ species which adds to the aromatic ring. Similar reactions are performed to "juice up" other potential substituents (i.e. alkyl, acyl, iodine, etc.) to become powerful electrophiles to add to the aromatic ring.

When groups are attached to the aromatic ring, the intermediate charge delocalization is affected. There are two classes of substituents: ortho-para (o-p) directors and meta directors. As implied, these groups indicate where most of the electrophile will end up in the reaction.

5.2.1 O-P Directors

If a substituted benzene reacts more rapidly than a benzene alone, the substituent group is said to be an <u>activating group</u>. Activating groups can *donate* electrons to the ring. Thus the ring is more attractive to an electrophile. All activating groups are o/p directors. Some examples are -OH,-NH$_2$,-OR,-NR$_2$, and alkyl groups.

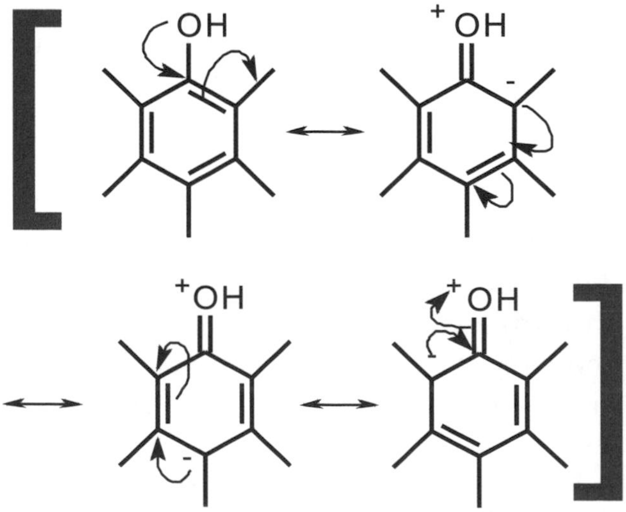

Good stabilization results with a substituent at the ortho or para positions:

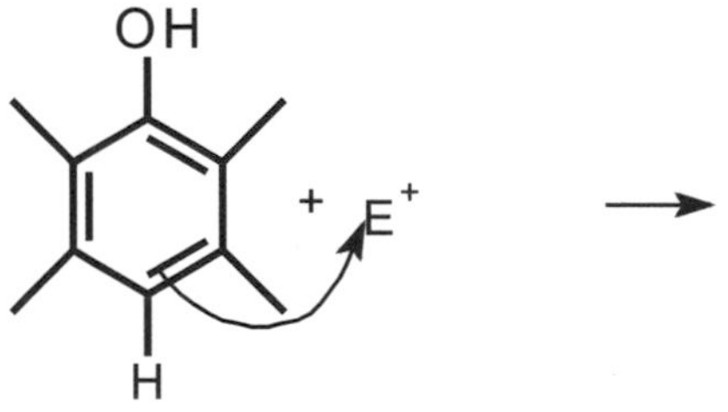

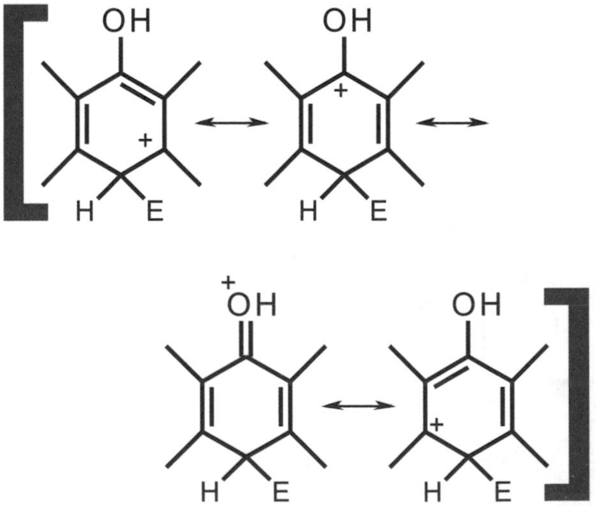

Note that the partial electron density (δ-) is at the ortho and para positions, so the electrophile favors attack at these positions.

When there is a substituent at the meta position, the -OH can no longer help to delocalize the positive charge, so the o-p positions are favored over the meta:

Note that even though the substituents are o-p directors, probability suggests that there will still be a small percentage of the electrophile that will add at the meta position.

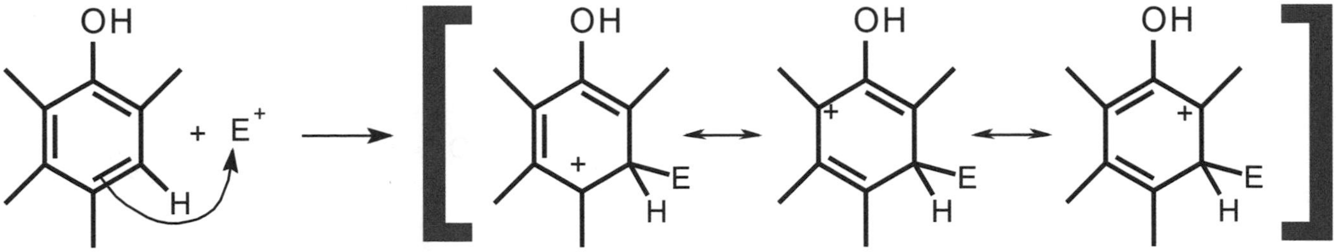

5.2.2 Meta Directors

If a substituted benzene reacts more slowly than the benzene alone, the substituent group is said to be a deactivating group. Deactivating groups can *withdraw* electrons from the ring. Thus the ring is less attractive to an electrophile. All deactivating groups are meta directors, with the exception of the weakly deactivating halides which are o-p directors. Some examples of meta directors are $-NO_2$, $-SO_2$, $-CN$.

Without any substituents, the partial positive charge density (δ^+) will be at the o-p positions. Thus the electrophile avoids the positive charge and favors attack at the meta position:

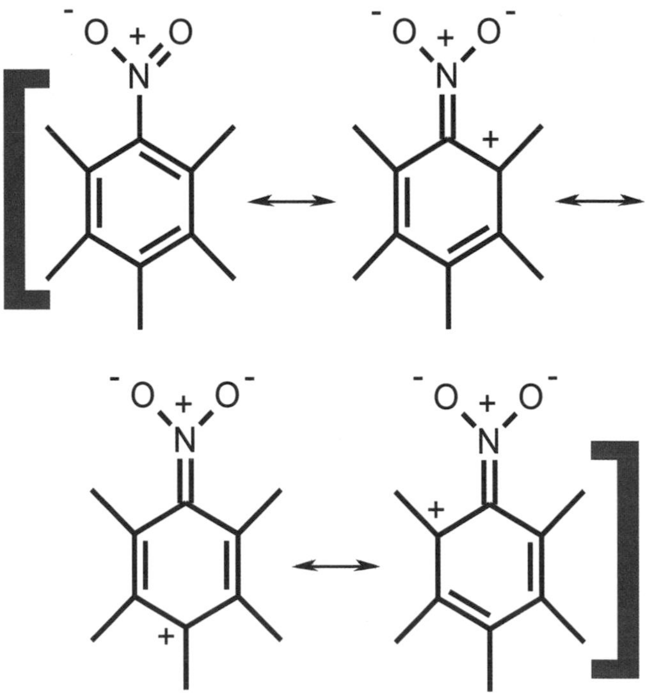

With a substituent at the meta position:

Note that even though the substituents are meta directors, probability suggests that there will still be a smaller percentage of the electrophile that will add at the o-p positions.

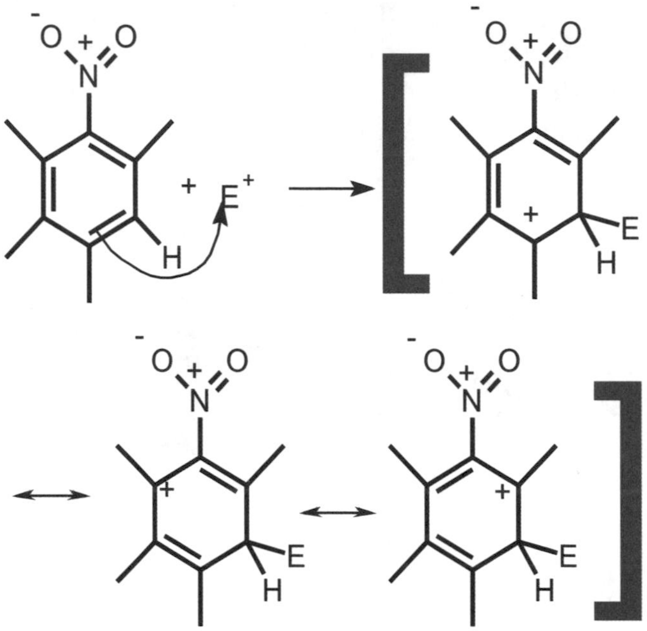

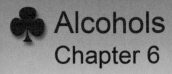

Alcohols
Chapter 6

Memorize	Understand	Not Required*
* IUPAC nomenclature * Physical properties * IR absorption of -OH * Products of oxidation * Define: steric hindrance	* Trends based on length, branching * Effect of hydrogen bonds * Mechanisms of reactions * Nucleophilic substitution	* Advanced level college info * Dehydration/alkene production * Elimination reactions/alkenes

MCAT-Prep.com

Introduction

An alcohol is any organic compound in which a hydroxyl group (-OH) is bound to a carbon atom of an alkyl or substituted alkyl group. Spectroscopy is discussed in Chapter 14 but, because it comes up frequently on the MCAT, you should memorize that 3200 - 3650 is the approximate IR absorbance of -OH.

Additional Resources

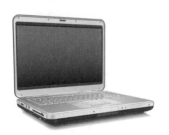

Free Online Q & A

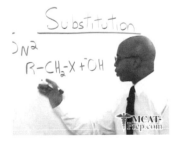

Video: DVD Discs 2,3,4

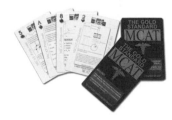

Flashcards

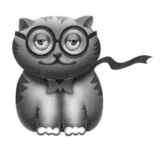

Special Guest

6.1 Description and Nomenclature

The systematic naming of alcohols is accomplished by replacing the -e of the corresponding alkane with -ol. As with alkanes, special names are used for branched groups:

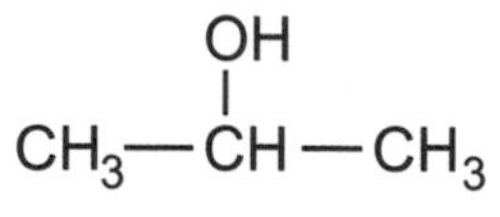

OH
|
$CH_3 — CH — CH_3$

isopropanol
(isopropyl alcohol)

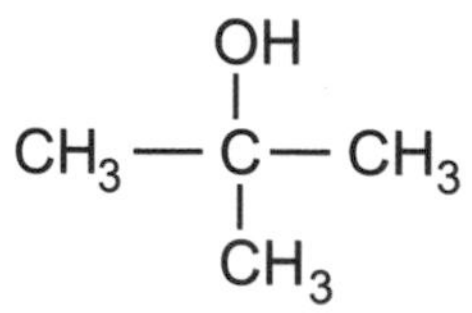

OH
|
$CH_3 — C — CH_3$
|
CH_3

tert - butanol
(tert - butyl alcohol)

The alcohols are always numbered to give the carbon with the attached hydroxy (-OH) group the lowest number:

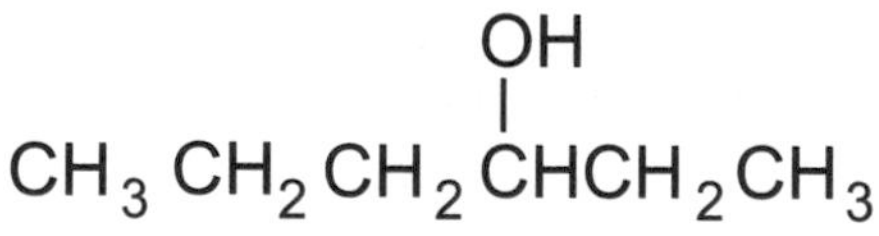

OH
|
$CH_3\ CH_2\ CH_2\ CHCH_2\ CH_3$

3- hexanol

CH_3 \quad OH \quad CH_3
| \qquad | \qquad |
$CH_3\ CH_2\ CH_2\ CHCH_2\ CHCH_2\ CHCH_3$

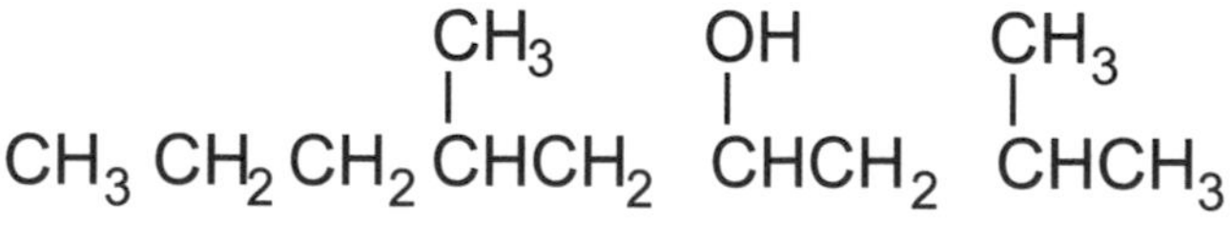

2,6 - dimethyl- 4- nonanol

The shorthand for methanol is MeOH, and the shorthand for ethanol is EtOH. Alcohols are weak acids ($K_a \approx 10^{-18}$), being weaker acids than water. Their conjugate bases are called alkoxides, very little of which will be present in solution:

$$C_2H_5OH + OH^- \rightleftharpoons C_2H_5O^- + H_2O$$
ethanol \qquad\qquad *ethoxide*

The acidity of an alcohol decreases with increasing number of attached carbons. Thus CH_3OH is more acidic than CH_3CH_2OH; and CH_3CH_2OH (a primary alcohol) is more acidic than $(CH_3)_2CHOH$ (a secondary alcohol), which is, in turn, more acidic than $(CH_3)_3COH$ (a tertiary alcohol).

Alcohols have higher boiling points and a greater solubility than comparable alkanes, alkenes, aldehydes, ketones and alkyl halides. This greater solubility is due to the greater polarity and hydrogen bonding of the alcohol. In alcohols, hydrogen bonding is a weak association of the -OH proton of one molecule, with the oxygen of another. To form the hydrogen bond, both a donor, and an acceptor are required:

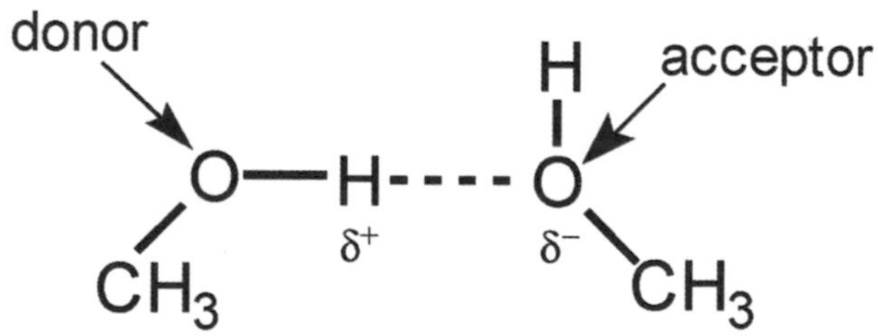

Sometimes an atom may act as both a donor and acceptor of hydrogen bonds. One example of this is the oxygen atom in an alcohol:

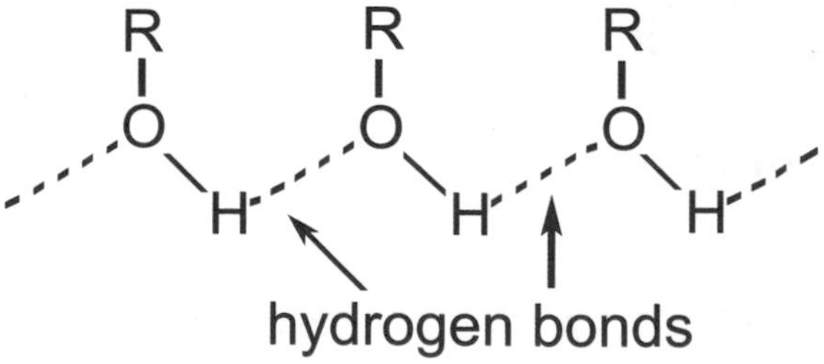

As the length of the carbon chain of the alcohol molecule increases, the nonpolar chain becomes more meaningful, and the alcohol becomes less water soluble. The hydroxyl group of a primary alcohol is able to form hydrogen bonds with molecules such as water more easily than the hydroxyl group of a tertiary alcohol. The hydroxyl group of a tertiary alcohol is crowded by the surrounding methyl groups and thus its ability to participate in hydrogen bonds is lessened. As well, in solution, primary alcohols are more acidic than secondary alcohols, and secondary alcohols are more acidic than tertiary alcohols. In the gas phase, however, the order of acidity is reversed.

6.2 Important Reactions of Alcohols

6.2.1 Dehydration

Dehydration (= *loss of water*) reactions of alcohols produce alkenes. The general dehydration reaction is shown in Figure IV.B.6.1.

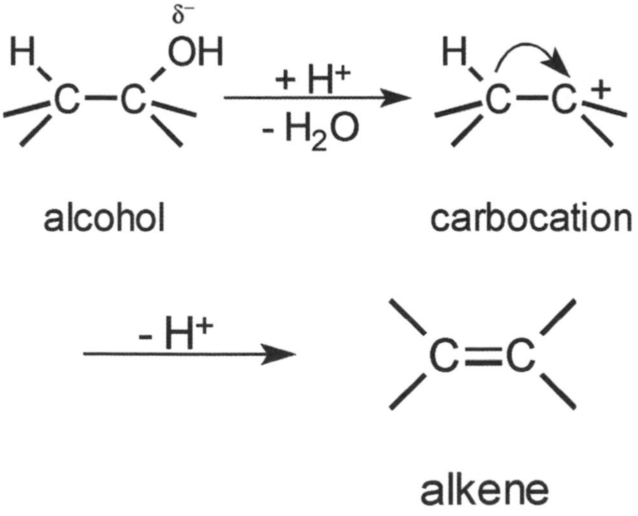

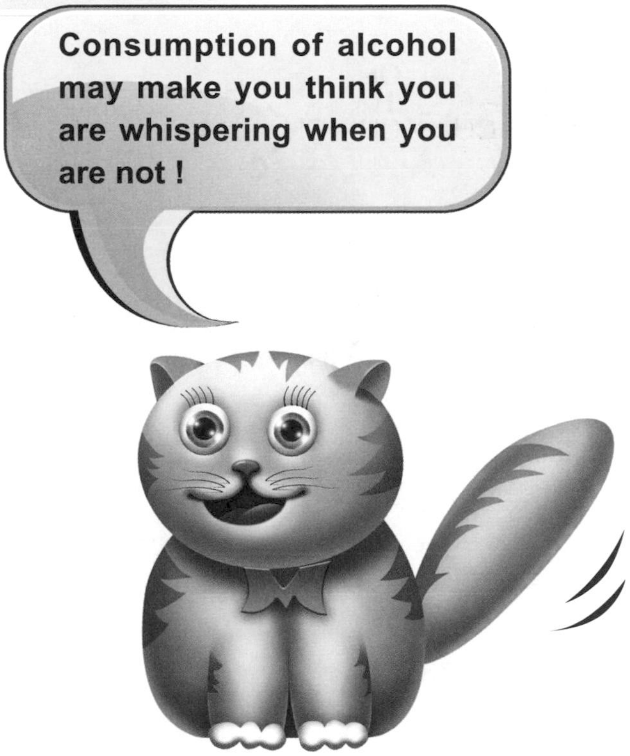

> **Consumption of alcohol may make you think you are whispering when you are not !**

alcohol   carbocation

alkene

Figure IV.B.6.1: Dehydration of an alcohol. The proton (H^+) is attracted to the partial negative charge of -OH thus water is formed which is a good leaving group. Then electrons are attracted to the positively charged carbon causing a proton to leave. Thus the acid is a catalyst.

For the preceding reaction to occur, the temperature must be between 300 and 400 degrees Celsius, and the vapors must be passed over a metal oxide catalyst. Alternatively, strong, hot acids, such as H_2SO_4 or H_3PO_4 at 100 to 200 degrees Celsius may be used.

The reactivity depends upon the type of alcohol. A tertiary alcohol is more reactive than a secondary alcohol which is, in turn, more reactive than a primary alcohol. The faster reactions have the most stable carbocation intermediates. The alkene that is formed is the most stable one. A phenyl group will take preference over one or two alkyl groups, otherwise the most substituted double bond is the most stable (= *major product*) and the least substituted is less stable (= *minor product*).

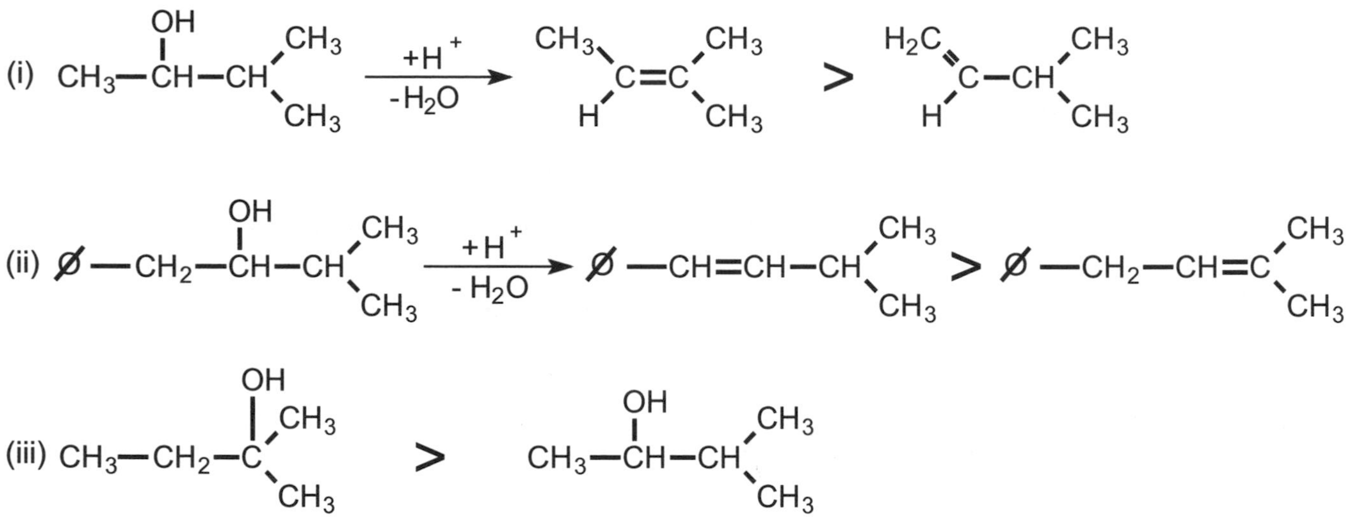

Figure IV.B.6.2: Dehydration of substituted alcohols. Major and minor products, respectively, are represented in reactions (i) and (ii). An example of a reactant with a greater reaction rate due to more substituents as an intermediate is represented by (iii). Ø = a phenyl group.

6.2.2 Oxidation

In oxidation reactions there is an increasing oxygen content or a decreasing hydrogen content. Primary alcohols are converted to aldehydes using the mild oxidizing agents CrO_3 or $K_2Cr_2O_7/H_2SO_4$ or by using the powerful oxidizing agent, $KMnO_4$, under mild conditions (i.e. room temperature, neutral pH). Primary alcohols can produce carboxylic acids in the presence of $KMnO_4$ under abrasive conditions (i.e.

increased temperature, presence of OH^-). Secondary alcohols are converted to ketones by any of the preceding oxidizing agents.

It is *very* difficult to oxidize a tertiary alcohol. Under acidic conditions, tertiary alcohols are unaffected; they may be oxidized under acidic conditions by dehydration and *then* oxidizing the double bond of the resultant alkene.

$$R-CH_2OH \xrightarrow{(O)} R-\overset{\overset{\displaystyle O}{\|}}{C}-H \xrightarrow{(O)} R-\overset{\overset{\displaystyle O}{\|}}{C}-OH$$

1° Alcohol   Aldehyde   Carboxylic acid

$$R-\overset{\overset{\displaystyle OH}{|}}{C}H-R' \xrightarrow{(O)} R-\overset{\overset{\displaystyle O}{\|}}{C}-R'$$

2° Alcohol   Ketone

6.2.3 Substitution

In a substitution reaction one atom or group is *substituted* or replaced by another atom or group. For an alcohol, the -OH group is replaced (*substituted*) by a halide (usually chlorine or bromine). A variety of reagents may be used, such as HCl, HBr or PCl_3. There are two different types of substitution reactions, S_N1 and S_N2.

In the S_N1 (*1st order or monomolecular nucleophilic substitution*) reaction, the transition state involves a carbocation, the formation of which is the rate-determining step. Alcohol substitutions that proceed by this mechanism are those involving benzyl groups, allyl groups, tertiary and secondary alcohols. The mechanism of this reaction is:

(i) $R-L \longrightarrow R^+ + L^-$
(ii) $Nu^- + R^+ \longrightarrow Nu-R$

The important features of this reaction are:

- The reaction is first order (this means that the rate of the reaction depends only on the concentration of one compound); the rate depends on [R-L], where R represents an alkyl group, and L represents a substituent or ligand.

- There is a racemization of configuration, when a chiral molecule is involved.

- A stable carbonium ion should be formed; thus in terms of reaction rate, benzyl groups = allyl groups > tertiary alcohols > secondary alcohols >> primary alcohols.

- The stability of alkyl groups is as follows: primary alkyl groups < secondary alkyl groups < tertiary alkyl groups.

The mechanism of the S_N2 (*2nd order or bimolecular nucleophilic substitution*) reaction is:

$$Nu^- + R\!-\!L \longrightarrow [Nu\text{----}R\text{----}L]^- \longrightarrow Nu\!-\!R + L^-$$

There are several important points to know about this reaction:

- The reaction rate is second order overall (the rate depends on the concentration of two compounds); first order with respect to [R-L] and first order with respect to the concentration of the nucleophile [Nu^-].

- Note that the nucleophile adds to the alkyl group by *backside displacement* (i.e. Nu must add to the *opposite* site to the ligand). Thus optically active alcohols react to give an inversion of configuration, forming the opposite enantiomer.

- Large or bulky groups near or at the reacting site may hinder or retard a reaction. This is called *steric hindrance*. Size or steric factors are important since they affect S_N2 reaction rates; in terms of reaction rates, CH_3- > primary alcohols > secondary alcohols >> tertiary alcohols.

The substitution reactions for methanol (CH_3OH) and other primary alcohols are by the S_N2 reaction mechanism.

6.2.4 Elimination

Elimination reactions occur when an atom or a group of atoms is removed (*eliminated*) from adjacent carbons leaving a multiple bond:

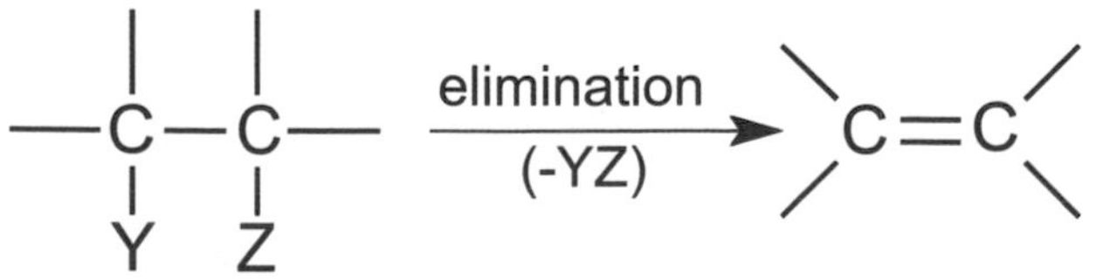

There are two different types of elimination reactions, E1 and E2. In the E1 (Elimination, 1st order) reaction, the rate of reaction depends on the concentration of one compound. E1 often occurs as minor products alongside S_N2 reactions. E1 can occur as major products in alkyl halides or, as in the following example, to an alcohol:

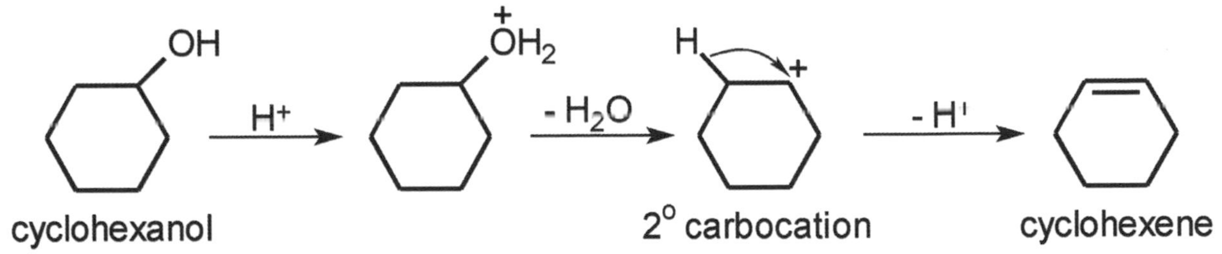
OH
H+
OH2
- H2O
H
- H'
cyclohexanol
2° carbocation
cyclohexene

In the E2 (Elimination, 2nd order) reaction the rate of reaction depends on the concentration of two compounds. E2 reactions require strong bases like KOH or the salt of an alcohol (i.e. *sodium alkoxide*). An alkoxide can be synthesized from an alcohol using either Na(*s*) or NaH (*sodium hydride*) as reducing agents. The hydride ion H- is a powerful base:

$$\text{R-OH} + \text{NaH} \longrightarrow \underset{\text{sodium alkoxide}}{\text{R-O}^-\text{Na}^+} + H_2$$

Now the alkoxide can be used as a proton acceptor in an E2 reaction involving an alkyl halide:

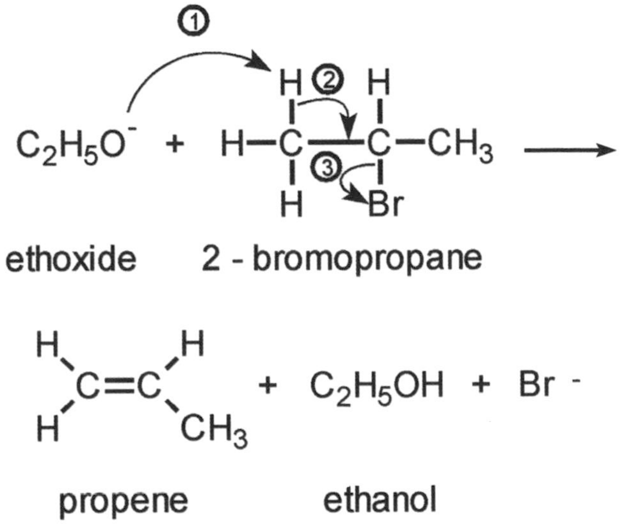
1
2
3
C2H5O-
H
C
CH3
Br
ethoxide
2 - bromopropane
C=C
CH3
C2H5OH
Br -
propene
ethanol

In the above reaction, the first step (1) involves the base (ethoxide) removing (*elimination*) a proton, thus carbon has a negative charge (*primary ca*rbanion, <u>very</u> *unstable*). The electron pair is quickly attracted to the δ^+ neighboring carbon (2) forming a double bond (note that the carbon was δ^+ because it was attached to the electronegative atom Br, *see* ORG 1.5). Simultaneously, Br (*a halide, which are good leaving groups*) is bumped (3) from the carbon as carbon can have only four bonds. {Notice that in organic chemistry the curved arrows always follow the movement of electrons}

The determination of the quality of a leaving group is quite simple: <u>good leaving groups</u> have *strong* conjugate acids. As examples, H_2O is a good leaving group because H_3O^+ is a strong acid, likewise for Br^-/HBr, Cl^-/HCl, HSO_4^-/H_2SO_4, etc.

Memorize	Understand	Not Required*
* IUPAC nomenclature * IR absorption of C=O * Redox reactions	* Effect of hydrogen bonds * Mechanisms of reactions * Acidity of the alpha H * Resonance, polarity * Grignards, organometallic reagents	* Advanced level college info * The Wittig reaction * Ozonolysis of alkenes * Friedel-Crafts Acylation

MCAT-Prep.com

Introduction ▀▀▀▀

An aldehyde contains a terminal carbonyl group. The functional group is a carbon atom bonded to a hydrogen atom and double-bonded to an oxygen atom (O=CH-) and is called the aldehyde group. A ketone contains a carbonyl group (C=O) bonded to two other carbon atoms: R(CO)R'. You should memorize that 1630 - 1780 is the approximate IR absorbance of C=O.

Additional Resources

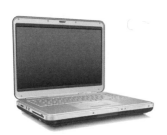

Free Online Q & A

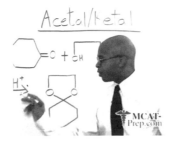

Video: DVD Discs 1, 2, 3, 4

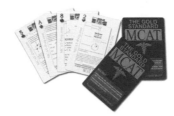

Flashcards

Special Guest

7.1 Description and Nomenclature

Aldehydes and ketones are two types of molecules, both containing the carbonyl group, C=O, which is the basis for their chemistry.

The general structure of aldehydes and ketones is:

$$\underset{\text{Aldehyde}}{R-\overset{\overset{\textstyle O}{\|}}{C}-H} \qquad \underset{\text{Ketone}}{R-\overset{\overset{\textstyle O}{\|}}{C}-R'}$$

Aldehydes have at least one hydrogen bonded to the carbonyl carbon, as well as a second hydrogen (= *formaldehyde*) or either an alkyl or an aryl group (= *benzene minus one hydrogen*). Ketones have two alkyl or aryl groups bound to the carbonyl carbon (i.e. the carbon forming the double bond with oxygen).

Systematic naming of these compounds is done by replacing the '-e' of the corresponding alkane with '-al' for aldehydes, and '-one' for ketones. For ketones the chain is numbered as to give the lowest possible number to the carbonyl carbon. Common names are given in brackets:

$$\underset{\substack{\text{Ethanal}\\\text{(acetaldehyde)}}}{CH_3\overset{\overset{\textstyle O}{\|}}{C}-H} \qquad \underset{\substack{\text{Propanone}\\\text{(acetone)}}}{CH_3\overset{\overset{\textstyle O}{\|}}{C}CH_3}$$

$$CH_3\overset{\overset{\textstyle O}{\|}}{C}CH_2CH_2CH_3$$

2-Pentanone
(methyl propyl ketone)

The important features of the carbonyl group are:

- Resonance: There are two resonance forms of the carbonyl group:

$$R-\overset{\overset{\textstyle \delta^-O}{\|}}{\underset{\delta^+}{C}}-R' \quad\longleftrightarrow\quad R-\overset{\overset{\textstyle {}^-O}{|}}{\underset{+}{C}}-R'$$

- Polarity: Reactions about this group may be either nucleophilic, or electrophilic. Since opposite charges attract, nucleophiles (Nu⁻) attack the δ^+ carbon, and electrophiles (E⁺) attack the δ^- oxygen. In both of these types of reactions, the character of the double bond is altered:

$$R-\overset{\overset{\textstyle O\delta^-}{\|}}{\underset{\delta^+}{C}}-R \quad\longrightarrow\quad E^+$$

Electrophilic

$$\left[\; R-\overset{\overset{\textstyle {}^+O{}^{\diagup E}}{\|}}{C}-R \quad\longleftrightarrow\quad R-\overset{\overset{\textstyle O{}^{\diagup E}}{|}}{\underset{+}{C}}-R \;\right]$$

$$\underset{Nu^-}{R-\overset{\overset{\textstyle O\delta^-}{\|}}{\underset{\delta^+}{C}}-R} \quad\longrightarrow\quad R-\overset{\overset{\textstyle O^-}{|}}{\underset{Nu}{C}}-R$$

Nucleophilic

- Acidity of the α-hydrogen: The α-hydrogen is the hydrogen attached to the carbon next to the carbonyl group (the α-carbon). The β-carbon is the carbon adjacent to the α-carbon. The α-hydrogen may be removed by a base. The acidity of this hydrogen is increased if it is between 2 carbonyl groups:

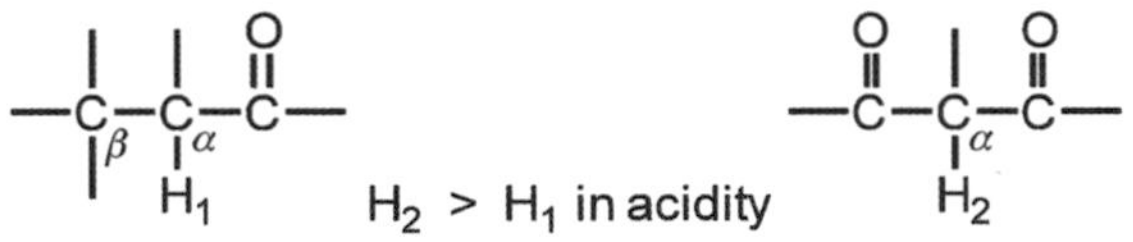

$H_2 > H_1$ in acidity

This acidity is a result of the resonance stabilization of the α-carbanion formed. This stabilization will also permit addition at the β-carbon in α-β unsaturated carbonyls (*those with double or triple bonds*):

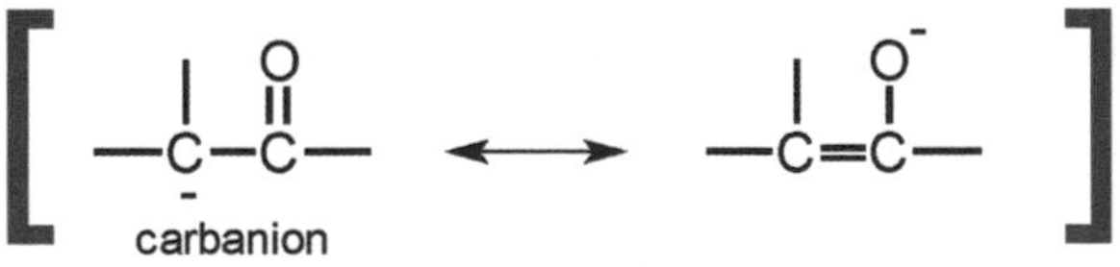

carbanion

resonance stabilization

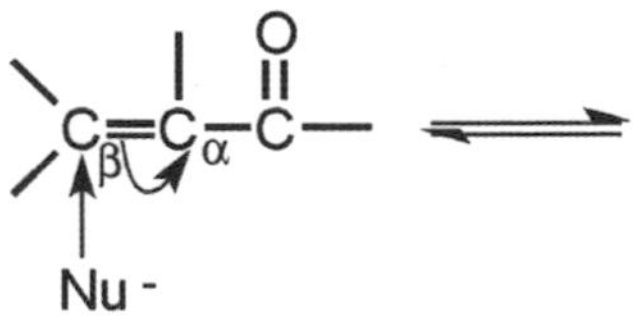

α, β unsaturated carbonyl

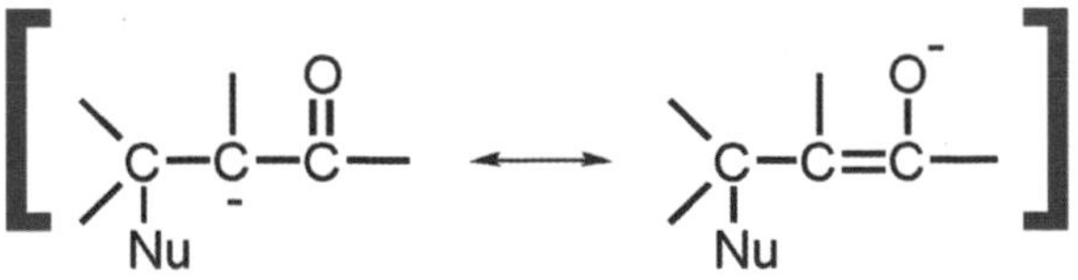

- Keto-enol tautomerization: The carbonyl exists in equilibrium with the enol form of the molecule. Although the carbonyl is usually the predominant one, if the enol double bond can be conjugated with other double bonds, it becomes stable (conjugated double bonds are those which are separated by a single bond):

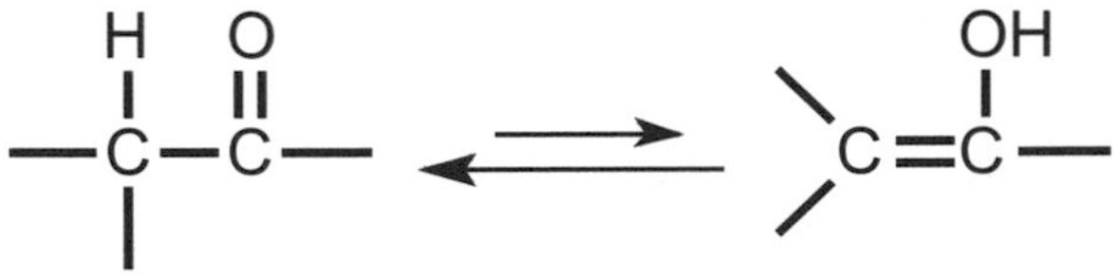

carbonyl   enol

- Hydrogen bonds: The O of the carbonyl forms hydrogen bonds with the hydrogens attached to other electronegative atoms, such as O's or N's:

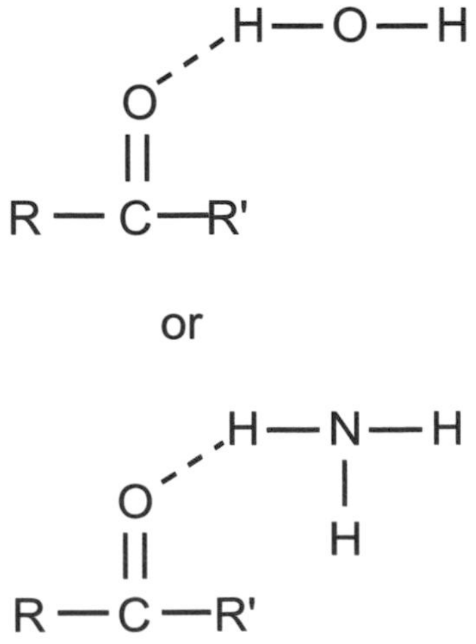

or

7.2 Important Reactions of Aldehydes & Ketones

7.2.1 Overview

Since the carbonyl group is the functional group of aldehydes and ketones, groups adjacent to the carbonyl group affect the rate of reaction for the molecule. For example, an electron withdrawing ligand adjacent to the carbonyl group will increase the partial positive charge on the carbon making the carbonyl group more attractive to a nucleophile. Conversely, an electron donating ligand would decrease the reactivity of the carbonyl group.

Generally, aldehydes oxidize easier, and undergo nucleophilic additions easier than ketones. This is a consequence of steric hindrance.

Aldehydes will be oxidized to carboxylic acids with the standard oxidizing agents. Ketones rarely oxidize. Carbonyls are also reduced using reducing agents (i.e. the hydrides $NaBH_4$ and $LiAlH_4$) forming alcohols. Aldehydes can be made by reacting an acetal with aqueous acid or by reacting a primary alcohol with $CrO_3/$ pyridine, or by reacting an acid chloride with $H_2/Pd/C$.

There are two classes of reactions that will be investigated: nucleophilic addition reactions at C=O bond, and reactions at adjacent positions.

7.2.2 Acetal (ketal) and Hemiacetal (hemiketal) Formation

Aldehydes and ketones will form hemiacetals and hemiketals, respectively, when dissolved in an excess of a primary alcohol. In addition, if this mixture contains a trace of an acid catalyst, the hemiacetal (hemiketal) will react further to form acetals and ketals.

An acetal is a composite functional group in which two ether functions are joined to a carbon bearing a hydrogen and an alkyl group. A ketal is a composite functional group in which two ether functions are joined to a carbon bearing two alkyl groups.

This reaction may be summarised:

$$\underset{\substack{\text{aldehyde (R' = H)}\\\text{or ketone (R' = alkyl)}}}{R-\overset{\displaystyle\overset{O}{\|}}{C}-R'} \quad + \quad \underset{\substack{\text{excess}\\\text{alcohol}}}{R''OH} \quad \underset{-\,H^+}{\overset{+\,H^+}{\rightleftharpoons}}$$

$$\underset{\substack{\text{hemiacetal}\\\text{or}\\\text{hemiketal}}}{R-\overset{\displaystyle OH}{\underset{\displaystyle OR''}{C}}-R'} \quad \underset{+\,H_2O}{\overset{+\,H^+/-\,H_2O}{\rightleftharpoons}} \quad \underset{\substack{\text{acetal}\\\text{or}\\\text{ketal}}}{R-\overset{\displaystyle OR''}{\underset{\displaystyle OR''}{C}}-R'}$$

The <u>first step</u> in the above reaction is that the most charged species (+, the hydrogen) attracts electrons from the δ⁻ oxygen, leaving a carbocation intermediate. The <u>second step</u> involves the δ⁻ oxygen from the alcohol *quickly* attracted to the current most charged species (+, carbon). A proton is lost which regenerates the catalyst, and produces the hemiacetal or hemiketal. Now the proton may attract electrons from -OH forming H_2O, a good leaving group. Again the δ⁻ oxygen on the alcohol is attracted to the positive carbocation. And again the alcohol releases its proton, regenerating the catalyst, producing an acetal or ketal.

7.2.3 Imine and Enamine Formation

Imines and enamines are formed when aldehydes and ketones are allowed to react with amines.

When an aldehyde or ketone reacts with a primary amine, an <u>imine</u> (or Schiff base) is formed. A primary amine is a nitrogen compound with the general formula $R-NH_2$, where R represents an alkyl or aryl group. In an imine the carbonyl group of the aldehyde or ketone is replaced with a C=N-R group.

When an aldehyde or ketone reacts with a secondary amine, an <u>enamine</u> is formed. A secondary amine is a nitrogen with the general formula R_2N-H, where R represents aryl or alkyl groups (these groups need not be identical).

Tertiary amines (of the general form R_3N) do not react with the aldehydes or ketones.

The reaction may be summarised:

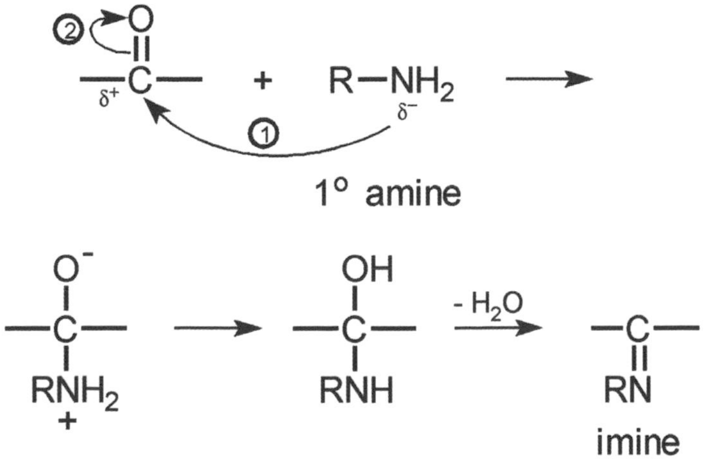

1° amine

imine

7.2.4 Aldol Condensation

Aldol condensation is a base catalized reaction of aldehydes and ketones that have α-hydrogens. The intermediate, an aldol, is both an aldehyde and a alcohol. The aldol undergoes a dehydration reaction producing a carbon-carbon bond in the condensation product, an enal (= alkene + aldehyde).

The reaction may be summarised:

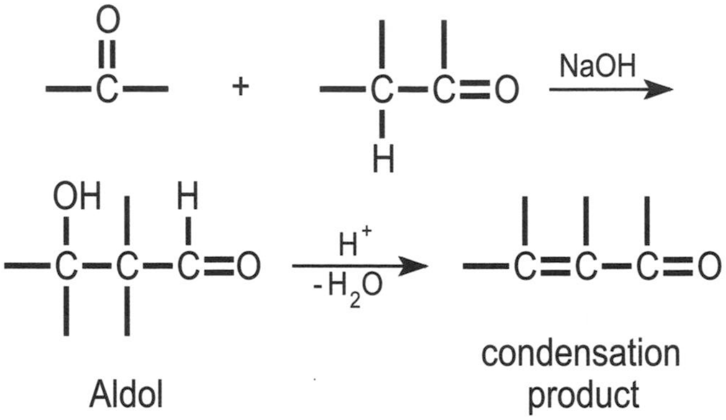

Aldol

condensation product

7.2.5 Conjugate Addition to α-β Unsaturated Carbonyls

α-β unsaturated carbonyls are unusually reactive with nucleophiles. This is best illustrated by example:

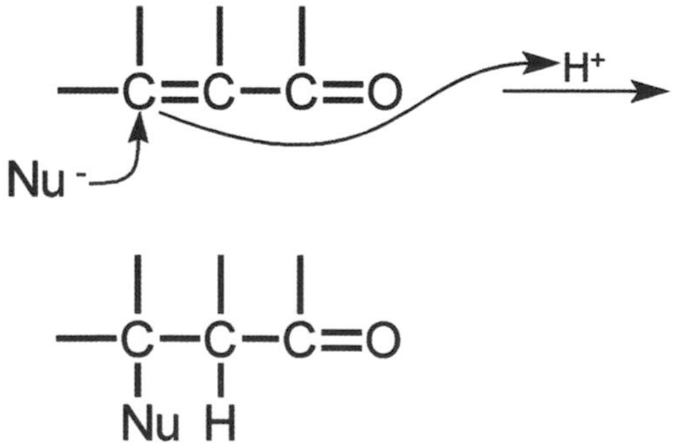

Examples of relevant nucleophiles includes CN⁻ from HCN, and R⁻ which can be generated by a Grignard Reagent (= RMgX) or as an alkyl lithium (= RLi).

CARBOXYLIC ACIDS
Chapter 8

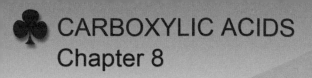

Memorize	Understand	Not Required*
* IUPAC nomenclature * IR absorption of C=O * Redox reactions	* Hydrogen bonding * Mechanisms of reactions * Relative acid strength * Resonance, inductive effects * Grignards, organometallic reagents	* Advanced level college info * Friedel-Crafts Acylation * Nitrile reaction mechanisms

MCAT-Prep.com

Introduction ▮▮▮▮

Carboxylic acids are organic acids with a carboxyl group, which has the formula -C(=O)OH, usually written -COOH or $-CO_2H$. Carboxylic acids are Brønsted-Lowry acids (proton donors) that are actually, in the grand scheme of chemistry, weak acids. Salts and anions of carboxylic acids are called carboxylates. You should memorize that 1630 - 1780 is the approximate IR absorbance of C=O.

Additional Resources

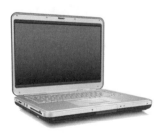

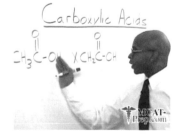

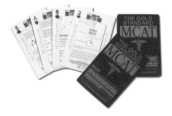

O
‖
R — C — OH

Free Online Q & A   Video: DVD Discs 2, 3   Flashcards   Special Guest

8.1 Description and Nomenclature

Carboxylic acids are molecules containing the *carboxylic group* (carbonyl + hydroxyl), which is the basis of their chemistry. The general structure of a carboxylic acid is:

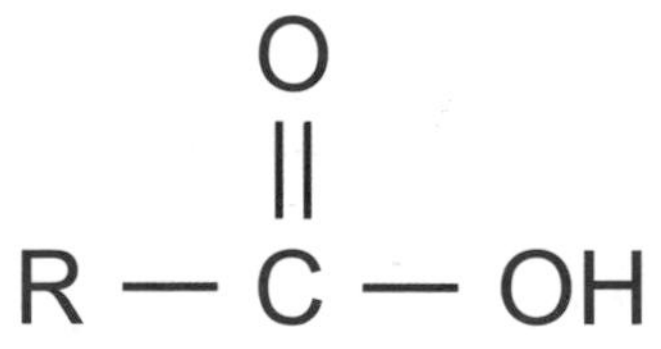

$$R - C(=O) - OH$$

Systematic naming of these compounds is done by replacing the '-e' of the corresponding alkane with '-oic acid'. The molecule is numbered such that the carbonyl carbon is carbon number one. Many carboxylic acids have common names by which they are usually known:

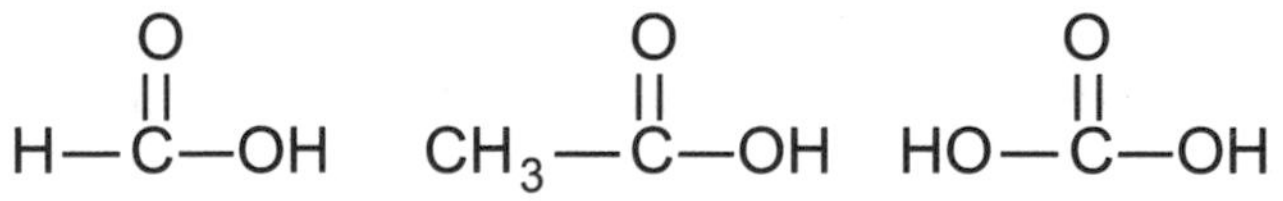

formic acid   acetic acid   carbonic acid

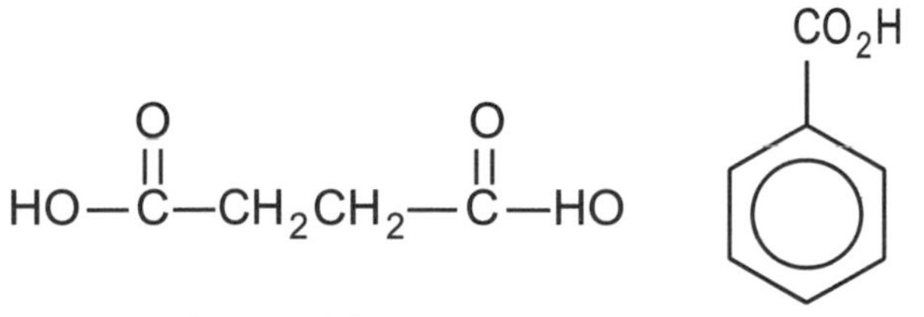

$$HO - C(=O) - CH_2CH_2 - C(=O) - HO$$

succinic acid   benzoic acid

Low molecular weight carboxylic acids are liquids with strong odours and high boiling points. The high boiling point is due to the polarity and the hydrogen bonding capability of the molecule. Because of this hydrogen bonding, these molecules are water soluble. As well, carboxylic acids are soluble in dilute bases (NaOH or $NaHCO_3$), because of their acid properties. The

carboxyl group is the basis of carboxylic acid chemistry, and there are four important features to remember. Looking at a general carboxylic acid:

- The hydrogen (H) is weakly acidic. This is due to its attachment to the oxygen atom, and because the carboxylate anion is resonance stabilized:

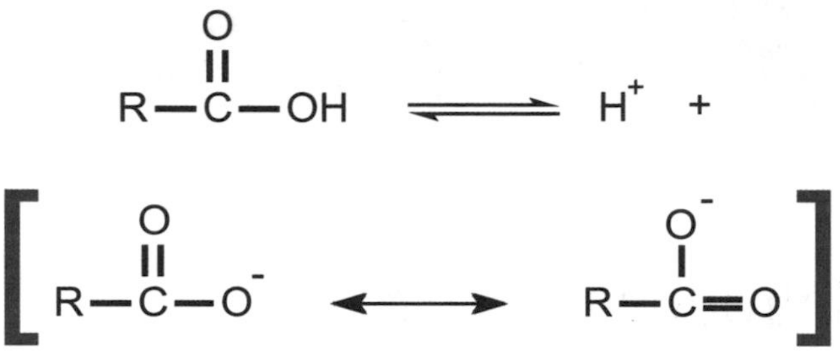

$$R - C(=O) - OH \rightleftharpoons H^+ +$$

$$\left[R - C(=O) - O^- \longleftrightarrow R - C(-O^-)=O \right]$$

resonance forms

- The carboxyl carbon is very susceptible to nucleophilic attack. This is due to the attached oxygen atom, and the carbonyl oxygen, both atoms being electronegative:

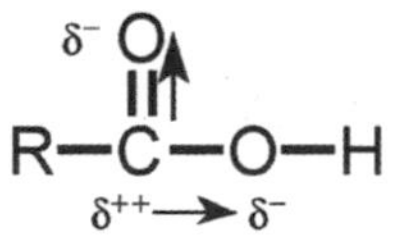

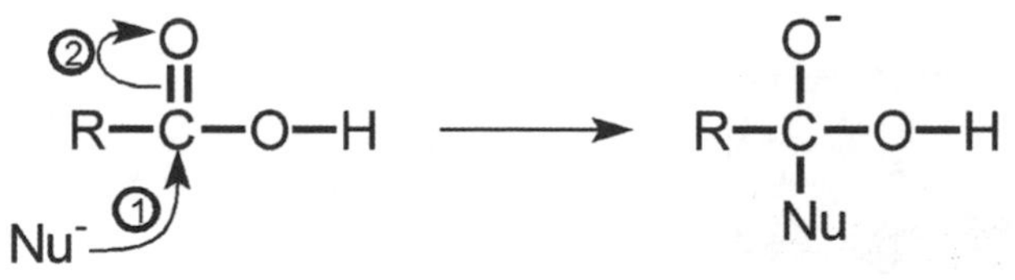

- In basic conditions, the hydroxyl group, as is, is a good leaving group. In acidic conditions, the protonated hydroxyl (i.e. water) is an excellent leaving group. This promotes nucleophilic substitution:

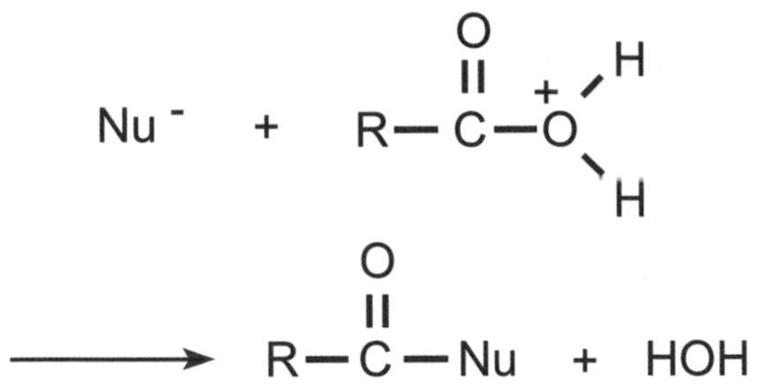

$$Nu^- \ + \ R-\overset{\overset{\displaystyle O}{\|}}{C}-\overset{+}{O}\overset{\diagup H}{\diagdown H}$$

$$\longrightarrow \ R-\overset{\overset{\displaystyle O}{\|}}{C}-Nu \ + \ HOH$$

- Because of the carbonyl and hydroxyl moieties (i.e. parts), hydrogen bonding is possible both inter- and intramolecularly:

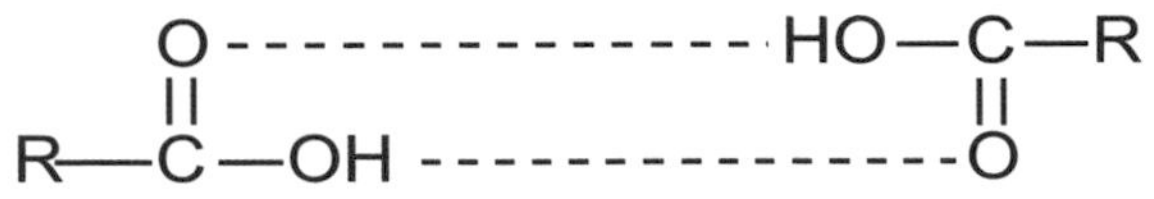

$$R-\overset{\overset{\displaystyle O}{\|}}{C}-OH \ ------- \ \overset{\overset{\displaystyle HO-C-R}{}}{\underset{O}{\|}}$$

intermolecular (dimerization)

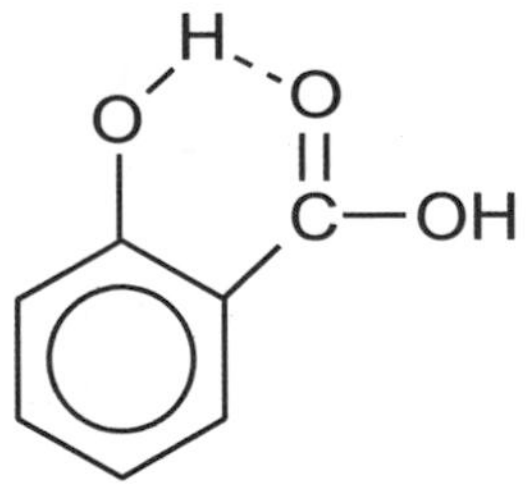

intramolecular

8.1.1 Carboxylic Acid Formation

As implied by their name, carboxylic acids are acidic; the most acidic of all organic compounds. In fact, they are colloquially known as *organic acids*. Organic classes of molecules in order of increasing acid strength are:

alkanes < ammonia < alkynes < alcohols < water < carboxylic acids

Substituted phenols may be stronger acids than water.

The relative acid strength among carboxylic acids depends on the <u>inductive effects</u> of the attached groups, and their proximity to the carboxyl. For example:

CH_3CH_2-$C(Cl)_2$-$COOH$ *is a stronger acid than* CH_3CH_2-$CH(Cl)$-$COOH$.

The reason for this is that chlorine, which is electronegative, withdraws electron density and stabilizes the carboxylate anion. Proximity is important, as:

CH_3CH_2-$C(Cl)_2$-$COOH$ *is a stronger acid than* CH_3-$C(Cl)_2$-CH_2COOH.

A carboxylic acid can be formed by reacting a Grignard reagent with carbon dioxide, or by reacting an aldehyde with $KMnO_4$. Carboxylic acids are also formed by reacting a nitrile (in which nitrogen shares a triple bond with a carbon) with aqueous acid.

8.2 Important Reactions of Carboxylic Acids

Carboxylic acids undergo nucleophilic substitution reactions with many different nucleophiles, under a variety of conditions:

$$Nu^- + R - \overset{\overset{\displaystyle O}{\|}}{C} - OH \longrightarrow R - \overset{\overset{\displaystyle O}{\|}}{C} - Nu + OH^-$$

If the nucleophile is -OR, the resulting compound is an ester. If it is $-NH_2$, the resulting compound is an amide. If it is Cl from $SOCl_2$, or PCl_5, the resulting compound is an acid chloride.

The typical esterification reaction may be summarized:

$$R'O^*H + R - \overset{\overset{\displaystyle O}{\|}}{C} - OH \longrightarrow$$

alcohol   acid

$$R - \overset{\overset{\displaystyle O}{\|}}{C} - O^*R' + H_2O$$

ester

The decarboxylation reaction involves the loss of the carboxyl group as CO_2:

$$HO - \overset{\overset{\displaystyle O}{\|}}{C} - \underset{\underset{\displaystyle R}{|}}{\overset{\overset{\displaystyle H}{|}}{C}} - \overset{\overset{\displaystyle O}{\|}}{C} - OH \xrightarrow[\text{heat}]{\text{base}} H - \underset{\underset{\displaystyle R}{|}}{\overset{\overset{\displaystyle H}{|}}{C}} - \overset{\overset{\displaystyle O}{\|}}{C} - OH + CO_2$$

β – diacid

$$R - \overset{\overset{\displaystyle O}{\|}}{C} - \underset{\underset{\displaystyle H}{|}}{\overset{\overset{\displaystyle H}{|}}{C}} - \overset{\overset{\displaystyle O}{\|}}{C} - OH \xrightarrow[\text{heat}]{\text{base}} R - \overset{\overset{\displaystyle O}{\|}}{C} - CH_3 + CO_2$$

β – keto acid

This reaction is not important for most ordinary carboxylic acids. There are certain types of carboxylic acids that decarboxylate easily, mainly:

- Those which have a keto group at the β position, known as β-keto acids.
- Malonic acids and its derivatives (i.e. β-diacids: those with two carboxyl groups, separated by one carbon).
- Carbonic acid and its derivatives.

Carboxylic acids are reduced to alcohols with lithium aluminum hydride, $LiAlH_4$, or H_2/metals. Sodium borohydride, $NaBH_4$, being a milder reducing agent, only reduces aldehydes and ketones. Carboxylic acids may also be converted to esters or amides first, and then reduced:

$$LiAlH_4 + R - \overset{\overset{\displaystyle O}{\|}}{C} - OH$$

$$\longrightarrow R - CH_2 - OH$$

alcohol

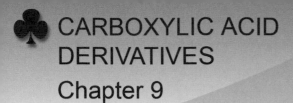

CARBOXYLIC ACID DERIVATIVES

Chapter 9

Memorize	Understand	Not Required*
* IUPAC nomenclature * IR absorption of C=O	* Mechanisms of reactions * Relative reactivity * Steric, inductive effects	* Advanced level college info * Friedel-Crafts Acylation * Nitrile reaction mechanisms

MCAT-Prep.com

Introduction ▮▮▮▮

Carboxylic acid derivatives are a series of compounds that can be synthesized using carboxylic acid. For the MCAT, this includes acid chlorides, anhydrides, amides and esters. You should memorize that 1630 - 1780 is the approximate IR absorbance of C=O.

Additional Resources

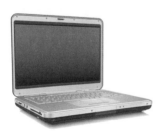

Free Online Q & A

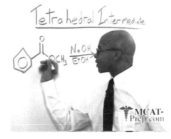

Video: DVD Disc 3

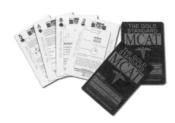

Flashcards

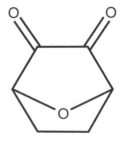

Special Guest

9.1 Acid Halides

The general structure of an acid halide is:

$$R — \overset{\overset{\textstyle O}{\|}}{C} — X \qquad X = Halide$$

These are named by replacing the 'ic acid' of the parent carboxylic acid with the suffix 'yl halide.' For example:

$$CH_3CH_2CH_2 — \overset{\overset{\textstyle O}{\|}}{C} — Br \qquad \text{Butanoyl bromide}$$

$$CH_3 — \overset{\overset{\textstyle O}{\|}}{C} — Cl \qquad \begin{array}{l}\text{Acetyl chloride} \\ \text{(ethanoyl chloride)}\end{array}$$

Acid chlorides are synthesized by reacting the parent carboxylic acid with PCl_5 or $SOCl_2$. Acid chlorides react with $NaBH_4$ to form alcohols. This can be done in one or two steps. In one step, the acid chloride reacts with $NaBH_4$ to immediately form an alcohol. In two steps, the acid chloride can react first with $H_2/Pd/C$ to form a carboxylic acid; reaction of the carboxylic acid with $NaBH_4$ then produces an alcohol.

Acid halides can engage in nucleophilic reactions similar to carboxylic acids (*see* ORG 8.2); however, acid halides are more reactive (*see* ORG 9.6).

9.2 Acid Anhydrides

The general structure of an acid anhydride is:

$$R — \overset{\overset{\textstyle O}{\|}}{C} — O — \overset{\overset{\textstyle O}{\|}}{C} — R$$

These are named by replacing the 'acid' of the parent carboxylic acid with the word 'anhydride.' For example:

$$CH_3 — \overset{\overset{\textstyle O}{\|}}{C} — O — \overset{\overset{\textstyle O}{\|}}{C} — CH_3 \qquad \text{acetic anhydride}$$

$$CH_3 — \overset{\overset{\textstyle O}{\|}}{C} — O — \overset{\overset{\textstyle O}{\|}}{C} — H \qquad \begin{array}{l}\text{acetic formic} \\ \text{anhydride}\end{array}$$

Both acid chlorides and acid anhydrides have boiling points comparable to esters of similar molecular weight.

9.3 Amides

The general structure of an amide is:

$$R-\overset{\overset{\displaystyle O}{\|}}{C}-NR'_2$$

These are named by replacing the '-ic (oic) acid' of the parent anhydride with the suffix '-amide.' If there are alkyl groups attached to the nitrogen, they are named as substituents, and designated by the letter N. For example:

$$CH_3-\overset{\overset{\displaystyle O}{\|}}{C}-N\overset{\displaystyle C_2H_5}{\underset{\displaystyle C_2H_5}{}}$$ N,N-diethylacetamide

$$CH_3CH_2-\overset{\overset{\displaystyle O}{\|}}{C}-NH_2$$ propanamide

Unsubstituted and monosubstituted amides form very strong intermolecular hydrogen bonds, and as a result, they have very high boiling and melting points. The boiling points of disubstituted amides are similar to those of aldehydes and ketones. Amides are essentially neutral (no acidity, as compared to carboxylic acids, and no basicity, as compared to amines).

Amides may be prepared by reacting carboxylic acids (or other carboxylic acid derivatives) with ammonia:

$$R-\overset{\overset{\displaystyle O}{\|}}{C}-OH + NH_3 + heat \xrightarrow{-H_2O} R-\overset{\overset{\displaystyle O}{\|}}{C}-NH_2$$

As well, amides undergo nucleophilic substitution reactions at the carbonyl carbon:

$$R-\overset{\overset{\displaystyle O}{\|}}{C}-NH_2 + NuH \longrightarrow R-\overset{\overset{\displaystyle O}{\|}}{C}-Nu + NH_3$$

Amides can be hydrolyzed to yield the parent carboxylic acid and amine. This reaction may take place under acidic or basic conditions:

$$\underset{\text{amide}}{R-\overset{\overset{\displaystyle O}{\|}}{C}-NHR} + H_2O \xrightarrow{H^+} \underset{\text{acid}}{R-\overset{\overset{\displaystyle O}{\|}}{C}-OH} + \underset{\text{amine}}{RNH_2}$$

$$\underset{\text{amide}}{R-\overset{\overset{\displaystyle O}{\|}}{C}-NHR} + H_2O \xrightarrow{OH^-}$$

$$\underset{\text{carboxylate}}{R-\overset{\overset{\displaystyle O}{\|}}{C}-O^-} + \underset{\text{amine}}{RNH_2} \xrightarrow{H^+} \underset{\text{acid}}{R-\overset{\overset{\displaystyle O}{\|}}{C}-OH}$$

Amides can also form amines by reacting with $LiAlH_4$.

The general structure of an ester is:

$$R - \overset{\overset{\displaystyle O}{\|}}{C} - O - R'$$

These are named by first citing the name of the alkyl group, followed by the parent acid, with the 'ic acid' replaced by 'ate.' For example:

$$CH_3 - \overset{\overset{\displaystyle O}{\|}}{C} - O - CH_3 \quad \text{methylacetate}$$

The boiling points of esters are lower than those of comparable acids or alcohols, and similar to comparable aldehydes and ketones, because they are polar compounds, without hydrogens to form hydrogen bonds. Esters with longer side chains (R-groups) are more nonpolar than esters with shorter side chains (R-groups). Esters usually have pleasing, fruity odors.

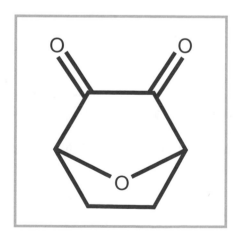

The Ester Bunny

NB: The Ester Bunny is NOT MCAT material. In fact for you super-keeners: is the Ester Bunny a real ester? Find out in our Forum!

Esters may be synthesized by reacting carboxylic acids or their derivatives with alcohols under either basic or acidic conditions:

$$\underset{\text{alcohol}}{R'O^*H} + \underset{\text{acid}}{R - \overset{\overset{\displaystyle O}{\|}}{C} - OH} \longrightarrow \underset{\text{ester}}{R - \overset{\overset{\displaystyle O}{\|}}{C} - O^*R'} + H_2O$$

As well, esters undergo nucleophilic substitution reactions at the carbonyl carbon:

$$R - \overset{\overset{\displaystyle O}{\|}}{C} - OR' + NuH \longrightarrow R - \overset{\overset{\displaystyle O}{\|}}{C} - Nu + R'OH$$

Esters may also be hydrolyzed, to yield the parent carboxylic acid and alcohol. This reaction may take place under acidic or basic conditions.

$$\underset{\text{ester}}{R - \overset{\overset{\displaystyle O}{\|}}{C} - O^*R'} + H_2O \quad \xrightarrow{\text{H}^+}$$

$$\underset{\text{acid}}{R - \overset{\overset{\displaystyle O}{\|}}{C} - OH} + \underset{\text{alcohol}}{R'O^*H}$$

9.4.1 Fats, Glycerides and Saponification

A special class of esters is known as fats (i.e. mono-, di-, and triglycerides). These are biologically important molecules, and they are formed in the following reaction:

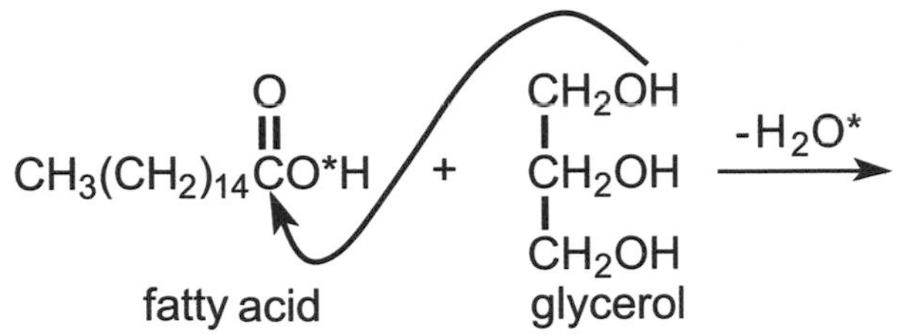

fatty acid   glycerol

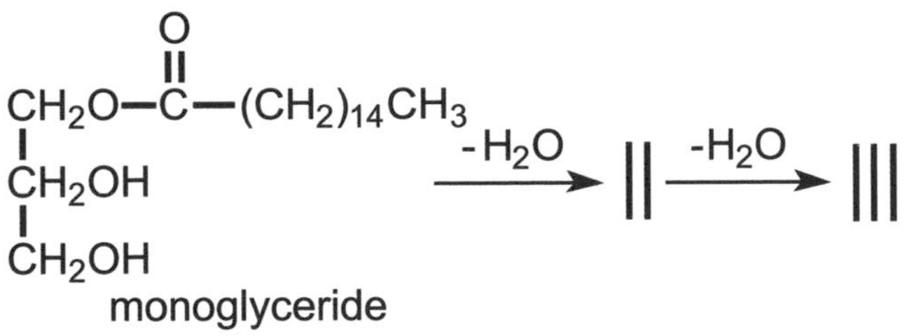

monoglyceride

Fatty acids (= *long chain carboxylic acids*) are formed through the condensation of C2 units derived from acetate, and may be added to the monoglyceride formed in the above reaction, forming diglycerides, and triglycerides. Fats may be hydrolyzed by a base to the components glycerol and the salt of the fatty acids. The salts of long chain carboxylic acids are called soaps. Thus this process is called *saponification*:

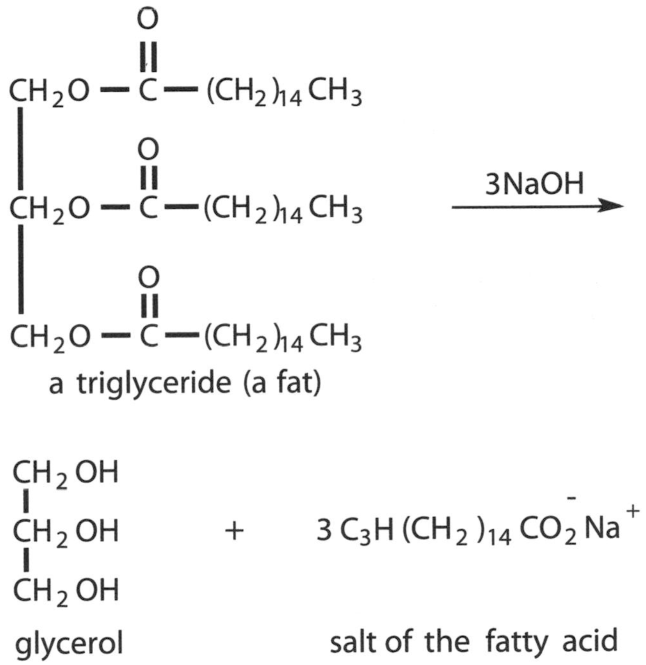

a triglyceride (a fat)

$$CH_2OH$$
$$CH_2OH \qquad + \qquad 3\, C_3H(CH_2)_{14}\, CO_2^-\, Na^+$$
$$CH_2OH$$

glycerol   salt of the fatty acid

9.5 β-Keto Acids

β-keto acids are carboxylic acids with a keto group (i.e. *ketone*) at the β position. Thus it is an acid with a carbonyl group one carbon removed from a carboxylic acid group. Upon heating the carboxyl group can be readily removed as CO_2. This process is called *decarboxylation*. For example:

$$R-\overset{\overset{\displaystyle O}{\|}}{C}-CH_2-\overset{\overset{\displaystyle O}{\|}}{C}-OH \xrightarrow{\text{heat}} \overset{\overset{\displaystyle O}{\|}}{R}CCH_3 + CO_2$$

β – keto acid   ketone

9.6 Relative Reactivity of Carboxylic Acid Derivatives

In terms of nucleophilic substitution, generally, carboxylic acid derivatives are more reactive than comparable non-carboxylic acid derivatives. One important reason for the preceding is that the carbon in carboxylic acids is also attached to the electronegative oxygen atom of the carbonyl group; therefore, carbon is more δ^+, thus being more attractive to a nucleophile. Hence an acid chloride (R-COCl) is more reactive than a comparable alkyl chloride (R-Cl); an ester (R-COOR') is more reactive than a comparable ether (R-OR'); and an amide (R-CONH$_2$) is more reactive than a comparable amine (R-NH$_2$).

Amongst carboxylic acid derivatives, the carbonyl reactivity in order from most to least reactive is:

acid chlorides > anhydrides >> esters > acids > amides > nitriles

The reasons for this may be attributed to resonance effects and inductive effects. The resonance effect is the ability of the substituent to stabilize the carbocation intermediate by delocalization of electrons. The inductive effect is the substituent group, by virtue of its electronegativity, to pull electrons away increasing the partial positivity of the carbonyl carbon.

Within each carboxylic acid derivative, steric or bulk effects also play an important role. The less the steric hindrance, the more access a nucleophile will have to attack the carbonyl carbon, and vice versa.

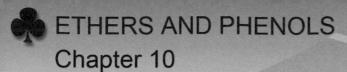

Memorize	Understand	Not Required*
* Nothing	* Nothing	* Ethers and phenols!

MCAT-Prep.com

Introduction

Ethers are composed of an oxygen atom connected to two alkyl or aryl groups of the general formula R–O–R'. A classic example is the solvent and anesthetic diethyl ether, often just called "ether." Phenol is a toxic, white crystalline solid with a sweet tarry odor often referred to as a "hospital smell"! Its chemical formula is C_6H_5OH and its structure is that of a hydroxyl group (-OH) bonded to a phenyl ring thus it is an aromatic compound. Ether and phenol chemistry are no longer required for the new MCAT.

Additional Resources

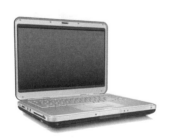

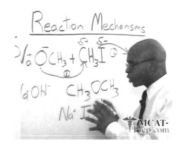

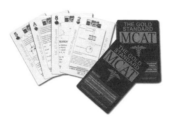

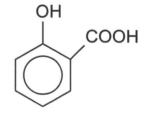

| Free Online Q & A | Video: DVD Discs 1, 4 | Flashcards | Special Guest |

10.1 Description and Nomenclature of Ethers

The general structure of an ether is R-O-R', where the R's may be either aromatic or aliphatic (= *containing only carbon and hydrogen atoms*). In the common system of nomenclature, the two groups on either side of the oxygen are named, followed by the word ether:

$$CH_3 - O - CH_3$$
dimethyl ether

$$CH_3 - O - \overset{\overset{\displaystyle CH_3}{|}}{CHCH_3}$$
methyl isopropyl ether

In the systematic system of nomenclature, the alkoxy (RO-) groups are always named as substituents:

$$CH_3 - O - CH_3$$
methoxy methane

$$CH_3 - O - \overset{\overset{\displaystyle CH_3}{|}}{CHCH_3}$$
methoxy isopropane

The boiling points of ethers are comparable to that of other hydrocarbons. Ethers are more polar than other hydrocarbons, but are not capable of forming intermolecular hydrogen bonds (those between two ether molecules). Ethers are similar to alcohols in water solubility, as they can form intermolecular hydrogen bonds between the ether and the water molecules.

Ethers are <u>good solvents</u>, as the ether linkage is inert to many chemical reagents. Ethers are weak Lewis bases and can be protonated to form positively charged conjugate acids. In the presence of a high concentration of a strong acid (especially HI or HBr), the ether linkage will be cleaved, to form an alcohol and an alkyl halide:

$$CH_3 - O - CH_3 + HI \longrightarrow$$
$$CH_3 - OH + CH_3 - I$$

Ether synthesis can proceed using alcohols or their derivatives. For example, the reverse of the preceding reaction would occur if $NaOCH_3$ (sodium methoxide) instead of $HOCH_3$ was in the reaction flask (the inorganic product would be $Na^+ I^-$).

$$Na^+\,{}^-OCH_3 + {}^{\delta+}CH_3\text{-}I^{\delta-} \longrightarrow$$
$$CH_3\text{-}O\text{-}CH_3 + Na^+I^-$$

10.2 Phenols

A phenol is a molecule consisting of a hydroxyl (-OH) group attached to a benzene (aromatic) ring. The following are some phenols and derivatives which are important to biochemistry, medicine and nature:

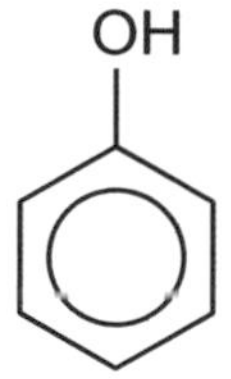

phenol

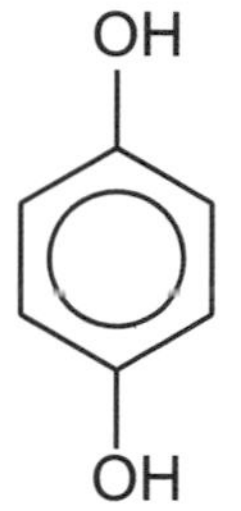

hydroquinone

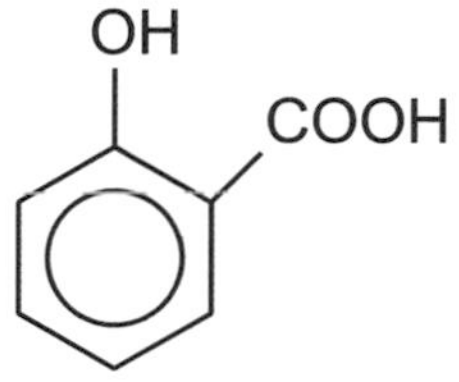

salicylic acid

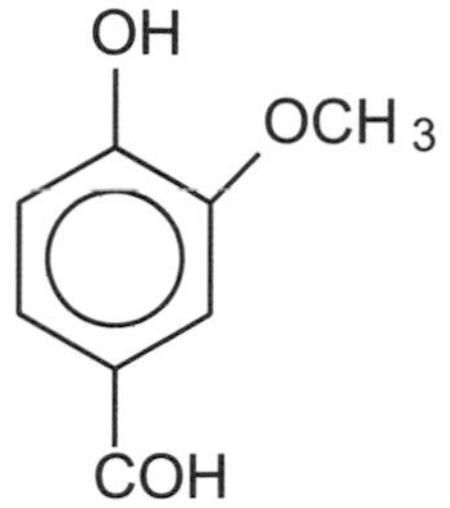

vanillin

Phenols are more acidic than their corresponding alcohols. This is due mainly to the electron withdrawing and resonance stabilization effects of the aromatic ring in the conjugate base anion (the phenoxide ion):

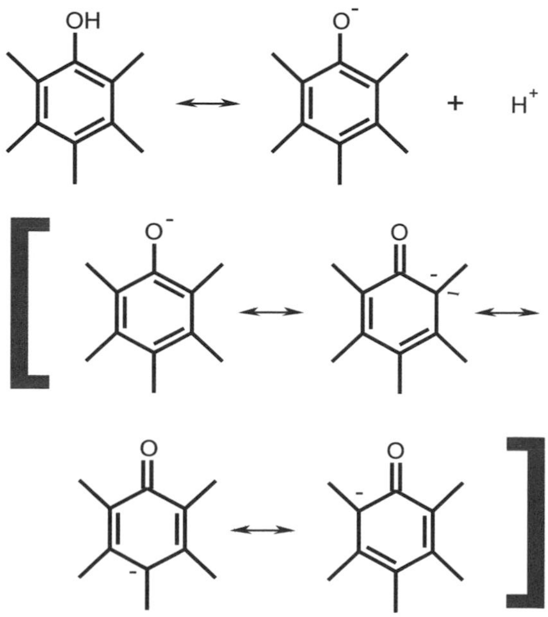

Substituent groups on the ring affect the acidity of phenols by both inductive effects (as with alcohols) and resonance effects. The resonance structures show that electron stabilizing (*withdrawing* or *meta directing*) groups at the ortho or para positions should increase the acidity of the phenol. Examples of these groups include the nitro group ($-NO_2$), -CN, $-CO_2H$, and the weakly deactivating o-p directors - the halogens. Destabilizing groups, such as alkyl groups, or other ortho-para directors, will make the compound less acidic. Phenols are ortho-para directors.

Phenols can form hydrogen bonds, resulting in fairly high boiling points. Their solubility in water, however, is limited, because of the hydrophobic nature of the aromatic ring. Ortho phenols have lower boiling points than meta and para phenols, as they can form intramolecular hydrogen bonds. However, the para and even the ortho compounds can sometimes form intermolecular hydrogen bonds:

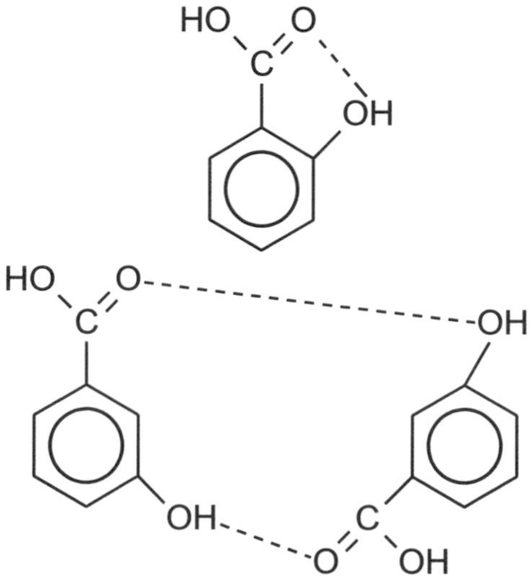

10.2.1 Electrophilic Aromatic Substitution for Phenols

Electrophilic aromatic substitution reactions of phenols may show some unusual effects, due to the hydroxyl group. For example, phenols are fairly unreactive in the Friedel-Crafts acylation reaction (*a reaction in which an acyl group*, R-C=O, *is added to another molecule using* $AlCl_3$ *as a catalyst*), because the -OH group reacts with the catalyst.

The hydroxyl group is a powerful activating group and an ortho-para director in electrophilic substitutions. Thus phenols can brominate three times in bromine water as follows:

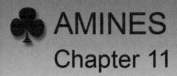

Memorize	Understand	Not Required*
* IUPAC nomenclature * IR absorption of N-H	* Effect of hydrogen bonds * Mechanisms of reactions * Trends in basicity * Resonance, delocalization of electrons	* Advanced level college info * Aromatic amine chemistry * Gabriel synthesis * Staudinger reduction

MCAT-Prep.com

Introduction ▮▮▮▮

Amines are compounds and functional groups that contain a basic nitrogen atom with a lone pair. Amines are derivatives of ammonia (NH_3), where one or more hydrogen atoms are replaced by organic substituents such as alkyl and aryl groups. You should memorize that 3300 - 3500 is the approximate IR absorbance of N-H.

Additional Resources

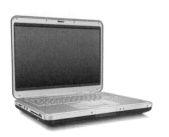

Free Online Q & A

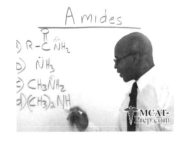

Video: DVD Disc 3

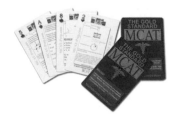

Flashcards

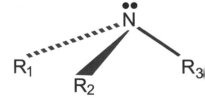

Special Guest

11.1 Description and Nomenclature

Organic compounds with a trivalent nitrogen atom bonded to one or more carbon atoms are called amines. These are organic derivatives of ammonia. They may be classified depending on the number of carbon atoms bonded to the nitrogen:

Primary Amine: RNH_2
Secondary Amine: R_2NH
Tertiary Amine: R_3N
Quaternary Salt: $R_4N^+ X^-$

In the common system of nomenclature, amines are named by adding the suffix '-amine' to the name of the alkyl group. In a secondary or tertiary amine, where there is more than one alkyl group, the groups are named as N-substituted derivatives of the larger group:

$$CH_3 - CH - N - CH_2 - CH_3$$

with CH₃ substituents:

$$\underset{CH_3}{CH} \quad \underset{CH_3}{N}$$

N,N - methyl ethyl isopropylamine

In the systematic system of nomenclature, amines are named analagous to alcohols, except the suffix '-amine' is used instead of the suffix '-ol'.

11.1.1 The Basicity of Amines

Along with the three attached groups, amines have an unbonded electron pair. Most of the chemistry of amines depends on this unbonded electron pair:

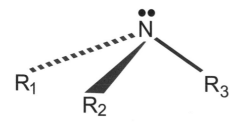

The electron pair is stabilized by the electron donating effects of alkyl groups. Thus the lone pair in tertiary amines is more stable than in secondary amines which, in turn, is more stable than in primary amines. As a result of this electron pair, amines are Lewis bases, and good nucleophiles. In aqueous solution, amines are weak bases, and can accept a proton:

$$R_3N + H_2O \longrightarrow R_3NH^+ + OH^-$$

The ammonium cation in the preceding reaction is stabilized, once again, by the electron donating effects of the alkyl groups. Conversely, should the nitrogen be adjacent to a carbocation, the lone pair can stabilize the carbocation by delocalizing the charge.

The relative basicity of amines is determined by the following:

- If the free amine is stabilized relative to the cation, the amine is less basic.
- If the cation is stabilized relative to the

free amine, the amine is more stable, thus the stronger base.

Groups that withdraw electron density (such as halides or aromatics) decrease the availability of the unbonded electron pair. Electron releasing groups (such as alkyl groups) increase the availability of the unbonded electron pair. The base strength then increases in the following series (where Ø represents a phenyl group):

$$NO_2\text{-}Ø\text{-}NH_2 < Ø\text{-}NH_2 < Ø\text{-}CH_2\text{-}NH_2 <$$
$$NH_3 < CH_3\text{-}NH_2 < (CH_3)_2\text{-}N\text{-}H < (CH_3)_3\text{-}N$$

Note that a substituent attached to an aromatic ring can greatly affect the basicity of the amine. For example, electron withdrawing groups (i.e. $-NO_2$) withdraw electrons from the ring which, in turn, withdraws the lone electron pair (*delocalization*) from nitrogen. Thus the lone pair is less available to bond with a proton; consequently, it is a weaker base. The opposite occurs with an electron donating group, making the amine, relatively, a better base.

11.1.2 More Properties of Amines

- The nitrogen atom can <u>hydrogen bond</u> (using its electron pair) to hydrogens attached to other N's or O's. It can also form hydrogen bonds from hydrogens attached to it with electron pairs of N, O, F or Cl:

$$\begin{array}{c} H \\ | \\ -N-H\cdots\cdots\cdots O-H \\ | \end{array}$$

$$\text{or} \quad \begin{array}{c} \overset{\cdot\cdot}{-N-}\cdots\cdots\overset{\displaystyle H}{\underset{\displaystyle O-H}{|}} \\ | \end{array}$$

Note that primary or secondary amines can hydrogen bond with each other, but tertiary amines cannot. This leads to boiling points which are higher than would be expected for compounds of similar molecular weight, like alkanes, but lower than similar alcohols or carboxylic acids. The hydrogen bonding also renders low weight amines soluble in water.

- A <u>dipole moment</u> is possible:

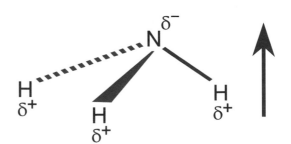

- The nitrogen in amines can contribute its lone pair electrons to activate a benzene ring. Thus amines are ortho-para directors.

- The solubility of quaternary salts decreases with increasing molecular weight. The quaternary structure has steric hindrance and the lone pair electrons on N is not available for H-bonding, thus their solubility is much less than other amines or even alkyl ammonium salts (i.e. $R\text{-}NH_3^+X^-$, $R_2\text{-}NH_2^+X^-$, $R_3\text{-}NH^+X^-$). Quaternary ammonium salts can be synthesized from ammonium hydroxides which are very strong bases.

$$(CH_3)_4N^+OH^- + HCl \longrightarrow$$
Quaternary hydroxide

$$(CH_3)_4N^+Cl^- + H_2O$$
Quaternary salt

11.2 Important Reactions of Amines

- Amide formation is an important reaction for protein synthesis. Primary and secondary amines will react with carboxylic acids and their derivatives to form *amides*:

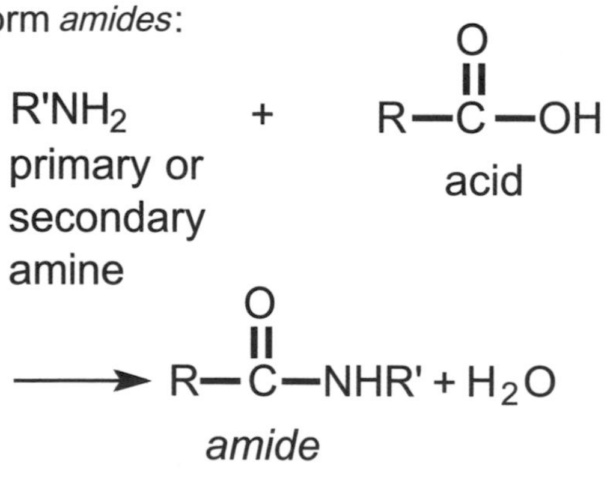

R'NH$_2$ + R—C(=O)—OH

primary or secondary amine   acid

⟶ R—C(=O)—NHR' + H$_2$O

amide

Amides can engage in resonance such that the lone pair electrons on the nitrogen is delocalized. Thus amides are by far less basic than amines.

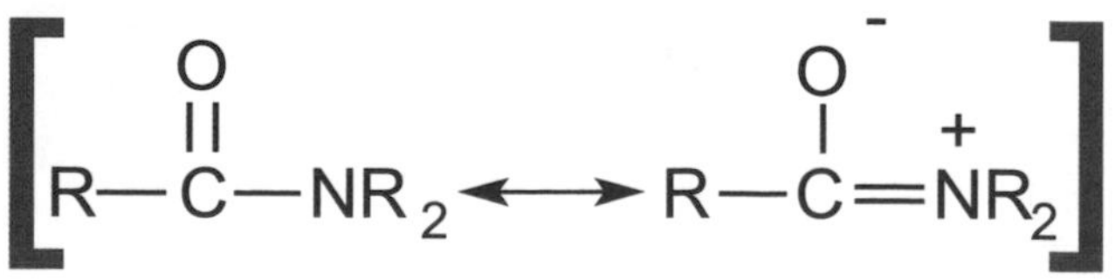

$$\left[R-\overset{\overset{\displaystyle O}{\|}}{C}-NR_2 \longleftrightarrow R-\overset{\overset{\displaystyle O^-}{|}}{C}=\overset{+}{N}R_2 \right]$$

As can be seen, the C-N bond has a partial double bond character. Thus there is restricted rotation about the C-N bond.

- Alkylation is another important reaction which involves amines with alkyl halides:

$$RCH_2Cl + R'NH_2 \longrightarrow RCH_2NHR' + HCl$$
1°, 2° or 3° amine

Both amide formation and alkylation make use of the nucleophilic character of the electrons on nitrogen.

Memorize	Understand	Not Required*
* Basic structures * Isoelectric point equation * Define: amphoteric, zwitterions	* Effect of H, S, hydrophobic bonds * Basic mechanisms of reactions * Effect of pH, isoelectric point * Protein structure * Different ways of drawing structures	* Advanced level college info * Memorizing all the names of amino acids * Detailed mech. specific to bio mole

MCAT-Prep.com

Introduction

Biological molecules truly involve the chemistry of life. Such molecules include amino acids and proteins, carbohydrates (glucose, disaccharides, polysaccharides), lipids (triglycerides, steroids) and nucleic acids (DNA, RNA).

Additional Resources

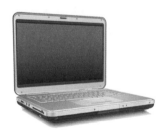 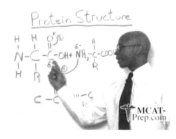 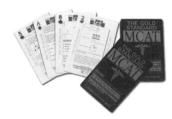 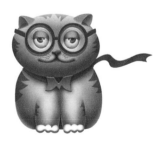

| Free Online Q & A | Video: DVD Disc 3 | Flashcards | Special Guest |

12.1 Amino Acids

Amino acids are molecules that contain a side chain (*R*), a carboxylic acid, and an amino group at the α carbon. Thus the general structure of α-amino acids is:

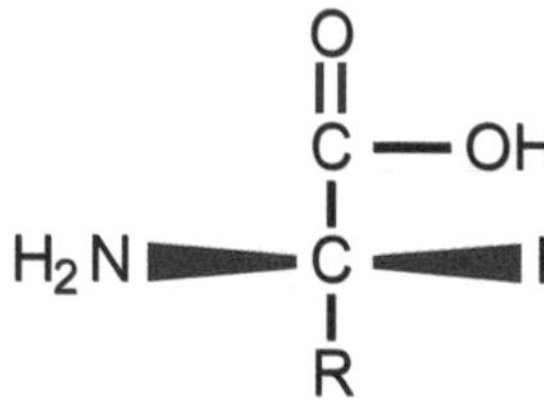

L - amino acid 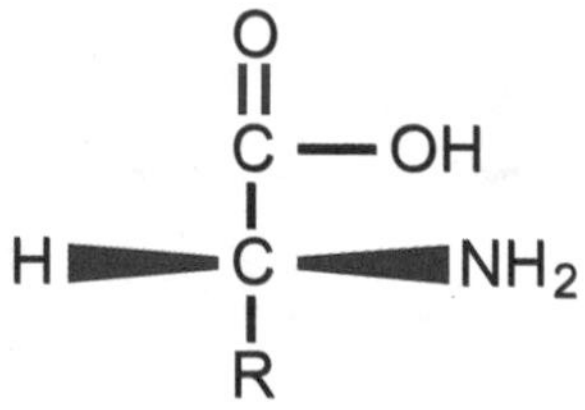   D - amino acid

Amino acids may be named systematically as substituted carboxylic acids, however, there are 20 important α-amino acids that are known by common names. These are naturally occurring and they form the building blocks of most proteins found in humans. The following are a few examples of α-amino acids:

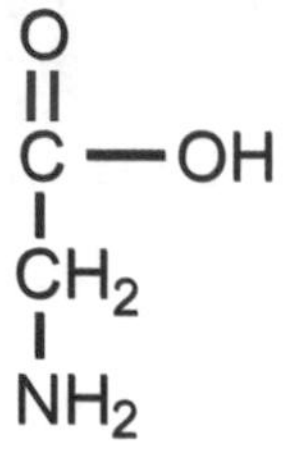

Glycine 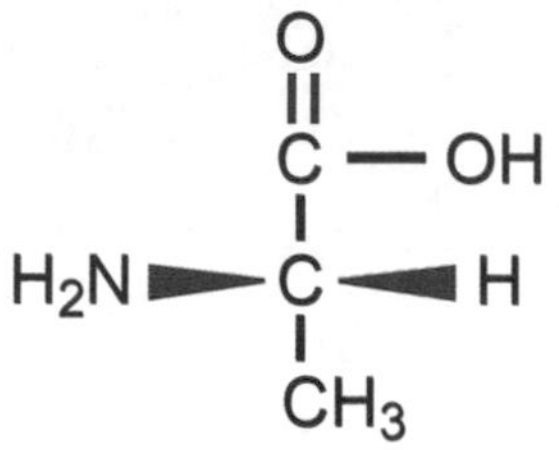   Alanine

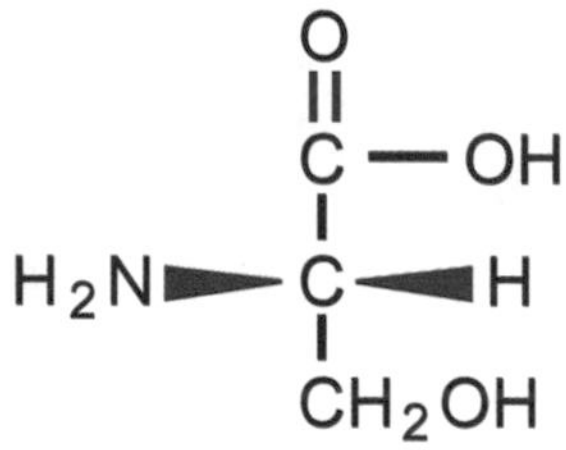

Serine 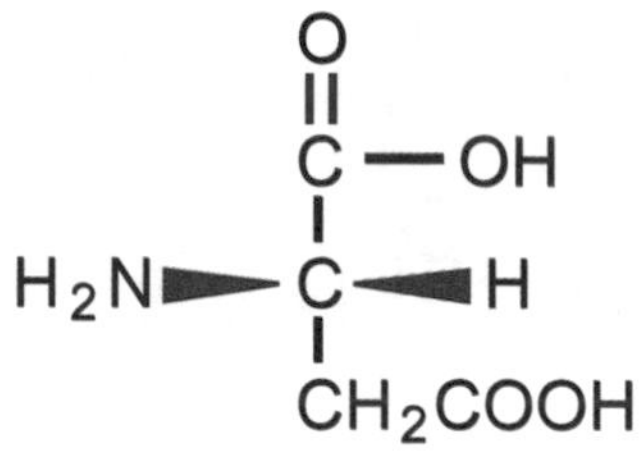   Aspartic acid

Note that all amino acids have the same relative configuration, the L-configuration. However, the absolute configuration depends on the priority assigned to the side group (*see* ORG 2.3.1 *for rules*). In the preceding amino acids, the S-configuration prevails (*except glycine which cannot be assigned any configuration since it is not chiral*).

12.1.1 Hydrophilic vs. Hydrophobic

Different types of amino acids tend to be found in different areas of the proteins that they make up. Amino acids which are ionic and/or polar are hydrophilic, and tend to be found on the exterior of proteins (i.e. *exposed to water*). These include aspartic acid and its amide, glutamic acid and its amide, lysine, arginine and histidine. Certain other polar amino acids are found on either the interior or exterior of proteins. These include serine, threonine, and tyrosine. Hydrophobic amino acids which may be found on the interior of proteins include methionine, leucine, tryptophan, valine and phenylalanine. Hydrophobic molecules tend to cluster in aqueous solutions (= *hydrophobic bonding*). Alanine is a nonpolar amino acid which is unusual because it is less hydrophobic than most nonpolar amino acids. This is because its nonpolar side chain is very short.

Glycine is the smallest amino acid, and the only one that is not optically active. It is often found at the 'corners' of proteins. Alanine is small and, although hydrophoblc, is found on the surface of proteins.

12.1.2 Acidic vs. Basic

Amino acids have both an acid and basic components (= *amphoteric*). The amino acids with the R group containing an amino ($-NH_2$) group, are basic. The two basic amino acids are lysine and arginine. Amino acids with an R group containing a carboxyl (-COOH) group are acidic. The two acidic amino acids are aspartic acid and glutamic acid. One amino acid, histidine, may act as either an acid or a base, depending upon the pH of the resident solution. This makes histidine a very good physiologic buffer. The rest of the amino acids are considered to be neutral.

The basic $-NH_2$ group in the amino acid is present as an ammonium ion, $-NH_3^+$. The acidic carboxyl -COOH group is present as a carboxylate ion, $-COO^-$. As a result, amino acids are dipolar ions, or *zwitterions*. In an aqueous solution, there is an equilibrium present between the dipolar, the anionic, and the cationic forms of the amino acid:

Therefore the charge on the amino acid will vary with the pH of the solution, and with the isoelectric point. This point is the pH where a given amino acid will be neutral (i.e. have no net charge). This isoelectric point is the average of the two pK_a values of an amino acid (*depending on the dissociated group*):

$$\text{isoelectric point} = pI = (pK_{a1} + pK_{a2})/2$$

Above the isoelectric point (basic conditions), the amino acids will have a net negative charge. Below the isoelectric point (acidic conditions), the amino acids will have a net positive charge.

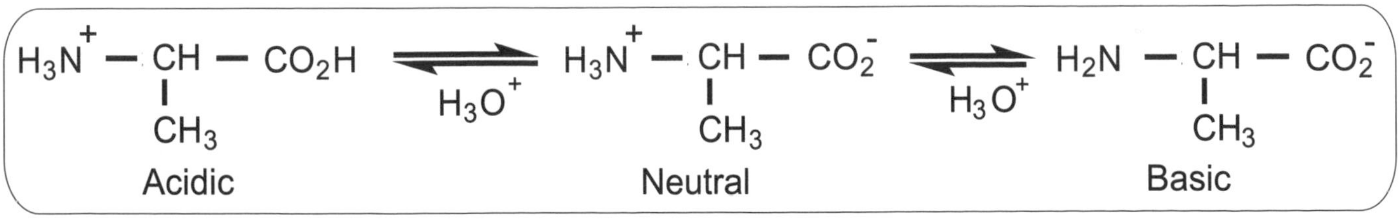

12.2 Proteins

12.2.1 General Principles

Proteins are long chain polypeptides which often form higher order structures. Polypeptides are polymers of 40 to 1000 α-amino acids joined together by amide (*peptide*) bonds. These peptide bonds are derived from the amino group of one amino acid, and the acid group of another. When a peptide bond is formed, a molecule of water is released (*condensation*). The bond can be broken by adding water (*hydrolysis*).

Since proteins are polymers of amino acids, they also have isoelectric points. Classification as to the acidity or basicity of a protein depends on the numbers of acidic and basic amino acids it contains. If there is an excess of acidic amino acids, the isoelectric point will be at a pH of less than 7. At pH = 7, these proteins will have a net negative charge. Similarly, those with an excess of basic amino acids will have an isoelectric point at a pH of greater than 7. Therefore, at pH = 7, these proteins will have a net positive charge.

12.2.2 Protein Structure

Protein structure may be divided into primary, secondary, tertiary and quaternary structures. The primary structure is the sequence of amino acids as determined by the DNA and the location of covalent bonds (*including disulfide bonds*). This structure determines the higher order structures.

The secondary structure is the orderly inter- or intramolecular *hydrogen bonding* of the protein chain. The resultant structure may be the more stable α-helix (e.g. keratin), or a β-pleated sheet (e.g. silk). Proline is an amino acid which cannot participate in the regular array of H-bonding in an α-helix. Proline disrupts the α-helix, thus it is usually

12.3.2 Important Reactions of Carbohydrates

A disaccharide is a molecule made up of two monosaccharides, joined by a *glycosidic bond* between the hemiacetal carbon of one molecule, and the hydroxyl group of another. The glycosidic bond forms an α-1,4-glycosidic linkage if the reactant is an α anomer. A β-1,4-glycosidic linkage is formed if the reactant is a β anomer. When the bond is formed, one molecule of water is released (condensation). In order to break the bond, water must be added (hydrolysis):

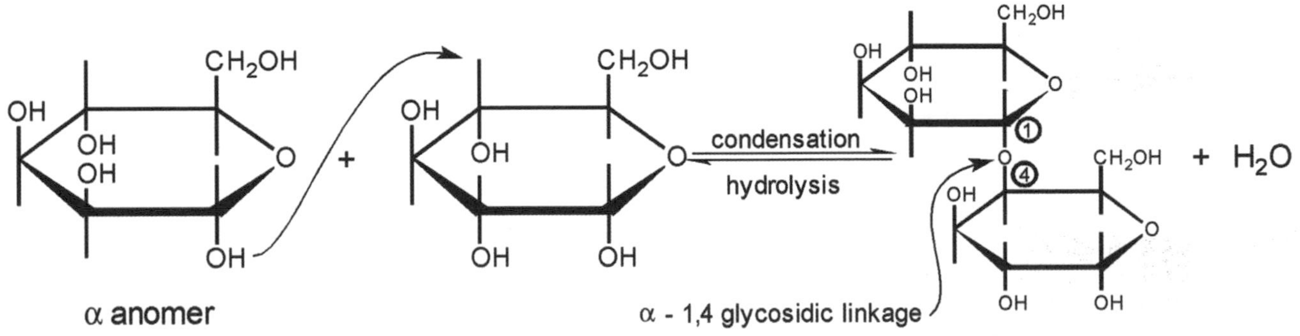

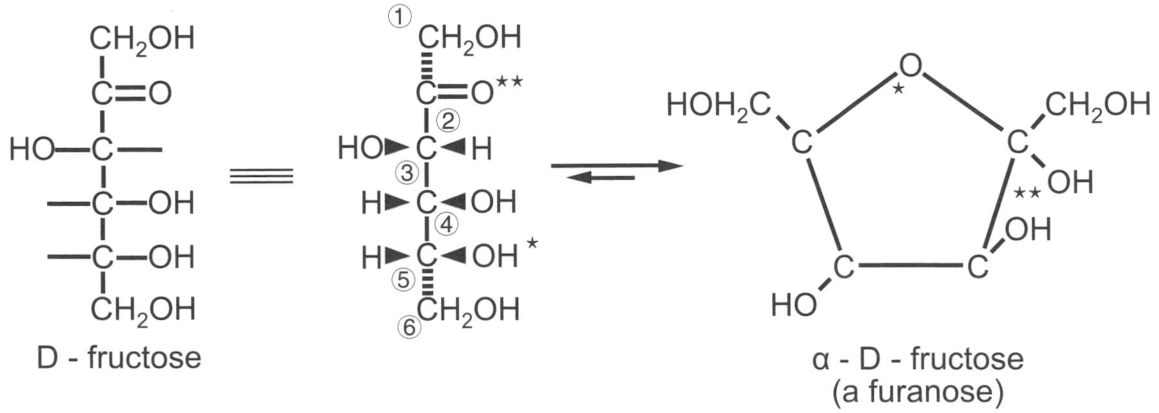

Figure IV.B.12.1 Part I: Names, structures and configurations of common sugars.

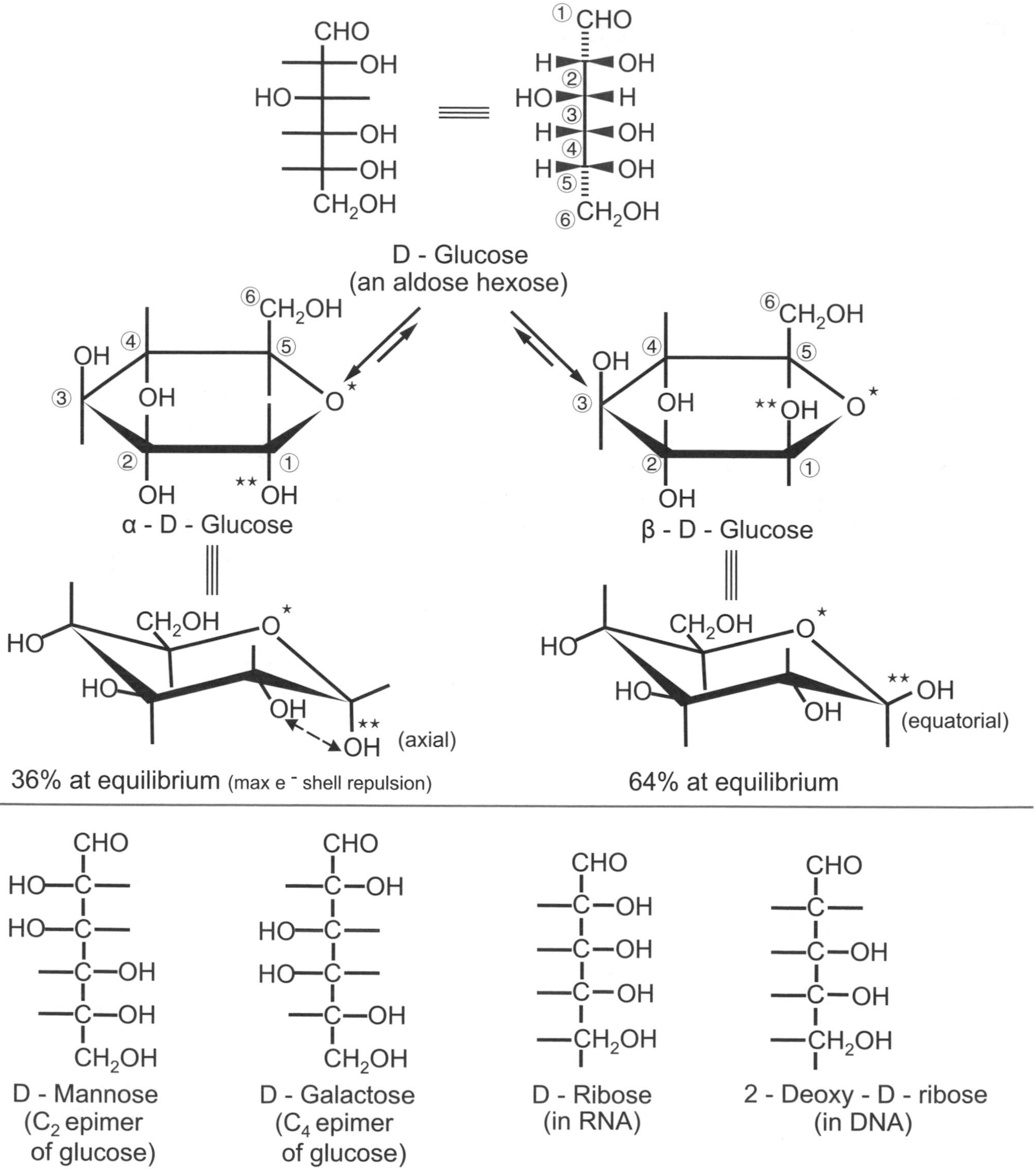

CHO
—OH
HO—
—OH
—OH
CH$_2$OH

$\equiv$

① CHO
H—OH ②
HO—H ③
H—OH ④
H—OH ⑤
⑥ CH$_2$OH

D - Glucose
(an aldose hexose)

α - D - Glucose

β - D - Glucose

36% at equilibrium (max e⁻ shell repulsion)

64% at equilibrium

CHO
HO—C—
HO—C—
—C—OH
—C—OH
CH$_2$OH

D - Mannose
(C$_2$ epimer
of glucose)

CHO
—C—OH
HO—C—
HO—C—
—C—OH
CH$_2$OH

D - Galactose
(C$_4$ epimer
of glucose)

CHO
—C—OH
—C—OH
—C—OH
—CH$_2$OH

D - Ribose
(in RNA)

CHO
—C—
—C—OH
—C—OH
—CH$_2$OH

2 - Deoxy - D - ribose
(in DNA)

Figure IV.B.12.1 Part II: Names, structures and configurations of common sugars.

- Sucrose (common sugar) = glucose + fructose
- Lactose (milk sugar) = glucose + galactose
- Maltose (α-1,4 bond) = glucose + glucose
- Cellobiose (β-1,4 bond) = glucose + glucose

Sugars can undergo <u>oxidation</u>. When aldoses are treated with bromine water, the aldehyde is oxidized to a carboxylic acid group, resulting in a product known as an *aldonic acid*:

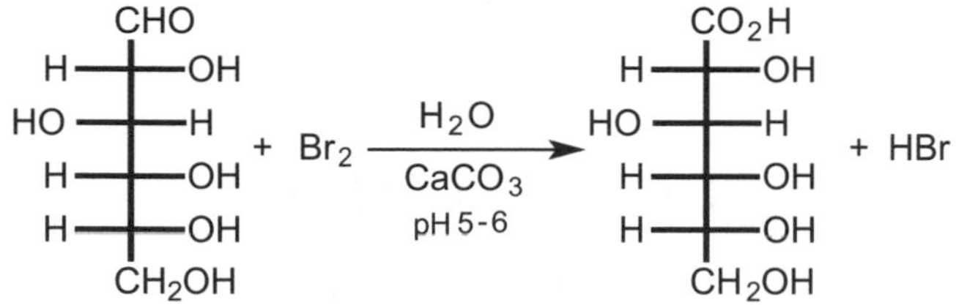

Aldoses treated with dilute nitric acid will have both the primary alcohol and aldehyde groups oxidize to carboxylic acid groups, resulting in a product known as an *aldaric acid*:

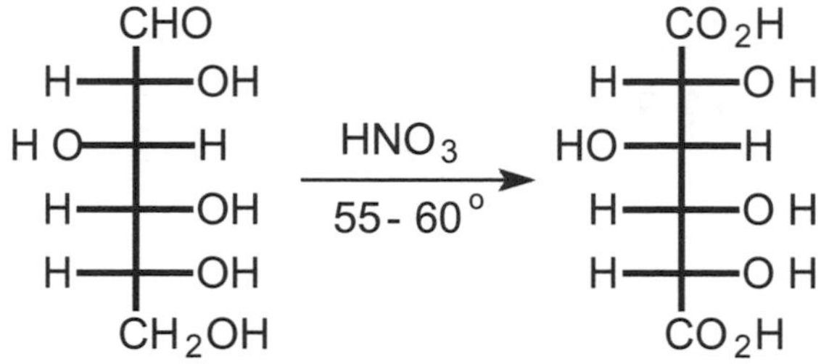

$$CHO \xrightarrow[55-60°]{HNO_3} CO_2H$$

D-glucose (an aldose)

D-Gluconic acid (an aldonic acid)

D-glucose (an aldose)

D-Glucaric acid (an aldaric acid)

12.3.3 Polysaccharides

Polymers of many monosaccharides are called <u>polysaccharides</u>. As in disaccharides, they are joined by glycosidic linkages. They may be straight chains, or branched chains. Some common polysaccharides are:

- Starch (plant energy storage)
- Cellulose (plant structural component)
- Glycocalyx (associated with the plasma membrane)
- Glycogen (animal energy storage in the form of glucose)
- Chitin (structural component found in shells or arthropods)

Carbohydrates are the most abundant organic constituents of plants. They are the source of chemical energy in living organisms, and, in plants, they are used in making the support structures.

12.4 Lipids

Lipids are a class of organic molecules containing many different types of substances, such as fatty acids, fats, waxes, triacyl glycerols, terpenes and steroids.

Triacyl glycerols are oils and fats of either animal or plant origin. In general, fats are solid at room temperature, and oils are liquid at room temperature. The general structure of a triacyl glycerol is:

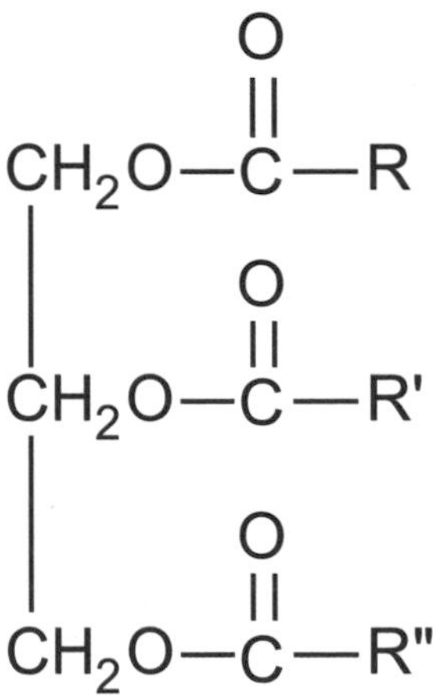

The R groups may be the same or different, and are usually long chain alkyl groups. Upon hydrolysis of a triacyl glycerol, the products are three fatty acids and glycerol (*see* ORG 9.4.1). The fatty acids may be saturated (= no multiple bonds, i.e. *palmitic acid*) or unsaturated (= containing double or triple bonds, i.e. *oleic acid*). Unsaturated fatty acids are usually in the cis configuration. Saturated fatty acids have a higher melting point than unsaturated fatty acids. Some common fatty acids are:

$$CH_3(CH_2)_{14}COOH$$
palmitic acid

$$CH_3(CH_2)_{16}COOH$$
stearic acid

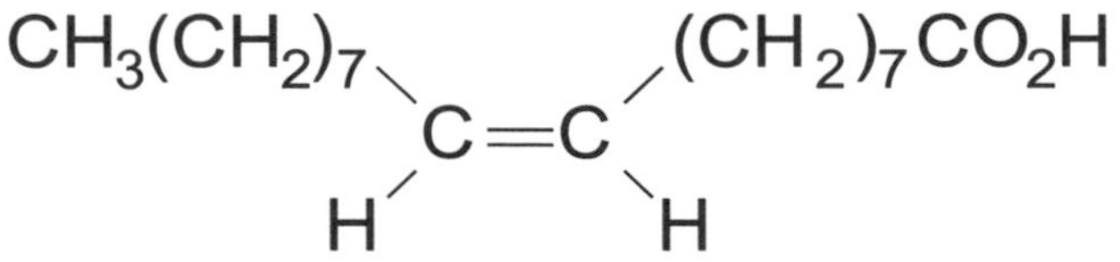

$$CH_3(CH_2)_7 \diagdown \atop C=C \diagup (CH_2)_7CO_2H$$
$$H \diagup \qquad \diagdown H$$
oleic acid

12.4.1 Steroids

Steroids are derivatives of the basic ring structure:

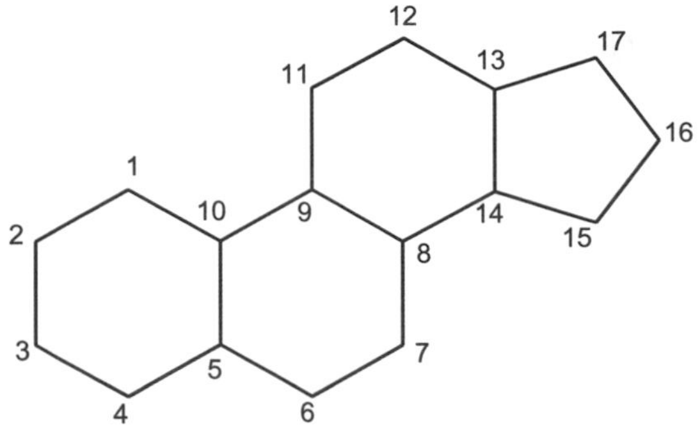

The carbon atoms are numbered as shown. Many important substances are steroids, some examples include: cholesterol, D vitamins, bile acids, adrenocortical hormones, and male and female sex hormones.

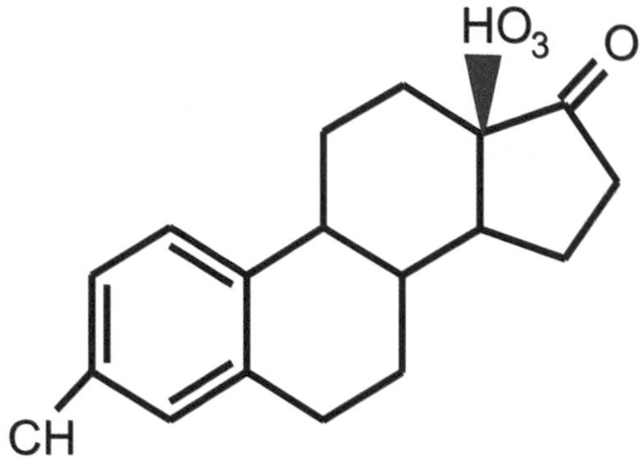

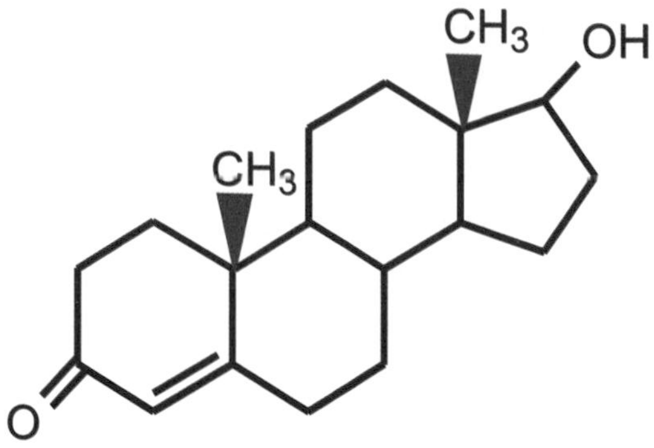

Testosterone
(an androgen)

Estradiol
(an estrogen)

Since such a significant portion of a steroid contains hydrocarbons, which are hydrophobic, steroids can dissolve through the hydrophobic interior of a cell's plasma membrane. Furthermore, steroid hormones contain polar side groups which allow the hormone to easily dissolve in water. Thus steroid hormones are well designed to be transported through the vascular space, to cross the plasma membranes of cells, and to have an effect either in the cell's cytosol or, as is usually the case, in the nucleus.

12.5 Phosphorous in Biological Molecules

Phosphorous is an essential component of various biological molecules including adenosine triphosphate (ATP), phospholipids in cell membranes, and the nucleic acids which form DNA. Phosphorus can also form phosphoric acid and several phosphate esters:

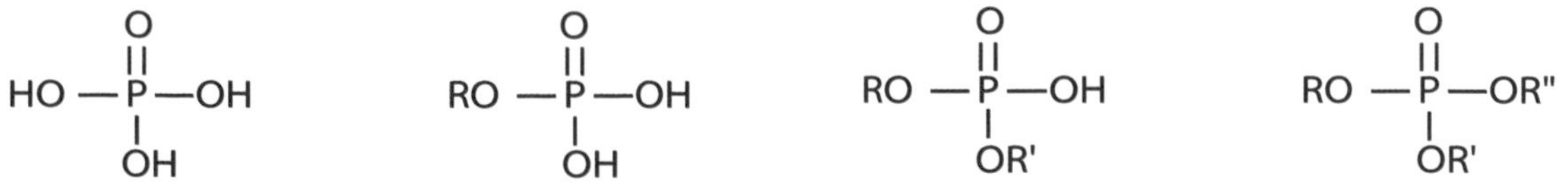

phosphoric acid

phosphate esters

A phospholipid is produced from three ester linkages to glycerol. Phosphoric acid is ester linked to the terminal hydroxyl group and two fatty acids are ester linked to the two remaining hydroxyl groups of glycerol (*see Biology Section 1.1 for a schematic view of a phospholipid*).

In DNA the phosphate groups engage in two ester linkages creating phosphodiester bonds. It is the 5' phosphorylated position of one pentose ring which is linked to the 3' position of the next pentose ring (*see BIO 1.1.2*):

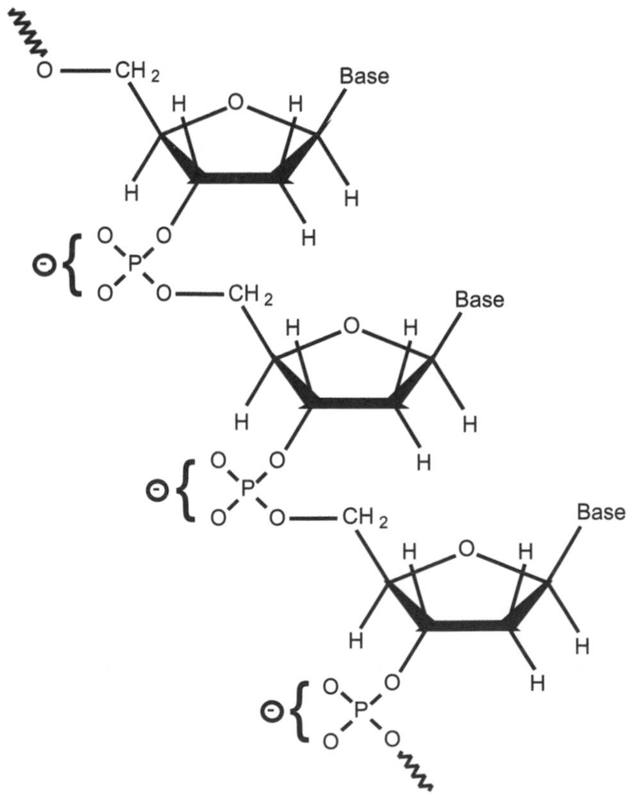

In Biology Chapter 4, the production of ATP was discussed. In each case the components ADP and P_i (= *inorganic phosphate*) combined using the energy generated from a coupled reaction to produce ATP. The linkage between the phosphate groups are via *anhydride bonds*:

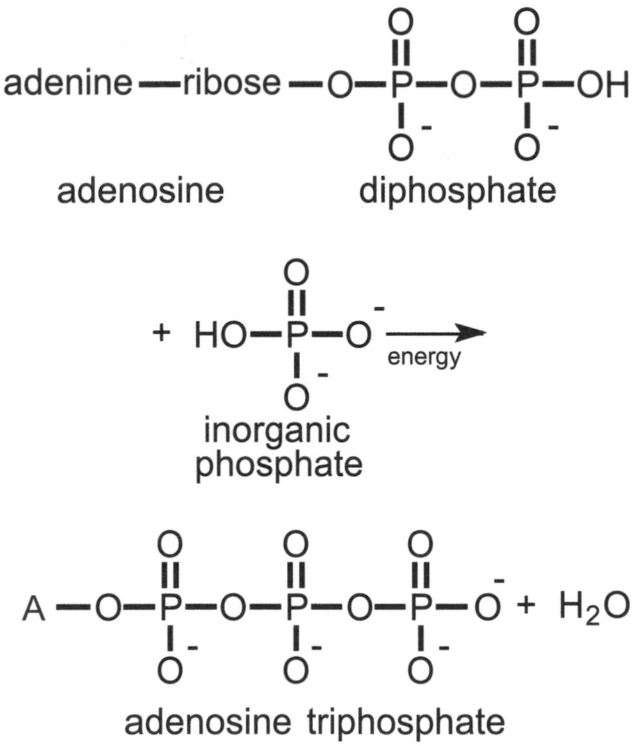

adenine —ribose —O—P—O—P—OH

adenosine   diphosphate

+ HO—P—O⁻ ——→ energy

inorganic phosphate

A —O—P—O—P—O—P—O⁻ + H_2O

adenosine triphosphate

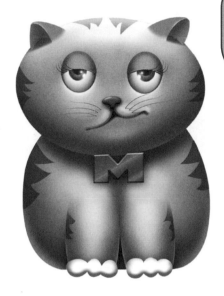

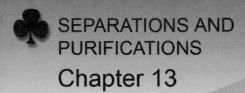

SEPARATIONS AND PURIFICATIONS
Chapter 13

Memorize	Understand	Not Required*
* Definitions of the major techniques * Interactions between organic molecules	* Different phases in the various techniques * How to improve separation, purification * How to avoid overheating (distillation)	* Advanced level college info * Electrolysis, affinity purification * Refining, smelting

MCAT-Prep.com

Introduction

Separation techniques are used to transform a mixture of substances into two or more distinct products. The separated products may be different in chemical properties or some physical property (i.e. size). Purification in organic chemistry is the physical separation of a chemical substance of interest from foreign or contaminating substances.

Additional Resources

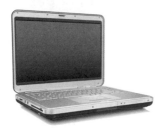

Free Online Q & A

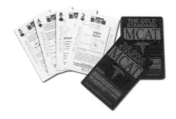

Flashcards

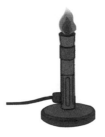

Special Guest

13.1 Extraction

Extraction is the process by which a solute is transferred (*extracted*) from one solvent and placed in another. This procedure is possible if the two solvents used cannot mix (= *immiscible*) and if the solute is more soluble in the solvent used for the extraction.

For example, consider the extraction of solute A which is dissolved in solvent X. We choose solvent Y for the extraction since solute A is highly soluble in it and because solvent Y is immiscible with solvent X. We now add solvent Y to the solution involving solute A and solvent X. The container is agitated. Solute A begins to dissolve in the solvent where it is most soluble, solvent Y. The container is left to stand, thus the two immiscible solvents separate. The phase containing solute A can now be removed.

In practice, solvent Y would be chosen such that it would be sufficiently easy to evaporate (= *volatile*) after the extraction so solute A can be easily recovered. Also, it is more efficient to perform several extractions using a small amount of solvent each time, rather than one extraction using a large amount of solvent.

13.2 Chromatography

Chromatography is the separation of a mixture of compounds by their distribution between two phases: one stationary and one moving. Molecules are separated based on differences in polarity and molecular weight.

13.2.1 Gas-Liquid Chromatography

In gas-liquid chromatography, the *stationary phase* is a liquid absorbed to an inert solid. The liquid can be polyethylene glycol, squalene, or others, depending on the polarity of the substances being separated.

The mobile phase is a gas (i.e. He, N_2) which is unreactive both to the stationary phase and to the substances being separated. The sample being analyzed can be injected in the direction of gas flow into one end of a column packed with the stationary phase. As the sample migrates through the column certain molecules will move faster than others. As mentioned the separation of the different types of molecules is dependent on size (*molecular weight*) and charge (*polarity*). Once the molecules reach the end of the column special detectors signal their arrival.

13.2.2 Thin-Layer Chromatography

Thin-layer chromatography is a solid-liquid technique, based on adsorptivity and solubility. The *stationary phase* is a type of finely divided polar material, usually silica gel or alumina, which is thinly coated onto a glass plate.

There are several types of interactions that may occur between the organic molecules in the sample and the silica gel, in order from weakest to strongest:

- Van der Waals force (nonpolar molecules)
- Dipole-dipole interaction (polar molecules)
- Hydrogen bonding (hydroxylic compounds)
- Coordination (Lewis bases)

Molecules with functional groups with the greatest polarity will bind more strongly to the stationary phase and thus will not rise as high on the glass plate.

Organic molecules will also interact with the *mobile phase* (= a solvent), or *eluent* used in the process. The more polar the solvent, the more easily it will dissolve polar molecules. The mobile phase usually contains organic solvents like ethanol, benzene, chloroform, acetone, etc.

As a result of the interactions of the organic molecules with the stationary and moving phases, for any adsorbed compound there is a dynamic distribution equilibrium between these phases. The different molecules will rise to different heights on the plate. Their presence can be detected using special stains (i.e. pH indicators, $KMnO_4$) or uv light (*if the compound can fluoresce*).

13.3 Distillation

Distillation is the process by which compounds are separated based on differences in boiling points. A classic example of simple distillation is the separation of salt from water. The solution is heated. Water will boil and vaporize at a far lower temperature than salt. Hence the water boils away leaving salt behind. Water vapor can now be condensed into pure liquid water (*distilled water*).

As long as one compound is more volatile, the distillation process is quite simple. If the difference between the two boiling points are low, it will be more difficult to separate the compounds by this method. Instead, fractional distillation can be used in which, for example, a column is filled with glass beads which is placed between the distillation flask and the condenser. The glass beads increase the surface area over which the less volatile compound can condense and drip back down to the distillation flask below. The more volatile compound boils away and condenses in the condenser. Thus the two compounds are separated.

The efficiency of the distillation process in producing a pure product is improved by repeating the distillation process, or, in the case of fractional distillation, increasing the length of the column and avoiding overheating. Overheating may destroy the pure compounds or increase the percent of impurities. Some of the methods which are used to prevent overheating include boiling slowly, the use of boiling chips (= *ebulliator*, which makes bubbles) and the use of a vacuum which decreases the vapor pressure and thus the boiling point (cf. CHM 4.3.2).

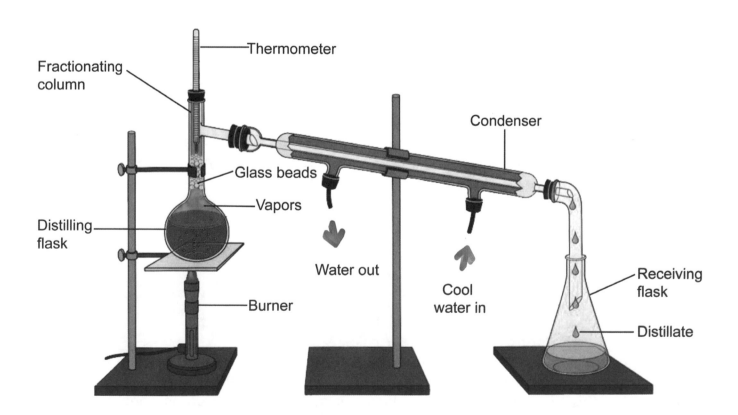

Figure IV.B.13.1: Standard distillation apparatus

13.4 Recrystallization

Recrystallization is a useful purification technique. A solid organic compound with some impurity is dissolved in a hot solvent, and then the solvent is slowly cooled to allow the pure compound to reform or *recrystallize*, while leaving the impurities behind in the solvent. This is possible because the impurities do not normally fit within the crystal structure of the compound.

In choosing a solvent, solubility data (e.g. K_{sp} at various temperatures, etc.) regarding both the compound to be purified and the impurities should be known. The data should be analyzed such that the solvent would:

- have the capability to dissolve alot of the compound (to be purified) at or near the boiling point of the solvent, while being able to dissolve little of the compound at room temperature. As well, the impurities should be soluble in the cold solvent.
- have a low boiling point, so as to be easily removed from the solid in a drying process.
- not react with the solid.

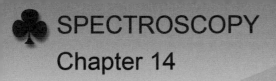

SPECTROSCOPY
Chapter 14

Memorize	Understand	Not Required*
* IR abs. values of basic functional groups * At minimum recall these: C=O, -OH * Basic rules to interpret NMRs	* Basic theory: IR spect., NMR * Very basic spectrum (graph) analysis * Deuterium exchange	* Advanced level college info * mass spectrometry, x-ray, Raman * NMR other than proton NMR * Interpreting complex proton NMRs

MCAT-Prep.com

Introduction ▪▪▪▪

Spectroscopy is the use of the absorption, emission, or scattering of electromagnetic radiation by matter to study the matter or to study physical processes. The matter can be atoms, molecules, atomic or molecular ions, or solids. For MCAT organic chemistry, spectroscopy is used to determine the presence of functional groups (IR spect.) or the kinds/types of H's in a molecule (proton NMR).

Additional Resources

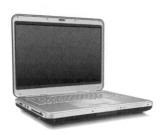

Free Online Q & A

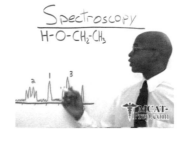

Video: DVD Disc 4

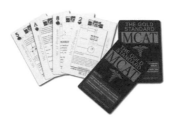

Flashcards

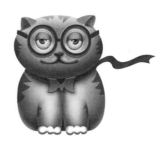

Special Guest

14.1 IR Spectroscopy

In an infrared spectrometer, a beam of infrared (IR) radiation is passed through a sample. The spectrometer will then analyze the amount of radiation transmitted (= % *transmittance*) through the sample as the incident radiation is varied. Ultimately, a plot results as a graph showing the transmittance or absorption (*the inverse of transmittance*) versus the frequency or wavelength of the incident radiation.

The location of an IR absorption band (*or peak*) can be specified in *frequency units* by its wave number, measured in cm^{-1}. As the wave number decreases, the wavelength increases, thus the energy decreases (recall from physics: $v = \lambda f$ and $E = hf$). A schematic representation of the IR spectrum of octane is:

Electromagnetic radiation consists of discrete units of energy called *quanta* or *photons*. All organic compounds are capable of absorbing many types of electromagnetic energy. The absorption of energy leads to an increase in the amplitude of intramolecular rotations and vibrations.

Intramolecular rotations are the rotations of a molecule about its center of gravity. The difference in rotational energy levels is inversely proportional to the moment of inertia of a molecule. Rotational energy is quantized and gives rise to absorption spectra in the microwave region of the electromagnetic spectrum.

Intramolecular vibrations are the bending and stretching motions of bonds

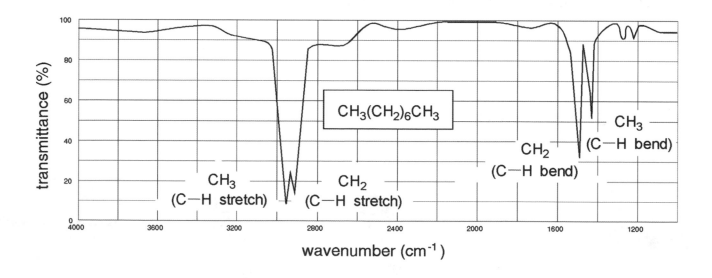

within a molecule. The relative spacing between vibrational energy levels increases with the increasing strength of an intramolecular bond. Vibrational energy is quantized and gives rise to absorption spectra in the infrared region of the electromagnetic spectrum.

Thus there are two types of bond vibration: stretching and bending. That is, after exposure to the IR radiation the bonds stretch and bend (or contract) to a greater degree once energy is absorbed. In general, bending vibrations will occur at lower frequencies (higher wavelengths) than stretching vibrations of the same groups. So, as seen in the sample spectra for octane, each group will have two characteristic peaks, one due to stretching, and one due to bending.

Different functional groups will have transmittances at characteristic wave numbers, which is why IR spectroscopy is useful. Some examples (approximate values) of characteristic absorbances are:

Group	Frequency Range (cm^{-1})
Alkyl (C-H)	2850 - 2960
Alkene (C=C)	1620 - 1680
Alkyne (C≡C)	2100 - 2260
Alcohol (O-H)	3200 - 3650
Benzene (Ar-H)	3030
Carbonyl (C=O)	1630 - 1780
▶ Aldehyde	1680 - 1750
▶ Ketone	1735 - 1750
▶ Carboxylic Acid	1710 - 1780
▶ Amide	1630 - 1690
Amine (N-H)	3300 - 3500
Nitriles (C≡N)	2220 - 2260

By looking at the characteristic transmittances of a compound's spectrum, it is possible to identify the functional groups present in the molecule.

14.2 NMR Spectroscopy

Nuclear Magnetic Resonance (NMR) spectroscopy can be used to examine the environments of the hydrogen atoms in a molecule. In fact, using a (proton) NMR or ^{1}HNMR, one can determine both the number and types of hydrogens in a molecule. The basis of this stems from the magnetic properties of the hydrogen nucleus (proton). Similar to electrons, the hydrogen proton has a nuclear spin, able to take either of two values. These values are designated as +1/2 and -1/2. As a result of this spin, the nucleus will respond to a magnetic field by being oriented in the direction of the field. NMR spectrometers measure the absorption of energy by the hydrogen nuclei in an organic compound.

A schematic representation of an NMR spectrum, that of dimethoxymethane is shown:

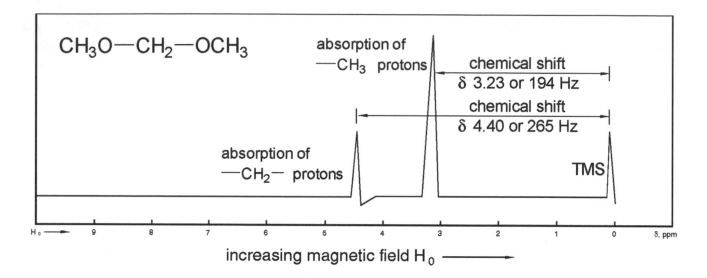

The small peak at the right is that of TMS, tetramethylsilane, shown here:

$$CH_3 - Si - CH_3$$

with CH_3 groups above and below the Si.

This compound is added to the sample to be used as a reference, or standard. It is volatile, inert and absorbs at a higher field than most other organic chemicals.

The position of a peak relative to the standard is referred to as its *chemical shift*. Since NMR spectroscopy differentiates between types of protons, each type will have a different chemical shift, as shown. Protons in the same environment, like the three hydrogens in $-CH_3$, are called *equivalent protons*.

Dimethoxymethane is a symmetric molecule, thus the protons on either methyl group are equivalent. So, in the example above, the absorption of $-CH_3$ protons occurs at one peak (*a singlet*) 3.23 ppm downfield from TMS. In most organic molecules, the range of absorption will be in the 0-10 ppm (= *parts per million*) range.

The area under each peak is directly related to the number of protons contributing to it, and thus may be used to determine the relative number of protons in the molecule. Accurate measurements of the area under the two peaks above yield the ratio 1:3 which represents the relative number of hydrogens (i.e. 1:3 = 2:6).

Let us now examine a schematic representation of the NMR spectrum of ethyl bromide:

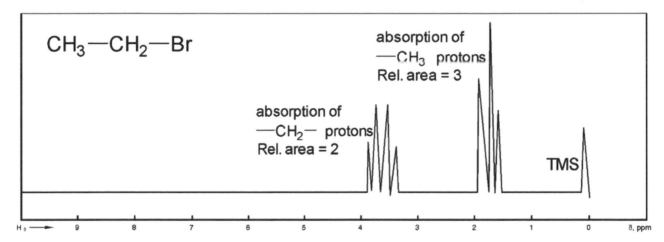

It is obvious that something is different. Looking at the molecule, one can see that there are two different types of protons (*either far from Br or near to Br*). However, there are more than two signals in the spectrum. As such, the NMR signal for each group is said to be split. This type of splitting is called spin-spin splitting (= *spin-spin coupling*) and is caused by the presence of neighboring protons (*protons on an adjacent or vicinal carbon*) that are not equivalent to the proton in question.

The number of lines in the splitting pattern for a given set of equivalent protons depends on the number of adjacent protons according to the following rule: if there are n equivalent protons in adjacent positions, a proton NMR signal is split into $n + 1$ lines.

Therefore the NMR spectrum for ethyl bromide can be interpreted thus:

- There are two groups of lines (*two split peaks*), therefore there are two different environments for protons.
- The relative areas under each peak is 2:3, which represents the relative number of hydrogens in the molecule.
- There are 4 splits (*quartet*) in the peak which has relatively two hydrogens ($-CH_2$). Thus the number of adjacent hydrogens is n + 1 = 4; therefore, there are 3 hydrogens on the carbon adjacent to $-CH_2$.
- There are 3 splits (*triplet*) in the peak which has relatively three hydrogens ($-CH_3$). Thus the number of adjacent hydrogens is $n + 1 = 3$; therefore, there are 2 hydrogens on the carbon adjacent to $-CH_3$.

The relative areas under each peak may be expressed in three ways: (i) the information may simply be provided to you (*too easy!*); (ii) the integers may be written above the signals (=*integration integers*, i.e. 2,3 in the previous example); or (iii) a step-like *integration curve* above the signals where the relative height of each step equals the relative number of hydrogens.

14.2.1 Deuterium Exchange

Deuterium, the hydrogen isotope ^2H or D, can be used to identify substances with readily exchangeable or acidic hydrogens. Rather than H_2O, D_2O is used to identify the chemical exchange:

$$ROH + DOD \rightleftharpoons ROD + HOD$$

The previous signal due to the acidic -O$\boxed{H}$ would now disappear. However, if excess D_2O is used, a signal as a result of HOD may be observed.

Solvents may also be involved in exchange phenomena. The solvents carbon tetrachloride (CCl_4) and deuteriochloroform ($CDCl_3$) can also engage in exchange-induced decoupling of acidic hydrogens (usu. in alcohols).

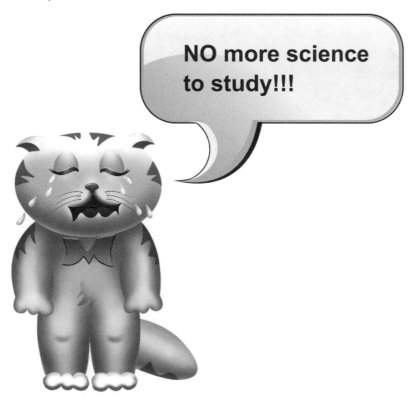

NO more science to study!!!

THE SILVER BULLET

Real MCATs Explained

MCAT*

with Verbal Reasoning Prep

- Answers and explanations to AAMC Tests 3 and 4**
- Clear, complete explanations like having a personal tutor
- Pre-study suggestions, Test-taking skills analysis
- Powerful Verbal strategies for the new computer based test
- Learn "MCAT Reasoning" from the MDs who teach MCAT teachers

Dr. James L. Flowers, M.D.
Dr. Brett Ferdinand, M.D.

2010 EDITION

Real MCAT Experts!

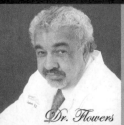

Dr. James L. Flowers, a graduate of the Harvard Medical School, wrote the first comprehensive MCAT book ever in the 1970s. He has since taught thousands of premeds personally, as well as through his books and DrFlowersMCAT.com. Dr. Brett Ferdinand, trained surgeon, wrote 16 editions of The Gold Standard MCAT, developed the first premed multimedia website at MCAT-prep.com and has also taught thousands of students from coast to coast.

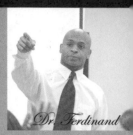

Real MCATs Explained!

If you want to ace the real MCAT*, you must practice using real past MCAT exams under real test conditions in order to assess your progress and improve. The Gold Standard provides the complete science review you need. The AAMC provides real past MCAT exams. The Silver Bullet provides detailed, cross-referenced explanations to these real past MCAT exams and much, much more!

Real MCAT Explanations!

Some books just repeat the answer. Others make assumptions about what you may know. We provide clear explanations - to both right and wrong answers - for hundreds of challenging questions. Each question is analyzed for learning opportunities including test taking skills and content. And furthermore, each question is cross-referenced to a passage, graphic or to The Gold Standard MCAT textbook for further information. We've got you covered.

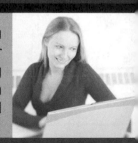

ISBN 978-0-9784638-1-6

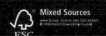

Appendix

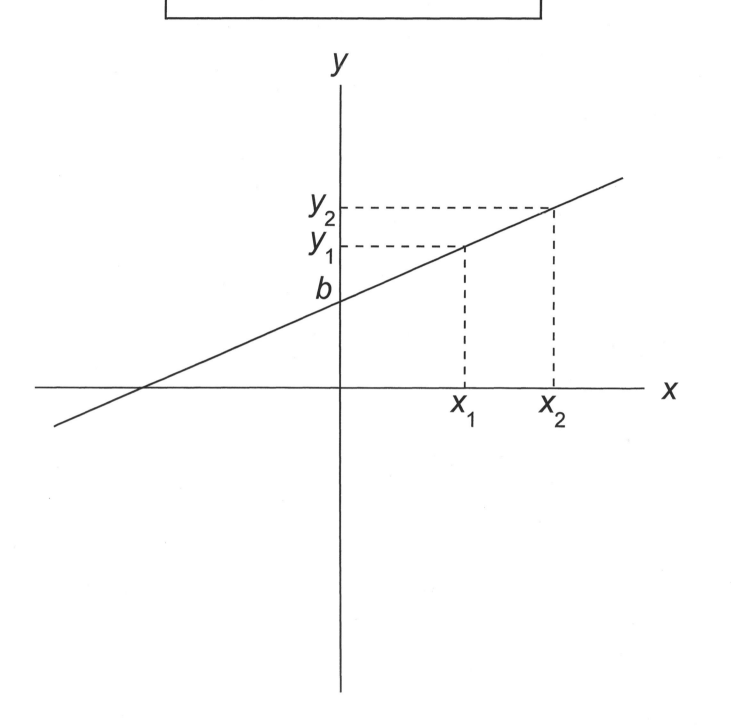

Appendix A

MCAT MATH REVIEW

In the preceding science review sections, several mathematical concepts were presented (i.e. MCAT trigonometry, vectors, rules of logarithms, the quadratic equation, the right hand rule, etc.). The purpose of this section is to review the MCAT mathematical concepts *not* presented elsewhere, though there may be some overlap for emphasis.

A.1 Probability and Statistics for the MCAT

No calculations of correlation coefficients or standard deviations is required for the MCAT. However, an understanding of these concepts is necessary.

A.1.1 The Correlation Coefficient

The correlation coefficient r indicates whether two sets of data are associated or *correlated*. The value of r ranges from -1.0 to 1.0. The larger the absolute value of r, the stronger the association. Given two sets of data X and Y, a positive value for r indicates that as X increases, Y increases. A negative value for r indicates that as X increases, Y decreases.

Imagine that the weight (X) and height (Y) of everyone in the entire country was determined. There would be a strong positive correlation between a person's weight and their height. In general, as weight increases, height increases (*in a population*). However, the correlation would not be perfect (i.e. $r \neq 1.0$). After all, there would be some people who are very tall but very thin, and others who would be very short but overweight. We might find that $r = 0.7$. This would suggest there is a strong positive association between weight and height, but it is not a perfect association.

If two sets of data are correlated, does that mean that one *causes* the other? Not necessarily; simply because weight and height are correlated does not mean that if you gained weight you will necessarily gain height! Thus association does not imply causality.

A.1.2 The Standard Deviation

When given a set of data, it is often useful to know the average value, *the mean*, and the *range* of values. The <u>mean</u> is simply the sum of the data values divided by the number of data values. The <u>range</u> is the numerical difference between the largest value and the smallest value.

Another useful measurement is the *standard deviation*. The <u>standard deviation</u> indicates the dispersion of values around the mean. Given a bell shaped distribution of data (i.e. the height and weight of a population, the GPA of undergraduate students, etc), each standard deviation (SD) includes a given percentage of data. For example, the mean $\pm$ 1 SD includes approximately 68% of the data values, the mean $\pm$ 2 SD includes 95% of the data values, and the mean $\pm$ 3 SD includes 99.7% of the data values.

For example, imagine that you read that the mean GPA required for admission to Belcurve University's Medical School is 3.5 with a standard deviation of 0.2 (SD = 0.2). Thus approximately 68% of the students admitted have a GPA of 3.5 $\pm$ 0.2, which means between 3.3 and 3.7. We can also conclude that approximately 95% of the students admitted have a GPA of 3.5 $\pm$ 2(0.2), which means between 3.1 and 3.9. Therefore the standard deviation becomes a useful measure of the dispersion of values around the mean 3.5.

A.1.3 Simple Probability

If a phenomenon or experiment has n equally likely outcomes, s of which are called successes, then the probability P of success is given by $P = s/n$. Examples: i) if "heads" in a coin toss is considered a success, then P(success) = 1/2; ii) if a card is drawn from a deck and diamonds are considered successes, then P(success) = 13/52. It follows that P(success) = 1 - P(failure).

A.1.4 Permutations

Suppose n is a positive integer. The symbol $n!$, read *n-factorial*, is defined as follows:

$$n! = (n)(n - 1)(n - 2) \ . \ . \ . \ (3)(2)(1)$$

By definition $0! = 1$.

A <u>permutation</u> of a set is an *ordered* arrangement of the elements in that set. The number of permutations of n objects is $n!$. For example, using 5 different amino acids, the number of possible permutations creating different outcomes (*oligopeptides*) is: 5! = (5)(4)(3)(2)(1) = 120.

Suppose you have 7 books and place 3 on a shelf. The first slot can be filled by any of 7 choices, the second slot can be filled by one less or 6 choices, and again there is one less choice for the third slot leaving 5 books from which to choose. The total number of ways to fill the 3 slots on the shelf is thus (7)(6)(5) = 210.

The general rule is that the number of permutations of n things taken r at a time is n_r, where $n_r = n!/(n - r)!$. In the preceding example, $n = 7$ and $r = 3$ thus,

$$n_r = 7!/(7 - 3)! = (7)(6)(5)(4!)/(4!) = (7)(6)(5) = 210.$$

A.1.5 Combinations

Permutations are important when the *order* of selection matters (e.g. *simply by changing the order of the amino acids, the activity of the oligopeptide or the* outcome *changes*). Combinations are important when the order of selection does not matter (e.g. *as long as there is a red book, a green book, and a blue book on the shelf, the order does not matter*).

Since the order does not matter, there are fewer combinations than permutations. In fact, the combination C_r is given by:

$$C_r = n_r/r! = n!/[r!(n - r)!].$$

For example, once again consider a total of 7 books where there are only 3 slots on the shelf. This time you are told that the order the books appear on the shelf is not relevant. The number of different combinations is therefore

$$C_r = n_r/r! = n!/[r!(n - r)!] = 7!/[3!(7 - 3)!] = 210/3! = 210/6 = 35.$$

A.2 Scientific Notation

Numbers with many zeroes on either side of a decimal can be written in *scientific notation*. For example, a number which is an integer power of ten, the number of zeroes equals the exponent; thus $10^0 = 1$, $10^1 = 10$, $10^2 = 10 \cdot 10 = 100$, $10^3 = 10 \cdot 10 \cdot 10 = 1000$, and so on.

Conversely, the negative exponent corresponds to the number of places to the right of the decimal point; thus $10^{-1} = 1/10 = 0.1$, $10^{-2} = 1/(10 \cdot 10) = 0.01$, $10^{-3} = 1/(10 \cdot 10 \cdot 10) = 0.001$, and so on.

Scientific notation allows us to express a number as a product of a power of ten and a number between 1 and 10. For example, the number 5,478,000 can be expressed as 5.478×10^6; 0.0000723 can be expressed as 7.23×10^{-5}.

A.3 Basic Graphs

A.3.1 The Graph of a Linear Equation

Equations of the type $y = ax + b$ are known as *linear equations* since the graph of y (= *the ordinate*) versus x (= *the abscissa*) is a straight line. The value of y where the line intersects the y axis is called the *intercept b*. The constant a is the *slope* of the line. Given any two points (x_1, y_1) and (x_2, y_2) on the line, we have:

$$y_1 = ax_1 + b$$

and

$$y_2 = ax_2 + b.$$

Subtracting the upper equation from the lower one and dividing through by $x_2 - x_1$ gives the value of the slope,

$$a = (y_2 - y_1)/(x_2 - x_1).$$

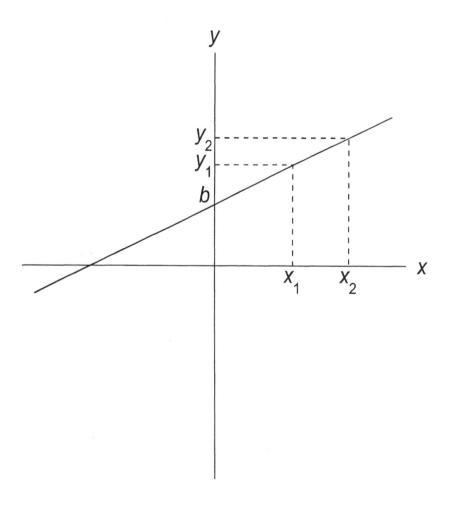

A.3.2 Reciprocal Curve

For any real number x, there exists a unique real number called the multiplicative inverse or *reciprocal* of x denoted $1/x$ or x^{-1} such that $x \, (1/x) = 1$. The graph of the reciprocal $1/x$ for any x is:

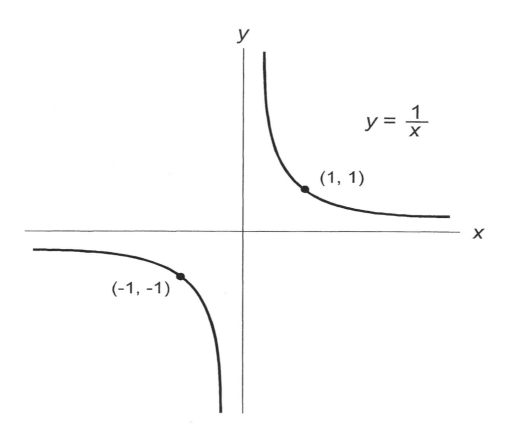

A.3.3 Miscellaneous Graphs

There are classical curves which are represented or approximated in the science text as follows: sigmoidal curve (CHM 6.9.1, BIO 7.5.1), sinusoidal curve (PHY 7.1.1 and 7.1.2), and hyperbolic curves (CHM 9.7 Fig III.A.9.3, BIO 1.1.2).

If you were to plot a set of experimental data, often one can draw a line (A.3.1) or curve (A.3.2/3, A.4.2) which can "best fit" the data. The preceding defines a *regression* line or curve. The main purpose of the regression graph is to predict what would likely occur outside of the experimental data.

A.4 Exponents and Logarithms

A.4.1 Rules of Exponents

$$a^0 = 1 \qquad\qquad\qquad a^1 = a$$
$$a^n \, a^m = a^{n+m} \qquad\qquad a^n/a^m = a^{n-m}$$
$$(a^n)^m = a^{nm} \qquad\qquad a^{1/n} = \sqrt[n]{a}$$

{See Chemistry Section 6.5.1 for rules of logarithms}

A.4.2 Exponential and Logarithmic Curves

The exponential and logarithmic functions are *inverse functions*. That is, their graphs can be reflected about the $y = x$ line.

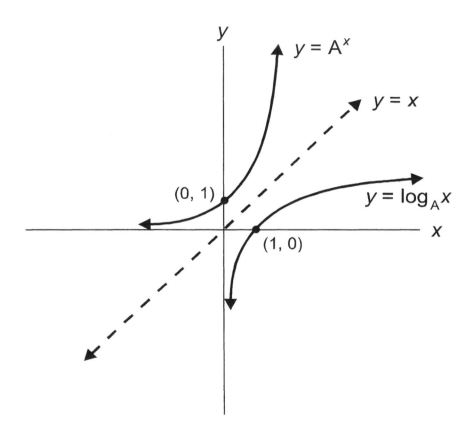

Figure A.2: Exponential and Logarithmic Graphs. $A > 0$, $A \neq 1$.

A.4.3 Logarithmic Scales

The graphs commonly seen in this text, including the preceding one, are drawn to a unit or *arithmetic scale*. In other words, each unit on the *x* and *y* axes represents exactly *one* unit. This scale can be adjusted to accomodate rapidly changing curves. For example, in a unit scale the numbers 1 (= 10^0), 10 (= 10^1), 100 (= 10^2), and 1000 (= 10^3), are all far apart with varying intervals. Using a <u>logarithmic scale</u>, the sparse values suddenly become separated by one unit: log 10^0 = 0, log 10^1 = 1, log 10^2 = 2, log 10^3 = 3, and so on.

In practice, logarithmic scales are often used to convert a rapidly changing curve (e.g. an exponential curve) to a straight line. It is called a *semi-log* scale when either the abscissa *or* the ordinate is logarithmic. It is called a *log-log* scale when both the abscissa *and* the ordinate are logarithmic.

A.5 Simplifying Algebraic Expressions

Algebraic expressions can be factored or simplified using standard formulae:

$$a(b + c) = ab + ac$$

$$(a + b)(a - b) = a^2 - b^2$$

$$(a + b)(a + b) = (a + b)^2 = a^2 + 2ab + b^2$$

$$(a - b)(a - b) = (a - b)^2 = a^2 - 2ab + b^2$$

$$(a + b)(c + d) = ac + ad + bc + bd$$

A.6 Significant Digits, Experimental Error

If we divide 2 by 3 on a calculator, the answer on the display would be 0.6666666667. The leftmost digit is the *most significant digit* and the rightmost digit is the *least significant digit*. The number of digits which are really significant depends on the accuracy with which the values 2 and 3 are known.

For example, suppose we wish to find the sum of two numbers *a* and *b* with <u>experimental errors</u> (or *uncertainties*) Δa and Δb, respectively. The uncertainty of the sum *c* can be determined as follows:

$$c \pm \Delta c = (a \pm \Delta a) + (b \pm \Delta b) = a + b \pm (\Delta a + \Delta b)$$

thus

$$\Delta c = \Delta a + \Delta b.$$

The sign of the uncertainties are not correlated, so the same rule applies to subtraction. Therefore, *the uncertainty of either the sum or difference is the sum of the uncertainties*.

Now we will apply the preceding to significant digits. The number 3.7 has an implicit uncertainty. Any number between 3.65000... and 3.74999... rounds off to 3.7, thus 3.7 really means 3.7 ± 0.05. Similarly, 68.21 really means 68.21 ± 0.005. Adding the two values and their uncertainties we get: $(3.7 \pm 0.05) + (68.21 \pm 0.005) = 71.91 \pm 0.055$. The error is large enough to affect the first digit to the right of the decimal point; therefore, the last digit to the right is not significant. The answer is thus 71.9.

The <u>rule for significant digits</u> states that *the sum or difference of two numbers carries the same number of significant digits to the right of the decimal as the number with the least significant digits to the right of the decimal.* For example, $105.64 - 3.092 = 102.55$.

Multiplication and division is somewhat different. Through algebraic manipulation, the uncertainty or experimental error can be determined:

$$c \pm \Delta c = (a \pm \Delta a)(b \pm \Delta b)$$

after some manipulation we get

$$\Delta c/c = \Delta a/a + \Delta b/b.$$

The preceding result also holds true for division. Thus for $(10 \pm 0.5)/(20 \pm 1)$, the fractional error in the quotient is:

$$\Delta c/c = \Delta a/a + \Delta b/b = 0.5/10 + 1/20 = 0.1 \ (10\% \ error)$$

Thus the quotient including its absolute error is $c \pm \Delta c = 0.5(1 \pm 0.1) = 0.5 \pm 0.05$.

The <u>rule for significant digits</u> can be derived from the preceding and it states that *the product or quotient of two numbers has the same number of significant digits as the number with the least number of significant digits (see Physics Sections 4.4.1 and 8.5.1).*

Appendix B

THE IMPERIAL AND METRIC SYSTEMS

B.1 The Basic Units

The basic units for the *British* or Imperial System are the foot (length), the slug (mass), the pound (weight, force), and the second (time). The Metric System includes the SI System (*le Systeme International*) and the CGS System (*centimeter-gram-second*). The basic units for the SI System are the meter (length), the kilogram (mass), the newton (weight, force), and the second (time). The basic units for the CGS System are the centimeter, the gram, the dyne (weight, force) and the second.

The metric system uses prefixes to indicate the power of 10. For example: *giga* = 10^9, *mega* = 10^6, *kilo* = 10^3, *hecto* = 10^2, *deka* = 10^1, *deci* = 10^{-1}, *centi* = 10^{-2}, *milli* = 10^{-3}, *micro* = 10^{-6}, *nano* = 10^{-9}. Thus one kilogram is 10^3 grams.

B.2 Conversion Factors

Length
1 m = 39.4 in = 3.23 ft
1 in = 2.54 cm
1 km = 0.62 mi
1 mi = 5280 ft = 1.609 km

Mass
1 kg = 10^3 gm = 6.9×10^{-2} slug
1 slug = 14.6 kg
1 kg = 2.2 lb (*where g* = 9.8 m/s²)

Time
1 min = 60 s
1 hour = 3600 s
1 day = 8.64×10^4 s

Volume
1 L = 1000 cm³ (or *cc, ml*) = 3.5×10^{-2} ft³
1 dm³ = 1 L
1 gallon = 3.8 L = 230 in³

Force
1 N = 0.23 lb = 10^5 dynes
1 lb = 4.45 N
1 dyne = 10^{-5} N = 2.25×10^{-6} lb

Work and Energy
1 J = 10^7 erg = 0.74 ft· lb = 0.24 cal
1 cal = 4.18 J
1 ft· lb = 1.36 J
1 Btu = 1.054×10^3 J = 252 cal
1 J = 6.24×10^{18} eV
1 eV = 1.60×10^{-19} J
1kW· h = 3.60×10^6 J

Pressure
1 atm = 1.013×10^5 N/m² (or Pa)
     = 14.7 lb/in² (or psi)
     = 1.013 bar
1 Pa = 1 N/m² = 1.45×10^{-4} lb/in²

Note: *many conversion factors involve approximations.*

Appendix C

THE EXPERIMENT

C.1 Introduction

There is no one page in this book that will affect your MCAT score more than this one! Unless, of course, you have been involved in research in which case your time would be best spent reading anything else...

Many MCAT questions, particularly in the Biological Sciences section, will present experiments which you have never heard of and which you are not responsible for knowing. The point of the experiment is to test your ability to read scientific material, understand what is being tested, and determine if the hypothesis has been proved, refuted or neither. When a hypothesis survives rigorous testing, it graduates to a *theory*.

Observation, formulation of a theory, and testing of a theory by additional observation is called the <u>scientific method</u>. In biology, a key aspect to evaluate the validity of a trial or experiment is the presence of a *control group*. Generally, treatment is withheld from the control group but given to the *experimental group*.

First we will make an observation and then use deductive reasoning to create an appropriate hypothesis which will result in an experimental design. Consider the following: trees grow well in the sunlight. Hypothesis: exposure to light is directly related to tree growth. Experiment: two groups of trees are grown in <u>similar</u> conditions except one group (*experimental*) is exposed to light while the other group (*control*) is not exposed to light. Growth is carefully measured and the two groups are compared. Note that tree growth (*dependent variable*) is <u>dependent</u> on light (*independent variable*).

There are experiments where it is important to expose the control group to some factor different from the factor given to the experimental group (= *positive control*; as opposed to not giving the control group any exposure at all = *negative control*). Exposure for a control group is used in medicine because of the "Placebo Effect."

Experiments have shown that giving a person a pill that contains no biologically active material will cure many illnesses in up to 30% of individuals. Thus if Drug X is developed using a traditional control group, and the "efficacy" is estimated at 32%, it may be that the drug is no more effective than a sugar pill! In this case, the control group must be exposed to an unmedicated preparation to negate the Placebo Effect. To be believable the experiment must be well-grounded in evidence (= *valid,* based on the scientific method) and then one must be able to reproduce the results.

C.2 The Experiment

A lab in Houston reports 15% cell death when maximally stimulating the APO-1 receptor. In order to appropriately interpret the results, it must first be compared to:

A. data from other labs.
B. the attrition rate of other cell types.
C. the actual number of APO-1 cells dying in the tissue culture.
D. the rate of cell death without stimulation of APO-1.

- The experiment: stimulating a specific receptor on cells led to a 15% rate of cell death.

- Treatment is the stimulation of a receptor.

- The control (*group without treatment*): under the same conditions, do not stimulate the receptor (choice **D.**).

Choice **C.** does not answer the question. Choices **A.** and **B.** are most relevant if the initial data is shown to be significant. To prove that the data is significant or valid, one must first compare to a control group (choice **D.**).

Appendix D

STUDY AIDS FOR THE MCAT

Many students use The Gold Standard and the AAMC materials as the cornerstone to their MCAT and premed preparation. Some students seek some additional help in order to supplement what they get from these sources. This appendix is for those students.

D.1   The Silver Bullet: Real MCATs Explained

AAMC Exams are available from the AAMC. Test III is currently free. Here comes a detailed analysis in 640 pages for 2 full length real past MCATs. We've gone through these past exams, and provided the answers as well as clear, complete explanations on how they were solved. This study guide also includes equation lists to memorize for the exam, eight pages of new 3D color diagrams, and an organic chemistry summary. In addition, verbal reasoning is analyzed along with detailed verbal reasoning strategies. On top of all this, everything is cross-referenced to The Gold Standard. For more details concerning The Silver Bullet, please refer to the MCAT Store: www.mcat-bookstore.com.

D.2   The Gold Standard Video MCAT Science Review DVDs

We've produced 20 hours of video content covering the science subjects required for the MCAT. Across 16 DVDs, all the important Physics, Biology, General and Organic Chemistry topics are covered in the necessary detail. The material is covered using clear, lecture-style teaching methods. The videos contain explanations and cross-references to the current edition of The Gold Standard, where applicable. The videos are available in several different formats, either all together as a set of 16 DVDs or by individual sets of 4 DVDs on the separate subjects of Physics, Biology, General and Organic Chemistry. Some topics covered by the DVDs are also available and streamed online. For more information about the DVDs and what's available online, please refer to the MCAT Store: www.mcat-bookstore.com.

D.3   The Gold Standard MCAT CBT Flashcards (Science Review)

Another trick for studying is using flashcards. We've condensed over 200 of the most frequently tested concepts on the MCAT into 54 high quality poker sized cards in color. You can use them as flashcards or to play games with your MCAT buddies! For more information about them, go to MCAT-bookstore.com.

D.4   The Gold Standard MCAT CBT Practice Tests

The MCAT is a Computer Based Test (CBT, not on paper). The only way to properly practice taking the test is by taking it on computer, just like you will be taking the real MCAT. The Gold Standard (published by MCAT-prep.com) has an incredible 10 full length NEW 2012-2013 format MCAT CBTs. These tests are interactive, timed, and instantly corrected. After taking these exams, you can review the answers in detail, get suggestions for further study and even reference online videos. You can even participate in our online forums discussing each question. You can find these practice tests online at MCAT-prep.com.

D.5   The Silver Bullet High Yield Audio

Using The Gold Standard as a reference, we compiled 4 hours of audio notes into a single CD. We go over the major points of what you should know for the MCAT exam. Repetition of this material over and over, just by listening to it, should make your studying more efficient. Listen on your iPod, mp3 player or car stereo on the way to school, etc. Please make sure that your CD player is capable of playing an mp3 CD. For more details, you can go to MCAT-bookstore.com.

D.6   MCAT Camp

Every year, Dr. Ferdinand gives MCAT courses in different cities, each running for a week. Over the week, students go through an intensive MCAT prep course, taught by the MCAT Master himself: Dr. Brett Ferdinand (who just happened to write the book that you have in your hands now). Dr. Ferdinand developed methods for studying for the MCAT when he took it as a student, and ended up acing the test. He turned this method into an intensive course that many students have successfully used over the years to become MCAT Masters themselves. The plan for 2012-2013 is to have these camps in both Montreal and Las Vegas. To get further information on these MCAT Camps, and to see where future ones will occur, just check for details at MCAT-bookstore.com.

D.7 Online Resources

MCAT-Prep.com & *MCAT-bookstore.com* – great resources for premed students, as well as our online store of MCAT products.

MCAT-Prep.com/forum – become a member and participate as part of our online community; discuss everything from MCAT questions to what you should wear to the exam!

MCATscoring.com – determine your chances of getting into medical school.

MCATchanges.com – Keep up to date with the changes in the MCAT effective 2015.

FutureDoctor.net - a treasure-trove of information for students planning a career in medicine. Everything from study tips to when to take your MCAT exam.

StudentDoctor.net – the Student Doctor Network is a non-profit educational organization for pre-health and health professional students in the US and Canada. Visit us in their forums at our *Gold Standard MCAT Headquarters*.

AAMC.org – The website for the people that actually run the MCAT, the Association of American Medical Colleges.

Gold Standard
MCAT* Exams

THE GOLD STANDARD MCAT

Introduction

Prior to doing these exams, section 2.3 from Part II - The *new* MCAT - should be reviewed.

The following exams are designed to challenge you and to reach you at a whole new level. You will need to take the tools you have learned and build new structures and create new paths to solving problems. The problems will range from very simple to very challenging, but they will all be very helpful for your MCAT preparation. Do not be afraid of making mistakes - it is part of the learning process. The student who makes the most mistakes has the greatest learning potential!

Timing is critical. Many students do not complete various sections of the exams. If you decide to do a few problems from time to time then you have never practiced for the MCAT. A full day exam is a rigorous event. It requires practice that simulates exam conditions. An important aspect of the latter is timing. Practice according to the prescribed exam schedule.

Upon finishing the exam, the next challenge is the equally important thorough review. Mistakes, and even correct answers for which some doubt existed, should be examined without time restrictions for maximum learning benefit.

Preparing the Tests

To write these super-length paper MCATs, you will need a pen with black ink for the Writing Sample. Books, notes, slide rulers, electronic devices or aids including calculators are forbidden. Calculations or notations are made in the test booklet.

For each MCAT there are four test booklets and two answer documents. To create your test booklets tear your sheets out gently and systematically. Place the front of the book flat on a table and open to the pages just after the three exams where you will find Answer Document 1 and Answer Document 2 for the exam you wish to write. Tear along the perforation.

The page numbers reflect the exam to which the page belongs. For example, GS 2-8 is the 8th page of the 2nd Gold Standard (GS2) MCAT. Skim to the last page of the exam you would like to write. Begin pulling out pages while paying close attention to the page numbers. Once a complete exam is removed, you will require a stapler. Each of the four test sections has a cover page with a light gray line extending down the left margin. Staple on the line 5 times: the topmost and bottommost parts of the line, once in between the two, and finally, staple once between the top and the middle staple, and again between the middle and the bottom staple. You should now have four test booklets.

Now you can use Answer Document 1 for multiple choice questions. Answer Document 2 will be used for the Writing Sample. Answer Document 2 should be stapled together forming a booklet similar to the other exam booklets.

Exam Schedule

The test day schedule pre-2007 was such you expect to arrive at the designated exam center by 8 am, local time. Usually logistics were settled and students were writing the exam by 9 am. About 8 hours later, the exam would have ended. Here is your exam day schedule:

Table 1: MCAT schedule

Section	Number of Questions	Time in Minutes
Physical Sciences	77	100
(BREAK)	-	(10)
Verbal Reasoning	60	85
(LUNCH BREAK)	-	(60)
Writing Sample	2	60
(BREAK)	-	(10)
Biological Sciences	77	100

Answer Key Information

The answer keys to the exams are fully cross-referenced. In other words, if you make a mistake, the answer key will direct you either to a specific area in a passage or to a specific section in the science review of this manual. Alternatively, a key word, concept or equation might be written. If a problem strictly relies on reasoning skills, "deduce" may be written in the answer key without a cross-reference, or, with a cross-reference but only for background information. The hope is that you will find these new answer keys informative and helpful. Please feel free to get in touch with Dr. Ferdinand with your comments about any part of The Gold Standard by clicking on Forum at www.MCAT-prep.com.

Table 2: Identification of abbreviations and symbols for GS MCAT Answer Keys. Note: answers marked "deduce" may be explained in greater detail in the "Understanding" sections at the back of The Gold Standard.

Ap	Appendix	PT	Periodic Table
B	Background Information	Q	Question
C	Concept	R	Reaction
cf.	Compare	T	Table
D.A.	Dimensional Analysis (*see* Part II, 2.3, #16)	X.	Answer Choice X
		X. = ba	emphasizes Choice X as being the *best* answer
E	Equation		
EN	Electronegativity	X.:T/F	Choice X is true but does not answer Q
endo	Endothermic		
ESR	Electron Shell Repulsion	X. ↔ ...	Choice X is wrong because...
exo	Exothermic		
F	Figure	Δ	Change, difference in
G	Graph	↑	Increase, higher
info	Information	↓	Decrease, lower
KS	Key Step	→	Proceeds to... , next step...
KW	Key Word	∴	Therefore
L	Line(s) where info can be found	*	Important!
		10.5-7	Section 10.5 to 10.7
P	Paragraph where info can be found	10.5/7	Section 10.5 and 10.7
PoE	Process of Elimination		

Conversion Tables

The following represent conversion tables for The Gold Standard MCAT exams. You will soon notice the power of the bell curve! For example, 15 mistakes in Verbal Reasoning results in a scaled score of barely 8/15, whereas the same number of mistakes in Physical Sciences results in a scaled score of 12/15. Your performance is important. Your performance compared to other students is *more* important.

Your raw score is simply the number of correct answers in a given section. Using the table you can estimate your scaled score and percentile rank. The power of these estimates is in monitoring your progress which includes understanding, memorization, speed, etc.

Table 3: Approximate conversions of percentile ranks to scaled scores for the GS MCAT exams.

Verbal Reasoning			Physical Sciences			Biological Sciences		
Scaled Score	Percentile Rank Range	Raw Score	Scaled Score	Percentile Rank Range	Raw Score	Scaled Score	Percentile Rank Range	Raw Score
> 12	> 97	58-60	> 12	> 97	70-77	> 12	> 99	73-77
12	95-97	56-57	12	95-97	62-69	12	96-99	67-72
11	88-94	53-55	11	89-94	58-61	11	90-95	64-66
10	76-87	51-52	10	79-88	55-57	10	77-89	61-63
9	60-75	48-50	9	68-78	50-54	9	62-76	54-60
8	45-59	45-47	8	51-67	44-49	8	43-61	47-53
7	33-44	42-44	7	33-50	41-43	7	31-42	41-46
6	19-32	37-41	6	17-32	35-40	6	19-30	36-40
5	12-18	28-36	5	7-16	29-34	5	10-18	31-35
< 5	< 11	0-27	< 5	< 7	0-28	< 5	< 10	0-30

TEST GS-1

Physical Sciences
Questions 1-77
Time : 100 Minutes

OPEN BOOKLET ONLY WHEN TIMER IS READY.

The Gold Standard MCAT* has been designed exclusively to test knowledge and thinking skills. The exam may contain hypothetical statements and/or express controversial ideas. Statements contained herein do not necessarily reflect the policy, position, or view of RuveneCo Publishing.

* MCAT is a registered service mark of the Association of American Medical Colleges, which is not associated with this product.

PHYSICAL SCIENCES

INSTRUCTIONS: Of the 77 questions in the Physical Sciences test, 62 are organized into groups preceded by a passage. After evaluating the passage, select the best answer to each question in the group. Fifteen questions are independent of any descriptive passage or each other. Similarly, select the best answer to these questions. If you are unsure of an answer, eliminate the alternatives that you know to be incorrect and select an answer from the remaining alternatives. To indicate your selection, blacken the corresponding oval on Answer Document 1, GS-1. A periodic table is provided for your use during the test.

PERIODIC TABLE OF THE ELEMENTS

1 H 1.008																	2 He 4.003
3 Li 6.941	4 Be 9.012											5 B 10.81	6 C 12.011	7 N 14.007	8 O 15.999	9 F 18.998	10 Ne 20.179
11 Na 22.990	12 Mg 24.305											13 Al 26.982	14 Si 28.086	15 P 30.974	16 S 32.06	17 Cl 35.453	18 Ar 39.948
19 K 39.098	20 Ca 40.08	21 Sc 44.956	22 Ti 47.90	23 V 50.942	24 Cr 51.996	25 Mn 54.938	26 Fe 55.847	27 Co 58.933	28 Ni 58.70	29 Cu 63.546	30 Zn 65.38	31 Ga 69.72	32 Ge 72.59	33 As 74.922	34 Se 78.96	35 Br 79.904	36 Kr 83.80
37 Rb 85.468	38 Sr 87.62	39 Y 88.906	40 Zr 91.22	41 Nb 92.906	42 Mo 95.94	43 Tc (98)	44 Ru 101.07	45 Rh 102.906	46 Pd 106.4	47 Ag 107.868	48 Cd 112.41	49 In 114.82	50 Sn 118.69	51 Sb 121.75	52 Te 127.60	53 I 126.905	54 Xe 131.30
55 Cs 132.905	56 Ba 137.33	57 *La 138.906	72 Hf 178.49	73 Ta 180.948	74 W 183.85	75 Re 186.207	76 Os 190.2	77 Ir 192.22	78 Pt 195.09	79 Au 196.967	80 Hg 200.59	81 Tl 204.37	82 Pb 207.2	83 Bi 208.980	84 Po (209)	85 At (210)	86 Rn (222)
87 Fr (223)	88 Ra 226.025	89 **Ac 227.028	104 Unq (261)	105 Unp (262)	106 Unh (263)												

*	58 Ce 140.12	59 Pr 140.908	60 Nd 144.24	61 Pm (145)	62 Sm 150.4	63 Eu 151.96	64 Gd 157.25	65 Tb 158.925	66 Dy 162.50	67 Ho 164.930	68 Er 167.26	69 Tm 168.934	70 Yb 173.04	71 Lu 174.967
**	90 Th 232.038	91 Pa 231.036	92 U 238.029	93 Np 237.048	94 Pu (244)	95 Am (243)	96 Cm (247)	97 Bk (247)	98 Cf (251)	99 Es (254)	100 Fm (257)	101 Md (258)	102 No (259)	103 Lr (260)

Passage I (Questions 1-6)

The four forces that act on a plane are lift, weight, drag or air resistance, and thrust, the last of which is produced by the plane's engine.

Impact pressure produces 30% of the lift. It results from the fact that wings are given a *dihedral* angle where the distance from the tip of the wing to the ground is greater than that from the root of the wing to the ground.

The other 70% of lift can be accounted for by the Bernoulli effect. A cross-section of an airplane's wing reveals greater surface area above the wing compared to a flatter, lower surface. Thus air, moving in streamline flow, must move more rapidly over the top of the wing.

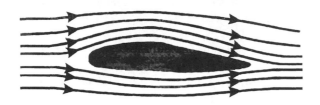

Bernoulli's equation, $P + 1/2\rho v^2 + \rho gh$ = constant, is often modified when discussing an airplane's wing. The "ρgh" component is usually left out since the difference in distance from the top of the wing to the ground compared to the bottom of the wing to the ground is usually negligible.

1. Newton's Third Law states that for every action there must be an equal and opposite reaction. This is applicable to lift and the dihedral angle because:
   A. the fast moving air above the wing increases the pressure.
   B. drag must be as low as possible to improve forward motion.
   C. there is a large pressure difference between the wings.
   D. the wing deflects the air downward and the air in turn deflects the wing upward.

2. Compared to the wing's upper surface, the air moving along the undersurface has:
   A. greater velocity, greater pressure.
   B. greater velocity, lower pressure.
   C. lower velocity, greater pressure.
   D. lower velocity, lower pressure.

3. A plane flies from low to high altitude at constant velocity. Which of the following is true?
   A. At the lower altitude the plane will experience greater lift.
   B. At the higher altitude the plane will experience greater lift.
   C. The lift the plane experiences is not dependent on altitude.
   D. At low altitudes Bernoulli's effect is not applicable.

4. An airplane is encircling an airport with DECREASING speed. When the airplane reaches point P, what is the general direction of its acceleration?

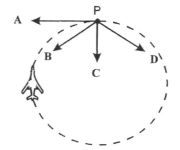

5. The following represents an incompressible fluid in laminar flow through pipes. Where is the pressure highest?

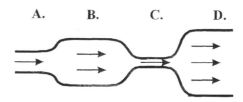

6. Concerning the preceding diagram, what can be determined regarding the flow?
   A. It is highest at C.
   B. It is highest at D.
   C. It cannot be determined.
   D. It is constant throughout.

Passage II (Questions 7-14)

The essential stages in the manufacture of H_2SO_4 and H_2SO_3 involve the burning of sulfur or roasting of sulfide ores in air to produce SO_2. This is then mixed with air, purified and passed over a vanadium catalyst (either VO_3^- or V_2O_5) at 450 degrees Celsius. Thus the following reaction occurs.

$$2SO_2(g) + O_2(g) \rightleftharpoons 2SO_3 \ (g) \quad \Delta H = \text{-197 kJ mol}^{-1}$$

Reaction I

If the SO_2 is very carefully dissolved in water, sulfurous acid (H_2SO_3) is obtained. The first proton of this acid ionizes as if from a strong acid while the second ionizes as if from a weak acid.

$$H_2SO_3 + H_2O \rightarrow H_3O^+ + HSO_3^-$$

Reaction II

$$HSO_3^- + H_2O \rightleftharpoons H_3O^+ + SO_3^{2-} \quad K_a = 5.0 \times 10^{-6}$$

Reaction III

The concentration of H_2SO_3 in cleaning fluid was determined by titration with 0.10 M NaOH (strong base) as shown in Fig.1. Two equivalence points were determined using 30 ml and 60 ml of NaOH respectively:

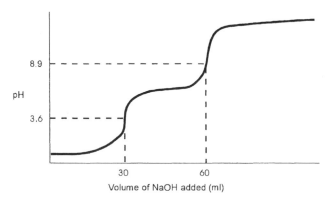

Figure 1

7. What is the oxidation number of sulfur in sulfurous acid?
   A. +3
   B. +4
   C. +5
   D. +6

8. What is the percent by mass of oxygen in sulfurous acid?
   A. 31.9%
   B. 19.7%
   C. 39.0%
   D. 58.5%

9. Which of the following acid-base indicators is most suitable for the determination of the first end point of the titration shown in Figure 1?
   A. Cresol red (color change between pH = 0.2 and pH = 1.8)
   B. p-Xylenol blue (color change between pH = 1.2 and pH = 2.8)
   C. Bromophenol blue (color change between pH = 3.0 and pH = 4.6)
   D. Bromocresol green (color change between pH = 3.8 and pH = 5.4)

10. H_2SO_3 acts as a Lewis acid probably because sulfurous acid:
    A. is a proton donor.
    B. accepts a pair of electrons from another species.
    C. reacts with NaOH which is a strong base.
    D. possesses oxygen atoms.

11. If no catalyst was used in Reaction I, which of the following would experience a change in its partial pressure when the same system reaches equilibrium?
    A. There will be no change in the partial pressure of any of the reactants
    B. $SO_3 \ (g)$
    C. $SO_2 \ (g)$
    D. $O_2 \ (g)$

12. If the temperature was decreased in Reaction I, which of the following would experience an increase in its partial pressure when the same system reaches equilibrium?
A. There will be no change in the partial pressure of any of the reactants
B. SO_3 (g)
C. SO_2 (g)
D. O_2 (g) and SO_2 (g)

13. Reaction I is usually carried out at atmospheric pressure. During the reaction, before equilibrium was reached, the mole fractions of SO_2 (g) and SO_3 (g) were ½ and 1/6 respectively. What was the partial pressure of O_2 (g)?
A. 0.66 atm
B. 0.16 atm
C. 0.50 atm
D. 0.33 atm

14. What is the pH of 0.01 M H_2SO_3?
A. 1.0
B. 2.0
C. 3.0
D. 4.0

Passage III (Questions 15-20)

The phenomenon of refraction has long intrigued scientists and was actually used to corroborate one of the major mysteries of early science: the determination of the speed of light.

The refractive index of a transparent material is related to a number of the physical properties of light. In terms of velocity, the refractive index represents the ratio of the velocity of light in a vacuum to its velocity in the material. From this ratio, it can be seen that light is retarded when it passes through most types of matter. It is worth noting that prisms break up white light into the seven "colors of the rainbow" because each color has a slightly different velocity in the medium.

Snell's law allows one to follow the behavior of light in terms of its path when moving from a material of one refractive index to another with the same, or different refractive index. It is given by: $n_1\sin\theta_1 = n_2\sin\theta_2$, where "1" refers to the first medium through which the ray passes, "2" refers to the second medium, and the angles refer to the angle of incidence in the first medium (θ_1) and the angle of refraction in the second (θ_2).

A ship went out on a search for a sunken treasure chest. In order to locate the chest, they shone a beam of light down into the water using a high intensity white light source as shown in Fig.1. The refractive index for sea water is 1.33 while that for air is 1.00.

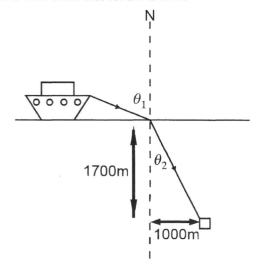

Figure 1

15. From the information in the passage, how would you expect the speed of light in air to compare with the speed of light in a vacuum (which is given by "c")?
   A. It would be the same (=c).
   B. It would be greater than c.
   C. It would be less than c.
   D. This cannot be determined from the information given.

16. Using the information in the passage, what must the approximate value of θ_2 be such that it hits the chest as shown in Figure 1?
   A. 15.2°
   B. 30.4°
   C. 45.6°
   D. 63.4°

17. How does the refractive index in water for violet light compare with that of red light given that violet light travels more slowly in water than red light?
   A. $n_{violet} = n_{red}$
   B. $n_{violet} < n_{red}$
   C. $n_{violet} > n_{red}$
   D. This depends on the relative speeds of the different colors in a vacuum.

18. Total internal reflection first occurs when a beam of light travels from one medium to another medium which has a smaller refractive index at such an angle of incidence that the angle of refraction is 90°. This angle of incidence is called the critical angle. What is the value of the sine of this angle when the ray moves from water towards air?
   A. 2π
   B. 0.75
   C. 0.50
   D. 0

19. What would happen to the critical angle, in the previous question, if the beam of light was travelling from water to a substance with a greater refractive index than air, but a lower refractive index than water?
   A. It would increase.
   B. It would decrease.
   C. It would remain the same.
   D. Total internal reflection would not be possible.

20. Which of the following would you expect to remain constant when light travels from one medium to another and the media differ in their refractive indices?
A. velocity
B. frequency
C. wavelength
D. intensity

The enthalpy of solution (ΔH_{soln}) of a salt depends on two other quantities: the energy released when free gaseous ions of the salt combine to give the solid salt (lattice energy: ΔH_{latt}) and the energy released when free gaseous ions of the salt dissolve in water via solute-solvent interactions to yield the solvated ions (enthalpy of hydration: ΔH_{solv}) where:

$$\Delta H_{soln} = \Delta H_{solv} - \Delta H_{latt} \quad \textbf{Equation I}$$

From the formal definition of the quantities, it can be seen that both ΔH_{latt} and ΔH_{solv} are exothermic. Although these values seem to be in competition, the factors that affect ΔH_{latt} and ΔH_{solv} do so in the same way. Firstly, the smaller the ion, the closer the association of the ion with either other ions in the crystal lattice, or, with water molecules and thus the more negative ΔH_{latt} and ΔH_{solv} become. Also, the greater the charge on the ion, the greater the increase in electrostatic forces of attraction between itself and other ions or water molecules, and the more negative ΔH_{latt} and ΔH_{solv} become.

Although ΔH_{latt} and ΔH_{solv} undergo similar changes, the change in ΔH_{solv} up or down a group is much more profound than that of ΔH_{latt}. A good example of this is seen in the solubility changes of the Group II carbonates.

However, there is one exception to these general rules. If the cation of the salt is approximately the same size as the anion, the arrangement of ions in the crystal lattice is more uniform and hence the lattice is more stable and ΔH_{latt} is more negative.

Table 1

Group II Carbonate	Solubility (mol L^{-1} H_2O)
$MgCO_3$	1.30×10^{-3}
$CaCO_3$	0.13×10^{-3}
$SrCO_3$	0.07×10^{-3}
$BaCO_3$	0.09×10^{-3}

21. The solubility product for $MgCO_3$ is:
    A. 1.3×10^{-4}
    B. 2.6×10^{-4}
    C. 1.7×10^{-6}
    D. 6.7×10^{-8}

22. $Ca(OH)_2$ has approximately the same K_{sp} as $CaSO_4$. Which of them has the greater solubility in terms of mol L^{-1}?
    A. They both have the same solubility.
    B. $Ca(OH)_2$
    C. $CaSO_4$
    D. It depends on the temperature at the time.

23. The CO_3^{2-} anion is approximately the same size as
    A. Mg^{2+}.
    B. Ca^{2+}.
    C. Sr^{2+}.
    D. Ba^{2+}.

24. The ΔH_{solv} for a doubly charged anion X^{2-} was found to be more negative than that for the carbonate anion. Which of the following is the most likely explanation?
    A. X^{2-} is the same size as the carbonate anion.
    B. X^{2-} is larger than the carbonate anion.
    C. X^{2-} is smaller than the carbonate anion.
    D. It depends on the H_{latt} for the salt containing the anion.

25. A solution of $SrCO_3$ in water boils at a higher temperature than pure water. Why is this?
    A. $SrCO_3$ increases the density of water.
    B. $SrCO_3$ decreases the vapor pressure of the water.
    C. $SrCO_3$ has a low solubility in water.
    D. $SrCO_3$ decreases the surface tension of the water.

26. The following system includes a frictionless pulley and a cord of negligible mass. Since the system is at rest, what can be said about the force of friction between the platform and the large weight?

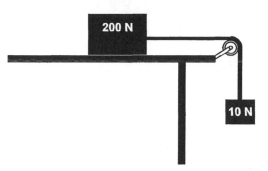

A. It is 200 N.
B. It is 10 N.
C. It is 190 N.
D. In this case, the force of friction is not necessarily present.

27. Which of the following describes the orbital geometry of an sp^2 hybridized atom?
A. Trigonal planar
B. Linear
C. Tetrahedral
D. Octahedral

28. Two charged particles are a distance x apart. If the charges on the two particles remains the same while the distance between them is doubled, how does the force between the particles change?
A. It stays the same
B. It decreases by a factor of 4
C. It decreases by a factor of 2
D. It decreases by a factor of $\sqrt{2}$

29. The intensity level of sound X is 1000 times that of sound Y. What is the difference in the intensity levels of X and Y in terms of decibels?
A. 1000
B. 3
C. 100
D. 30

30. A mass of 100 kg is placed on a uniform bar at a point 0.5 m to the left of a fulcrum. Where must a 75 kg mass be placed relative to the fulcrum in order to establish a state of equilibrium given that the bar was in equilibrium before any weights were applied?
A. 0.66 m to the right of the fulcrum
B. 0.66 m to the left of the fulcrum
C. 0.38 m to the right of the fulcrum
D. 0.38 m to the left of the fulcrum

Passage V (Questions 31-35)

A 1200 kg car is travelling at 7.5 m s⁻¹ in a northerly direction on an icy road. It crashes into a 8000 kg truck moving in the same direction as the car with a velocity of 3.0 m s⁻¹ before the collision. The speed of the car after the collision is 3.0 m s⁻¹ in its original direction.

31. Which of the following is true regarding the relationship between energy and momentum in the passage?
     A. The collision is not perfectly elastic, both momentum and energy are not conserved.
     B. The collision is inelastic, kinetic energy is conserved but momentum is not.
     C. The collision is not perfectly elastic, momentum is conserved but total energy is not.
     D. The collision is not perfectly elastic, momentum is conserved but kinetic energy is not.

32. What is the velocity of the truck after the collision?
     A. 7.5 m s⁻¹
     B. 3.7 m s⁻¹
     C. 3.0 m s⁻¹
     D. 1.1 m s⁻¹

33. The car then proceeds to a garage. To get there, the driver turns off onto a smooth road with a coefficient of friction = ⅓. He then stops for a snack and then tries to drive off. What is the value of frictional force when the force the car exerts is 300 N?
     A. 0 N
     B. 100 N
     C. 300 N
     D. 4000 N

34. After leaving the garage, the driver of the car follows the same road and eventually has to go up a hill. How does the frictional force on the car now compare to the value when the car was driving on level ground?
     A. No change
     B. It increased.
     C. It decreased.
     D. The direction of change depends on the angle of elevation.

35. If the car is moving up the hill at 5 m s⁻¹ and the car is 40 m up the hill as shown in the diagram, how much potential energy does the car possess at that point?

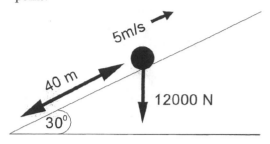

$$g = 9.8 \text{ m s}^{-2}$$

A. 2.40×10^5 J
B. 2.40×10^4 J
C. 4.95×10^5 J
D. 4.95×10^4 J

Passage VI (Questions 36-41)

It is well known that there are two major forms of carbon, that is, carbon has two main allotropes: graphite and diamond. These differ greatly from each other with respect to their physical properties as shown in Table 1. The physical properties of silicon are also shown in Table 1 for comparison as carbon and silicon belong to the same group in the periodic table.

Table 1

Physical properties	Graphite	Diamond	Silicon
Density (g cm^{-3})	2.26	3.51	2.33
Enthalpy of combustion to yield oxide (ΔHc) kJ mol^{-1}	-393.3	-395.1	-910
Melting point (°C)	2820	3730	1410
Boiling point (°C)		4830	2680
Conductivity (electrical)	Fairly good	Non-conductor	Good

Graphite possesses what is commonly known as a layer structure: carbon atoms form three covalent bonds with each other to yield layers of carbon assemblies parallel with each other. These layers are held together via weak Van der Waals' forces which permit some movement of the layers relative to one another.

The most common compound of carbon is carbon dioxide which makes up 0.03% of the atmosphere. The triple point of carbon dioxide occurs at 217 K and 515 kPa.

One of the unique properties of carbon is that it can form multiple bonds between itself and other atoms, including other carbon atoms. Thus, large polymers involving carbon atoms are possible.

36. Which of the following is a correct representation of the phase diagram for carbon dioxide?

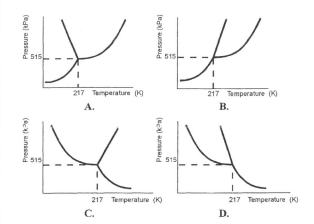

37. The properties of the layer-like structure of solid graphite stated in the passage would lend it to which of the following industrial uses?
   A. Insulator
   B. Structural
   C. Corrosive
   D. Lubricant

38. Using the information in the table, calculate the enthalpy change for the following process:

$$C_{graphite} \rightarrow C_{diamond}$$

   A. +1.8 kJ mol^{-1}
   B. -1.8 kJ mol^{-1}
   C. +1.0 kJ mol^{-1}
   D. -1.0 kJ mol^{-1}

39. It is possible to convert graphite into diamond via various chemical processes. Based on the information in the passage, which of the following would facilitate increased amounts of diamond assuming that the system is in equilibrium?
   A. High pressures
   B. High temperatures
   C. A catalyst
   D. None of the above

40. Diamond consists of tetrahedral arrangements of carbon atoms, with each atom covalently bound to four others to yield a giant molecular structure. What is the hybridization state of carbon in diamond?
A. It is not hybridized
B. sp
C. sp^2
D. sp^3

41. Carbon is in Group IV of the periodic table, along with such elements as silicon. However, compared with silicon, carbon forms more stable covalent bonds with itself. Why is a C-C bond stronger than a Si-Si bond?
A. Because carbon is not as good an electrical conductor.
B. Because carbon has a smaller atomic number.
C. Because carbon has a smaller atomic radius.
D. Because carbon has a smaller relative atomic mass.

Passage VII (Questions 42-46)

Most of the energy of the sun which reaches this planet is "wasted," that is, not harnessed by any system, natural or artificial. It has been theorized that if just 10% of the sun's radiant energy incident on the planet Earth could be perfectly harnessed, there would be enough energy to sustain all life on the planet.

The solar collector represents the first step in man's attempt to harness solar energy. It is a relatively simple apparatus, consisting of mainly a glass covered collector which contains a system of copper pipes coated with black paint and connected to a power supply. The entire inside of the collector is coated with the same black paint as the copper pipes.

The sun radiates energy at a rate of about 3.9×10^{26} W and the solar energy incident on our planet is received at a rate of approximately 1600 W m^{-2}. A solar collector measuring 20 m by 20 m is exposed to the sun. Approximately 4 L of water is passed through the solar collector per second. The specific heat capacity of water is 4.2 J g^{-1} °C^{-1} and the combined heat capacity of the collector walls and copper pipes is negligible.

42. The black paint prevents heat loss via which of the following processes?
   A. Conduction of radiant energy
   B. Convection of radiant energy
   C. Absorption of radiant energy
   D. All of the above

43. It was found that 1 L of water from the supplying pipes to the collector weighed more than 1 L of water from the draining pipes from the collector when an accurate weighing apparatus was used. Why is this?
   A. The density of the water in the supplying pipes is less than that of the water in the draining pipes.
   B. The density of the water in the supplying pipes is greater than that of the water in the draining pipes.
   C. The pressure of the water in the supplying pipes is less than that of the water in the draining pipes.
   D. The pressure of the water in the supplying pipes is greater than that of the water in the draining pipes.

44. By which process does the energy of the sun reach Earth?
   A. Conduction only
   B. Convection only
   C. Radiation only
   D. Conduction and radiation

45. Assuming that the thermal conductivity of the copper is large enough to allow almost instantaneous energy transfer, what is the temperature difference between the water in the supplying pipes and the water in the draining pipes using the data in the passage? (Assume that the water covers the whole area of the collector)

   Density of water = 1 g cm^{-3}

   A. 38,100.0 °C
   B. 38.1 °C
   C. 76.2 °C
   D. 9.5 °C

46. The amount of electricity that can be generated from the fluid coming from the draining pipe of the collector is dependent upon its temperature. Therefore, it might be more efficient to use a fluid with which of the following properties?
   A. A lower thermal conductivity
   B. A higher thermal conductivity
   C. A higher specific heat capacity
   D. A lower specific heat capacity

Passage VIII (Questions 47-52)

In the strictest sense, *crystal lattice* refers to an orderly arrangement of particles. Thus, any substance which solidifies forms its own crystal lattice, with orderly arrangements of atoms or molecules. Each atom, molecule or ion is said to occupy a lattice site as shown below in Figure 1.

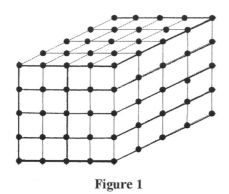

Figure 1

Usually, solidification or freezing occurs when the distance between individual particles is closer than in the liquid state. This leads to the mutual electrostatic attractive forces between the particles overcoming the mutual electrostatic forces of repulsion between the particles and the change from the liquid state to the solid state. In some substances, however, the distance over which the intermolecular forces act in the crystal lattice is greater than in the liquid state. This is due to certain intermolecular forces existing in the liquid state which become "fixed" in the lattice. An example of these types of bonds is the hydrogen bond. Thus, solid water (ice) floats on "liquid" water. The phenomenon gives rise to a phase diagram similar to that shown in Figure 2.

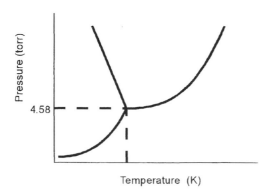

Figure 2

47. Why does "solid" water (ice) float on "liquid" water?
   A. Because it is less dense.
   B. Because it occupies less volume.
   C. Because it exists at lower temperatures.
   D. Because it is a solid.

48. From Figure 2, what do you expect to happen to the melting point of solid water (ice) if an increased external pressure is applied to the system?
   A. The melting point would increase.
   B. The melting point would decrease.
   C. The melting point would remain at the same value.
   D. The direction of change in the value of the melting point depends on the magnitude of the applied pressure.

49. Which of the following molecules would yield a similar phase diagram to that of water?
   A. CO_2
   B. CH_4
   C. NH_3
   D. H_2

50. 50 grams of glucose ($C_6H_{12}O_6$) and 50 grams of sucrose ($C_{12}H_{22}O_{11}$) were each added to beakers of water (beaker 1 and beaker 2, respectively). Which of the following would be true?
   A. Boiling point elevation for beaker 1 would be greater than the boiling point elevation for beaker 2.
   B. Boiling point elevation for beaker 1 would be less than the boiling point elevation for beaker 2.
   C. The same degree of boiling point elevation will occur in both beakers.
   D. No boiling point elevation would be observed in either of the beakers.

51. What would the freezing point in Kelvin of a solution which is 0.50 molal in sucrose and 0.50 molal in acetic acid be?
   (K_f of water = 2.0 °C mol^{-1} and freezing point of water = 0 °C)
   A. -1.0 K
   B. -2.0 K
   C. 272 K
   D. 271 K

52. The density of solid water (i.e. ice) at 25 °C is 0.98 g cm^{-3} while that of liquid mercury at the same temperature is 13.60 g cm^{-3}. What percentage of the height of the ice would be above the surface of a container filled with mercury?

    A. 93%

    B. 81%

    C. 19%

    D. 7%

53. 20 mL of 0.05 M Mg^{2+} in solution is desired. It is attempted to achieve this by adding 5 mL of 0.005 M $MgCl_2$ and 15 mL of $Mg_3(PO_4)_2$. What is the concentration of $Mg_3(PO_4)_2$?
    A. 0.065 M
    B. 0.022 M
    C. 0.150 M
    D. 0.100 M

54. Which of the following is the strongest reducing agent?

Electrochemical reaction	E° value (V)
$MnO_2 + 4H^+ + 2e^- \rightleftharpoons Mn^{2+} + 2H_2O$	+1.23
$Fe^{3+} + e^- \rightleftharpoons Fe^{2+}$	+0.771
$N_2 + 5H^+ + 4e^- \rightleftharpoons N_2H_5^+$	-0.230
$Cr^{3+} + e^- \rightleftharpoons Cr^{2+}$	-0.410

    A. Cr^{3+}
    B. Cr^{2+}
    C. Mn^{2+}
    D. MnO_2

55. As the atomic number increases as one moves across the periodic table, electron affinity generally:
    A. becomes more positive because of the increasing atomic radius.
    B. becomes more positive because of the decreasing effective nuclear charge.
    C. becomes more negative because of the increasing effective nuclear charge.
    D. becomes more negative because of the increasing atomic radius.

56. A 0.2 kg ball accelerates from rest at 5 m s^{-2} for five seconds. It then collides with a 0.5 kg ball which is initially at rest. The smaller ball stops moving while the larger ball begins its motion. After the collision, how fast is the larger ball initially moving?
    A. 2.0 m s^{-1}
    B. 10 m s^{-1}
    C. 2.5 m s^{-1}
    D. 5.0 m s^{-1}

57. A vertically oriented spring is stretched by 0.50 m when a mass of 1 kg is suspended from it. What is the work done on the spring?
    A. 5.0 J
    B. 2.5 J
    C. 0.5 J
    D. 20.0 J

Passage IX (Questions 58-61)

The viscosity of a fluid, that is, a gas, a pure liquid or a solution is an index of its resistance to flow. The viscosity of a fluid in a cylindrical tube of radius R and length L is given by:

$$n = \pi \Delta P R^4 t/(8VL) \quad \textbf{Equation I}$$

where n = viscosity of fluid, ΔP = change in pressure, t = time, V = volume of fluid and V/t = rate of flow of fluid. This equation can be applied to the study of blood flow in our bodies. The heart pumps blood through the various vessels in our bodies to supply all of its tissues. At rest, the rate of blood flow is about 80 cm^3 s^{-1} and this is maintained in all blood vessels. However, the radii of the blood vessels decreases the further away blood moves from the heart. Therefore, in order to maintain the rate of blood flow, a pressure drop occurs as one moves from one blood vessel to another of smaller radius.

A great number of physiological conditions can be explained using Equation I, for example, hypertension.

58. What would be the pressure drop per cm of the blood in the first blood vessel leaving the heart if the blood vessel is of unit radius and the body is at rest?

$$n_{blood} = 0.04 \text{ dyn s cm}^{-3}$$

   A. 25.6/π dyn cm^{-3}
   B. 16000/π dyn cm^{-3}
   C. π/25.6 dyn cm^{-3}
   D. π/16000 dyn cm^{-3}

59. Which of the following has the greatest effect on the viscosity of a fluid per unit change in its value?
   A. Volume of the fluid
   B. Length of the tube
   C. Pressure of the fluid
   D. Radius of the tube

60. The equation for the rate of flow of a fluid (from Equation I) has often been compared to Ohm's law. Given that P can be likened to the voltage and flow rate can be likened to the current, which of the following can be likened to resistance?
   A. πR^4
   B. $\pi R^4/(8Ln)$
   C. $8Ln/(\pi R^4)$
   D. $8Ln$

61. Hypertension involves the decrease in the radius of certain blood vessels. If the radius of a blood vessel is halved, by what factor must the pressure increase to maintain the normal rate of blood flow, all other factors being constant?
   A. 2
   B. 4
   C. 8
   D. 16

Passage X (Questions 62-67)

In the simple model of a gas as described by the kinetic molecular theory, a gas is pictured as an assembly of particles travelling at high velocities in straight lines in all directions. The particles are constantly colliding, but they are supposed to be perfectly elastic so that no momentum is lost on impact. They are also supposed to be point masses, that is, they have mass but occupy no space. In addition, no attractive or repulsive forces are exerted between particles.

From this theory, and the work of other great scientists like Boyle and Charles, the ideal gas law was devised: $PV = nRT$ where P = pressure of the gas, V = volume of the gas, n = number of moles of gas particles present, T = Kelvin temperature of the gas and R = universal gas constant.

However, no "real" gas conforms to this "ideal" gas theory, that is, no real gas obeys all of these laws at all temperatures and pressures. These deviations were investigated by the French physicist Amagat, who used pressures up to 320 atmospheres and a range of temperatures to investigate these deviations. The following diagram shows how the PV/nRT value varies with pressure for certain gases at 50 °C.

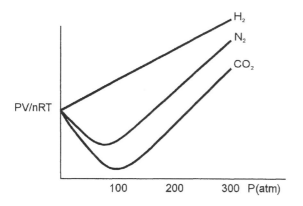

The deviations of real gases from ideality confers a number of properties on the gas which could not be explained by the kinetic molecular theory.

62. What would the PV/nRT versus P graph look like for an ideal gas?

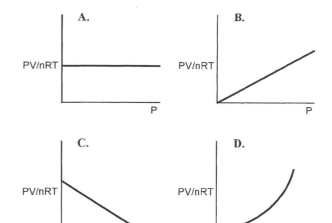

63. From the information in the passage, if 1 dm³ of H_2 gas initially at 50 atmospheres had its pressure increased to 100 atmospheres at a constant temperature, which of the following would be true?
A. Volume = 500 cm³
B. Volume > 500 cm³
C. Volume < 500 cm³
D. The change in volume will depend on the rate of increase of the external pressure.

64. Which of the following does not contribute to the explanation of the deviation of "real" gases from ideality?
A. Gas particles occupy space.
B. Gas particles have an attraction for each other.
C. Gas particles possess mass.
D. Gas particles do not undergo elastic collisions.

65. A sample of N_2, known to contain traces of water, occupied a volume of 200 dm³ at 25 °C and 1 atm. When passed over solid Na_2SO_4 (drying agent), the increase in mass of the salt was 35.0 grams. What was the partial pressure of the N_2 in the sample? (Assume ideality and molar volume at 25 °C = 24 dm³)
A. 0.1 atm
B. 0.2 atm
C. 0.4 atm
D. 0.8 atm

66. Which of the following would cause a gas to more closely resemble an ideal gas?
    A. Decreased pressure
    B. Decreased temperature
    C. Decreased volume
    D. None of the above

67. If a gas behaved ideally, which of the following would be expected on cooling the gas to 1 K ?
    A. It would remain a gas.
    B. It would liquify.
    C. It would solidify.
    D. Cannot be determined from the information given.

Natural uranium contains two isotopes: ^{238}U and the much rarer ^{235}U. The latter is the isotope responsible for the vast release of energy during nuclear fission. The two major uses of ^{235}U are in nuclear reactors and in atomic bombs. Both of these processes rely on self-sustaining fission reactions.

The radioactive disintegration of ^{235}U involves, as a first step, the incorporation of a slow moving neutron into its nucleus. All of the neutrons released during nuclear fission are capable of splitting another ^{235}U nucleus. Each reaction produces three neutrons and provided that the chain can build up rapidly enough, there is an enormous release of energy and this is the basis for the action of the atomic bomb. This will only occur if the ^{235}U sample present is larger than a certain mass known as the *critical size*. In the atomic bomb, two pieces of pure ^{235}U or ^{239}Pu each below the critical size are brought together and the two pieces form one larger piece larger than the critical size and this leads to the explosion observed.

In the nuclear reactor, the *atomic pile* consists of rods of uranium inserted into channels surrounded by blocks of graphite. The temperature of the pile can be controlled by the use of movable boron or cadmium rods. The heat generated during the fission process is removed by a stream of carbon dioxide. The hot gas is then used to produce steam which drives a turbine and so produces electrical energy.

68. Why must the uranium rods be stored well apart before use in the reactor?
   A. Because a fusion reaction would begin while in storage.
   B. Because an explosion could occur.
   C. Because they are then easier to transport.
   D. Because conversion of ^{235}U to non-fissionable ^{238}U would occur.

69. In an atomic bomb, the chain reaction depends on:
   A. all three neutrons produced from a ^{235}U nucleus splitting other ^{235}U nuclei.
   B. at least four neutrons produced from a ^{235}U nucleus splitting other ^{235}U nuclei.
   C. at least two neutrons produced from a ^{235}U nucleus splitting another ^{235}U nucleus.
   D. none of the above.

70. Given the following reactions, identify X.

$$^{1}_{0}n + {}^{238}_{92}U \rightarrow {}^{239}_{92}U + X$$

$$^{239}_{92}U \rightarrow {}^{239}_{93}Np + {}^{0}_{-1}e$$

$$^{239}_{93}Np \rightarrow {}^{239}_{94}Pu + {}^{0}_{-1}e$$

   A. α - particle
   B. β - particle
   C. γ - ray
   D. proton

71. The Dounreay Nuclear Power Station has been in operation for quite some time. Over the last six years, they have turned out a total of two megawatt-years of energy. Assuming that operations were continuous over the six year period at a constant rate, what was its power in watts?
   A. 3.3×10^5 W
   B. 6.6×10^5 W
   C. 3.3×10^2 W
   D. 6.6×10^2 W

72. Nuclear reactors are usually surrounded by lead and concrete. Which of the following is this safety precaution particularly for?
   A. α - particle
   B. β - particle
   C. γ - ray
   D. proton

73. Which of the following is NOT characteristic of hydrogen bonding?
- **A.** The hydrogen atom involved must be covalently bonded to a very electronegative atom.
- **B.** The hydrogen bonds are typically weaker than ionic or covalent bonds.
- **C.** The other atom involved in the hydrogen bond (not the hydrogen atom) must be covalently bonded to a hydrogen atom.
- **D.** The other atom involved in the hydrogen bond (not the hydrogen atom) must possess at least one lone pair of electrons.

74. A current of 2.0 A is passed through a wire for 1.5 minutes. How many electrons passed through the wire?
(Charge on electron = 1.6×10^{-19} C)
- **A.** 1.1×10^{21}
- **B.** 2.5×10^{19}
- **C.** 1.1×10^{17}
- **D.** 2.5×10^{15}

75. Which of the following s-block elements is NOT in one of the first two groups in the periodic table?
- **A.** $1s^2\ 2s^2\ 2p^6\ 3s^2\ 3p^6\ 4s^2$
- **B.** $1s^2\ 2s^2\ 2p^6\ 3s^2$
- **C.** $1s^2\ 2s^2$
- **D.** $1s^2$

76. The data in Table 1 were collected for Reaction I:

$$2X + Y \rightarrow Z \qquad \textbf{Reaction I}$$

Table 1

Exp.	[X] in M	[Y] in M	Initial rate of reaction
1	0.050	0.100	2×10^{-4}
2	0.050	0.200	8×10^{-4}
3	0.200	0.100	8×10^{-4}

What is the rate law for the reaction?
- **A.** Rate = $k[X]^2[Y]$
- **B.** Rate = $k[X]^2[Y]^2$
- **C.** Rate = $k[X][Y]^2$
- **D.** Rate = $k[X][Y]$

77. The freezing point of a solution of sucrose was noted and then a *dissacharidase*, which degrades sucrose, was added to the solution. The enzyme was subsequently removed. How would the freezing point of this final solution compare to that of the original solution?
- **A.** It would be lower.
- **B.** It would be higher.
- **C.** It would be the same.
- **D.** It cannot be determined from the information given.

END OF PHYSICAL SCIENCES. IF TIME REMAINS, YOU MAY GO BACK AND CHECK YOUR WORK IN THIS TEST BOOKLET.

THE GOLD STANDARD MCAT*

TEST GS-1

Verbal Reasoning
Questions 78-137
Time : 85 Minutes

OPEN BOOKLET ONLY WHEN TIMER IS READY.

The Gold Standard MCAT* has been designed exclusively to test knowledge and thinking skills. The exam may contain hypothetical statements and/or express controversial ideas. Statements contained herein do not necessarily reflect the policy, position, or view of RuveneCo Publishing.

* MCAT is a registered service mark of the Association of American Medical Colleges, which is not associated with this product.

VERBAL REASONING

INSTRUCTIONS: The Verbal Reasoning test contains nine passages, each of which is followed by several questions. After reading the passage, select the best answer to each question. If you are unsure of the answer, eliminate the alternatives you know to be false then select an answer from the remaining alternatives. Indicate your answer by blackening the corresponding oval on Answer Document 1, GS-1.

Passage I (Questions 78-84)

"What is art?" Few questions provoke such heated debate and provide so few satisfactory answers. If we cannot come to any definitive conclusions, there is still a good deal we can say. Art is first of all a *word* - one that acknowledges both the idea and the fact of art. Without it, we might well ask whether art exists in the first place. The term, after all, is not found in every society. Yet art is *made* everywhere. Art, therefore, is also an object, but not just any kind of object. Art is an *aesthetic object.* It is meant to be looked at and appreciated for its intrinsic value. Its special qualities set art apart, so that it is often placed away from everyday life - in museums, churches, or caves... [Its] absolute qualities elude us, [so] that we cannot escape viewing works of art in the context of time and circumstance, whether past or present...

We all dream, that is imagination at work. To imagine means simply to make an image - a picture - in our minds. Human beings are not the only creatures who have imagination. Even animals dream. Cats' ears and tails may twitch as they sleep and sleeping dogs may whine and growl and paw the air, as if they were having a fight. Even when awake, animals "see" things. For no apparent reason, a cat's fur may rise on its back as it peers into a dark closet, just as you or I may get goose bumps from phantoms we neither see nor hear. Clearly, however, there is a profound difference between human and animal imagination. Humans are the only creatures who can tell one another about imagination in stories or pictures. The urge to make art is unique to us. No other animal has ever been observed to draw a recognizable image spontaneously in the wild. In fact, their only images have been produced under carefully controlled laboratory conditions that tell us more about the experimenter than they do about art. There can be little doubt, on the other hand, that people possess an aesthetic faculty. By the age of five every normal child has drawn a moon pie-face. The ability to make art is one of our most distinctive features, for it separates us from all other creatures across an evolutionary gap that is unbridgeable.

Just as an embryo retraces much of the human evolutionary past, so budding artists reinvent the first stages of art. Soon, however, they complete that process and begin to respond to the culture around them. Even children's art is subject to the taste and outlook of the society that shapes his or her personality...

Given the many factors that feed into it, art must play a very special role in the artist's personality. Sigmund Freud, the founder of modern psychiatry, conceived of art primarily in terms of sublimation outside of consciousness. Such a view hardly does justice to artistic creativity, since art is not simply a negative force at the mercy of our neuroses but a positive expression that integrates diverse aspects of personality...

In a larger sense art, like science and religion, fulfils our innate urge to comprehend ourselves and the universe. This function makes art especially significant and, hence, worthy of our attention. Art has the power to penetrate to the core of our being, which recognizes itself in the creative act. For that reason, art represents its creator's deepest understanding and highest aspirations. At the same time, artists often play an important role as the articulators of our shared beliefs and values, which they express through an ongoing tradition to us, their audience. A masterpiece, then, is a work that contributes to our vision of life and leaves us profoundly moved. Moreover, it can bear the closest scrutiny and withstand the test of time.

Adapted from H.W. Janson, *History of Art.* ©1991, 1995 Harry N. Abrams, Inc.

78. According to the passage, what important characteristic separates humans from other creatures?
A. Humans can dream, but other creatures cannot.
B. Humans have the urge and ability to make art, but other creatures do not.
C. Humans have imaginations, but other creatures do not.
D. Humans develop from an embryo, but other creatures do not.

79. Based on the passage, if one were to describe the author's ideal artist, which of the following qualities would he/she possess?
A. A highly developed aesthetic faculty
B. The ability to see and hear phantoms that are not there
C. An acute awareness of his/her subconscious impulses
D. An abnormal imagination

80. The passage suggests that one's appreciation for art might be heightened if one:
A. views art in the context of the time in which it was produced.
B. knows the artist and can get a detailed explanation firsthand.
C. regularly visits museums, churches and caves.
D. has had a happy childhood.

81. The passage suggests that a budding artist is like an embryo in that he/she:
A. grows slowly, nurtured by a mother's care.
B. begins with basic elements and evolves into more complex forms.
C. has begun to be influenced by cultural forces.
D. has the ability to produce recognizable images.

82. According to the passage, the author does not agree with Sigmund Freud's concept of art because the author:
A. does not think psychiatry is scientific enough.
B. believes that a young artist must develop creativity to be a good artist as an adult.
C. believes that art is not primarily derived from the unconscious.
D. does not think art is the result of repressed aggression and diverse aspects of personality.

83. According to the passage, art combines which of the following aspects of the artist's human experience?
A. Reason and emotion
B. Deep understanding and high aspirations
C. Happiness and suffering
D. Dream and reality

84. Which of the following best expresses the main idea of the passage?
A. Art is an aesthetic object, little understood by psychiatrists.
B. Art allows us to see a great deal that reminds us of life.
C. Art is an expressive form that has perpetuated since the beginning of man.
D. Art is one of the greatest forms of expression available exclusively to humans.

Almost everyone has had experiences that are cause for some slight wonder... It is of course possible to attribute any of these and thousands of similar events to coincidence. And yet, so many instances of apparent knowledge have accumulated throughout history - some of them very difficult to explain away as simple quirks of fate - that millions of people have come to believe humans possess more than five senses...

All ESP phenomena, because they seem beyond the limits of our present understanding, are said to be paranormal; serious investigators describe their research field as the science of parapsychology...

Parapsychologists face two basic challenges: proving that psychic powers exist and, if so, explaining how they work. Most psi researchers have quite logically devoted themselves to the first problem, however, the absence of a coherent theory of ESP has cast doubt on the entire field. Critics point out that psychic powers are so unlikely from a scientific point of view that any other explanation for positive experimental results, including fraud, must be considered first.

Indeed, telepathy, clairvoyance, and precognition seem to contradict the elementary physical laws that govern our lives. How can information travel from person to person, or from event to person, without following known sensory channels? Standard physics dictates that no signals of any kind can travel faster than the speed of light and that as they travel, they lose strength. How then can parapsychologists account rationally for precognition, in which information from an event is said to reach the subject before the event occurs? How can they explain the way in which a telepathic message allegedly arrives at its target undiminished by intervening distances?

Some psychic researchers have responded to these questions with theories, or at least interpretations of theories... Such researchers speculate that some physical descriptions of the universe might serve as models, or metaphors, for the way psychic phenomena behave. Among these models are electromagnetism and multidimensional geometry.

The nineteenth-century discovery of electromagnetism, which described how some signals travel in waves from a source to a receiver, provided one of the earliest models for ESP. Physicists found that light, the infrared energy of heat, and other phenomena fit into an electromagnetic spectrum. At one end are extremely short, high-frequency waves, such as X rays, and, at the other end, extremely long, low-frequency waves, such as radio waves from distant galaxies.

With a few exceptions, such as light and heat, humans cannot sense electromagnetic radiation. Perhaps, said early researchers, psychic information also travels invisibly, like radio waves, and is accessible only to those people who can tune in their psychic receivers. Speculation generally located "psi waves" in the low-frequency end of the spectrum.

Psi waves, however, have never been found, and this model still fails to account for the faster-than-light speeds and undiminished power suggested by reports of precognition and telepathy. Most parapsychologists now believe that electromagnetism is a naive model for extrasensory perception.

Another, more recent model for supposed psychic effects places them in a dimension outside of - but interacting with - the four dimensions of space and time we can perceive... If a line, with only the single dimension of height, moves through space, its shape over time is a plane - a shape in the two dimensions of height and width. The plane, moved through space and time to gain depth, will form the outlines of a three-dimensional cube as it travels.

These three dimensions are the only ones we can see, but we experience the dimension of time no less clearly. The existence of the cube over time adds a fourth coordinate to the shape, creating a new configuration known as a hypercube - invisible to human eyes but not to the vision of mathematics.

Some mathematicians have suggested the universe may contain even more than four dimensions - as many as eleven, or even twenty-six. A few psychic theorists speculate that human consciousness itself belongs to one of these additional dimensions intersecting our four-dimensional world. If so, the four "hard" coordinates of space-time would be joined by a fifth, "soft" coordinate of psi. If our minds could somehow tap into this extra dimension, the way information travels outside of the natural laws we presently know might be explained. However, with no physical evidence to support extra dimensions, the idea of a consciousness plane remains nothing more than fascinating speculation.

Adapted from *Mysteries of the Unknown, Psychic Powers.*
Copyright © 1987 Time-Life Books Inc.

85. According to the passage the greatest evidence for the existence of ESP phenomena comes from:
   A. the nineteenth century discovery of electromagnetism.
   B. the discovery by mathematicians that the universe may contain more than four dimensions.
   C. the number of instances of ESP phenomena reported throughout history.
   D. the number of scientists willing to devote time to parapsychological research.

86. The passage suggests that according to the laws of physics, one would expect that precognitive signals:
   A. travel faster than the speed of light.
   B. cannot travel over large distances uninterrupted.
   C. have properties similar to those of gamma rays.
   D. can neither be created nor destroyed.

87. Given what the author writes about critics of parapsychology, one would expect that critics:
   A. want scientific proof of the existence of psychic powers.
   B. have very limited imaginations.
   C. think all parapsychologists are frauds.
   D. have never had any paranormal experiences.

88. According to the electromagnetic theory for the way psychic powers behave, one could expect psychic information to:
   A. exist as high frequency waves from distant galaxies.
   B. be able to penetrate several centimeters of lead.
   C. be near the visible region of the electromagnetic spectrum.
   D. be long, low-frequency waves.

89. Consider the following: "The existence of the cube over time adds a fourth coordinate... creating a new configuration, known as the hypercube - invisible to human eyes, but not to the vision of mathematics." Psychic theorists might use this phenomenon to speculate that:
   A. many theories of mathematics belong to the realm of the paranormal.
   B. perhaps, like the hypercube, psychic signals do exist, but are invisible to the human eye.
   C. psychic signals are not waves similar to those of the electromagnetic spectrum, but shapes with several dimensions.
   D. scientists should show the field of mathematics the same scepticism that they do the field of parapsychology.

90. According to the passage, which of the following claims about the two models described is inaccurate?
   A. The invisible wave theory of electromagnetism is naive and has been abandoned by most psychic theorists.
   B. There is greater supporting evidence for the psi dimension theory than the electromagnetic theory.
   C. There is no physical evidence to support the existence of extra dimensions in the universe.
   D. None of the above.

91. "Prior to the sinking of the Titanic, nearly seventy people reported having had 'visions' of the event." Given this statement, which of the following is most consistent with the theme of the passage?
   A. The seventy people were frauds seeking attention from the media.
   B. The seventy people belonged to the select group who can tune in their psychic receivers and access psychic information in the form of waves.
   C. While the high number of reports makes it hard to attribute the visions to coincidence, there is as yet no scientific explanation to account for this phenomenon.
   D. Psychic signals travelling faster than the speed of light reached these seventy people, allowing them to experience the visions.

It was a travelling exhibit for schoolchildren. Titled "Population: The Problem Is Us," it toured the country at government expense in the mid-1970s... It told the children that "the birth rate must decrease and/or the death rate must increase" since resources were all but exhausted and mass starvation loomed. It warned that, "driven by starvation, people have been known to eat dogs, cats, bird droppings, and even their own children," and it featured a picture of a dead rat on a dinner plate as an example of future "food sources." Overpopulation, it threatened, would lead not only to starvation and cannibalism but to civil violence and nuclear war.

The exhibit was created at the Smithsonian Institute, the national museum of the U.S. government, using federal funds provided by the National Science Foundation, an agency of the U.S. government.

Concurrently, other American schoolchildren were also being treated to federally funded "population education," instructing them of "the growing pressures on global resources, food, jobs, and political stability." They read Paul Ehrlich's book, *The Population Bomb*. They were taught, falsely, that "world population is increasing at a rate of 2 percent per year whereas the food supply is increasing at a rate of 1 percent per year," and equally falsely, that "population growth and rising affluence have reduced reserves of the world's minerals." They viewed slides of the "biological catastrophes" that would result from overpopulation and held class discussions on "what responsible individuals in a 'crowded world' should or can do about population growth." They learned that the world is like a spaceship or a crowded lifeboat, to deduce the fate of mankind, which faces a "population crisis"... They were told to "say good-bye" to numerous wildlife species doomed to extinction as a result of the human population explosion.

This propaganda campaign in the public schools, which indoctrinated a generation of children, was federally funded, despite the fact that no law had committed the United States to this policy. Nor, indeed, had agreement been reached among informed groups that the problem of "overpopulation" even existed. To the contrary, during the same period the government drive against population was gaining momentum, contrary evidence was proliferating. One of the world's most prominent economic demographers, Colin Clark of Oxford University, published a book titled *Population Growth: the Advantages;* and economists Peter Bauer and Basil Yamey of the London School of Economics discovered that the population scare "relies on misleading statistics... misinterprets the causalities in changes in fertility and changes in income" and "envisages children exclusively as burdens." Moreover, in his major study of *The Economics of Population Growth,* Julian Simon found that population growth was economically beneficial. Other economists joined in differing from the official antinatalist position.

Commenting on this body of economic findings, Paul Ehrlich, the biologist author of *The Population Bomb,* charged that economists "continue to whisper in the ears of politicians all kinds of nonsense." If not on the side of the angels, Ehrlich certainly found himself on the side of the U.S. government, which since the mid-1960s has become increasingly committed to a worldwide drive to reduce the growth of population. It has absorbed rapidly increasing amounts of public money, as well as the energies of a growing number of public agencies and publicly subsidized private organizations.

The spirit of the propaganda has permeated American life at all levels, from the highest reaches of the federal bureaucracy to the chronic reporting of overpopulation problems by the media and the population education being pushed in public schools. It has become so much a part of daily American life that its presuppositions and implications are scarcely examined: though volumes are regularly published on the subject, they rarely do more than restate the assumptions as a prelude to proposing even "better" methods of population planning.

Adapted from Jacqueline Kasun, *The War Against Population.*
© Ignatius Press, San Francisco, 1988.

92. Based on the passage, the attitude of the United States government, as reflected by their funding of population education programs in schools, was that it:
A. saw population growth as a crisis which should be eliminated.
B. was committed to determining the actual effects of population growth.
C. was indifferent to population growth.
D. was determined to follow United States policy.

93. Paul Ehrlich's book *The Population Bomb,* probably:
   A. contained similar opinions to those expressed in *Population Growth: The Advantages.*
   B. contained an ambivalent perspective on the issue of population growth.
   C. described the negative effects of population growth on food and jobs.
   D. was a favorite of the author of the passage.

94. The author claims that on the question of population growth, economists were:
   A. in agreement with biologists.
   B. convinced that its effects could only be disadvantageous.
   C. supportive of government programs.
   D. producing evidence of its possible economic benefits.

95. According to the passage, which of the following was NOT a result of the government's drive?
   A. Chronic reporting of overpopulation problems by the media
   B. Increasing amounts of public money were absorbed by government programs
   C. A decrease in population growth
   D. Children were viewed more and more as burdens

96. When the author says "If not on the side of angels" (paragraph 5), she implies that:
   A. angels and the government can never be on the same side.
   B. Ehrlich was supporting the wrong side of the issue.
   C. religion was also being affected as a result of the propaganda campaign.
   D. the angels were on the side of the biologists.

97. The passage suggests that the author is most disappointed by the government because:
   A. the author is an economist.
   B. of the government's commitment to reducing population growth.
   C. the government disregarded available evidence supporting population growth.
   D. it indoctrinated a generation of children with the propaganda campaign.

98. In the passage, government money was used to:
   I. Aid the publication of *The Population Bomb*.
   II. Fund an exhibition created at the Smithsonian Institute.
   III. Research the effects of population growth.

   A. II only
   B. III only
   C. I and III only
   D. II and III only

99. The passage claims that the United States government took the stand it did with respect to population growth:
   A. because a law committed them to their official position.
   B. because the government was embarrassed to alter its position when contrary evidence surfaced.
   C. because the economists were from England.
   D. it is not explicitly stated in the passage why the government took the stand it did.

100. The "crowded lifeboat" analogy used in the passage (paragraph 3), is most effective when:
   A. one considers that a crowded lifeboat is dangerous.
   B. one considers the infinite size of a lifeboat.
   C. one considers the limited resources available in a crowded lifeboat.
   D. The analogy is ineffective.

101. The attitude of the author at the end of the passage is best described as:
   A. hopeful.
   B. practical.
   C. indifferent.
   D. disheartened.

Passage IV (Questions 102-107)

In recent years two apparently unconnected events have had a revolutionary impact on meteorology. One of these is the emergence of high speed electronic computers capable of providing sufficiently rapid numerical solutions to the mathematical equations used to describe atmospheric motions...

The other noteworthy event is the development of the artificial earth satellite. The launching of the first weather satellite TIROS I in April 1960 surprisingly quickly showed that the latest technological devices could be used profitably by the meteorologist. The potential value of this unique new platform for global observations was no doubt one of the prime reasons why the United Nations General Assembly twenty months later adopted a decision which in meterological circles is accorded historic importance and which led to the concept of the World Weather Watch.

What is the World Weather Watch?

The main purpose of the World Weather Watch (WWW) is to establish a system by which all countries can be provided with the weather data and other information they need to carry out their national obligations. All nations participate actively in the system both by receiving and by transmitting weather information. In addition, some countries have specific international functions; thus there are three World Meterological Centres and 21 Regional Meteorological Centres...

These large meterological centres carry out numerical forecasts of the future state of the atmosphere, making use of physical laws expressed in mathematical equations called "models." In addition to the problem of developing suitable "models," there are three major conditions which must be satisfied:

- We must know the actual state of the entire atmosphere preferably at a chosen hour (i.e. by making representative observations of temperature, pressure, humidity, wind and so on) and also the conditions at the lower and upper boundaries of the atmosphere;

- We must have the facilities to process this vast quantity of observational data very quickly in order to reduce to a minimum the time of delay between the hour of observation and the hour of issuing the forecast;

- We must be able to transmit the original observations rapidly to suitable forecasting centres and to distribute quickly the products of such centres (weather analyses, prognoses, forecasts, warnings, etc.) to their users.

One of the first goals of the WWW is to plan and develop a truly global observational system. The most promising new techniques to fill the gaps are meterological satellites and the so-called constant-level balloons... the automatic buoy weather station should also be mentioned as a promising supplementary of obtaining data from ocean areas.

Adapted from Kaare Langlo, *Unlocking The Secrets of Tomorrow's Weather*, (8)'73 The Unesco Courier.

102. According to the passage, which of the following events has had a revolutionary impact on meteorology?
   I. The development of mathematical equations which can be used to describe atmospheric motion
   II. The development of the weather satellite TIROS I
   III. The development of the concept of the World Weather Watch by the United Nations General Assembly

   A. II only
   B. I and II only
   C. II and III only
   D. I, II and III

103. "In September 1961, Hurricane "Carla" was discovered in time for 500 000 people to be evacuated from the threatened area in Texas and Louisiana." This remarkable event was likely most influential in:
   A. proving that technological devices such as weather satellites have great potential value.
   B. stimulating the development of automatic buoy weather stations.
   C. stimulating the development of mathematical models for use in forecasting.
   D. allowing the major conditions that need to be satisfied for proper forecasting to occur, to be defined for the first time.

104. Many land areas in developing countries, particularly where the climatic conditions are harsh, still lack adequate observing networks. Which of the major conditions for proper forecasting, would this problem leave unsatisfied?
   A. The actual state of the entire atmosphere at a chosen hour must be known.
   B. The WWW must be made aware of any problems discovered by the public as soon as possible.
   C. Observational data must be processed very quickly.
   D. Observations must be transmitted to suitable forecasting centres for distribution.

105. According to the passage, the main purpose of the WWW is to:
   A. encourage and fund the development of new technological devices for use by the meteorologist.
   B. determine the reliability of the data obtained from the three World Meterological Centres.
   C. coordinate the flow of weather information between the different countries of the world.
   D. investigate whether or not the three major requirements for accurate weather forecasting are being fulfilled.

106. According to the passage, the WWW is made up of:
   A. three World Meterological Centres.
   B. twenty-one Regional Meterological Centres.
   C. all the countries of the world.
   D. both A and B.

107. The passage indicates that all of the following fields are important for the proper functioning of the WWW EXCEPT:
   A. telecommunications.
   B. computer technology.
   C. chemistry.
   D. space technology.

Passage V (Questions 108-114)

The modern "Seven Wonders of the World" have been controversial since their inception. Unlike the wonders of the ancient world which were based on architecture and sculpture, modern wonders are based on technology. Since technology is continually evolving, there can be no permanence to a definition of the modern wonders. On the other hand, the ancient wonders have a precise definition; though their structures have had no permanence - except for the pyramids of Egypt.

Six of the seven wonders had been iterated as early as the 2nd century B.C. in an epigram of Antipater of Sidon. A list dating from about the 6th century A.D. has since been considered the gold standard: (1) the pyramids of Egypt; (2) the Hanging Gardens of Babylon; (3) the statue of Zeus at Olympia; (4) the Colossus of Rhodes; (5) the Mausoleum of Halicarnassus; (6) the temple of Artemis at Ephesus; and (7) Pharos of Alexandria.

The ancient pyramids of Egypt are truly a wonder! They are the oldest of the seven, yet the only one which remains substantially in existence. The most famous of these venerable tombs lie along a 70 kilometer expanse of the Nile Valley and date from the Old Kingdom, 2700-2300 B.C. It is fascinating to allow one's imagination to explore the awesome nature of such a construction in its own era. Four thousand years ago a young African man courted a Nubian princess, they strolled along the Nile Valley, a darkness enveloped the land revealing points of lights above. They watched in awe as the moon shone brightly displaying three Great Pyramids, rising from the landscape as high as 480 feet. They loved their land, they loved each other. The man would one day be Pharaoh...

The second wonder, the Hanging Gardens of Babylon, has left no traces with any certainty. These gardens were not truly "hanging," rather they were laid out on a series of terraces irrigated by water pumped from the Euphrates. The legend is that in the 6th century B.C., King Nebuchadnezzar built the enticing gardens to console his Median wife who missed the mountains of her homeland.

The next two wonders represent majestic statues. The statue of Zeus at Olympia, Greece, was constructed of ivory and gold and stood 40 feet high. It was likely destroyed in the 5th century about 800 years after its construction. The Colossus of Rhodes was a huge bronze statue standing over 100 feet high. It represented the sun god Helios who was brought to his knees by an earthquake in 225 B.C. When the Arabs invaded Europe 800 years later, Helios became scraps of metal for a Muslim dealer. Legend has it that over 1000 camels were required to transport the numerous pieces of metal.

The fifth wonder, the Mausoleum of Halicarnassus in Asia Minor, was built in the 4th century B.C. in memory of King Mausolus by his sister and widow, Artemisia. This beautifully constructed monument included a great rectangular pile of masonry, surmounted by columns cradling a rooflike pyramid. To this day the word *mausoleum* refers to a monumental tomb.

The next ancient wonder also stood in Asia Minor, the Temple of Artemis at Ephesus. Few remains of the 4th century temple, once 110 by 55 m^2, are on display at the British Museum. Legend has it that the huge temple was burned to the ground in 356 B.C., the night Alexander the Great was born.

The seventh wonder of the ancient world stood in Egypt - Pharos of Alexandria - forerunner of the modern lighthouse. The name was derived from an island off the Egyptian coast. The structure was said to be almost 150 meters high with a spiral ramp leading to the top where a fire burned at night.

108. According to the passage, all of the following may be considered wonders of the modern world EXCEPT:
   A. the computer.
   B. Niagara Falls.
   C. the radio.
   D. the airplane.

109. Antipater of Sidon (paragraph 2) was likely a (an):
   A. general in a powerful army.
   B. local physician.
   C. sociologist.
   D. accountant.

110. The "points of lights" mentioned in paragraph 3, likely refer to:
   A. the sun.
   B. the stars.
   C. the moon.
   D. comets.

111. The Hanging Gardens of Babylon likely acquired its name because:
   A. they were named after King Nebuchadnezzar's Median wife.
   B. the gardens were suspended with nothing below.
   C. water pumped from the Euphrates irrigated the gardens.
   D. the gardens were on an incline so that some of the foliage hung over each terrace.

112. The passage indicates which of the following concerning King Nebuchadnezzar's wife?
   A. The King had married an equal number of wives before and after her.
   B. Her native land, Media, was mountainous but Babylon was not.
   C. She was an average wife.
   D. She was a midwife.

113. According to the passage, the wonders of the ancient world were found in which of the following:
   I. Africa
   II. Asia
   III. Europe

   A. I only
   B. III only
   C. II and III only
   D. I, II and III

114. The passage suggests that of all the reasons a great construction would be built in ancient times, the LEAST likely would be:
   A. a shrine to commemorate the death of a leader.
   B. a structure that represented a god.
   C. an edifice to be used as living quarters for the masses.
   D. a building with a practical use.

There are images behind the two rather different criticisms of Taso's life history to which I have referred. The first such image has to do with science. Scientific objectivity is possible. It requires either that the ethnographer ignore the fact that he/she, too, is a human being; or so completely "prosthetize" the method that he/she becomes invisible. Then the life history is pushed out in front of the reader with a long stick, from offstage. One objectifies the data collection by becoming a camera, a lens, near-transparent; one capitalizes on nondirectiveness, neutrality, stranger value. The second such image has to do with self. Objectivity, in this image, is impossible. The ethnographer remembers that there is no such thing as a fact; there are only interpretations because he or she, as well as the informant, is a human being. One must deobjectify the data collection because one is part of the data and the data are part of one; one never separates oneself from one's own thoughts, during the data collection.

The contrast has, I think, political implications but they may not be apparent. Both the scientist and the self-person may be of the Right or the Left; for instance, either may believe in self-determination for dependent peoples, or its opposite. Neither is bound naturally to any particular political ideology. It is not that anthropology as a field, or in its viewpoints, has moved in any particular direction on the political spectrum. It is merely that 40 years ago there seem to have been more scientists; now there appear to be more selves.

Some political implications do enter, but by a different route. Anthropology began as a Western project. It had to become aware of its limitations as a form of objective inquiry, and thus to understand better the conditions under which ethnographer and informant work together. To the extent that its practitioners may fail to recognize this, anthropology can serve as handmaiden for other forms of Western penetration of the rest of the world. Then its role in projects of the sort Taso and I undertook together can be to conceal, rather than reveal, a history of oppression. But that is the politics of understanding how nation, societies, and peoples are related to each other. It is a different matter from the ways in which individuals - say, the informant and the ethnographer - are related to each other.

If one defends the possibility that anthropology, in spite of its limitations, may play a part in documenting what the West has done to other societies, then giving people like Taso voice (while admitting that by our errors or bad intentions, we deform and distort what they say) is better than leaving them mute. Some readers of *Worker in the Cane*, though they may admire the remarkable human being who tells his story there, have probably wished that he could have told it without the proddings and cockeyed imaginings of some foreign social scientist (most of all one coming from the colonial power that rules Puerto Rico). But Taso's story was "there" all along - he just had not told it to anyone. He may not even have known that he was ready to tell it; and then I came along. The kind of person he is, the conditions under which he lived, his place in his society, the point at which we became friends, all figured in the writing of the book. Its story always was, and still is, Taso's story. I do not know by what means other than our joined intent it could have become something others might read and think about.

Adapted from American Ethnologist volume 16, *The Sensation of Moving While Standing Still* by Sidney W. Mintz.

115. In the context of the passage, "prosthetize" (paragraph 1), means:
A. prostitute.
B. teach.
C. master.
D. understand.

116. The passage suggests that it is impossible to be objective when the ethnographer uses the "self-person" approach because:
A. the ethnographer's own personal experience impacts on the interpretation of the informant's information.
B. anthropology is a social science.
C. of the political implications of adopting an objective approach.
D. distortion of data inevitably results.

117. According to the passage, an ethnographer could be like a camera in that he/she:
A. captures accurately a moment in history that would otherwise be forgotten.
B. serves as a tool to be used by politicians.
C. records information accurately, without interpretation.
D. deobjectifies data collection by capitalizing on nondirectiveness.

118. Taso is most probably:
   A. an ethnographer.
   B. an anthropologist.
   C. a worker on a Puerto Rican sugar cane plantation.
   D. a Western politician.

119. The limitations of anthropology described by the author include which of the following?
   I. Compared to years ago, there are more 'selves' in the field
   II. The extent to which the field can be considered completely objective
   III. The possible political implications of the field

   A. II only
   B. III only
   C. I and II only
   D. II and III only

120. The author implies that anthropology can be regarded as a handmaiden for other forms of Western penetration of the rest of the world because:
   A. of our desire for domestic help from citizens of other nations.
   B. many other fields of science do not consider anthropology scientific enough.
   C. anthropology is looked down upon by other forms of Western penetration.
   D. it can allow Western influence to affect the rest of the world with a clear conscience by misrepresenting information.

The carbon dioxide theory of climatic change was widely accepted fifty years ago, then generally discredited, but new research suggests that the reasons for rejecting the theory may not be valid...

Because of the relatively low temperatures at the earth's surface and in the atmosphere, nearly all the outgoing radiation from the earth is in the infrared region of the spectrum. Three gases occur in the atmosphere that, although present in small amounts, do absorb strongly over a portion of the infrared spectrum. These are carbon dioxide, water vapor, and ozone. The action of carbon dioxide may be compared to a greenhouse where the transparent glass admits the rays of the sun with their heat but prevents the escape of the outgoing heat waves from the plants and earth...

In order to estimate the change of carbon dioxide in the atmosphere, the so-called carbon dioxide balance must be understood. The atmosphere loses carbon dioxide today, owing to photosynthesis in plants, in the amount of about 60 billion tons per year. If the balance is steady, precisely the same amount is returned by the processes of respiration and decay of organic material. In times of great coal and oil formation some may be retained by the earth...

Carbon dioxide may be added from the interior of the earth by hot springs, fumaroles, and volcanoes. At times great volumes of the gas have been taken from the atmosphere by the formation of extensive limestone and dolomite deposits. These two factors, one that adds and one that subtracts, may upset the balance momentarily and change the amount in the atmosphere... Man has recently added a new factor and upset the balance. The combustion of fossil fuels in 1954 added 6 billion tons of carbon dioxide gas to the atmosphere, and the amount is doubling every ten years...

Now the theory's first premise is that, during times of continental elevation of mountain uplift, the weathering processes were greater, and greater amounts of carbonates were laid down in the shallow oceans. This reduced the carbon dioxide content of the atmosphere sufficiently so that a glacial stage was brought on. The second premise is that, once the atmosphere has been prepared for a glacial epoch by the reduction of carbon dioxide, there will follow a series of oscillations of cold and warm climates... As soon as the total [carbon dioxide] is restored to the pre-glacial amount, the oscillations cease, and the glacial epoch is over.

This theory has been criticized on the grounds that it assumes that a colder climate is accompanied by increased precipitation. If the sun's radiation is decreased, the earth's surface becomes cooler, and the energy available to drive the general circulation of the atmosphere is reduced. A decreased circulation means, presumably, less precipitation. Hence colder climates, although contributing to greater snow preservation, will also result in less snow, and the condition necessary for a glaciation does not necessarily develop. The several theories of variable solar energy definitely run afoul of this conclusion.

The carbon dioxide theory in new dress offers a plausible explanation of the desired situation of greater precipitation with cooler climates and lesser precipitation with warmer climates. It is pointed out that with a lesser amount of carbon dioxide in the atmosphere the upper surface of a cloud loses heat energy faster to space and is cooler. Furthermore, the upward flux of radiation from the earth that strikes the lower surface of the cloud is greater. These two factors contribute to a greater temperature difference between the top and bottom of a cloud and increases convection in the cloud. This makes for greater precipitation. Thus with decreased carbon dioxide in the atmosphere there will be colder climates and greater precipitation.

Adapted from A.J. Eardley, *General College Geology*. © 1965 by A.J. Eardley.

121. The passage asserts that all of the following factors will upset the balance of carbon dioxide in the same direction EXCEPT:
   A. photosynthesis.
   B. oil formation.
   C. the formation of dolomite deposits.
   D. volcanic eruptions.

122. According to the passage, the carbon dioxide theory of climatic change states that:
   A. during times of continental elevation, there was a decrease in carbonate deposition which caused an increase in carbon dioxide concentration that brought on a glacial stage.
   B. once there is an increase in carbon dioxide concentration, a glacial stage necessarily follows.
   C. once there is a decrease in carbon dioxide concentration, a series of oscillations of warm and cold climates results
   D. a colder climate is accompanied by decreased precipitation and a warmer climate by increased precipitation.

123. Based on the modified carbon dioxide theory of climate change, it could be reasonably inferred that man's contribution to the carbon dioxide concentration of the atmosphere, will result in:
   A. increased carbon dioxide concentrations, warmer climates and less precipitation.
   B. increased carbon dioxide concentrations, cooler climates and more precipitation.
   C. decreased carbon dioxide concentrations, warmer climates and less precipitation.
   D. decreased carbon dioxide concentrations, cooler climates and more precipitation.

124. The author describes the effect of the sun's radiation on the general circulation of the atmosphere (paragraph 6), in order to counter the claim that:
   A. colder climates may result in decreased precipitation.
   B. high carbon dioxide concentrations contribute to greater precipitation.
   C. when weathering processes are greater, carbonate deposition increases.
   D. a colder climate is accompanied by increased precipitation and a warmer climate by decreased precipitation.

125. The passage suggests that the action of carbon dioxide and a greenhouse are comparable in that:
   A. they are both necessary for plant growth.
   B. they both facilitate the entry of heat, but inhibit heat loss.
   C. they are both associated with two other gases, water vapor and ozone.
   D. they both contribute to the rising temperature of the atmosphere.

126. Which of the following would challenge the modified carbon dioxide theory of climatic change put forward in the passage?
   I. The discovery that, with a lesser amount of carbon dioxide in the atmosphere, the upper surface of a cloud gains heat faster from space and is hotter.
   II. Evidence that the temperature difference between the top and bottom of a cloud is always negligible.
   III. Evidence supporting the claim that, with increased carbon dioxide concentration in the atmosphere, colder climates and greater precipitation inevitably result.

   A. I only
   B. III only
   C. I and II only
   D. I, II and III

Passage VIII (Questions 127-131)

A popular delusion widely prevalent holds that books are inanimate, ineffective, peaceful objects, belonging to the cloistered shades and academic quiet of monasteries, universities, and other retreats from a materialistic, evil world. According to this curious misconception, books are full of impractical theory, and of slight significance for the hard-headed man of affairs.

A more realistic understanding is given to the jungle savage, as he bows down before the printed page, with its apparently supernatural power to convey messages. Throughout history, the evidence is piled high that books, rather than being futile, harmless, and innocent, are frequently dynamic, vital things, capable of changing the entire direction of events - sometimes for good, sometimes for ill.

In the dictators of every era is found a shrewd insight into the potentialities of books... No one realizes better than the despot the enormous explosive forces pent up in books. Occasionally the same point is forcefully brought home to democratic nations. An instance is the widespread sense of shock and incredulity among the American people and their friends abroad a few years ago at the news that the U.S. State Department, in its information libraries abroad, was engaged in a widespread program of book censorship. Instinctively, people everywhere perceived that books are as basic to modern culture and civilization as they have been in past centuries...

As one reviews books, there is always a question present: Did the times make the book, or vice versa, i.e. was a particular book influential chiefly because the period was ripe for it? Would the book have been equally significant in another era, or could it even have been written at another date? It is impossible to escape the conclusion that the times produced the book in nearly every instance. In some other historical epoch, the work would either not have been produced at all, or if it had appeared would have attracted little attention.

Examples are on every hand. Machiavelli's *The Prince* was written for the express purpose of freeing his beloved Italy from foreign aggression. England was ready for a vast expansion of her commercial and industrial economy when Adam Smith was writing his *Wealth of Nations*. Thomas Paine's *Common Sense* triggered the American Revolution, already primed for explosion; and Harriet Beecher Stowe's *Uncle Tom's Cabin* did likewise for the Civil War. Except for dreadful conditions prevailing in European industry, especially the English factory system, in the mid-nineteenth century, Karl Marx would have lacked ammunition for *Das Kapital*. Inauguration of a naval race among world powers after 1890 was inspired by Admiral Mahan's *Influence of Sea Power Upon History*, but the pressure for expansion and imperialistic adventure already existed. Adolf Hitler might well have remained an unknown Austrian house painter except for the chaos in Germany following World War I.

On the other hand, like slow fuses, there are books which did not make their full impact until years after their initial publication. Adam Smith and Karl Marx, to illustrate, were dead when the importance of their books was perceived. Thoreau had been gone half a century when his doctrine of civil disobedience was applied by Mahatma Ghandi in India and South Africa. Not until the rise of the German school of geopoliticians under Haushofer's direction did Mackinger's theories, formulated several decades earlier, receive the notice they deserved. These are among the names of pioneering thinkers who knew the disappointment of having their first editions go begging.

Also a recurring question in the back of one's mind... is this: how can influence be measured? Frequently, a book has attempted to find a solution to problems in a limited field at some particular period. Dealing as they do, therefore, with timely and topical matters, such books inevitably tend to date more rapidly than the great works of religion, philosophy, or literature.

Adapted from Robert B. Downs, *Books That Changed The World*. © 1956 by Robert B. Downs

127. Elsewhere in his writing, the author states: "Wherever tyrants have wanted to suppress opposition, their first thought, almost invariably has been to destroy books..." This would most support the claim that:
   A. books are of slight significance for the hard-headed man of affairs.
   B. historically, only dictators have realized the potential of books.
   C. books are peaceful objects which provide retreats from a materialistic world.
   D. no one realizes better than the despot, the enormous explosive forces pent up in books.

128. Implicit in the passage is the assumption that the reaction of the American people to the action of the U.S. State Department, stemmed from:
   A. a strong belief in the precepts of democracy.
   B. the fact that the masses had been irreversibly indoctrinated by books.
   C. the naive belief that all published material must be good.
   D. their support for censorship of morally questionable books only.

129. According to the passage, throughout history, different books have been influential in:
   I. triggering the American Revolution and Civil War.
   II. readying England for a vast expansion of her commercial and industrial economies.
   III. fuelling Hitler's rise to power.

   A. I only
   B. I and II only
   C. II and III only
   D. I, II and III

130. The author's comparison of books which make their full impact years after their initial publication, is most effective when one considers:
   A. the first edition of many magazines and comics increase in value over time.
   B. publishing in America is a multibillion dollar industry.
   C. Karl Marx published *The Communist Manifesto* in 1848, by 1920 there were millions of communists.
   D. more books are printed today than ever before.

131. The author's discussion of books in the last paragraph, suggests that he believes that:
   A. a science textbook would become outdated faster than a text on philosophy.
   B. religious texts are never outdated.
   C. books dealing with a limited field have little value.
   D. books should be written as to maximize influence.

Passage IX (Questions 132-137)

It was a rainy day in August, 1995, Mayor Takashi Hiraoka shed some light: "Until now, Hiroshima has been a symbol of tragedy, but we have a vision to become a city that gives others hope and courage to live."

The ceremonies, the dedications, the interviews have come and gone. However, the atomic bomb that exploded at 8:15 am on August 6, 1945, released a blast that continues to reverberate today. Compassion is stirred by images of civilians buried under glass and debris, heat that scorched everything within a three mile radius, infants on the periphery whose skin simply melted committing them to bleed to death or succumb slowly and painfully to overwhelming infection. One day, one bomb, one hundred thousand civilians died. "Little Boy" ushered in the atomic age.

Of course one cannot forget that Japan was not simply a benign victim of American aggression. We cannot make the mistake of forgetting Pearl Harbor. Japan was one of the Axis powers which, like Germany, had malignant and destructive intentions, attitudes, and weapons. Only now a few politicians in Japan are admitting to the thousands of young Korean women and girls enslaved by the Japanese Imperial Army for sexual gratification. The brunt of Japanese terror was felt in China where millions died. Now the retired army medics have slowly come forth describing gruesome experiments performed on Chinese civilians, including vivisections (live dissections without anaesthetic).

President Harry S. Truman had much to consider the day he ordered Enola Gay to drop Little Boy. Incendiary bombing had laid waste to many Japanese cities, including Tokyo, where conventional bombing had killed 100 000 people. The Japanese refused an unconditional surrender. To make matters more complex, Soviet leader Joseph Stalin, knowing the outcome in Germany, was free to turn his communist gaze towards Japan. In fact, when Truman and Stalin met in Potsdam in July, 1945, it appears Stalin proclaimed his interest in entering the war on or about August 15...

The most openly debated issue concerning the use of the bomb is the preservation of American lives. Thousands of American lives had already been sacrificed in Asia and Europe. How many more would die? Some said as few as 25 000, others suggested over 500 000 Americans would die in an invasion of Japan. Little Boy would prevent their deaths.

Even after August 6 had passed, the Japanese would not surrender. Nagasaki followed. Even in the face of certain defeat diehard generals argued against surrender and had to be overruled by Emperor Hirohito. Surrender came August 14, the peace treaty was signed September 2. The debate would soon mushroom.

Was the A-bomb necessary? Many historians feel that the Japanese commitment to war meant more Japanese and American lives would be spared even if one factors in the use of both atomic weapons. Was Little Boy the necessary evil which hastened the end of World War II?

Ultimately, death and destruction are replaced by birth and rebuilding. They are always looking for more English teachers in Japan. Baseball is very popular. Michael Jackson sang before thousands in sold-out stadiums. Hiroshima is a budding metropolis of 1.1 million people, with wide, tree-lined streets. Mayor Takashi was quite correct.

132. Which of the following could be reasonably inferred by the author's writing:
    A. one should keep in mind the human suffering which accompanies war.
    B. war is usually necessary.
    C. history books should stick to objective facts and avoid subjective commentary.
    D. specific dates, times and other numbers are unimportant.

133. The author refers to "Little Boy" and "Enola Gay" which are likely code names for:
    A. the atomic bomb and the plane that delivered it to Hiroshima, respectively.
    B. the Axis and the Allies, respectively.
    C. the name of the plan and the target site, respectively.
    D. the bombing plane and the A-bomb, respectively.

134.	In paragraph 4, the author suggests that Stalin may have been interested in the war in Japan since:
A. he did not like the Japanese.
B. he wanted to help his American friends.
C. the war in Germany had been won, he had troops available for further conquests.
D. the war in Germany was hopeless, he wanted to try elsewhere.

135.	The author implies that President Truman's position on the Soviets' intent to enter the war:
A. was positive, since it might lower American casualties.
B. may have influenced the timing of when the A-bomb was used.
C. was negative, Stalin likely supported the Axis powers.
D. was marked by bewilderment and great surprise.

136.	The author explored the following main conflicts EXCEPT:
I.	modern Japan vs. American culture.
II.	imperialist Japan vs. images of suffering Japanese.
III.	lives preserved vs. lives sacrificed.

A. I only
B. II only
C. III only
D. None of the above.

137.	The main theme of the passage is:
A. the atomic bomb should be used as often as necessary.
B. war is terrible for all, but hope lets humans prosper.
C. the Japanese are violent people.
D. the Soviets could not be trusted.

END OF VERBAL REASONING. IF TIME REMAINS, YOU MAY GO BACK AND CHECK YOUR WORK IN THIS TEST BOOKLET.

TEST GS-1

Writing Sample
Questions : 2
Time : 60 Minutes
Two 30 Minute Prompts,
Timed Separately

OPEN BOOKLET ONLY WHEN TIMER IS READY.

The Gold Standard MCAT* has been designed exclusively to test knowledge and thinking skills. The exam may contain hypothetical statements and/or express controversial ideas. Statements contained herein do not necessarily reflect the policy, position, or view of RuveneCo Publishing.

* MCAT is a registered service mark of the Association of American Medical Colleges, which is not associated with this product.

WRITING SAMPLE

INSTRUCTIONS: This test is designed to evaluate your writing skills. There are two writing assignments. You will have 30 minutes to complete each part.

Your answers for the Writing Sample should be written in ANSWER DOCUMENT 2. Your response to Part 1 must be written only on answer sheets marked " 1 ," and your response to Part 2 on answer sheets marked " 2 ." The first 30 minutes may be used to respond to Part 1 only. The second 30 minutes may be used to respond to Part 2 only. If you finish writing before time is up, you may review your work ONLY on the response you have just completed.

Use your time in an efficient manner. Prior to writing your response, read the assignment carefully. The space below each writing assignment may be used to make notes in planning a response.

Since this is a test of your writing skills, you should use complete sentences as well organized as you can make them in the allotted time. Corrections or additions can be made neatly between the lines but there should be no writing in the margins of the answer booklet.

There are three pages in the answer document for each part of the test. Though you are not expected to use each page, do not skip lines.

Use a black pen to write your response.

Illegible essays cannot be scored.

PART I

Consider the following statement:

A politician's role should be that of a nation's leader, not a public servant.

Write a unified essay performing the following tasks. Explain the meaning of the statement. Describe a specific situation in which a politician's role should be that of a public servant. Discuss what you think determines whether a politician's role should be that of a nation's leader or a public servant.

DO NOT TURN TO THE NEXT PAGE UNTIL TIME PERMITS.

PART II

Consider the following statement:

If science could create anything, it should do so freely.

Write a unified essay performing the following tasks. Explain the meaning of the statement. Describe a specific situation in which science should not create freely. Discuss what you think determines whether or not science should create anything freely.

END OF WRITING SAMPLE.
DO NOT RETURN TO PART I.

TEST GS-1

Biological Sciences
Questions 143-219
Time : 100 Minutes

OPEN BOOKLET ONLY WHEN TIMER IS READY.

The Gold Standard MCAT* has been designed exclusively to test knowledge and thinking skills. The exam may contain hypothetical statements and/or express controversial ideas. Statements contained herein do not necessarily reflect the policy, position, or view of RuveneCo Publishing.

* MCAT is a registered service mark of the Association of American Medical Colleges, which is not associated with this product.

BIOLOGICAL SCIENCES

INSTRUCTIONS: Of the 77 questions in the Biological Sciences test, 62 are organized into groups preceded by a passage. After evaluating the passage, select the best answer to each question in the group. Fifteen questions are independent of any descriptive passage or each other. Similarly, select the best answer to these questions. If you are unsure of an answer, eliminate the alternatives that you know to be incorrect and select an answer from the remaining alternatives. To indicate your selection, blacken the corresponding oval on Answer Document 1, GS-1. A periodic table is provided for your use during the test.

PERIODIC TABLE OF THE ELEMENTS

1 H 1.008																	2 He 4.003
3 Li 6.941	4 Be 9.012											5 B 10.81	6 C 12.011	7 N 14.007	8 O 15.999	9 F 18.998	10 Ne 20.179
11 Na 22.990	12 Mg 24.305											13 Al 26.982	14 Si 28.086	15 P 30.974	16 S 32.06	17 Cl 35.453	18 Ar 39.948
19 K 39.098	20 Ca 40.08	21 Sc 44.956	22 Ti 47.90	23 V 50.942	24 Cr 51.996	25 Mn 54.938	26 Fe 55.847	27 Co 58.933	28 Ni 58.70	29 Cu 63.546	30 Zn 65.38	31 Ga 69.72	32 Ge 72.59	33 As 74.922	34 Se 78.96	35 Br 79.904	36 Kr 83.80
37 Rb 85.468	38 Sr 87.62	39 Y 88.906	40 Zr 91.22	41 Nb 92.906	42 Mo 95.94	43 Tc (98)	44 Ru 101.07	45 Rh 102.906	46 Pd 106.4	47 Ag 107.868	48 Cd 112.41	49 In 114.82	50 Sn 118.69	51 Sb 121.75	52 Te 127.60	53 I 126.905	54 Xe 131.30
55 Cs 132.905	56 Ba 137.33	57 *La 138.906	72 Hf 178.49	73 Ta 180.948	74 W 183.85	75 Re 186.207	76 Os 190.2	77 Ir 192.22	78 Pt 195.09	79 Au 196.967	80 Hg 200.59	81 Tl 204.37	82 Pb 207.2	83 Bi 208.980	84 Po (209)	85 At (210)	86 Rn (222)
87 Fr (223)	88 Ra 226.025	89 **Ac 227.028	104 Unq (261)	105 Unp (262)	106 Unh (263)												

*	58 Ce 140.12	59 Pr 140.908	60 Nd 144.24	61 Pm (145)	62 Sm 150.4	63 Eu 151.96	64 Gd 157.25	65 Tb 158.925	66 Dy 162.50	67 Ho 164.930	68 Er 167.26	69 Tm 168.934	70 Yb 173.04	71 Lu 174.967
**	90 Th 232.038	91 Pa 231.036	92 U 238.029	93 Np 237.048	94 Pu (244)	95 Am (243)	96 Cm (247)	97 Bk (247)	98 Cf (251)	99 Es (254)	100 Fm (257)	101 Md (258)	102 No (259)	103 Lr (260)

Passage I (Questions 143-148)

The process of depolarization triggers the cardiac cycle. The electronics of the cycle can be monitored by an electrocardiogram (EKG). The cycle is divided into two major phases, both named for events in the ventricle: the period of ventricular contraction and blood ejection, *systole*, followed by the period of ventricular relaxation and blood filling, *diastole*.

During the very first part of systole, the ventricles are contracting but all valves in the heart are closed thus no blood can be ejected. Once the rising pressure in the ventricles becomes great enough to open the aortic and pulmonary valves, the ventricular ejection or systole occurs. Blood is forced into the aorta and pulmonary trunk as the contracting ventricular muscle fibers shorten. The volume of blood ejected from a ventricle during systole is termed *stroke volume*.

During the very first part of diastole, the ventricles begin to relax, and the aortic and pulmonary valves close. No blood is entering or leaving the ventricles since once again all the valves are closed. Once ventricular pressure falls below atrial pressure, the atrioventricular (AV) valves open. Atrial contraction occurs towards the end of diastole, after most of the ventricular filling has taken place. The ventricle receives blood throughout most of diastole, not just when the atrium contracts.

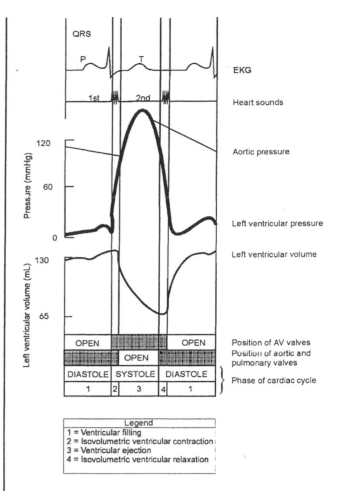

Figure 1: Electronic and pressure changes in the heart and aorta during the cardiac cycle.

143. Position P on the EKG of Fig. 1 probably corresponds to:
    A. atrial contraction.
    B. ventricular contraction.
    C. the beginning of ventricular systole.
    D. the beginning of ventricular diastole.

144. The first heart sound represented in Fig. 1 is probably made when:
    A. during ventricular systole, blood in the ventricle is forced against the closed atrioventricular valve.
    B. during ventricular diastole, blood in the arteries is forced against the aortic and pulmonary artery pocket valves.
    C. during ventricular diastole, blood in the ventricle is forced against the closed atrioventricular valve.
    D. during ventricular systole, blood in the arteries is forced against the aortic and pulmonary artery pocket valves.

145. Would the walls of the atria or ventricles expected to be thicker?
    A. Atria, because blood ejection due to atrial contraction is high.
    B. Atria, because blood ejection due to atrial contraction is low.
    C. Ventricles, because ventricular stroke volume is high.
    D. Ventricles, because ventricular stroke volume is low.

146. The graph below shows the effects on stroke volume of stimulating the sympathetic nerves to the heart.

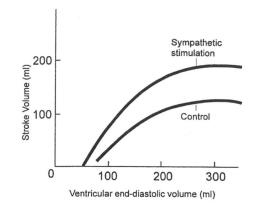

According to the graph, the net result of sympathetic stimulation on stroke volume is to:

A. approximately double stroke volume at any given end-diastolic volume.

B. decrease stroke volume at any given end-diastolic volume.

C. increase stroke volume at any given end-diastolic volume.

D. leave stroke volume relatively unchanged.

147. The wall of the left ventricle is at least three times as thick as that of the right ventricle. This feature aids circulation by assuring that:

A. blood entering the pulmonary artery is at a much higher pressure than blood entering the aorta.

B. blood entering the aorta is at a much higher pressure than blood entering the pulmonary artery.

C. the left ventricle has a higher blood capacity than the right ventricle at all times.

D. the right ventricle has a higher blood capacity than the left ventricle at all times.

148. According to Fig. 1, the opening of the aortic and pulmonary valves is NOT associated with:

A. ventricular systole.

B. a rise and fall in aortic pressure.

C. a drop and rise in left ventricular volume.

D. the third phase of the cardiac cycle.

Sweat is a watery fluid containing between 0.1 and 0.4% sodium chloride, sodium lactate and urea. It is less concentrated than blood plasma and is secreted by the activity of sweat glands under the control of pseudomotor neurons. These neurons are part of the sympathetic nervous system and they relay impulses from the hypothalamus.

When sweat evaporates from the skin surface, energy as latent heat of evaporation is lost from the body and this reduces body temperature. Experiments have now confirmed that sweating only occurs as a result of a rise in core body temperature. Blood from the carotid vessels flows to the hypothalamus and these experiments have indicated its role in thermoregulation. Inserting a thermistor against the eardrum gives an acceptable estimate of hypothalamic temperature.

149. The transport of electrolytes in sweat from blood plasma to the sweat glands is best accounted for by which of the following processes?
A. Osmosis
B. Simple diffusion
C. Active transport
D. All of the above

150. Drinking iced water results in a lowering of core body temperature. Thus, exposing the skin to heat while drinking iced water would result in which of the following?
A. An increase in sweating
B. A decrease in sweating
C. An increase in sweating followed by a decrease in sweating
D. No change in sweat production

Questions 151-153 refer to Fig. 1

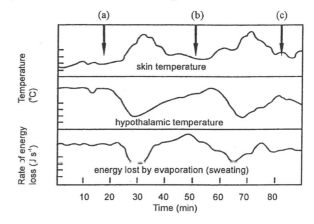

Figure 1: The relation between skin temperature, hypothalamic temperature and rate of evaporation for a human in a warm chamber (45 °C). Iced water is swallowed at points labelled (a), (b) and (c).

151. During the first 20 minutes the temperature and evaporation rate remain relatively constant because during this time:
A. evaporation was at a minimum.
B. the energy loss was not constant.
C. the subject was allowed to equilibrate with his surroundings.
D. 45 °C was considerably higher than the mean body temperature.

152. The relationship between hypothalamic temperature and rate of sweating could be best described as:
A. direct, suggesting that the rate of sweating is controlled by hypothalamic activity.
B. direct, suggesting that hypothalamic activity is controlled by the rate of sweating.
C. inverse, suggesting that changes in the rate of sweating occur in the opposite direction to changes in hypothalamic temperature.
D. independent, suggesting that the rate of sweating and hypothalamic activity change independently of each other.

153. Shortly after ingestion of the iced water, skin temperature rises. This can best be explained by which of the following?

   A. As the evaporation rate falls, latent heat is no longer being lost from the skin, causing a rise in skin temperature.

   B. The unusually high temperature of the chamber over the 30 minute period caused the rise in temperature.

   C. The skin temperature rose to counteract the disturbance in body temperature caused by ingestion of the iced water.

   D. Change in skin temperature always occurs in the opposite direction to change in hypothalamic temperature.

Passage III (Questions 154-159)

Yeast are single-celled organisms of the *Saccharomyces* genus. There exists an obligate anaerobic mutant of yeast. These "petite" mutants inherit the wild-type or petite mitochondrial phenotype in a nonchromosomal fashion. Thus a mutable substance in the cytoplasm is implicated in the synthesis of a mitochondrion.

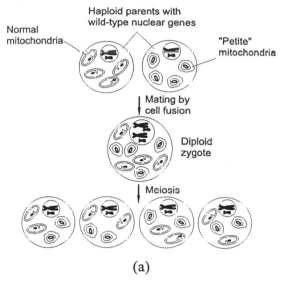

(a)

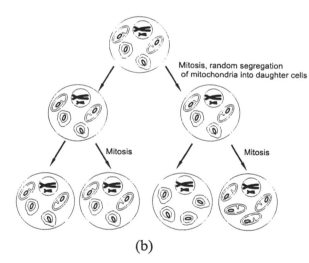

(b)

Figure 1: Cytoplasmic inheritance in yeast. (a) Haploid cells fuse producing a diploid cell that undergoes meiosis. All products of meiosis usually contain both normal and petite mitochondria. (b) As these cells divide mitotically, the cytoplasm, including mitochondria, is randomly distributed to the daughter cells.

154. Wild-type mutants are probably called "petite" mutants because:
    A. the size of the chromosomes in the mutants are smaller than normal.
    B. the size of the mutant colonies are smaller than normal.
    C. the size of the nuclear envelope of the mutants is smaller than normal.
    D. the daughter cells produced by the mutants are smaller than the mitochondria of normal yeast cells.

155. The most probable cause of the mutation in the wild-type mutant is:
    A. an inversion in the nuclear DNA.
    B. a deletion in the mitochondrial DNA.
    C. endomitosis.
    D. translocation of a chromosome.

156. The passage indicates that "petite" mutants differ from regular cells in terms of their:
    A. ability to produce ATP.
    B. ability to ferment glucose to ethanol.
    C. ability to carry out cell fusion.
    D. relative sizes.

157. During which of the following processes can complete cytoplasmic inheritance of the "petite" mutation occur?
    A. Meiotic division
    B. Mitotic division
    C. The time gap between the meiotic and mitotic divisions
    D. Metaphase

158. In which of the following cells, could a respiratory deficiency be present?
    A. The diploid zygote resulting after fusion
    B. The daughter cells of the meiotic division
    C. The daughter cells of the mitotic division
    D. The parent cell with the normal mitochondria

159. In humans, a cancer cell loses its ability to divide in a normal fashion. The source of this abnormality is likely in the cell's:
    A. lysosomes.
    B. Golgi apparatus.
    C. DNA.
    D. tRNA.

Questions 160-164 are NOT based on a descriptive passage.

160. Benzene reacts with bromine to form bromobenzene, but the reaction requires the use of an appropriate Lewis acid catalyst such as ferric bromide.

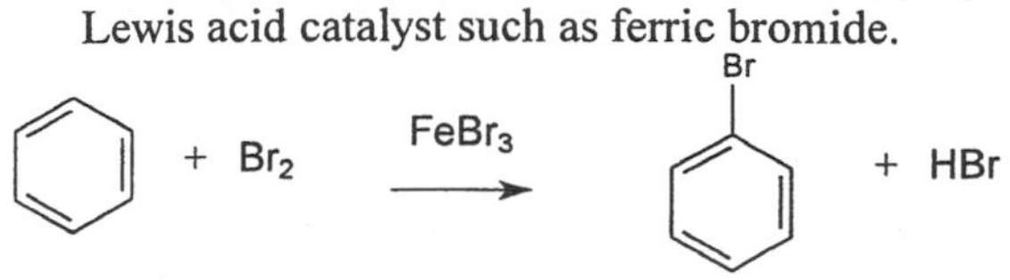

Reaction I

It is reasonable to assume that Reaction I will proceed via which of the following reaction mechanisms?

A. Nucleophilic substitution first order
B. Nucleophilic substitution second order
C. Electrophilic substitution first order
D. Electrophilic substitution second order

161. A biologically active agent, which completely diffuses through capillary beds, is injected into the brachiocephalic vein of the left arm. Which of the following would be most affected by the agent?

A. Heart
B. Lung
C. Left arm
D. Right arm

162. Which of the following does NOT follow normal anatomic sequence?

I. gametogenesis → seminal vesicles → seminiferous tubules
II. seminiferous tubules → epididymis → vas deferens
III.vas deferens → ejaculatory duct → urethra

A. I only
B. II only
C. I and II only
D. II and III only

163. Acid catalysts such as *p*-toluensulfonic acid are often used to dehydrate alcohols. The role of the acid catalyst is to:

A. increase $\Delta G°$ and increase the activation energy for the dehydration reaction.
B. increase $\Delta G°$ and lower the activation energy for the dehydration reaction.
C. maintain $\Delta G°$ at the same value and lower the activation energy for the dehydration reaction.
D. lower $\Delta G°$ and increase the activation energy for the dehydration reaction.

164. The reaction between a secondary alkyl halide and a base would tend to yield a higher percentage of elimination product by treatment with:

A. a very weak base which is also a very hindered electrophile.
B. a very weak base which is also a very hindered nucleophile.
C. a very strong base which is also a very hindered electrophile.
D. a very strong base which is also a very hindered nucleophile.

Proteins are frequently adorned by straight-chain or branched oligosaccharides, in which case they are called glycoproteins. This type of modification can serve a variety of functions. It can stabilize the protein, facilitate its correct folding, be part of a lipid anchor for attaching the protein to a membrane, or provide the protein with surface characteristics that facilitate its recognition.

The carbohydrate group or *moiety* in a glycoprotein is attached to the polypeptide chain by a covalent connection to certain amino acid side chains. Two types of glycosidic linkages are commonly found: the O-glycosidic linkage involves attachment of the carbohydrate to the hydroxyl group of serine, threonine, or hydroxylysine; the N-glycosidic linkage involves attachment to the amide group of asparagine.

Glycoproteins are found in all cellular compartments and are also secreted from the cell. Collagen, a secreted glycoprotein of the extracellular matrix, has simple carbohydrates - the disaccharide Glcβ(1,2) Gal linked to hydroxylysine.

Glycolipids are lipids modified with carbohydrate attachments. They fit into the structure of the membrane because of their long hydrophobic tails. There are various places where they occur particularly concentrated, one of which is on the surface of nerve cells. The myelin sheath is composed of specific lipids that are crucial to insulate nerve cells. It is also found on the synapse of the nerve ending and has particular lipids attached.

165. In which of the following cellular components would the greatest proportion of glycoproteins be expected?
   A. Lysosomes
   B. Microfilaments
   C. Mitochondria
   D. Phospholipid bilayer

166. Oligosaccharide modification most likely occurs in the:
   A. smooth endoplasmic reticulum.
   B. Golgi apparatus.
   C. lysosomes.
   D. cytosol.

167. Glycoprotein formation would be most affected by treating a protein with an agent which destroyed its:
   A. hydrophobic bonds.
   B. Van der Waals bonds.
   C. covalent bonds.
   D. electrostatic bonds.

168. If a base mutation occurred in cells so that all the hydroxylysine residues were replaced by asparagine residues in the amino acid side chains, which of the following would result?
   A. Glycoprotein formation would cease.
   B. The strength of loose connective tissue might be affected.
   C. Protein folding could not occur.
   D. Protein recognition would be impossible.

169. Which of the following processes would be LEAST affected by a reduction in a cell's ability to produce glycolipids?
   A. The passage of nervous impulses from one neuron to another.
   B. The passage of nervous impulses along the length of the axon.
   C. The initial generation of a nerve impulse as a result of depolarization.
   D. The passage of nervous impulses along the length of the dendrite.

170. The passage indicates that the functions of which of the following cells or cellular components would be most affected by an irregularity in glycolipid production?
   A. Nerves lying in grooves on the surface of the neurolemma of glial cells
   B. The nodes of Ranvier
   C. Schwann cells
   D. Cell bodies of neurons

Passage V (Questions 171-176)

Sickle cell anemia in humans is an example of a mutation affecting a base in one of the genes involved in the production of hemoglobin. Hemoglobin, in adults, is made up of four polypeptide chains attached to the prosthetic group heme. The polypeptide chains influence the oxygen-carrying capacity of the molecule. A change in the base sequence of the triplet coding for one amino acid out of the normal 146 amino acids in the β chains gives rise to the production of sickle cell hemoglobin. The physiological effect of this is to lower the oxygen-carrying capacity of these red blood cells. In the heterozygous condition individuals show the sickle-cell trait. The red blood cells appear normal and only about 40% of the hemoglobin is abnormal.

A gene represented by two or more alleles within a population is said to be *polymorphic*. Allelic differences are caused by sequence differences, that is, the DNA itself is polymorphic and results in sequence differences between homologous regions of DNA in different individuals. These differences can be detected even when no other differences can be found and knowledge of this polymorphism could be used for the pre- or postnatal diagnosis for the sickle-cell gene.

Rather than directly sequencing a gene, differences called restriction fragment length polymorphisms (RFLPs) can be used to highlight the regions of sequence differences between individuals. The technique depends on a restriction enzyme making a cut at a site on the gene for normal hemoglobin, not present on sickle-cell hemoglobin, causing fragments cut by the given enzyme to be smaller than it is in individuals not possessing the site.

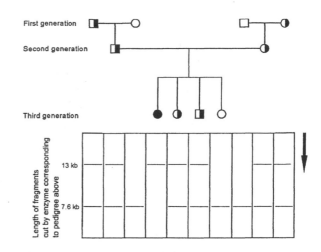

Figure 1: Inheritance pattern of an RFLP associated with sickle-cell disease. Males are represented by squares and females by circles. An open square or circle indicates an individual who is homozygous normal. A half-filled square or circle indicates an individual with sickle-cell trait. A filled square or circle indicates a homozygous individual with sickle-cell disease. The direction of electrophoresis is indicated by an arrow.

171. The passage suggests that sickle-cell anemia involves a point mutation involving:
  A. the inversion of a valine residue with a glutamic acid residue in one of the polypeptide chains of hemoglobin.
  B. the deletion of a valine residue from a polypeptide chain in hemoglobin.
  C. the insertion of a valine residue into a polypeptide chain of hemoglobin.
  D. the substitution of a valine residue for a glutamic acid residue in a polypeptide chain of hemoglobin.

172. Which of the following biological processes will be most affected by the presence of the mutant gene for sickle cell anemia in an individual?
  A. Fermentation of pyruvate to lactate and ATP
  B. Production of pyruvate and ATP in glycolysis
  C. The production of carbon dioxide, water and ATP during the Kreb's cycle and oxidative phosphorylation
  D. The production of carbon dioxide and ATP from ADP in the electron transport chain

173. If the heterozygous male in the first generation in Fig. 1 was substituted with a homozygous male for the normal condition, the phenotypes of the third generation would be expected to be in the ratio of:
A. 1 normal : 2 sickle-cell trait : 1 sickle-cell.
B. 1 normal : 1 sickle-cell trait.
C. 2 normal : 1 sickle-cell trait : 1 sickle-cell.
D. 1 sickle-cell trait : 1 sickle-cell.

174. Fig. 1 indicates that the fragment cut by the restriction enzyme in an individual who is homozygous for the sickle-cell condition is:
A. 7.6 kb long.
B. 13 kb long.
C. 20.0 kb long.
D. 5.4 kb long.

175. The passage indicates that an area in which information from restriction fragment length polymorphism could have the most practical value is:
A. criminology.
B. epidemiology.
C. genetic counselling.
D. forensic research.

176. In parts of the world where malaria is endemic, individuals with sickle-cell trait cannot contract the disease. Which of the following is the most likely explanation for this?
A. The protozoan which causes malaria needs the amino acid altered by the point mutation to survive.
B. A closely linked gene to the mutated gene in anemic patients confers resistance to malaria.
C. The protozoan which causes malaria cannot live in red blood cells containing the abnormal hemoglobin.
D. There is too little oxygen in sickle cell patients to support the protozoan which causes malaria.

When a compound reacts with the solvent the process is referred to as a *sovolysis* reaction. A chemist studied the mechanisms of the solvolysis reactions of t-butyl bromide (t-BuBr) in pure ethanol, and in a mixed solvent system containing 80% ethanol and 20% water.

In Reaction I, t-BuBr was refluxed in ethanol containing an added portion of sodium ethoxide. The reaction was exceedingly rapid with a half life of only a few minutes. The solvolysis product A was produced along with a significant amount of product B. Compound A was found to be an ether that had a molecular formula of $C_6H_{14}O$. Compound B had a molecular formula of C_4H_8 and the ^1HNMR revealed the presence of vinylic protons.

The rate of reaction of t-butyl bromide is given by the following expression:

$$rate = k_1 [t\text{-BuBr}] + k_2 [t\text{-BuBr}][C_2H_5O^-]$$

Gaseous hydrogen chloride was bubbled slowly into a solution of Compound B in methylene chloride at 0 °C. This reaction yielded t-butyl chloride (Compound D).

In Reaction II, t-BuBr was refluxed in the mixed solvent system of 80% ethanol and 20% water. Three compounds were isolated: A, B and C.

The IR spectrum of Compound C indicated a very intense stretch centered at about 3,600 cm^{-1}. Compound C had a molecular formula of $C_4H_{10}O$. A mixture of Compound C and PBr_3 was allowed to react further, resulting in the reformation of t-BuBr.

177. What is the IUPAC name of Compound B?
A. 3,4-dimethyl propane
B. 2-methyl-1-propene
C. 2-methyl-2-butene
D. propene

178. What functional group is present in Compound C?
A. Ether
B. Carboxylic acid
C. Hydroxyl
D. Ketone

179. The rates of solvolysis of t-butyl chloride, bromide, and iodide are predicted to be different. Which of the following series best represents the arrangement of these tertiary alkyl halides in order of decreasing rates of solvolysis?
A. t-BuBr > t-BuI > t-BuCl
B. t-BuCl > t-BuI > t-BuBr
C. t-BuCl > t-BuBr > t-BuI
D. t-BuI > t-BuBr > t-BuCl

180. The solvolysis reaction of t-butyl bromide in pure ethanol to produce Compound A can be classified mechanistically as:
A. bimolecular nucleophilic substitution.
B. bimolecular electrophilic substitution.
C. unimolecular electrophilic substitution.
D. unimolecular nucleophilic substitution.

181. What type of intermediate was formed in both reactions I and II?
A. A carboxylic anion
B. A free radical
C. A carbocation
D. A carbanion

182. In Reaction II, t-butyl bromide gave 3 products via 3 reaction mechanisms.

$$(CH_3)_3 C\ Br \xrightarrow[\substack{H_2O \\ 25\,°C}]{EtOH}
\begin{cases}
\text{I} & A\ (29\%) \\
\text{II} & B\ (13\%) \\
\text{III} & C\ (58\%)
\end{cases}$$

Which of the following series is an acceptable mechanistic rationalization for processes I, II and III, leading to the formation of compounds A, B, and C, respectively?
A. S_N1, S_N1, E2
B. S_N1, E2, S_N1
C. S_N2, S_N1, E1
D. S_N2, S_N2, S_N1

183. Which of the following is the most accurate representation of the reaction coordinate diagram for the solvolysis of t-butyl bromide?

A.

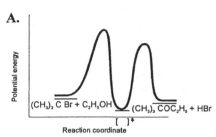

B.

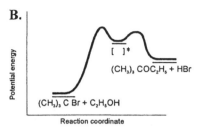

C.

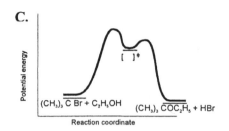

D.

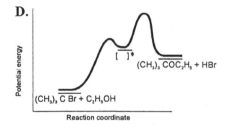

The combination of hemoglobin with oxygen can be affected not only by oxygen tension but also by pH, CO_2, and glycerate 2,3-biphosphate (GBP). GBP binds preferentially to the deoxygenated form of hemoglobin with a dissociation constant of about 10^{-5} M^{-1}. Its dissociation constant with HbO_2 is only about 10^{-3} M^{-1}. Since the concentrations of GBP and hemoglobin are both about 5 mM in the erythrocyte, we would expect most of the deoxy form to be complexed with GBP and most of the oxyhemoglobin to be free of GBP. The net effect of the GBP is to shift the oxygen-binding curve to higher oxygen tensions. This shift is not sufficient to lower the binding of oxygen at the high oxygen tensions in the capillaries of the lungs, but it is sufficient to cause a substantially greater release of oxygen at the lower oxygen tensions that exist where it is needed, that is, in the rest of the body tissues.

The myoglobin molecule is widely distributed in animals. It displays a great affinity for oxygen and in fact only begins to release oxygen when the partial pressure of oxygen is below 20 mmHg. In this way it acts as a store of oxygen, only releasing it when supplies of oxyhemoglobin have been exhausted.

184. Which of the following graphs represents the oxygen-binding curve in the presence of GBP?

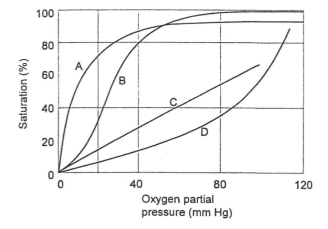

185. Glycerate 2,3-biphosphate functions to shift the oxygen binding curve by:
   A. increasing the carbon-dioxide concentration in the red blood cells.
   B. altering the pH of the tissue fluid surrounding the red blood cells.
   C. reducing the affinity between oxygen and hemoglobin at low oxygen concentrations.
   D. forming a complex with oxygen at low oxygen concentrations.

186. Which of the following graphs would you expect to represent the oxygen dissociation curve for myoglobin?

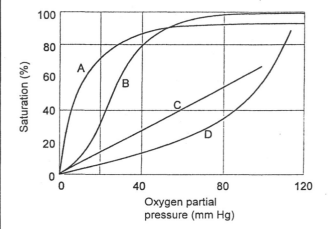

187. Which of the following tissues most benefits from the shifts in the oxygen-binding curves caused by GBP and myoglobin?
   A. Cardiac muscle tissue
   B. Skeletal muscle tissue
   C. Loose connective tissue
   D. Intestinal wall tissue

188. In regions with an increased partial pressure of carbon dioxide the oxygen dissociation curve is shifted to the right. This is known as the Bohr effect or shift. What is the physiological significance of this shift?
   A. It counteracts the shift in the oxygen-binding curve caused by the presence of GBP.
   B. It counteracts the shift in the oxygen-binding curve caused by the presence of myoglobin.
   C. It increases the pH of actively respiring tissue.
   D. It facilitates the delivery of increased quantities of oxygen from the blood to cells which produce energy.

189. Protons, like GBP, bind preferentially to deoxyhemoglobin. Thus, which of the following equations best explains the Bohr shift ?

A. $CO_2 + H_2O \rightleftharpoons H_2CO_3 \rightleftharpoons H^+ + HCO_3^-$ (tissues)

B. $H^+ + HbO_2 \rightleftharpoons HHb^+ + O_2$ (tissues)

C. $HCO_3^- + H^+ \rightleftharpoons H_2CO_3 \rightleftharpoons CO_2 + H_2O$ (lungs)

D. $HHB^+ + O_2 + HCO_3^- \rightleftharpoons HBO_2 + CO_2 + H_2O$
(lungs)

190. During embryogenesis, the three primary germ layers are first seen in which of the following?
    A. The morula
    B. The blastula
    C. The gastrula
    D. The neurula

191. A collection of nerve cell bodies in the central nervous system is generally referred to as a:
    A. nerve.
    B. conus.
    C. ganglion.
    D. nucleus.

192. Which is the dominant feature found in a newborn whose ductus arteriosus failed to obliterate?
    A. Increased O_2 partial pressure in pulmonary arteries
    B. Decreased CO_2 partial pressure in pulmonary arteries
    C. Increased O_2 partial pressure in systemic arteries
    D. Decreased O_2 partial pressure in systemic arteries

193. Which of the following is true about muscle contraction?
    A. Troponin and tropomyosin slide past one another allowing the muscle to shorten.
    B. Decreased intracellular $[Ca^{++}]$ enhances the degree of muscular contraction.
    C. Cardiac muscle fibers contain centrally located nuclei.
    D. Neither actin nor myosin change length during muscle contraction.

194. Which of the following represents the amino acid methionine at its isoelectric point?

A. $CH_3-S-CH_2-CH_2-\underset{\underset{NH_3^+}{|}}{\overset{\overset{H}{|}}{C}}-COO^-$

B. $CH_3-S-CH_2-CH_2-\underset{\underset{NH_3^+}{|}}{\overset{\overset{H}{|}}{C}}-COOH$

C. $CH_4^+-S-CH_2-CH_2-\underset{\underset{NH_2}{|}}{C}-COOH$

D. $CH_4^+-S-CH_2-CH_2-\underset{\underset{NH_3^+}{|}}{C}-COO^-$

Passage VIII (Questions 195-199)

The volume of air that flows into or out of an alveolus per unit time is directly proportional to the pressure difference between the atmosphere and alveolus and inversely proportional to the resistance to flow caused by the airways. During normal relaxed breathing, about 500 ml of air flows in and out of the lungs. This is the *tidal volume*. After expiration, approximately 2.5 liters of air remains in the lungs which is referred to as the *functional residual capacity*.

Airway resistance is: i) directly proportional to the magnitude of the viscosity between the flowing gas molecules; ii) directly proportional to the length of the airway; and iii) inversely proportional to the fourth power of the radius of the airway.

Resistance to air flow in the lung is normally small thus small pressure differences allow large volumes of air to flow. Physical, neural and chemical factors affect airway radii and therefore resistance. *Transpulmonary pressure* is a physical factor which exerts a distending force on the airways and alveoli. Such a force is critical to prevent small airways from collapsing.

The rate of respiration is primarily dependent on the concentration of carbon dioxide in the blood. As carbon dioxide levels rise, chemoreceptors in blood vessels are stimulated to discharge neuronal impulses to the respiratory center in the medulla oblongata in the brain stem. The respiratory center would then send impulses to the diaphragm causing an increase in the rate of contraction thus increasing the respiratory rate.

195. The *minute ventilation* is the tidal volume multiplied by the respiratory rate. Given a resting respiratory rate of 12 breaths per minute, what is the minute ventilation?
   A. 2.5 L/min
   B. 5.0 L/min
   C. 6.0 L/min
   D. 30 L/min

196. During inspiration, transpulmonary pressure should:
   A. increase, increasing airway radius and decreasing airway resistance.
   B. increase, increasing airway radius and increasing airway resistance.
   C. decrease, decreasing airway radius and decreasing airway resistance.
   D. decrease, decreasing airway radius and increasing airway resistance.

197. Lateral traction refers to the process by which connective tissue fibers maintain airway patency by continuously pulling outward on the sides of the airways. As the lungs expand these fibers become stretched. Thus during inspiration lateral traction acts:
   A. in the same direction as transpulmonary pressure, by increasing the viscosity of air.
   B. in the opposite direction to transpulmonary pressure, by decreasing the viscosity of air.
   C. in the same direction as transpulmonary pressure, by increasing the airway radius.
   D. in the opposite direction to transpulmonary pressure, by increasing the airway radius.

198. The chemoreceptors referred to in the passage are likely located in the:
   A. vena cava.
   B. pulmonary artery.
   C. femoral vein.
   D. aorta.

199. The Heimlich Maneuver is used to aid individuals who are choking on matter caught in the upper respiratory tract through the application of a sudden abdominal pressure with an upward thrust. The procedure probably works by:
   A. forcing the diaphragm downward, increasing thoracic size and causing a passive expiration.
   B. forcing the diaphragm upward, increasing thoracic size and causing a forced expiration.
   C. forcing the diaphragm upward, reducing thoracic size and causing a forced expiration.
   D. forcing the diaphragm upward, increasing thoracic size and causing a passive expiration.

Figure 1 illustrates a solubility based characterization procedure, often used by organic chemists, for the qualitative analysis of monofunctional organic compounds.

Table 1 lists the organic compounds comprising the various solubility classes of Fig. 1.

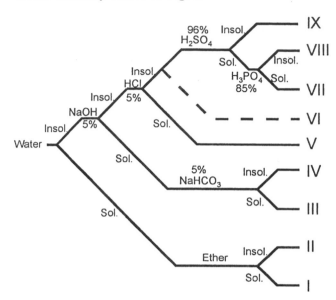

Figure 1

Table 1

Group	Compounds
I	Salts of organic acids, amino acids, amine chlorides Sugars (carbohydrates) and other polyfunctional compounds with hydrophilic groups
II	Arenesulfonic acids Monofunctional carboxylic acids, alcohols, ketones, aldehydes, esters, amides and nitriles with 5 or less carbon atoms Monofunctional amines with 6 or less carbon atoms
III	Phenols with ortho- and/or para- electron withdrawing groups, β-diketones Carboxylic acids with 6 or more carbon atoms
IV	Sulfonamides, nitro-compounds with α-hydrogens Phenols, oximes, enols, imides and thiophenols with 6 or more carbon atoms
V	Some oxy-ethers, anilines, aliphatic amines with 8 or more carbon atoms
VI	Neutral compounds containing sulfur or nitrogen with 6 or more carbon atoms
VII	Ethers with 7 or less carbon atoms Monofunctional esters, aldehydes, ketones, cyclic ketones, methyl ketones with between 6 and 8 carbon atoms; epoxides
VIII	Ethers, most other ketones Unsaturated hydrocarbons, aromatic compounds, particularly those which possess activating groups

200. Phenols are soluble in a strongly basic sodium hydroxide solution, and insoluble in dilute sodium bicarbonate. Phenol has a $pK_a = 10.0$. The introduction of an ortho bromine atom into the phenol would have the effect of:
   A. lowering the pK_a and thus decreasing the acidity of the phenol.
   B. lowering the pK_a and thus increasing the acidity of the phenol.
   C. increasing the pK_a and thus decreasing the acidity of the phenol.
   D. increasing the pK_a and thus increasing the acidity of the phenol.

201. A certain water insoluble compound is insoluble in 5% sodium hydroxide, insoluble in 5% HCl, and insoluble in concentrated H_2SO_4 and soluble in 5% sodium bicarbonate. In which class should this compound be classified?
   A. III
   B. IV
   C. VIII
   D. IX

202. Benzoic acid should be soluble in which of the following solvent pairs?
A. Water and 5% HCl
B. 5% NaOH and 5% $NaHCO_3$
C. 5% HCl and 5% NaOH
D. 85% H_3PO_4 and 5% NaOH

203. Low molecular weight amino acids fall into group I in Table 1. This is most likely due to the fact that low molecular weight amino acids are:
A. hydrophilic and basic.
B. hydrophobic and amphoteric.
C. hydrophobic and lipophilic.
D. hydrophilic and amphoteric.

204. A critical step in acid-catalyzed ester hydrolysis is the attack of water molecules on the protonated ester. If the water molecules are replaced with an alcohol, then the reaction will involve:
A. transesterification of one ester to another.
B. reduction to the corresponding aldehyde.
C. base-protonated ester hydrolysis to the corresponding acid.
D. decarboxylation to the corresponding C-H unit.

Carbohydrate intake per day ranges from about 300 to 800 grams in a typical American diet. About two-thirds of this carbohydrate is the plant polysaccharide starch, and most of the remainder consists of the disaccharides sucrose and lactose. Only small amounts of monosaccharides are normally present in the diet. Cellulose and certain other complex polysaccharides found in vegetable matter are not broken down in the small intestine. They are passed on to the large intestine, where they are partially metabolized by bacteria.

Starch digestion by salivary amylase begins in the mouth and continues in the upper part of the stomach before amylase is destroyed by gastric acid. Starch digestion is completed in the small intestine by pancreatic amylase. The products produced by both amylases are the disaccharide maltose and a mixture of short, branched chains of glucose molecules. These products, along with ingested sucrose and lactose, are then broken down into monosaccharides - glucose, galactose, and fructose - by enzymes located on the brush border membranes of the small intestine epithelial cells and transported across the intestinal epithelium into the blood.

205. All of the following could account for the large number of carbohydrates which exist in nature EXCEPT:
A. the ability of pentoses and hexoses to form furanose and pyranose rings.
B. the ability of monosaccharides to exhibit tautomerism.
C. the ability of monosaccharides to form optical isomers.
D. the existence of alpha and beta forms of glucose.

206. Cellulose is likely not broken down in the small intestine because:
A. it is actively transported from the lumen of the intestine, across the epithelial lining, in the polysaccharide form.
B. mastication, salivary amylase and enzymes in the upper part of the stomach completely break it down before it reaches the small intestine.
C. humans do not possess the enzymes that break down cellulose.
D. it is needed to propagate the necessary bacterial population in the large intestine.

207. In addition to starch, which of the following substances is also broken down by enzymes in the stomach?
A. Glucose
B. Fatty acids
C. Protein
D. Glycerol

208. After a meal rich in carbohydrates, monosacharides are likely transported across the epithelium primarily by:
A. diffusion.
B. exocytosis.
C. endocytosis.
D. carrier mediated transport.

209. From the lumen of the small intestine, fat products are absorbed by and transported to:
A. bile salts and the liver, respectively.
B. bile salts and the lymphatic system, respectively.
C. lacteals and the liver, respectively.
D. lacteals and the lymphatic system, respectively.

210. Along with gastric acid, a zymogen exists in the stomach. The enzyme exists in this form in order to:
A. prevent the enzyme's degradation while the stomach is empty.
B. prevent the enzyme from neutralizing the gastric acid in the stomach.
C. enhance the enzyme's activity.
D. prevent the enzyme from digesting the cells which produce it.

Testosterone, a steroid androgen, or male sex hormone, is synthesized according to the following pathway.

211. What is the product of the following reaction?

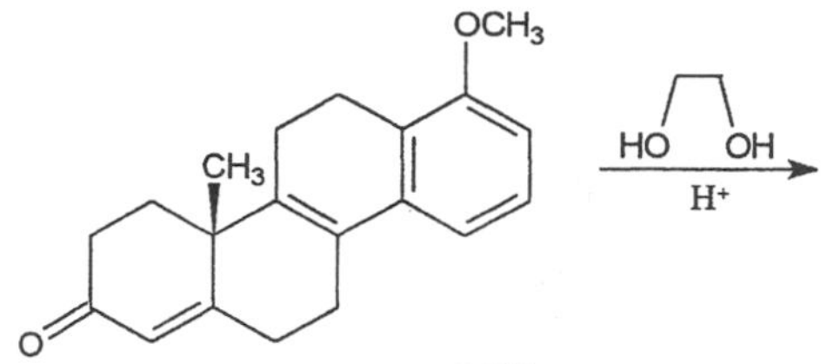

A.

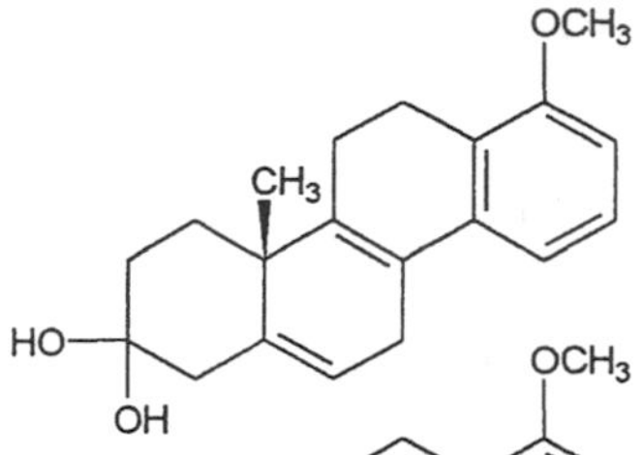

B.

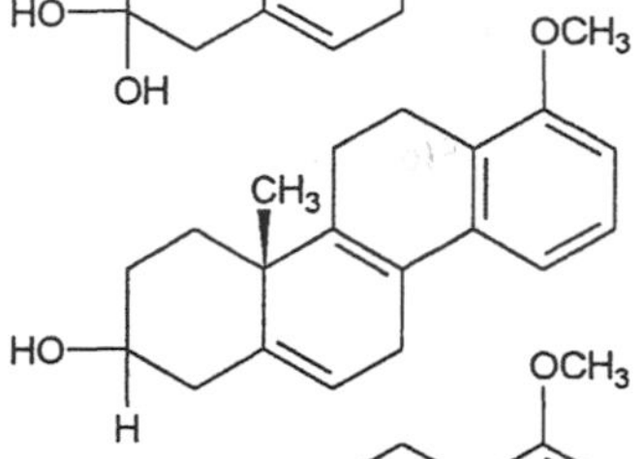

C.

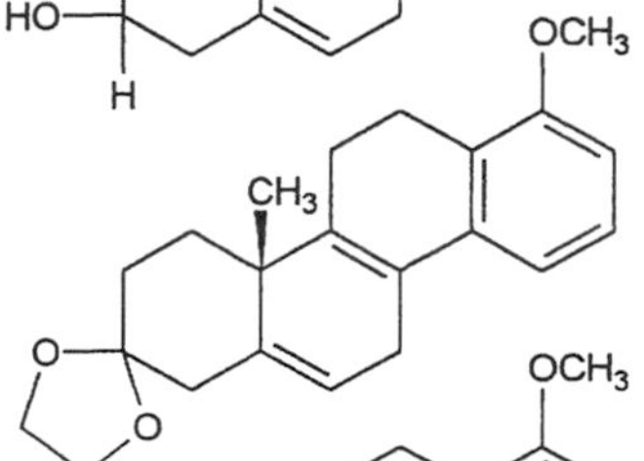

D.

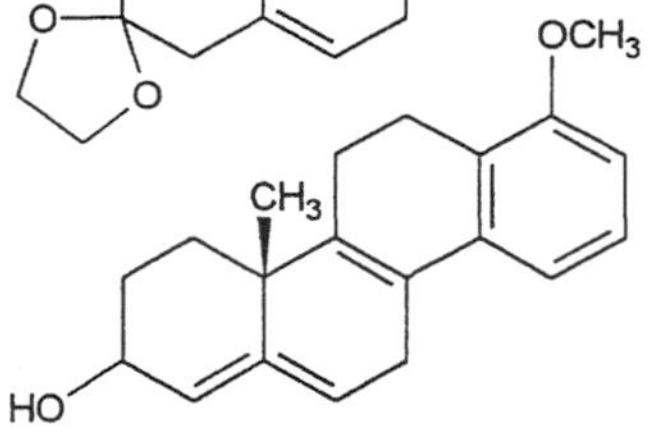

212. The synthesis of testosterone from the following precursor has been reported.

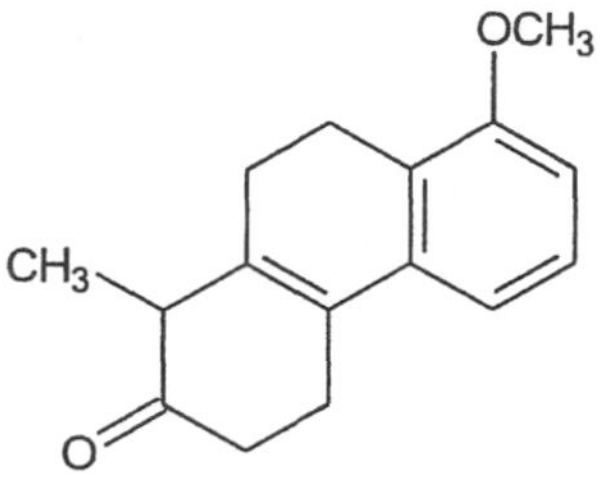

Which of the following is formed when a solution of the above compound is treated with lithium diisopropylamide (LDA), given that LDA is a hindered molecule whose conjugate acid has a pK_a of approximately 40?
A. A hemi-acetal
B. An enolate ion
C. A radical anion
D. A ketal

213. Step 1 generated a mixture of cyclohexene derivatives A and B. Products A and B can most easily be distinguished from each other by ¹HNMR because:
A. Product A has fewer vinylic protons than Product B.
B. Product A has more vinylic protons than Product B.
C. Product A has more protons than Product B.
D. Product A has more sigma bonds than Product B.

214. In the synthesis of testosterone, Step IX is what type of reaction?
A. A catalytic hydrogenation reaction
B. A reduction reaction
C. A saponification reaction
D. A dehydration reaction

215. The structure of 1,1-dichloroethane is shown below.

    If a beam of plane polarized light is passed through a large collection of 1,1-dichloroethane molecules, it would emerge with the plane of polarization having rotated:
    A. 0°
    B. 90°
    C. 60°
    D. 180°

216. Cartilage is likely to be found in all the following adult tissues EXCEPT:
    A. bronchus.
    B. tendons and ligaments.
    C. pinna of the ear.
    D. between the epiphysis and diaphysis of long bones.

217. *Apoptosis* refers to programmed cell death. The subunits of the component of a cell likely responsible for apoptosis are:
    A. proteins
    B. fatty acids
    C. nucleotides
    D. monosaccharides

218. Which of the following hormones, found in the human menstrual cycle, are produced in the ovary?

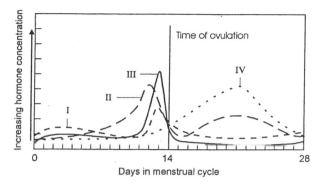

    A. I and II
    B. II and III
    C. III and IV
    D. II and IV

219. The structure of D-glucose is shown below:

    An alternative projection system, often used in carbohydrate chemistry is the Fischer system. Fischer projections are particularly useful devices for depicting the absolute configuration at the various stereocenters of a compound. Which of the following most accurately represents the modified Fischer projection of D-glucose?

    A.   B.   C.   D.

END OF BIOLOGICAL SCIENCES. IF TIME REMAINS, YOU MAY GO BACK AND CHECK YOUR WORK IN THIS BOOKLET.

TEST GS-2

Physical Sciences
Questions 1-77
Time : 100 Minutes

OPEN BOOKLET ONLY WHEN TIMER IS READY.

The Gold Standard MCAT* has been designed exclusively to test knowledge and thinking skills. The exam may contain hypothetical statements and/or express controversial ideas. Statements contained herein do not necessarily reflect the policy, position, or view of RuveneCo Publishing.

* MCAT is a registered service mark of the Association of American Medical Colleges, which is not associated with this product.

PHYSICAL SCIENCES

INSTRUCTIONS: Of the 77 questions in the Physical Sciences test, 62 are organized into groups preceded by a passage. After evaluating the passage, select the best answer to each question in the group. Fifteen questions are independent of any descriptive passage or each other. Similarly, select the best answer to these questions. If you are unsure of an answer, eliminate the alternatives that you know to be incorrect and select an answer from the remaining alternatives. To indicate your selection, blacken the corresponding oval on Answer Document 1, GS-2. A periodic table is provided for your use during the test.

PERIODIC TABLE OF THE ELEMENTS

1 H 1.008																		2 He 4.003
3 Li 6.941	4 Be 9.012											5 B 10.81	6 C 12.011	7 N 14.007	8 O 15.999	9 F 18.998	10 Ne 20.179
11 Na 22.990	12 Mg 24.305											13 Al 26.982	14 Si 28.086	15 P 30.974	16 S 32.06	17 Cl 35.453	18 Ar 39.948
19 K 39.098	20 Ca 40.08	21 Sc 44.956	22 Ti 47.90	23 V 50.942	24 Cr 51.996	25 Mn 54.938	26 Fe 55.847	27 Co 58.933	28 Ni 58.70	29 Cu 63.546	30 Zn 65.38	31 Ga 69.72	32 Ge 72.59	33 As 74.922	34 Se 78.96	35 Br 79.904	36 Kr 83.80
37 Rb 85.468	38 Sr 87.62	39 Y 88.906	40 Zr 91.22	41 Nb 92.906	42 Mo 95.94	43 Tc (98)	44 Ru 101.07	45 Rh 102.906	46 Pd 106.4	47 Ag 107.868	48 Cd 112.41	49 In 114.82	50 Sn 118.69	51 Sb 121.75	52 Te 127.60	53 I 126.905	54 Xe 131.30
55 Cs 132.905	56 Ba 137.33	57 *La 138.906	72 Hf 178.49	73 Ta 180.948	74 W 183.85	75 Re 186.207	76 Os 190.2	77 Ir 192.22	78 Pt 195.09	79 Au 196.967	80 Hg 200.59	81 Tl 204.37	82 Pb 207.2	83 Bi 208.980	84 Po (209)	85 At (210)	86 Rn (222)
87 Fr (223)	88 Ra 226.025	89 **Ac 227.028	104 Unq (261)	105 Unp (262)	106 Unh (263)												

*	58 Ce 140.12	59 Pr 140.908	60 Nd 144.24	61 Pm (145)	62 Sm 150.4	63 Eu 151.96	64 Gd 157.25	65 Tb 158.925	66 Dy 162.50	67 Ho 164.930	68 Er 167.26	69 Tm 168.934	70 Yb 173.04	71 Lu 174.967
**	90 Th 232.038	91 Pa 231.036	92 U 238.029	93 Np 237.048	94 Pu (244)	95 Am (243)	96 Cm (247)	97 Bk (247)	98 Cf (251)	99 Es (254)	100 Fm (257)	101 Md (258)	102 No (259)	103 Lr (260)

Passage I (Questions 1-6)

The invention of the compound microscope by Jansen in the late 1500's truly revolutionized the world of science, particularly the field of cellular and molecular biology. The discovery of the cell as the fundamental unit of living organisms and the insight into the bacterial world are two of the contributions of this instrument to science.

It is unseemly that such a relatively simplistic apparatus took generations to be developed. Its main components are two convex lenses: one acts as the main magnifying lens and is referred to as the objective, and another lens called the eyepiece. The two lenses act independently of each other when bending light rays. The actual lens set-up is depicted in Fig. 1.

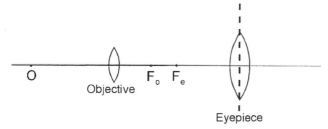

F_o = focal point of objective
F_e = focal point of eyepiece

Figure 1

Light from the object (O) first passes through the objective and an enlarged, inverted first image is formed. The eyepiece then magnifies this image. Usually the magnification of the eyepiece is fixed (either ×10 or ×15) and three rotating objective lenses are used: ×10, ×40 and ×60. The most recent development in microscope technology is the electron microscope which uses a beam of electrons instead of light. Photographic film must be used otherwise no image would be formed on the retina. This microscope has a resolution about a hundred times that of the light microscope.

1.   Based on the passage, what type of image would have to be produced by the objective magnification?
   A. Either virtual or real
   B. Virtual
   C. Real
   D. It depends on the focal length of the lens

2.   Where would the first image have to be produced by the objective relative to the eyepiece such that a second, enlarged image would be generated on the same side of the eyepiece as the first image (first image distance = d_i)?
   A. $d_i < F_e$
   B. $d_i = F_e$
   C. $2 \times F_e > d_i > F_e$
   D. $d_i > 2 \times F_e$

3.   Two compound microscopes A and B were compared. Both had objectives and eyepieces with the same magnification but A gave an overall magnification that was greater than that of B. Which of the following is a plausible explanation?
   A. The distance between objective and eyepiece in A is greater than the corresponding distance in B.
   B. The distance between objective and eyepiece in A is less than the corresponding distance in B.
   C. The eyepiece and objective positions were reversed in A.
   D. The eyepiece and objective positions were reversed in B.

4. A student attempted to make a compound microscope. However, when she tried to view an object through the apparatus, no image was seen. Which of the following could explain the mishap?
   I   The object distance = focal length of objective
   II   The object distance for eyepiece = focal length of eyepiece
   III The student used a diverging lens as her eyepiece
   IV The student used a converging lens as her objective

   A. I, II, III, and IV
   B. I, II, III
   C. I, II, IV
   D. II, III, IV

5. The magnification of the eyepiece of a compound microscope is ×15. The image height is 25 mm and the magnification of the objective is ×40. What is the object height?
    A. 1.67 mm
    B. 0.60 mm
    C. 0.38 mm
    D. 0.04 mm

6. What is the refractive power of an objective lens with a focal length of 0.50 cm?
    A. 0.2 diopters
    B. 2.0 diopters
    C. 20 diopters
    D. 200 diopters

Passage II (Questions 7-13)

1. When in the gaseous phase, hydrogen and chlorine react explosively in bright sunlight (slowly in the dark) to yield hydrogen chloride gas.

$$H_2 + Cl_2 \rightleftharpoons 2HCl$$

Reaction I

It is quite interesting to note that although this method of producing hydrogen chloride is both inexpensive and has a low energy requirement, it is not the method preferred in industry.

The HCl can be separated from the excess hydrogen and chlorine by either liquifying the HCl, which has a higher boiling point than the other two gases, or by dissolving the hydrogen chloride in water because it is more soluble than the other two gases.

Hydrochloric acid, produced when the HCl is dissolved in water, acts as a strong acid in solution. Because of this, it is often used to determine the concentration of bases, especially weak ones such as aniline which dissolves in water as shown in Reaction II.

$$C_6H_5NH_2 + H_2O \rightleftharpoons C_6H_5NH_3^+ + OH^-$$

Reaction II

A 20.00 mL aliquot of aniline was titrated with 0.01 M HCl and a few of the values of the titration are shown in Table 1.

Table 1

Volume of HCl added (mL)	pH
0.0	8.8
15.0	4.6
30.0	2.8

7. In the manufacture of HCl, 10 grams of chlorine gas were used. If the reaction went to completion and the hydrogen gas was in excess, how many grams of HCl were obtained?
A. 2.5
B. 5.1
C. 10.3
D. 20.0

8. Which of the following graphs accurately depicts the change in pH in Reaction II with increasing volumes of hydrochloric acid?

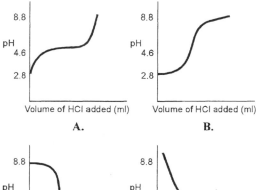

A.   B.

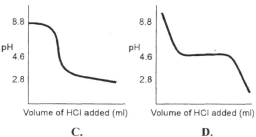

C.   D.

9. Aniline acts as a Lewis base because aniline:
A. exhibits hydrogen bonding.
B. has a lone pair of electrons on its nitrogen atom.
C. is an electron pair acceptor.
D. produces OH⁻ when in solution.

10. The most suitable acid/base indicator for the determination of the end point of the titration would probably have a pH range of:
A. 2.1-3.2.
B. 3.0-5.0.
C. 4.8-6.4.
D. 6.2-7.4.

11. The pH of the reaction mixture drops sharply near the equivalence point of the titration because:
A. the concentration of $C_6H_5NH_2$ decreases sharply.
B. the concentration of $C_6H_5NH_3^+$ decreases sharply.
C. the concentration of H^+ increases sharply.
D. the concentration of H^+ decreases sharply.

12. The passage states that HCl is expected to have a higher boiling point than either H_2 or Cl_2. The likely reason is that HCl:
A. exhibits hydrogen bonding, unlike H_2 and Cl_2.
B. has a greater molecular mass than either H_2 or Cl_2.
C. is less polar than either H_2 or Cl_2.
D. is a smaller molecule than H_2 and Cl_2.

13. Reaction I was carried out in the dark and stopped before equilibrium was reached. The partial pressure of Cl_2 was found to be 35 atm and the mole fraction of HCl found to be 0.40. If the total pressure of the system is 100 atm, what is the partial pressure of H_2?
A. 10 atm
B. 25 atm
C. 65 atm
D. 75 atm

Until 1940, the heaviest known atomic nucleus was that of uranium, with its atomic number of 92. However, with the advent of modern technology and some significant leaps of scientific deduction, thirteen new elements have been artificially manufactured, all from uranium and all with atomic numbers greater than 92. The first eight were prepared by successive neutron bombardments of uranium:

$$^{238}_{97}U \ + \ ^{1}_{0}n \ \rightarrow \ ^{239}_{93}Np \ + \ \beta^- \ + \ \overline{\nu} \qquad \textbf{Equation I}$$

This kind of reaction is not new. Transmutations such as this have been occurring in the stratosphere for thousands of years. Here, nitrogen is converted to carbon via a similar mechanism to that shown in Equation I.

$$^{14}_{7}N \ + \ ^{1}_{0}n \ \rightarrow \ ^{14}_{6}C \ + \ p \qquad \textbf{Equation II}$$

The only difference between these reactions is that a beta particle and another subatomic species called a *neutrino* are evolved from the former reaction while only a proton is obtained from the latter. This reaction, however, forms the basis of radiocarbon dating of organic remains. When organisms die, they stop replenishing their body's carbon-14 and a reverse process occurs.

$$^{14}_{6}C \ \rightarrow \ ^{14}_{7}N \ + \ \beta^- \ + \ \overline{\nu} \qquad \textbf{Equation III}$$

14. Why would a neutron be preferred to a proton for bombarding atomic nuclei?
    A. It is smaller than a proton.
    B. It weighs less than a proton.
    C. It has no charge.
    D. It can be obtained from a nucleus.

15. Which of the following types of radioactive emissions involves the emission of a helium nucleus?
    A. alpha decay
    B. beta decay
    C. gamma ray
    D. None of the above

16. A fossil was discovered in the forests of Africa and when examined, it was found that it had a carbon-14 activity of 10.8 disintegrations per minute per gram (dpm g^{-1}). If the average activity of carbon-14 in a living organism is 43.0 dpm g^{-1}, approximately how many half-lives have passed since the death of the organism?
    A. 8
    B. 4
    C. 3
    D. 2

17. A radioactive substance A was placed in a lead-lined container and the radiation it emitted was allowed to pass through a small aperture in the container and below a positively charged plate. The path of the particle changed such that it angled up toward the plate. Which of the following could it be?
    A. alpha particle
    B. beta particle
    C. proton
    D. gamma ray

18. The transmutation of ^{238}U to Np involves the formation of a compound nucleus of ^{239}U. What type of energy transfer is this?
    A. Mass to electrical
    B. Mass to potential
    C. Kinetic to mass
    D. Potential to kinetic

19. ^{238}U is also radioactive in and of itself. One of the intermediates in its decay is obtained via 3 alpha emissions, 2 beta emissions and 3 gamma emissions. What is the identity of this intermediate?
    A. $^{232}_{84}Po$
    B. $^{232}_{88}Ra$
    C. $^{226}_{84}Po$
    D. $^{226}_{88}Ra$

Passage IV (Questions 20-25)

When one thinks of structural abnormalities in metals, invariably the first thing to come to mind is rusting. The rusting of iron in particular is a remarkable phenomenon, especially from the electrochemical point of view. Consider the following diagram.

Drop of Water

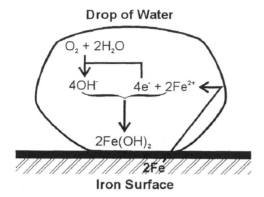

Iron Surface

Metals have a tendency to "throw off" ions into solution (referred to as the *solution pressure*). Therefore, one would expect the metal to exert its full solution pressure at the center of the drop. There is then an excess of electrons at the center of the drop and a flow of electrons occurs from the inside to the outside of the drop. Here, since the outside of the drop is exposed to the atmosphere, oxygen reacts with the electrons to yield hydroxide ions.

$2Fe \rightleftharpoons 2Fe^{2+} + 4e^-$	$E° = +0.440$ V	**Equation I**
$O_2 + 2H_2O + 4e^- \rightleftharpoons 4OH^-$	$E° = +0.401$ V	**Equation II**

The Fe^{2+} and OH^- then react to produce iron (II) hydroxide. Further oxidation and subsequent dehydration eventually give rise to the hydrated iron (III) oxide ($Fe_2O_3 \cdot xH_2O$) which is not closely adhering and tends to "flake off."

Many processes can be used to reduce rusting. One involves coating the iron with "galvanizing" zinc. When the surface is scratched and water enters, zinc hydroxide forms and this is a closely adhering salt which protects the iron underneath from further attack. Another method is the addition of bicarbonate (HCO_3^-) to remove the hydroxide ions produced before they can react with the iron.

$$HCO_3^- + OH^- \rightarrow CO_3^{2-} + H_2O \quad \textbf{Equation III}$$

Paints containing phosphoric acid are often used, the iron (III) ions produced react to form iron (III) phosphate which clings to the surface of the metal. The most common method of combatting rust is the use of alloys, especially those containing chromium. The chromium reacts before the iron to produce an oxide which adheres to the metal surface.

20. Although HCO_3^- acts as an acid in Equation III, it could also be referred to by another term because of its action on one of the reactions involved. How can its action be described?
    A. Anodic inhibitor
    B. Cathodic inhibitor
    C. Anodic promoter
    D. Cathodic promoter

21. For galvanizing to be effective, which of the following must be true?
    A. K_{sp} $Zn(OH)_2 < K_{sp}$ $Fe(OH)_2$
    B. K_{sp} $Zn(OH)_2 > K_{sp}$ $Fe(OH)_2$
    C. $E°$ (Zn^{2+}/Zn) > $E°$ (Fe^{2+}/Fe)
    D. $E°(Zn^{2+}$/Zn) < $E°(Fe^{2+}$/Fe)

22. From the information in the passage, determine the $E°$ for the overall reaction:

    $2Fe$ *(s)* $+ O_2$ *(g)* $+ 2H_2O$ *(l)* $\rightarrow 2Fe^{2+}$ *(aq)* $+ 4OH^-$ *(aq)*

    A. +0.382 V
    B. +0.841 V
    C. -0.058 V
    D. -1.702 V

23. A sample of iron was placed in a beaker of water and exposed to the atmosphere for one hour. After this, the iron that remained was removed from the beaker and a current of 0.2 A passed through the beaker which contained only Fe^{2+} in solution. After one hour and twenty minutes, all the iron present had been deposited on the cathode. Given that the Faraday constant F = 96000 C, what was the rate of rusting in grams per hour?
    A. 0.209
    B. 0.279
    C. 0.140
    D. 0.450

24. Why do you suppose that adding an electrolyte to the iron would increase its rate of rusting?
   A. It causes the $Fe_2O_3 \cdot xH_2O$ to flake off more rapidly.
   B. It increases the charge carrying capacity of the water.
   C. It increases the solution pressure of the iron.
   D. It inhibits the reactions involved.

25. Given that the K_{sp} of FeX_2 is 5.0×10^{-16} where "X" is an unknown anion, what is its solubility in moles per liter?
   A. 1.0×10^{-2}
   B. 2.1×10^{-3}
   C. 3.4×10^{-3}
   D. 5.0×10^{-6}

Questions 26-30 are NOT based on a descriptive passage.

26. Given the directions and magnitudes of current in the copper wires below, what is the magnitude of current in wire **R**?

Q = 7 A   T = 8 A
S = 4 A   U = 11 A

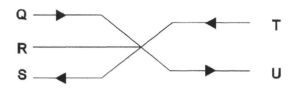

A. 0 A
B. 7 A
C. 15 A
D. 18 A

27. A mechanical wave has the following measured values.
amplitude = 0.50 N m^{-2}
speed = 7.5×10^3 m s^{-1}
intensity = 4.5×10^{-3} W m^{-2}
phase angle = $\pi/6$ radians
wavelength = 1.5 m

What is the frequency of this wave?
A. 1.1×10^4 Hz
B. 5.0×10^3 Hz
C. 3.7×10^3 Hz
D. 12.0 Hz

28. Which of the following describes the orbital geometry of an sp hybridized atom?
A. Octahedral
B. Tetrahedral
C. Linear
D. Trigonal planar

29. Two mechanical waves of the same frequency pass through the same medium. The range of amplitudes possible when the two waves pass through the medium is between four and twelve. Which of the following describes the possible amplitudes of the two waves?
A. 6 units and 2 units
B. 8 units and 4 units
C. 12 units and 4 units
D. 10 units and 2 units

30. A uniform plank is balanced on a pivot then a mass of 50 kg is placed 0.60 m to the left of the fulcrum. Equilibrium is maintained by a downward force applied at a position 0.30 m to the right of the fulcrum. What is the magnitude of that force? (g = 9.8 m s^{-2})
A. 250 N
B. 25 N
C. 100 N
D. 1000 N

Passage V (Questions 31-35)

Archimedes, one of the great mathematicians of all time, is famous for the story of how he managed to determine whether the king's crown was really made of gold. The mathematical law that he derived which enabled him to accomplish this challenge, states that any fluid applies a buoyant force to an object which is partially or completely immersed in it, the magnitude of which is equal to the weight of fluid the object displaces.

$$F_b = W_{fluid} \qquad \textbf{Equation 1}$$

where F_b = magnitude of the buoyant force and W_{fluid} = weight of fluid displaced. Once the maximum buoyant force possible is greater than or equal to the weight of the object, the object will float.

Consider the situation where a square block of pine wood is being immersed in water.

Density of water = 1.00×10^3 kg m^{-3}
Density of pine = 500 kg m^{-3}
Gravitational acceleration = 9.8 m s^{-2}
Length of side of block = 4.0 m

31. What is the maximum possible buoyant force that can be obtained when the block is held in water?
    A. 6.27×10^5 N
    B. 1.57×10^5 N
    C. 8.62×10^4 N
    D. 2.16×10^4 N

32. Given that the block of pine wood floats, how high is it out of the water?
    A. 0.5 m
    B. 1.0 m
    C. 2.0 m
    D. 4.0 m

33. The block is replaced by one with identical dimensions but greater density. Which of the following is true?
    A. The height of the block above the water is the same as before.
    B. The height of the block above the water is greater than before.
    C. The height of the block above the water is less than before.
    D. The height of the block above the water will depend on the temperature of the block.

34. Another block of identical dimensions to the first is held half immersed in the water. When released, it sinks. When the block was released, which of the following must be true?
    A. Weight of fluid displaced > weight of block
    B. Density of fluid < density of block
    C. Buoyant force < maximum buoyant force
    D. Maximum buoyant force = half the weight of the block

35. A student observes that when an ice cube floats in a glass of water, part of the ice cube projects above the surface of the water. When the ice cube melts, the level of the water surface will:
    A. go down slightly.
    B. go up slightly.
    C. remain the same.
    D. change depending on the weight of the ice cube.

Phosphorus is a Group V element and exhibits the phenomenon known as *allotropy:* - different forms of the same element, each form being a bit more stable than another under particular conditions. The following is a list of some of the physical properties of two of the allotropes of phosphorus (there is also a black phosphorus not listed in Table 1).

Table 1

Physical Property	White phosphorus	Red phosphorus
Melting point (°C)	44	Sublimes at 416
Boiling point (°C)	280	-
Enthalpy of formation of oxide (ΔH_{ox}) kJ mol^{-1}	-3020	-2900
Soluble in:		
benzene	yes	no
CS_2	yes	no
water	no	no
Structure	discrete P_4 molecules	polymer

Red phosphorus can be obtained by carefully heating white phosphorus to 400 degrees Celsius or via exposure of white phosphorus to ionizing radiation (usually visible light) in the absence of air.

Phosphorus vapor contains only P_4 molecules, regardless of the allotrope which was vaporized. This is due to the breakdown of the polymer-like structure of the other allotropes.

Although phosphorus is in Group V, black phosphorus does have a relatively significant degree of electrical conductivity. This is similar to the graphite allotrope of carbon.

36. Which of the following is a plausible structure for white phosphorus?

A.

B.

C.

D.

37. What is the standard enthalpy of formation of white phosphorus from red phosphorus?
A. 0 kJ mol^{-1}
B. -120 kJ mol^{-1}
C. -2900 kJ mol^{-1}
D. -3020 kJ mol^{-1}

38. Which of the following values do you think is closest to the bond angle in white phosphorus P_4 molecules?
A. 30°
B. 45°
C. 60°
D. 109.5°

39. A sample of white phosphorus was reacted with excess Cl_2 gas to yield 68.75 grams of phosphorus trichloride. How many discrete P_4 molecules were there in the sample?
A. 0.75×10^{23}
B. 1.50×10^{23}
C. 3.00×10^{-23}
D. 2.40×10^{-23}

40. At very high temperatures, P_4 molecules decompose to give rise to P_2 molecules. What type of bonding would you expect in these molecules?

A. Ionic with P^{3+} cations and P^{3-} anions

B. Covalent with no sigma bonds, 3 pi bonds and 2 lone pairs of electrons

C. Covalent with 1 sigma bonds, 2 pi bonds and 2 lone pairs of electrons

D. Covalent with 2 sigma bonds, 1 pi bonds and 2 lone pairs of electrons

41. One mole of an ideal gas with a molecular mass of 124.0 grams would have a lower density than one mole of P_4 because:

A. less particles are present.

B. it occupies a smaller volume.

C. it weighs less.

D. there are less strong intermolecular forces.

Passage VII (Questions 42-46)

Infrared spectroscopy is a powerful tool used in the field of organic chemistry. It is especially useful in detecting the functional groups present in a molecule, that is, those groups of atoms in a molecule which lend the compound its particular properties.

Infrared radiation comprises the portion of the electromagnetic spectrum in which the wavelengths range from 10^{-4} to 10^{-6} m. When a photon of infrared radiation is absorbed by a molecule, it results in a change in the vibrational energy state of a molecule due to stretching and/or bending of the bonds between atoms.

This phenomenon is very similar in principle to that of the model harmonic oscillator (a spring being stretched and compressed) where the frequency of vibration of a diatomic system comprised of two atoms with masses m_1 and m_2 is given by the following equation.

$$\nu = \frac{1}{2\pi}\sqrt{\frac{k}{m}}$$

where ν = frequency of vibration, k = force constant of the bond between two atoms and m = $(m_1+m_2)/(m_1m_2)$.

The absorption of infrared radiation, and hence the change in vibrational energy state of a diatomic system cannot occur unless there is a dipole, that is, an uneven distribution of charge between the two atoms. This can be determined from the electronegativities of the atoms involved since this gives a measure of the ability of an atom to draw electrons to itself. The electronegativities for a number of atoms according to Pauling's electronegativity scale is given in Table 1.

Table 1

Atom	Electronegativity
Carbon	2.5
Hydrogen	2.1
Oxygen	3.5
Fluorine	4.0
Sulphur	2.5

42. Which of the following types of radiation has a longer wavelength than infrared radiation?
   A. Radio waves
   B. Visible light
   C. Ultraviolet radiation
   D. Gamma rays

43. Which of the following diatomic systems will show no infrared absorption?
   A. C-H
   B. C-O
   C. C-F
   D. C-S

44. If the mass of each of the atoms in a diatomic system is doubled, what will be the effect on the frequency of vibration if all other physical properties of the system remain the same?
   A. It will decrease by a factor of 2
   B. It will increase by a factor of 2
   C. It will decrease by a factor of $\sqrt{2}$
   D. It will increase by a factor of $\sqrt{2}$

45. Given that the model harmonic oscillator operates in a similar fashion to a spring, and that the displacement is given by x, what would be the energy associated with the stretching of a chemical bond with force constant k?
   A. ½kx
   B. ½kx²
   C. ½k/x
   D. ½k/x²

46. Two atoms of masses 2 units each are joined by a chemical bond of force constant k = 4 units. What is the value for the frequency of vibration?
   A. $1/\pi$
   B. $1/\sqrt{2}\,\pi$
   C. $\sqrt{2}/\pi$
   D. $2/\pi$

Passage VIII (Questions 47-51)

From the ideal gas equation PV = nRT, it is possible to determine the molar mass of a gas once the other physical variables are known. One technique for doing this involves the production of a known volume of the gas from one of the reactions in which it is produced at a known temperature and pressure. In the reaction, stoichiometric amounts of the reactants are used, or more commonly, one reactant is used in large excess. For example, in order to determine the molar mass of carbon dioxide, one could utilize the reaction between carbonates and acid as shown in Reaction I.

$$MgCO_3 + 2HCl \rightarrow MgCl_2 + CO_2(g) + H_2O \quad \textbf{Reaction I}$$

The reaction is carried out in a closed vessel attached to a water manometer (a thin U-tube filled with water) where the difference in the height of the two levels in the two arms can be used to determine the pressure inside the vessel. This is due to the fact that the relative levels in the two arms gives the **difference** in pressure between the atmosphere and the vessel.

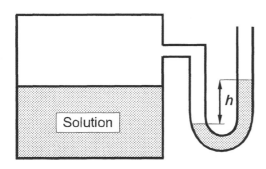

35.00 grams of $MgCO_3$ were placed into the reaction vessel and 150 mL of 5 M HCl were subsequently added. After all the $MgCO_3$ had reacted, the difference in height of the water in the two arms of the manometer was read.

47. Given that the density of water is 1000 kg m^{-3} and that gravitational acceleration g = 9.8 m s^{-2}, calculate the pressure inside the reaction vessel if the level of water in the right arm of the manometer was 50 cm higher than in the left arm.
    A. 4900 N m^{-2} + atmospheric pressure
    B. 490 N m^{-2} + atmospheric pressure
    C. 9800 N m^{-2} + atmospheric pressure
    D. 980 N m^{-2} + atmospheric pressure

48. How should the ideal gas equation be rearranged to allow for the determination of the molecular mass of the gas? (The mass of the gas is designated by "w" and the molar mass of the gas is designated by "M")
    A. M = wPT/(RV)
    B. M = RV/(wPT)
    C. M = wRT/(PV)
    D. M = PV/(wRT)

49. Regarding the experiment in the passage, how would you rate the efficiency of this method in measuring M?
    A. Low, because the intermolecular forces in CO_2 are greater than those in an ideal gas
    B. Low, because the intermolecular forces in CO_2 are less than those in an ideal gas
    C. High, because the intermolecular forces in CO_2 are greater than those in an ideal gas
    D. High, because the intermolecular forces in CO_2 are less than those in an ideal gas

50. If Reaction I was exothermic and the temperature of the reaction vessel ended up being higher than expected, if the initial temperature was used in the equation how would the recorded value of M compare to its predicted value?
    A. It would be higher than expected.
    B. It would be lower than expected.
    C. It would be the same.
    D. The direction of change of the value of M cannot be predicted from the data given.

51. CO_2 happens to be quite soluble in water. How would this affect the value of M obtained in the experiment?
    A. It would be higher than expected.
    B. It would be lower than expected.
    C. It would be the same.
    D. The direction of change of the value of M cannot be determined from the data given.

Questions 52-56 are NOT based on a descriptive passage.

52. What is the concentration of magnesium ions in a 0.1 M solution of magnesium phosphate?

A. 0.1 M
B. 0.4 M
C. 0.2 M
D. 0.3 M

53. If an object is made to resonate, which of the following properties of the system is not at its maximum?

A. Power
B. Energy
C. Amplitude
D. Speed

54. Which of the species in Table 1 is best suited to oxidize NO given that:

$$HNO_2 + H^+ + e^- \rightleftharpoons NO + H_2O \qquad E^\circ = +1.00\ V$$

Table 1

Electrochemical reaction	E° value (V)
$Ce^{4+} + e^- \rightleftharpoons Ce^{3+}$	+1.695
$H_2O_2 + 2e^- \rightleftharpoons 2OH^-$	+0.880
$MnO_4^- + e^- \rightleftharpoons MnO_4^{2-}$	+0.564
$Cd^{2+} + 2e^- \rightleftharpoons Cd$	-0.403

A. Ce^{4+}
B. Ce^{3+}
C. Cd^{2+}
D. Cd

55. Why is the first ionization energy of manganese (Mn) less than that of chromium (Cr)?

A. Because chromium has a half-filled d orbital.
B. Because manganese has a half-filled d orbital.
C. Because the relative atomic mass of chromium is greater than that of manganese.
D. Because the atomic radius of chromium is less than that of manganese.

56. A 1 kg ball moving at 12 m s^{-1} collides with and adheres to a 2 kg ball which is initially at rest. The balls stop moving after 10 seconds. What is the magnitude of the deceleration?

A. 10 m s^{-2}
B. 0.6 m s^{-2}
C. 1.2 m s^{-2}
D. 0.4 m s^{-2}

Keeping warm in cold climates and cool in tropical climates has been one of the earliest challenges man has faced in his attempts to explore the world. Thus the physics of heat transfer has interested scientists for many years. Summer and winter clothing, insulated houses and air conditioning are but a few of the technological advances that utilize the heat transfer properties of various materials.

When space exploration began, keeping the temperature of the space equipment relatively constant became of paramount concern since temperatures vary much more drastically in space than in an environment with an atmosphere. Thus, satellites and other artificial orbiting bodies such as the Hubble space telescope are covered with a highly reflective ("shiny") metal foil which reflects 90% of incident solar radiation.

Along with these types of measures, the possibility of using a circulating system of coolant built into the equipment and covering its sun-exposed area could also be used to aid in regulating temperature.

57. The metal foil would aid in preventing heat gain via which of the following processes?
    A. Reflecting radiant energy
    B. Conduction
    C. Convection
    D. Radiation and conduction

58. Down-filled winter clothing reduces heat losses by incorporating pockets of air into the material. Which type of heat transfer process do the air pockets limit?
    A. Radiation
    B. Conduction
    C. Convection
    D. Conduction and convection

59. Air-conditioning is usually used to lower the ambient temperature in an enclosed space. It is often said that for maximum efficiency, the unit should be placed near the ceiling. Why is this so?
    A. Cold air is heavier than warm air.
    B. Cold air is lighter than warm air.
    C. Cold air is less dense than warm air.
    D. Cold air is denser than warm air.

60. Three metal solids, X, Y, and Z, each of the same dimensions and made of the same material were placed into beakers filled with 500 grams of oil, water and ethanol, respectively. All the beakers were heated such that the liquids were given the same amount of energy. The solids were taken out after equilibrating with the liquids and their temperatures were noted. Which of the following is true?

Specific heat capacity of water = 4.2 J g^{-1} $°C^{-1}$
Specific heat capacity of oil = 2.9 J g^{-1} $°C^{-1}$

Specific heat capacity of ethanol = 3.1 J $g^{-1}°C^{-1}$

    A. Temperature of X > temperature of Y > temperature of Z
    B. Temperature of X > temperature of Z > temperature of Y
    C. Temperature of Y > temperature of X > temperature of Z
    D. Temperature of Y > temperature of Z > temperature of X

61. The total area of the Hubble telescope exposed to the sun is 70 000 m^2. The rate of solar energy incident on the telescope is 120 W m^{-2}. If a channel covering the entire exposed surface contains water and the temperature of the water must rise by at least 10 °C in order to keep the telescope cool, at what approximate rate must the water be made to flow assuming that energy transfer is instantaneous?

Specific heat capacity of water = 4.2 J g^{-1} $°C^{-1}$
Density of water = 1000 kg m^{-3}

    A. 200 L s^{-1}
    B. 3150 L s^{-1}
    C. 2.0×10^5 L s^{-1}
    D. 3.1×10^6 L s^{-1}

Passage X (Questions 62-67)

Metals can occur as ions - usually with positive oxidation states - in compounds with other species, or more rarely, in their elemental states. The more reactive a metal is, the more difficult it is to obtain as a free element. A number of metals have only one oxidation state, but quite a few have multiple oxidation states. Table 1 gives the standard reduction potentials for various metals in various oxidation states.

Table 1

Reaction	Standard reduction potential ($E°$)
$Zn^{2+} + 2e \rightleftharpoons Zn$	-0.76 V
$V^{3+} + e \rightleftharpoons V^{2+}$	-0.26 V
$SO_4^{2-} + 4H^+ + 2e \rightleftharpoons 2H_2O + SO_2$	+0.17 V
$VO^{2+} + 2H^+ + e \rightleftharpoons H_2O + V^{3+}$	+0.34 V
$Fe^{3+} + e \rightleftharpoons Fe^{2+}$	+0.77 V
$VO_2^+ + 2H^+ + e \rightleftharpoons H_2O + VO^{2+}$	+1.00 V
$Cr^{2+} + 2e \rightleftharpoons Cr$	-0.91 V
$Cr^{3+} + 3e \rightleftharpoons Cr$	-0.74 V
$Cr^{3+} + e \rightleftharpoons Cr^{2+}$	-0.41 V
$Cr_2O_7^{2-} + 14H^+ + 6e \rightleftharpoons 2Cr^{3+} + 7H_2O$	+1.33 V

Transition metals often form ions which are colored in solution. They also interact with a variety of species known as *ligands* forming a complex structure with the cation centrally located and the ligands forming bonds similar to coordinate covalent bonds with the cation. The transition metal ion can be associated with more than one different ligand species at a time.

62. If the ionization energies of the first row of transition metals is examined, it is observed that the third ionization energy of manganese is greater than expected from the trend across the period. Why is this?
   A. Because Mn^{2+} has a large relative molecular mass.
   B. Because Mn^{2+} has a relatively small charge.
   C. Because Mn^{2+} is less stable then Mn^{3+}.
   D. Because Mn^{2+} has a half-filled d-orbital system.

63. If a current was passed through a solution of sulfate ions and one mole of sulfur dioxide was obtained, how many moles of chromium metal would be obtained if the same current was passed through a solution of chromium (III) ions in solution?
   A. 0.33 moles
   B. 0.67 moles
   C. 1.00 moles
   D. 2.00 moles

64. Ligands, in order to associate with transition metal ions, must possess which of the following characteristics?
   A. A negative charge
   B. A positive charge
   C. A lone pair of electrons
   D. A vacant d-orbital

65. How many of the species in Table 1 could NOT reduce Fe^{3+} to Fe^{2+} ?
   A. 2
   B. 3
   C. 4
   D. 5

66. What would be the standard cell potential for the galvanic cell formed with the VO^{2+}/V^{3+} and VO_2^+/VO^{2+} half-cells?
   A. 0 V
   B. +0.66 V
   C. +1.34 V
   D. -1.34 V

67. What is the oxidation state of chromium in $Cr_2O_7^{2-}$?
   A. 6
   B. 7
   C. 8
   D. 12

Passage XI (Questions 68-72)

A truck of mass 5000 kg is transporting a load of goods of mass 1000 kg from Vancouver to San Francisco. Along the way, it has to ascend the side of a mountain which is inclined at an angle of 30° to the horizontal. The inclined surface is straight and 1.2 km long.

In order to go up the mountain, the truck accelerates from its initial velocity of 14 m s^{-1} uniformly at 6 m s^{-2} for five seconds. He then ascends the incline at a constant velocity and when he reaches the top he applies the brakes. Eight seconds later the truck has been brought to a stop via a uniform deceleration.

68. What is the potential energy of the truck when it has travelled a distance of 5 m up the inclined surface?

   Acceleration due to gravity = 9.8 m s^{-2}

   A. 2.25×10^5 J
   B. 2.94×10^5 J
   C. 1.47×10^5 J
   D. 2.45×10^5 J

69. What would the velocity versus time graph of the motion of the truck look like?

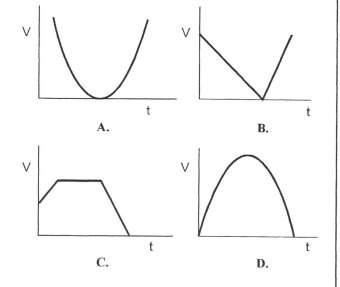

70. Given that the coefficient of friction of the surface is ⅓, what is the approximate maximum frictional force that can act on the truck when it is moving on level ground?
   A. 10 000 N
   B. 20 000 N
   C. 30 500 N
   D. 51 962 N

71. What is the ratio of the magnitude of the acceleration and the deceleration of the truck during its motion?
   A. 3 : 2
   B. 5 : 8
   C. 3 : 4
   D. 12 : 11

72. If the truck is on the incline, what would happen to the value of the normal force to the surface if the incline decreased to an angle less than the previous value of 30°?
   A. It will decrease.
   B. It will increase.
   C. It will stay the same.
   D. It depends on the coefficient if friction of the second surface.

Questions 73-77 are NOT based on a descriptive passage.

73. Why do chlorine atoms form anions more easily than they form cations?
   A. The valence electron shell of chlorine contains seven electrons.
   B. Attractive forces between halogen nuclei and valence electrons are weak.
   C. The valence electron shell of chlorine is vacant.
   D. Attractive forces between the valence electrons and the nuclei in halogens are strong.

74. A projectile is launched from a point on level ground with a velocity of 30 m s^{-1} at an angle of 45° to the horizontal. Which of the following is NOT true of the flight of the particle? (Ignore air resistance)
   A. The horizontal component of the velocity is constant.
   B. At the highest point in the projectile's flight, the vertical component of the velocity is zero.
   C. The path which the projectile traces is parabolic in nature.
   D. The initial horizontal and vertical components of the velocity are equal to half the initial velocity.

75. The equilibrium shown below was established within the confines of a closed system.

$4NH_3(g) + 5O_2(g) \rightleftharpoons 4NO(g) + 6H_2O(g)$ **Reaction I**
$$\Delta H_{rxn} = \text{-}1100 \text{ kJ mol}^{-1}$$

What effect will increasing the pressure have on this system?
   A. The equilibrium will shift to the left.
   B. The equilibrium will shift to the right.
   C. The equilibrium position will remain the same.
   D. The equilibrium position will depend on whether a catalyst is present or not.

76. A convex lens has a radius of curvature of 70 cm. An object was placed 35 cm away from the lens. What type of image will be formed?
   A. Real, inverted, enlarged
   B. Virtual, inverted, enlarged
   C. Real, inverted, same size
   D. No image will be formed.

77. Which of the following molecules can be involved in hydrogen bond formation but cannot form hydrogen bonds with molecules of its own kind?
   A. C_2H_5OH
   B. HCOOH
   C. CH_3OCH_3
   D. HF

END OF PHYSICAL SCIENCES. IF TIME REMAINS, YOU MAY GO BACK AND CHECK YOUR WORK IN THIS TEST BOOKLET.

BOOKLET GS2-II

THE GOLD STANDARD MCAT*

TEST GS-2

Verbal Reasoning
Questions 78-137
Time : 85 Minutes

OPEN BOOKLET ONLY WHEN TIMER IS READY.

The Gold Standard MCAT* has been designed exclusively to test knowledge and thinking skills. The exam may contain hypothetical statements and/or express controversial ideas. Statements contained herein do not necessarily reflect the policy, position, or view of RuveneCo Publishing.

* MCAT is a registered service mark of the Association of American Medical Colleges, which is not associated with this product.

VERBAL REASONING

INSTRUCTIONS: The Verbal Reasoning test contains nine passages, each of which is followed by several questions. After reading the passage, select the best answer to each question. If you are unsure of the answer, eliminate the alternatives you know to be false then select an answer from the remaining alternatives. Indicate your answer by blackening the corresponding oval on Answer Document 1, GS-2.

Passage I (Questions 78-84)

By adopting a cross-cultural perspective, social psychologists will be better able to explain human social behavior. In the following discussion, we shall review psychological differentiation theory to illustrate how the incorporation of culture in theory and empirical studies can enrich our understanding of social behavior.

According to the theory of psychological differentiation, psychological development involves a progression from undifferentiated to increasingly differentiated functioning. In this context, "differentiation" means, first, distinguishing between two or more phenomena; second, relating and integrating these distinguished phenomena.

There are two aspects to this progression - internal and external. Psychological processes such as feeling, perceiving, and thinking, are differentiated internally. For example, during the course of development, the individual learns to differentiate between various feelings, such as anger and shame. Externally, there is a clearer distinction between the self and nonself elements in the environment. For example, particularly in Western cultures, individuals learn to make sharp distinctions between events caused by factors "inside" themselves, as opposed to those caused by external factors. Thus, relative to the infant, the adult personality is a more complex structure, composed of differentiated, integrated elements.

Social differentiation theory proposes that differentiation is universal, in that all humans pass from a less to a more differentiated state during their development. However, the theory also focuses on *diversity* in social differentiation among different people, and sees culture as a major source of this diversity. In particular, the theory proposes that the culture influences differentiation through socialization practices, basically how children are "brought up." Generally speaking, more permissive socialization practices lead to greater differentiation, and stricter ones to less differentiation. This proposition has been particularly well studied through research on field dependence/independence.

The terms "field dependence" and "field independence" represent a continuum on which individuals can be placed, to indicate how dependent or independent on cues in the environment their perceptions are. Two experimental methods used to assess field dependence/independence are the Rod and Frame Test (RFT), and the Embedded Figures Test (EFT). In the RFT, respondents must adjust a tilted rod to a position that seems to them to be vertical. This rod is enclosed in a frame that is inclined by 28 degrees. "Field-independent" respondents are those who are more accurate in adjusting the rod; "field-dependent" respondents are distracted by the surrounding frame, so that they do this task less well. In the EFT, the task is to locate and recognize a simple figure contained in a relatively complex one. On this task, field-independent respondents are more successful at extracting a part of the figure from the whole.

John Berry reasoned that the ecocultural conditions of groups with different economic support systems, such as agriculturalists and hunters, should lead to differences in field dependence/independence. For example, hunters will depend to a greater degree than agriculturalists on their differentiation and reconstructing skills, so that they can pick out the relevant signs, tracks, odours, and sounds, from the surroundings. In order to survive, hunters must be able to sharply distinguish between different features of the environment, including the paths that lead them back to home. Agriculturalists, in contrast, have less need to wander into unfamiliar territory and, consequently, Berry predicted, and experimentally confirmed in a seventeen-culture study, greater field independence among hunters and higher dependence among agriculturalists.

Adapted from Foothill, Taylor and Wright, *Social Psychology in Cross Cultural Perspective*. ©1993 by W.H.Freeman and Company.

---

78. The passage suggests that human social behavior can best be understood by:
    A. administering the RFT and EFT tests.
    B. including culture as an integral part of social psychological theories.
    C. including cultural variables in empirical studies.
    D. both B and C.

79. The passage states that a difference between the adult and the infant lies in:
    A. their respective performances on the EFT test.
    B. how accurately they can differentiate between different feelings.
    C. their respective performances on the RFT test.
    D. the degree to which they are affected by cultural diversity.

80. Based on the passage, which of the following is NOT explained by social differentiation theory?
    A. An infant learns that mother and father are not the same.
    B. An elderly senator retires and shows no interest in the issues of the day.
    C. A girl in Calcutta sees the moon as powerful, while a girl in Iowa sees the moon as conquerable.
    D. A teen now knows what to look for to develop a successful relationship.

81. In the context of the passage, "field" represents:
    A. the personal history of an individual.
    B. the culture of an individual.
    C. the environmental cues available to an individual.
    D. the genetic make up of an individual.

82. Based on the information in the passage, a mother who discouraged independent decision making and encouraged conformity would most likely produce:
    A. a child who would perform well on the EFT test.
    B. a child who would perform poorly on the EFT test.
    C. a child who will grow up to be a hunter.
    D. a child who will grow up to be an agriculturalist.

83. According to John Berry, differences in field dependence/independence between hunters and agriculturalists are best explained by:
    A. their different economic support systems.
    B. their respective performances on the EFT and RFT tests.
    C. their respective degrees of dependence on their powers of differentiation.
    D. both A and C.

84. The main purpose of the passage was to:
    A. describe psychological differentiation theory and discuss some of the relevant research.
    B. show how two tests, the EFT and the RFT, have been influential in the field of social psychology.
    C. exemplify how the application of a theory across cultures can lead to a better understanding of social behavior.
    D. discuss how differences in field dependence/independence can influence one's choice of occupation.

Passage II (Questions 85-91)

To the sensational progress of science, what is generally called the general public reacts in different ways... Some admire and even act enthusiastic about the daring exploits of astrophysics and molecular biology... There is [another] attitude, however, which is wholly compounded of the anxiety and distrust inspired by scientific progress and at the same time by the attendant technical progress. Where are we heading with these machines and computers? Can we be sure that these atomic, space and genetic adventures are not going to end in disaster?

Thus, if the writer on scientific subjects is to cater for every category of reader, he must take care to reassure [both] groups. He must re-establish the naked truth stripped of the fantastic trappings with which it is all too often embellished by publicists - I dare not call them writers - who are either naive and ill-informed themselves or else unscrupulous popularity hunters.

There is no denying that this is a very difficult task. It is even regarded as an impossible one by some people of sound judgement who see the attempts of science writers to acquaint the general public with certain fields as leading simply to the creation of a new kind of mythology.

A word of warning however. It is essential that the mythical nature of such books be clearly indicated so that there is no mistake about what is being offered for public consumption. There has been too much talk of machines that think, and flying green men from outer space. From all this there seems to have been born a kind of myth which people are beginning to take as scientific fact.

... First of all, what distinguishes a scientific theory from a myth? Here I am using the word myth to signify an explanation or theory of natural or human phenomena and events...

The expression "scientific theory" is also used to signify explanations of natural - and, if need be, human phenomena, and although these explanations do not make use of human figures or animals, they nevertheless attribute specific properties to certain objects which secrete forces and are capable of generating phenomena and bringing about events...

I shall be told that the educated public of the developed countries will not fall prey to such confusion... [but] are we quite sure, that the information given by the popular science writers is always properly understood in the scientific sense? Is there not a tendency among the general public, simply to trust the presumably competent dispensers of information?... It is said quite commonly that space engineers have managed to put a satellite in orbit, or that it has gone off its trajectory and fallen into the sea. In this case, it seems clear that the orbit and the trajectory are thought of as abstract objects which the satellite may follow or leave just as a train does a track, or a car the road. This is understandable since we model our conceptions on familiar facts and events...

... A more general strategy must be adopted [and] in this connection, I would like to make a suggestion based on the concept of a "model." A model, which is basically nothing more than the concrete representation of an abstract theory, is a tool for thought which is very useful both in making scientific progress and in giving an account of such progress, scientists being no different from other men in the way they think...

Many models remain very useful, however, even when the knowledge they represent has been outdated by more general theories [and] this is one of the big differences between models and myths. The model is partial, incomplete and provisional, constructed to be useful for a time and then superseded. The myth, on the other hand, is total and definitive from the onset and in this draws close to belief.

Adapted from Pierre Auger, *Science and Myth*, The Unesco Courier, Feb. 1973.

85. In the second paragraph, the author does not want to refer to certain individuals as "writers." The books these individuals write are likely:
    A. romantic novels.
    B. science fiction novels.
    C. scientific textbooks.
    D. encyclopedias.

86. Based on the author's comments in the second paragraph, it is reasonable to conclude that those people who adopt an attitude of distrust towards scientific progress, do so because:
A. they can foresee the potential dangers that scientific progress will necessarily produce.
B. they are uneducated people who are wary of progress.
C. they have been misinformed about the true nature of scientific progress by publicists.
D. they, like the author, are aware of the mythical nature of science.

87. The author claims that myths and scientific theories are similar in that:
A. they both make use of figures with human characteristics.
B. they both make use of animals gifted with supernatural powers.
C. they both account for machines being able to think.
D. they both signify explanations of natural or human phenomena.

88. The example concerning the satellite (paragraph 7), best supports the author's claim that:
A. information given to the public is not always understood in the scientific sense.
B. from the mythical nature of books, there seems to have been born a myth which people are beginning to take as scientific fact.
C. there is an attitude towards scientific progress which is wholly compounded by anxiety and distrust.
D. atomic, space and genetic adventures will inevitably end in disaster.

89. According to the passage, a model:
I. is a concrete representation of an abstract theory.
II. is useful in both giving an account of scientific progress and in making scientific progress.
III. becomes useless, once the knowledge it represents has been outdated by more general theories.

A. I only
B. I and II only
C. I and III only
D. I, II and III

90. According to the author, the main difference between models and myths, is that:
A. models are incomplete, flexible and meant to be replaced, but myths are not.
B. myths remain useful when they have been outdated, but models do not.
C. myths make use of human figures or animals to signify explanations of human phenomena, but models do not.
D. myths are the result of popularity-hunting publicists, but models are not.

91. Based on the author's description of a model, it is reasonable to conclude that one characteristic of a model not mentioned by the author, is that it:
A. gives an account of the step by step development of a scientific accomplishment, rather than just the final product.
B. can usually only be understood by those knowledgeable in scientific fields.
C. has very specific applications.
D. is a device which is little used in the field of science today.

Passage III (Questions 92-98)

Television added a powerful new dimension to the developing mistrust between press and public, press and government. By the time Vietnam became a household concern in America, the television screen had transformed the news business. "The media," thereafter, would always outweigh "the press," and for several reasons.

One was the immediacy and power of the news when *seen*; no written or spoken story could convey the shock of Jack Ruby blasting the life out of Lee Harvey Oswald, or any of thousands of other happenings. But more important was the *reach* of television. By the 1960s, the networks, the local stations, and cable systems stretched into every corner of the nation. For news and public affairs, the effect was profound - remote areas long dependent on sketchy radio news and regional or local newspapers had come to be in live and frequent contact with Washington, Yankee Stadium, an Asian war, a revolution in Greece, a civil-rights melee in Alabama, with outer space and, later, the surface of the moon.

People who once had been too isolated to know much of what was happening in the great world had become engaged with public affairs; people who had found the news an irrelevant bore saw it transformed by the power of television into fascinating visual terms. Most newspapers could only benefit from the new interest generated by television...

And in the Vietnam years, the impact, reach, and omnipresence of television produced a situation no wartime government had faced before. The war's mushroom growth in 1966 and 1967 was visible to every American with a set, and it did not always look like the war that Lyndon Johnson and Robert McNamara and Dean Rusk claimed was being won. Even the television commentators, most of whom voiced views cautiously close to the official Washington attitude, could not make the pictures more palatable.

No amount of commentary could have countered that nightly parade of battlefield images through the American living room... Television made the war inescapable and finally sharpened to their intolerable points the questions: For what? To what end? No official source ever provided answers convincingly enough; but until the war's essential futility finally became clear to most Americans, television's graphic and unpalatable reports were another cause for the unease and mistrust with which many viewed the press...

The enormous importance of television news had started the process of change in the printed press. In the sixties and seventies every survey showed that most Americans got the news first from television and automobile radio. The broadcast media, therefore had taken over the front-page function of newspapers. The network evening-news broadcasts were illustrated front pages, compact and convenient, tuned to by most of the nation.

Reluctantly, sometimes not admitting even to themselves what they were doing, newspapers began to move beyond the front-page function - the summary of what happened yesterday. More analysis, background, and commentary began to appear in news columns - either as separate stories or as parts of regular news stories, sometimes even on the front page itself. This was not so much the choice of cautious editors as because of the necessary search for a role complementary to, rather than competing with, the nightly "front page" on television. Instead of "bringing the news," the printed press was evolving toward "explaining the news."

This creeping development was reasonably advanced when the "credibility gap" of the Johnson administration and the growing doubts of many reporters and commentators about the war in Vietnam added another element. To a greater degree than would have seemed possible in the Cold War days of Truman - Eisenhower, and Kennedy, the press - television included - found itself having to scrutinize official positions, challenge official statements, turn a sceptical eye and ear toward official spokesmen. Here and there reporters and editors began to speak openly of the "adversary function" of the press.

Adapted from Tom Wicker, *On Press*. © 1978 by Tom Wicker.

92. The overall point made by the author's comparison of the "press" and the "media" is that:
A. television, media and the press are all being transformed.
B. the press is an important part of the media.
C. the media is now dominated by television, no longer by the press.
D. the public trusts the press more than the media.

93. According to the passage, once television had become a fixture in many American homes all of the following events occurred EXCEPT:

 I. government officials became hostile towards both the press and the media.
 II. newspaper sales plummeted.
 III.the American people's interest in public affairs increased considerably.

 A. II only
 B. III only
 C. I and II only
 D. I, II and III

94. The passage suggests that the effect of television on newspapers was to:
 A. galvanize the industry to create a new role for itself.
 B. attract the best reporters to television news programs.
 C. encourage newspapers to place large color photos on the front page.
 D. reduce the number of printing presses across the country.

95. Robert McNamara and Dean Rusk were likely:
 A. reporters.
 B. broadcasters.
 C. government officials.
 D. members of the general public.

96. It could be reasonably inferred from the passage that television's graphic reports, caused mistrust towards the press because:
 A. the press never contained graphic reports.
 B. only the nation's elite read the press but television was available for everyone.
 C. the press could not present moving images.
 D. the press had often been conservative in their reporting but television allowed the public to judge for themselves.

97. Based on the passage, one would expect that a contemporary reporter's writings might differ from that of a "pre-television" reporter, in that the articles would be:
 A. more honest.
 B. more in line with government policy.
 C. less informative.
 D. more critical.

98. Which of the following events might reasonably have been influenced by the "adversary function" of the press alluded to by the author in the last paragraph?
 A. The press explores other forms of media.
 B. A senator retires when an article alleges he has links to organized crime.
 C. An editor agrees with the President's position on welfare.
 D. The reporting of a car accident leads to tougher safety legislation.

Passage IV (Questions 99-105)

Naturally occurring compounds known as semiochemicals influence the behavior of insects. They are part of the communications system of insects used, for example, to establish social hierarchies and in mating.

Semiochemicals can be employed as attractants, repellents and decoys, to lure pest species away from vulnerable plants and animals. Pheromones are particularly useful for this purpose. These are compounds by which an individual signals to others of the same species. For example, aphids release an alarm pheromone in response to attack; this causes them to disperse. A synthetic version of this pheromone has been produced for use in combination with pesticides. The pheromone increases the mobility of the aphids, thus increasing the chance that they will come into contact with the pesticides.

In some cases, the full alarm response requires the presence of metabolites originating from the plant host. Alarm pheromone synergists have been identified, and their use increases the range and effectiveness of formulations. Field trials have also been undertaken on a compound developed from chemical modification of the alarm pheromone. This has the potential to prevent aphid colonization of plants, and aphid transmission of plant viruses.

Sex pheromones allow males and females "to find and recognize each other" for mating. These can be used as bait to trap pests or as lures to direct them away from vulnerable species. The sex pheromone of the damson-hop aphid has been characterized and a synthetic form synthesised. In the autumn, asexual female aphids migrate from hop plants to *Prunus* species, mainly blackthorn and plum. There, sexual forms of the female produce the pheromone which attracts the males.

In field trials, very large numbers of male aphids were attracted to traps baited with the synthetic pheromone. Such traps might be used simply to immobilise the aphids, or they could contain a pathogen which the captives would pick up and subsequently spread to other aphids after they have escaped. A pheromone trap, baited with the fungal pathogen *Zoopthora radicans,* has been used to control the diamond-back moth that attacks brassica plants.

Egg-laying pheromones - signals by which individuals communicate the message "this is a safe place to lay eggs" are also potential decoys, attracting female pests to a site where they may safely be destroyed *en masse*. This approach is being used to develop a method to control mosquitoes. *Culex* mosquitoes carry various forms of encephalitis and filarial diseases, of which elephantiasis is an extremely unpleasant and debilitating example. The female mosquitoes lay their eggs on water. As the eggs mature they produce a chemical signal which attracts other egg-laying females to the site. This pheromone, identified as a fatty-acid like material, has been synthesized in the laboratory and formulated into effervescent tablets that release the compound when dropped into water. The tablets have been successfully field-tested in Kenya; an insecticide was incorporated into the tablets and larvae were killed as they hatched. Research is also in progress to use mating pheromones to lure biting midges away from areas used for forestry and recreation in the UK.

Semiochemicals also regulate the interactions between insects and their host plant. Insects do not find the plants on which they feed haphazardly; they respond to chemical attractants and repellents produced by the plants. Blocking these signals can help protect crops. Vulnerable species can also be protected by "hiding" them near others that repel pests; this is the rationale behind the idea of inter-planting onions with carrots to deter carrot fly.

Antifeedants are non-toxic compounds produced naturally by some wild plant species. They appear to interfere with tasting and cause pests to stop eating. Research is being carried out on the use of antifeedants against beetles and weevils that attack crops in the UK. One agent being investigated is Ajugarin 1, a diterpenoid from a plant relative of mint and thyme, that grows in Kenya.

Adapted from *The Biologist: Natural Weapons in the War against Pests* by Monica Winstanley. Volume 42, no.1, 1995.

99. According to the passage, which of the following would best explain how the synthesized version of the alarm pheromone works?
    A. It requires the presence of metabolites originating from the host plant.
    B. It is used in combination with herbicides.
    C. It fools the pests into dispersing, mobilizing them.
    D. It causes pests to stop eating.

100. Based on the passage, scientists would have assumed which of the following in their field tests in Kenya on *Culex* mosquitoes?
A. The egg-laying pheromone was the only thing responsible for attracting female pests to the site.
B. The egg-laying pheromone was not the only thing responsible for attracting female pests to the site.
C. All pheromones are fatty acid compounds.
D. *Zoopthora radicans* would kill the mosquitoes effectively.

101. Which of the following would be a possible negative effect of the tests in Kenya?
A. There would be a decrease in the number of *Culex* mosquitoes.
B. Other insects in the environment could be killed by the insecticides.
C. Less money would be available for the testing of Ajugarin 1.
D. The mobility of the *Culex* mosquitoes would increase.

102. If it were found that female aphids migrated from hop plants to blackthorn as a direct result of seasonal changes, which of the following possible conclusions from the passage would be challenged?
A. Semiochemicals regulate interactions between insects and their host plants.
B. Semiochemicals are part of the communications system of insects.
C. Pheromone synergists increase the range of formulations.
D. Antifeedants may cause pests to stop eating.

103. The passage suggests that carrots and onions are inter-planted because:
A. sex pheromones are released from the onion plant which deter the carrot fly.
B. a chemical repellent is produced by the onion plant which repels the carrot fly.
C. planting only one crop could result in a nutrient deficiency in the soil.
D. the onions contain the fungal pathogen *Zoopthora radicans*.

104. From the reasoning in the passage, one could conclude that Ajugarin 1 acts by:
A. releasing an insecticide which kills pests when they arrive on the host.
B. immobilizing the males of the pest species.
C. deterring the pest species through interference with tasting.
D. sending the message "this is a safe place to lay eggs" to individuals of the pest species.

105. Based on the information in the passage, a study in Denmark to control fly pests of animals, would most probably:
A. inter-plant onions and carrots where the animals feed.
B. investigate how antifeedants could be incorporated into animal coats.
C. seek to find compounds that act as host attractants and repellents.
D. drop insecticide containing tablets into the water sources of the hosts.

A virus is a remarkable structure. Some fear calling it an organism because it does not grow nor contain the extensive metabolic machinery as cells, and it cannot reproduce on its own. Whether or not a virus is considered to be "alive," its *existence* is not in doubt.

The virus is a parasite. It must gain admission to the inside of a cell, enslaving the cell to produce more parasites. In fact, so many may be produced that the cell may burst under the burden of their numbers. Equally insidious is the persistent or latent infection which may occur with little or no cell damage...

Fever is a generalized response to infection. Many mediators are involved in this response including interleukin-1 and tumour necrosis factor. Some viruses are inactivated at temperatures slightly above the hosts body temperature. Another important mediator is the protein interferon which can inhibit the reproduction of viruses in noninfected cells. Aside from the preceding generalized responses to viral infection, the immune system can *specifically* create protein molecules to bind to and aid in the destruction of the parasite. All these functions require white blood cells...

Viral illnesses are transmitted along two basic paths. In the more common *horizontal spread*, transmission occurs between individuals in a susceptible host population. Examples range from the benign "common cold" to the malignant Ebola virus. *Vertical spread* is when the parasite travels in the germ cells, or infects the placenta or birth canal thereby infecting the fetus. Hepatitis, herpes and rubella can be transmitted by vertical spread.

Of course, the creatures which have renewed interest in viral research are the human immunodeficiency viruses, HIV-1 and HIV-2, the former being the etiologic agent implicated in AIDS. It was the summer of 1981 when the Centers for Disease Control (CDC) reported the first cases of AIDS in the United States. The CDC was tipped off by the unusual occurrence of *Pneumocystis carinii* pneumonia in five previously healthy homosexual males in Los Angeles and Kaposi's sarcoma in 26 homosexual males in New York and Los Angeles. Twelve years later there were over 400 000 reported cases of AIDS and an estimated 1.5 million people infected in the United States. The cause is a microscopic particle that may not even be alive.

HIV transmission by sexual contacts outweighs other means of infection such as via blood from transfusions or from contaminated needles used for intravenous drug abuse. An infected mother transmits the virus to the developing fetus with an efficiency of 40%. If the infant survives birth unscathed, then survival may depend on avoiding a most intimate association with mother: the parasite awaits in breast milk.

HIV upsets the balance of the human immune system. Our most important guardians against infection, our white blood cells, are the focus. Specific cells, T-helper cells, are surreptitiously targeted and destroyed. T-helper cells have so many immunological functions that their wanton destruction places a defenceless person in an endless desert with ardent vultures. Though there are reports of exceptional cases, after the diagnosis of AIDS is made, the average survival is less than 3 years.

AIDS has thus far evaded definitive treatment. Consequently, prevention is critical. Education and behavior modification are the most potent forces in the current battle against HIV. Unfortunately, great battles have been created on social grounds and the losses are tremendous - time, money and human compassion. They may just be particles, but they sure look out for one another.

106. According to the author, a virus may not be considered an organism because:
    A. viruses cannot reproduce.
    B. organisms cannot cause infections.
    C. viruses do not exhibit growth and metabolism like cells do.
    D. the existence of viruses remains in doubt.

107. According to the passage, all of the following is true about the spread of viruses EXCEPT:
    A. viruses can be spread by one population to any other population of organisms.
    B. vertical spread occurs less frequently than horizontal spread.
    C. a newborn could have been infected by the father.
    D. both mother and father could infect a newborn by vertical or horizontal spread.

108. According to the passage, the virus responsible for AIDS is:
A. HIV-1.
B. HIV-2.
C. *Pneumocystis carinii*.
D. both A and B.

109. Based on the passage, the virus implicated in AIDS can be transmitted by:
I. vertical spread through breast milk.
II. horizontal spread via sexual contacts
III. both horizontal and vertical spread.

A. I only
B. II only
C. II and III only
D. I, II and III

110. The author refers to an "intimate association with mother" and infant (paragraph 6) which likely refers to:
A. hugging.
B. breast feeding.
C. kissing.
D. cradling.

111. With the analogy of the "defenceless person in an endless desert with ardent vultures" the author is suggesting:
A. everyone must defend themselves against HIV or they may be attacked by vultures.
B. the fact that the person is defenceless makes the future of AIDS research hopeless.
C. the vultures are HIV and the general public is defenceless.
D. if the immune system is ineffective, one can easily become infected by the parasites which are around us.

112. According to the author, an important response to individuals inflicted with HIV is:
A. more research.
B. compassion.
C. prevention.
D. anger.

The aftermath of the Gulf Crisis has shown that the success of the "blitzkrieg" of the Western Allies against the Iraqi Army has only had the limited success of ending the occupation of Kuwait... The UN role is a carefully limited one with the UN Secretary-General conscious all the time of the fact that the majority of his members, including veto-holding China and the Soviet Union, remain instinctively suspicious of the Western powers, their former "Imperialist" master...

On the Western side there are psychological twists too. Bob Woodward, the man who disclosed Watergate and thus prepared the ground for Richard Nixon's downfall, has just written another revealing book, *The Commanders*, about the background of the Gulf War. He describes in detail how decisions are made in the Bush White House. General Powell, he reveals, strongly favoured "containment" instead of the offensive and General Schwarzkopf had argued with the President that it would take eight to twelve months to be ready for an offensive. Secretary Baker was for raising the hostage issue... It was Bush himself, supported by the Security Advisor Air Force General Scowcroft, who took the decision to fight...

But in political terms Hussein has saved a great deal. He has, for the time being, eliminated Kuwait as an oil producer, and therefore competitor when sanctions are relaxed... He is successfully dealing with the Kurds and Shias but in different ways... He has been negotiating with the UN for months... Saddam has based his strategy of survival on his assessment that the US-led coalition against him that drove him out of Kuwait is noticeably disintegrating and that no majority in the UN for new effective measures against an Iraq, that is blandly, and sometimes vociferously, by-passing obligations entered into, will be found and that sanctions will wither away...

The other "super-power," the Soviet Union, has also suffered in status and prestige in the Gulf War and the continuing Gulf Crisis. In the first place in the war itself American and British arms, planes and, above all, electronic equipment without which no major action can be fought nowadays, have proved conspicuously superior. This must be kept in mind when evaluating the prestige President Gorbachev lost when President Bush turned down his last minute effort to prevent Western military action in which he refused to take part. The visit to Israel and to some Arab states by Soviet Foreign Minister Bessmertnykh also underlined the supportive and essentially minor role the Soviet Union has been forced to play in the Middle East.

This again must be seen against the continuing structural crisis in the Soviet Union. All Middle Eastern countries are aware of the fact that President Gorbachev had straightforwardly appealed for Western economic aid in the crises he faces, like any Third World leader...

The outcome of the Gulf crisis has also strengthened the international position of the most noticed contributors to the cost of the Gulf War, Germany and Japan. The most significant illustration of this is German Chancellor Kohl's message to President Bush, a warning almost, that his government is determined to bring about a United States of Europe by the next century.

Japan, again, has felt strong and secure enough to turn down President Gorbachev's appeal for financial aid and is steadily pursuing a policy of friendship with the Gulf states, as independent as present circumstances allow, from its relations with the US and the EEC.

The Gulf War, indeed continues to produce unexpected results, like every international conflict. It has significantly down-graded the superpowers.

Adapted from Contemporary Review, v.159(1991), *Still the Gulf Crisis* by Leo Muray.

113. The passage suggests that, in terms of ending the occupation of Kuwait, the Western Allies have been:
    A. generally successful.
    B. generally unsuccessful.
    C. constantly at loggerheads with each other.
    D. constantly at loggerheads with the UN.

114. According to the passage, during the Gulf Crisis, the decision makers in the White House were:
    A. in strong agreement with each other.
    B. in strong agreement with President Bush.
    C. not unanimously decided on how to proceed.
    D. committed to looking after the interests of the UN.

115. According to the passage, it is true of Saddam Hussein that he:

    I. is successfully dealing with the Kurds and Shias using similar strategies.

    II. is determined to respect the details of the provisions he accepted when hostilities were ended.

    III. has eliminated a major oil producing competitor.

    A. I only
    B. II only
    C. III only
    D. I and III only

116. Which of the following conclusions would be most in accord with a theme of the passage?

    A. The UN has become a useless organization.
    B. There was no successful purpose served by the Gulf War.
    C. International conflicts often redistribute power.
    D. Saddam Hussein is a power fanatic.

117. Based on the passage, one could reasonably conclude that President Gorbachev was:

    A. indifferent to the activities occurring in the Gulf.
    B. supportive of the actions of the Western Allies.
    C. opposed to Western military action in the Gulf.
    D. no more influential than the leader of a developing nation.

118. According to the passage, Japan and Germany's most significant contribution to the Gulf Crisis was their:

    A. pursuit of a policy of friendship with the Gulf states.
    B. military support.
    C. superior arms, planes and electronic equipment.
    D. economic support.

Passage VII (Questions 119-125)

We sometimes enjoy picturing the colonizer as a tall man, bronzed by the sun, wearing Wellington boots, proudly leaning on a shovel as he rivets his gaze far away on the horizon of his land. When not engaged in battles against nature, we think of him labouring selflessly for mankind, and spreading culture to the nonliterate. In other words, his pose is one of the noble adventurer, a righteous pioneer...

Today, leaving for a colony is not a choice sought because of its uncertain dangers, nor is it a desire of one tempted by adventure. It is simply a voyage towards an easier life. One need only ask a European living in the colonies what general reasons induced him to expatriate and what particular forces made him persist in his exile. He may mention adventure, the picturesque surroundings or the change of environment. Why then, does he usually seek them where his own language is spoken, where he does not find a large group of his fellow countrymen, an administration to serve him, an army to protect him? The change involved in moving to a colony, if one can call it a change, must first of all bring substantial profit... You go to a colony because jobs are guaranteed, wages high, careers more rapid and business more profitable. The young graduate is offered a position, the public servant a higher rank, the businessman substantially lower taxes, the industrialist raw materials and labour at attractive prices.

However, let us suppose that there is a naive person who lands just by chance. Would it take him long to discover the advantages of his new situation? The economic meaning of a colonial venture, even if it is realized after arrival, thrusts itself upon us no less strongly or quickly. Of course, a European in the colonies can also be fond of this new land and delight in its local color. But if he were repelled by its climate, lonely for his native country, the problem would be whether or not to accept these nuisances and this discomfort in exchange for the advantages of a colony.

Soon he hides it no longer... From then on, even though fed up, sick of the exotic, at times ill, he hangs on; he will be trapped into retirement or perhaps death. How can he return to his homeland if this would mean cutting his standard of living in half?

It is this simple reasoning which delays their return, even if life has become difficult, if not dangerous, during the recent past. Realizing that they have been away from their country long enough to have no more living acquaintances, we can understand them in part... But they exaggerate their anguish. In organizing their daily habits in the colonial community, they imported and imposed the way of life of their own country, where they regularly spend their vacations, from which they draw their administrative, political and cultural inspiration, and on which their eyes are constantly fixed...

Having found profit either by choice or by chance, the colonizer has nevertheless not yet become aware of the historic role which will be his. He is lacking one step in understanding his new status; he must also understand the origin and significance of this profit. Actually this is not long in coming. For how long could he fail to see the misery of the colonized and the relation of that misery to his own comfort? He realizes that this easy profit is so great only because it is wrested from others. In short, he finds two things in one: he discovers the existence of the colonizer as he discovers his own privilege.

Adapted from Albert Memmi, *The Colonizer and The Colonized.*
© 1965 by The Orion Press, Inc.

119. The passage suggests that historically, the attitude towards the colonizer, has been one of:
   A. reverance.
   B. scorn.
   C. appreciation.
   D. ambivilance.

120. The author rhetorically questions why the colonizer usually seeks a country where his language is spoken, in order to support the author's claim that:
   A. the colonizer is not searching for adventure.
   B. the colonizer will eventually want to return to his native land.
   C. the colonizer desires to spread his culture to the nonliterate.
   D. the colonized live in misery to support the comfort of the colonizer.

121. The passage asserts that the primary reason for leaving for a colony is:
   A. adventure.
   B. the need for a change of environment.
   C. a selfless desire to help mankind.
   D. economic profit.

122. The author argues that the unhappy colonizer is reluctant to leave the colony because:
   A. he has made many friends in the colony and enjoys the local color.
   B. he is unwilling to risk the financial security the colony provides.
   C. he visits his homeland often enough to enjoy the benefits of both countries.
   D. he does not want to be considered a failure by his acquaintances.

123. It may be reasonable to infer from the passage that the attitude of the colonizer to the colonized is one of:
   A. concern for cultural development.
   B. detachment; the colonized are relevant insofar as personal gain is involved.
   C. respect; the colonized were viewed as nobel adventurers.
   D. appreciation for helping to provide a better standard of living.

124. According to the passage, the success of a colonizer in a colony CANNOT be attributed to:
   I. the colonizer's adventurous nature.
   II. the colonizer's ability to grasp local customs and languages.
   III. the level of education of the colonizer.

   A. I only
   B. II only
   C. I and II only
   D. I, II, and III

125. According to the passage, what historic role will be accorded to the colonizer?
   A. International development
   B. Discovery of new lands and territories
   C. Draining resources and money from developing countries
   D. There is no historic role.

Englishmen have never cared for music as they care for football or film stars. They like singing, most of them, either making a noise themselves or listening to others. There is a long tradition both of religion and conviviality by which men and women who would not claim to be musical will gladly take part in a hymn or join in a chorus. There has been a tradition centuries old by which choral singing in parts has been a fairly widespread pastime. In Elizabethan times it was something more: for about forty years it appears to have been a fashionable craze among cultivated people, and, though it is easy to overestimate the excellence of their performance, the singers of those days conferred an incalculable benefit upon the art of music and a rich heritage upon English musical life by their assiduous practice, thereby stimulating to activity a whole school of first-rate composers. Assuredly England has never been a "land without music," as the reproachful German phrase went a couple of generations ago. But music, musical affairs, musical politics, new compositions, the status of individual artists, have never in this country been "front page news" : the bulk of the population does not really care how music gets along provided that on occasion it can obtain what it wants for ceremonial occasions, for occasional polite entertainment, for lubricating the wheels on which its theatrical or restaurant entertainment runs... Our festivals, our opera seasons, and the performance of our virtuosi, even our musical competitions, leave our national phlegm unmoved. The tantrums of a prima donna have a certain human interest for our popular newspapers, but by and large the great public does not care. Are we then a musical people?

... Are we a blue-eyed people? Some of us are blue-eyed and some of us are musical. The musical enthusiasts are a small minority, but the potentially musical are a much larger number. Perhaps five percent are definitely insusceptible to music... The rest are capable of having their interest, and perhaps ultimately their love, aroused for the art. There are many things in this beautiful world that compete for our attention, for our limited time, for our not unlimited mental energy, and for our pocket-money, and many will sacrifice music to fly-fishing or watching birds... many a gifted person with artistic abilities that run in several directions at once will devote himself to water-colors instead of the piano. But the coming of the wireless broadcasting has at least made numbers of people, running into the hundreds of thousands, aware of music as a factor in their experience of life.

The kind of satisfaction that comes from music... is one of the things that give value to life. Possibly it is the most perfect example of those higher disinterested values that give significance to life, in that it is unmixed with social, political and ethical purposes and so provides us with an instance of what is valuable in and for itself alone without further object. Not everyone will want this particular kind of satisfaction from music; some take a more hedonistic view of it and value it as just one more ingredient in the good life. Still others are content with the opiate of light music. But whichever of the many sorts of psychological satisfaction that can be got from music may be found by any individual, it is so far a part of his life's experience, and more and more people are coming to be aware of it as such and to value it as an enrichment of their lives.

Adapted from Frank Howes, *Fontana Guide to Orchestral Music*, © 1958 by Collins Clear Type Press.

126. According to the passage, the attitude of the English during the Elizabethan era was most influential in producing:
    A. an interest in musical affairs which had never been there previously.
    B. a revival in choral singing in parts.
    C. increased participation in hymn and choir singing in churches.
    D. great musical compositions by a new era of composers.

127. The passage suggests that the English might be less interested than Germans, in news concerning:
    A. the tantrums of a prima dona.
    B. the migration of a singer from one opera house to another.
    C. new forms of musical entertainment.
    D. football, and the newest developments in that sport.

128. According to the author, someone who is "insusceptible to music" is someone who:
    A. is uninterested in musical affairs, musical politics, and the state of individual artists.
    B. would rather not waste their time fly-fishing or bird-watching.
    C. is incapable of having their interest for music aroused.
    D. would rather devote their time to water-colors.

129. The passage indicates that the renewed musical awareness in England, can in part be attributed to:
   A. the assiduous practicing of singers over the years.
   B. the emergence of a whole new school for talented composers.
   C. the introduction of wireless broadcasting into society.
   D. a decline of interest in football that has occurred over the years.

130. Based on the passage, one could conclude that the author believes that music's greatest value lies in the fact that:
   A. it has a great ability to bring joy.
   B. it is a form of expression which is detached from politics, social and cultural issues.
   C. it is a component of the good life.
   D. it has the power to enrich the life of every individual who becomes aware of it.

131. Which of the following, best expresses the main idea of the passage?
   A. The English are an unmusical people who have never fully appreciated the value of the art.
   B. Music is an art which has never been developed to its full potential in England.
   C. Music is an art which has the power to enrich the lives of everyone it touches in different ways.
   D. The development of music in a society is wholly dependent on that society.

It was soon after Christmas, 1980. The women and the small boy with them had travelled to a town about fifteen miles from Houston for dinner: now, as they made their way home, the child noticed something strange in the sky. A blazing light was gliding toward them over the pines.

As it approached, the light resolved itself into a brilliant, diamond-shaped object. Flames shot out from its underside. In her fifty-one years, Betty Cash, the driver, had never seen anything like it. Nor had Vickie Landrum, who pulled her young grandson close to her as the object slowed and then hovered over the roadway as if preparing to land...

In its elusiveness, the so-called Cash-Landrum incident is typical of reports of mysterious objects flashing across the sky and, sometimes touching down on the surface of the earth. Indeed, the very term used to describe such phenomena, unidentified flying objects, or UFOs, shows how little is known about these sightings... David Jacobs, an American expert in the field, defines a UFO as "the report of an extraordinary airborne or landed object, or related experience, that remains anomalous after proper scientific analysis." The term is clearly not equivalent to the popular "flying saucer," although it can, in theory, include spaceships piloted by alien creatures. Using this definition, few people would dispute the existence of UFOs.

Disputes do arise, however, when investigators seek to determine exactly what a given UFO was... Most sightings of UFOs yield no tangible clues, only eyewitness accounts.

In these cases, two complicating factors come into play. The first is witness reliability. Even when those claiming to have seen UFOs are regarded as credible, it may be difficult to reconstruct exactly what it was that they saw. The objective, physical act of seeing can be vastly different from the subjective act of interpreting what is seen. The viewer forms judgements even in the act of observation...

The second complication in UFO cases is the bias of the investigator. Hard-core sceptics and ardent believers will inevitably reach different conclusions about an ambiguous case...

Sceptics frequently seek to portray UFO believers as fringe personalities and occultists who are unable to accept modern society. But surveys show that believers are, in fact, no more interested in the occult and no less satisfied with life than anyone else.

A sizeable number of people today envision UFOs exactly as the vehicles are portrayed in most science-fiction films and books - as spacecraft carrying extraterrestrial beings from technologically advanced worlds. This is, of course, a relatively recent conception that has been stimulated, perhaps, by our expanding knowledge of outer space as well as by the pervasive images of fiction and motion pictures. But strange sights appeared in the skies long before space flight - or manned flight of any kind - was possible. And in each century these visions took on identities that tell much about the world view of those who saw them. In antiquity, for example, people discerned angelic messengers; in the nineteenth century, they saw dirigibles. Today, awed observers look skyward and see glowing envoys from other worlds.

And yet, a common thread seems to link such sightings from earliest history through today. Gravity-bound humans, gazing at the endless sky, seem to have felt that there is more to existence than can be seen on the earth's surface, that life might come in more shapes than those we know, that we are not alone among the myriad stars sparkling in the boundless cosmos. The record of mysterious aerial sightings reaches back to the dawn of written history. Seen in the light of modern knowledge and theories, however, accounts of such incidents are far from conclusive. Clearly, if the modern and presumably scientific world has been unable to establish the nature of recent reports of UFOs, then conjectures that are based on ancient records can hardly be more conclusive. Even so, ancient and medieval chronicles of UFO-like sightings are fascinating and suggestive, and they often sound surprisingly like today's descriptions.

132. According to the passage, what was the attitude of Betty Cash and Vickie Landrum regarding the mysterious incident in 1980?
A. The incident was pleasant.
B. The incident was frightening and amazing.
C. The women were afraid to report the incident.
D. The incident was boring.

133. The author suggests that the term "flying saucer" is not equivalent to the definition of UFO proposed by David Jacobs because:
   A. there is clear evidence for the existence of UFOs but none for the existence of flying saucers.
   B. flying saucers are not extraordinary.
   C. flying saucers are piloted by alien creatures.
   D. a flying saucer is only one in a set of objects and experiences that the term UFO encompasses.

134. According to the passage, eyewitness accounts are complicated because:
   A. many witnesses lack credibility and do not accurately reconstruct what was seen.
   B. witnesses usually interpret their observations.
   C. investigators who are hard-core believers always confirm eyewitness reports.
   D. many eyewitnesses do not report their sightings at all.

135. The author claims that the way people envision UFOs today has been greatly influenced by which of the following?
   A. Books
   B. Motion pictures
   C. Space travel
   D. All of the above

136. The passage suggests that historical sightings of UFOs are far from conclusive because:
   A. they often sound surprisingly like today's descriptions.
   B. there is no way to scientifically establish the nature of these reports.
   C. historically, UFO believers have been occultists and fringe personalities.
   D. surveys have shown that people have only recently begun to believe that UFOs exist.

137. "In 1917, on October 13, fifty thousand people in Fatima watched in amazement as the clouds revealed a huge silver disk." This fulfilled a prophecy of the Virgin Mary and was declared a miracle by the Church. Ufologists thought the disk was a UFO. Which of the author's claims would this support?
   A. Sceptics frequently seek to portray believers as occultists who are unable to accept modern society.
   B. The objective physical act of seeing can be vastly different from the subjective act of interpreting what is seen.
   C. Humans, gazing at the endless sky, seem always to have known that there is more to existence.
   D. In antiquity, people discerned angelic messengers.

END OF VERBAL REASONING. IF TIME REMAINS, YOU MAY GO BACK AND CHECK YOUR WORK IN THIS TEST BOOKLET.

CANDIDATE'S
SIGNATURE _____
SOCIAL SECURITY NUMBER _____

BOOKLET GS2-III

TEST GS-2

Writing Sample
Questions : 2
Time : 60 Minutes
Two 30 Minute Prompts,
Timed Separately

OPEN BOOKLET ONLY WHEN TIMER IS READY.

The Gold Standard MCAT* has been designed exclusively to test knowledge and thinking skills. The exam may contain hypothetical statements and/or express controversial ideas. Statements contained herein do not necessarily reflect the policy, position, or view of RuveneCo Publishing.

* MCAT is a registered service mark of the Association of American Medical Colleges, which is not associated with this product.

WRITING SAMPLE

INSTRUCTIONS: This test is designed to evaluate your writing skills. There are two writing assignments. You will have 30 minutes to complete each part.

Your answers for the Writing Sample should be written in ANSWER DOCUMENT 2. Your response to Part 1 must be written only on answer sheets marked " 1 ," and your response to Part 2 on answer sheets marked " 2 ." The first 30 minutes may be used to respond to Part 1 only. The second 30 minutes may be used to respond to Part 2 only. If you finish writing before time is up, you may review your work ONLY on the response you have just completed.

Use your time in an efficient manner. Prior to writing your response, read the assignment carefully. The space below each writing assignment may be used to make notes in planning a response.

Since this is a test of your writing skills, you should use complete sentences as well organized as you can make them in the allotted time. Corrections or additions can be made neatly between the lines but there should be no writing in the margins of the answer booklet.

There are three pages in the answer document for each part of the test. Though you are not expected to use each page, do not skip lines.

Use a black pen to write your response.

Illegible essays cannot be scored.

PART I

Consider the following statement:

A nation cannot defend itself against the invasion of ideas.

Write a unified essay performing the following tasks. Explain the meaning of the statement. Describe a specific situation in which a nation can defend itself against the invasion of ideas. Discuss what you think determines whether a nation can or cannot defend itself against the invasion of ideas.

DO NOT TURN TO THE NEXT PAGE UNTIL TIME PERMITS.

PART II

Consider the following statement:

The right to do something means that doing it is right.

Write a unified essay performing the following tasks. Explain the meaning of the statement. Describe a specific situation in which the right to do something does not mean that doing it is right. Discuss what you think determines whether or not the right to do something means that doing it is right.

END OF WRITING SAMPLE.
DO NOT RETURN TO PART I.

TEST GS-2

Biological Sciences
Questions 143-219
Time : 100 Minutes

OPEN BOOKLET ONLY WHEN TIMER IS READY.

The Gold Standard MCAT* has been designed exclusively to test knowledge and thinking skills. The exam may contain hypothetical statements and/or express controversial ideas. Statements contained herein do not necessarily reflect the policy, position, or view of RuveneCo Publishing.

* MCAT is a registered service mark of the Association of American Medical Colleges, which is not associated with this product.

BIOLOGICAL SCIENCES

INSTRUCTIONS: Of the 77 questions in the Biological Sciences test, 62 are organized into groups preceded by a passage. After evaluating the passage, select the best answer to each question in the group. Fifteen questions are independent of any descriptive passage or each other. Similarly, select the best answer to these questions. If you are unsure of an answer, eliminate the alternatives that you know to be incorrect and select an answer from the remaining alternatives. To indicate your selection, blacken the corresponding oval on Answer Document 1, GS-2. A periodic table is provided for your use during the test.

PERIODIC TABLE OF THE ELEMENTS

1 H 1.008																	2 He 4.003
3 Li 6.941	4 Be 9.012											5 B 10.81	6 C 12.011	7 N 14.007	8 O 15.999	9 F 18.998	10 Ne 20.179
11 Na 22.990	12 Mg 24.305											13 Al 26.982	14 Si 28.086	15 P 30.974	16 S 32.06	17 Cl 35.453	18 Ar 39.948
19 K 39.098	20 Ca 40.08	21 Sc 44.956	22 Ti 47.90	23 V 50.942	24 Cr 51.996	25 Mn 54.938	26 Fe 55.847	27 Co 58.933	28 Ni 58.70	29 Cu 63.546	30 Zn 65.38	31 Ga 69.72	32 Ge 72.59	33 As 74.922	34 Se 78.96	35 Br 79.904	36 Kr 83.80
37 Rb 85.468	38 Sr 87.62	39 Y 88.906	40 Zr 91.22	41 Nb 92.906	42 Mo 95.94	43 Tc (98)	44 Ru 101.07	45 Rh 102.906	46 Pd 106.4	47 Ag 107.868	48 Cd 112.41	49 In 114.82	50 Sn 118.69	51 Sb 121.75	52 Te 127.60	53 I 126.905	54 Xe 131.30
55 Cs 132.905	56 Ba 137.33	57 *La 138.906	72 Hf 178.49	73 Ta 180.948	74 W 183.85	75 Re 186.207	76 Os 190.2	77 Ir 192.22	78 Pt 195.09	79 Au 196.967	80 Hg 200.59	81 Tl 204.37	82 Pb 207.2	83 Bi 208.980	84 Po (209)	85 At (210)	86 Rn (222)
87 Fr (223)	88 Ra 226.025	89 **Ac 227.028	104 Unq (261)	105 Unp (262)	106 Unh (263)												

*	58 Ce 140.12	59 Pr 140.908	60 Nd 144.24	61 Pm (145)	62 Sm 150.4	63 Eu 151.96	64 Gd 157.25	65 Tb 158.925	66 Dy 162.50	67 Ho 164.930	68 Er 167.26	69 Tm 168.934	70 Yb 173.04	71 Lu 174.967

**	90 Th 232.038	91 Pa 231.036	92 U 238.029	93 Np 237.048	94 Pu (244)	95 Am (243)	96 Cm (247)	97 Bk (247)	98 Cf (251)	99 Es (254)	100 Fm (257)	101 Md (258)	102 No (259)	103 Lr (260)

Passage I (Questions 143-148)

Following blastula formation the developing embryo undergoes gastrulation, a tremendous reshaping with little or no additional cell growth. Since the blastulas vary in shape between different animals, the geometry of the reshaping also varies. Regardless of the type of animal, gastrulation results in the same fundamental cell layers: the ectoderm, the endoderm and the mesoderm. These three tissue types or *primordial layers* will form every organ in the developing embryo.

Research has recently shed light on the cells responsible for the continuation of the life cycle - the gametes. Early in the development of all animals, certain cells undergo determination producing primordial germ cells. Experiments have demonstrated an area in the egg cytoplasm of some animals which appears to be responsible for the determination of the primordial germ cell. This special region is the *germ plasm*.

To clarify the importance of the germ plasm, experiments have been carried out using microinjection of the developing fruit fly *Drosophila melanogaster*. Under normal conditions, pregametic cells arise from the posterior end of the syncytial blastoderm. Irradiation of this end of the egg produces a sterile fly. If cytoplasmic material from the posterior part of the developing egg is suctioned with a micropipette and injected into the anterior part of another developing egg, germ cells are formed at this abnormal site as well as the normal position. No nuclei are transferred in this experiment thus the evidence points to non-genetic material in the germ plasm of the egg being responsible for germ cell formation.

143. Damage to the ectoderm during gastrulation will result in an embryo with an underdeveloped:
    A. reproductive system.
    B. nervous system.
    C. excretory system.
    D. digestive system.

144. Immediately prior to gastrulation, which of the following events take place?
    A. The sperm penetrates the corona radiata and zona pellucida so that fusion of the gametes occurs.
    B. The secondary oocyte becomes a mature ovum by completing its second meiotic division.
    C. Implantation in the endometrium occurs.
    D. Rapid mitotic divisions result in daughter cells, smaller than their parent cells, being formed.

145. After sexual maturation, the primordial germ cells in the testes are initially:
    A. called spermatids and are haploid.
    B. called primary spermatocytes and are haploid.
    C. called primary spermatocytes and are diploid.
    D. called spermatogonia and are diploid.

146. In the experiment described in the passage, which of the following materials in the germ plasm would likely be most functional in inducing germ cell function?
    A. Nuclear DNA
    B. Mitochondria
    C. RNA and protein molecules
    D. Microtubules

147. Which of the following experimental results would contradict the conclusion made from the experiment in the passage?
    A. The only subunits detected after digesting the germ plasm were nucleotides.
    B. Microinjection of the midportion of a developing egg with germ plasm resulted in germ cell production at an abnormal site.
    C. Microinjection of proteases into the posterior end of the syncytial blastoderm inhibited the production of germ cells.
    D. The irradiated egg which produced a sterile fly demonstrated no post-radiation genetic abnormalities.

148. The mechanism by which blastomeres differentiate into germ cells is referred to as:
    A. induction.
    B. determination.
    C. specialization.
    D. differentiation.

Muscular dystrophy is one of the most frequently encountered genetic diseases, affecting one in every 4000 boys (but much less commonly girls) born in America. Muscular dystrophy results in the progressive degeneration of skeletal and cardiac muscle fibers, weakening the muscle and leading ultimately to death from respiratory or cardiac failure.

The gene responsible for a major form of muscular dystrophy has been identified. This gene codes for a protein known as *dystrophin*, which is absent or present in a nonfunctional form in patients with the disease. Dystrophin is located on the inner surface of the plasma membrane in normal muscle protein.

The cloning of a fragment of DNA allows indefinite amounts of dystrophin to be produced from even a single original molecule. An insertion generates a hybrid or chimeric plasmid or phage, consisting in part of the additional "foreign" sequences. These chimeric elements replicate in bacteria just like the original plasmid or phage and so can be obtained in large amounts. Copies of the original foreign fragment can be retrieved from the progeny. Since the properties of the chimeric species usually are unaffected by the particular foreign sequences that are involved, almost any sequence of DNA can be cloned in this way. Because the phage or plasmid is used to "carry" the foreign DNA as an inert part of the genome, it is often referred to as the cloning vector.

149. Which of the following best explains the high incidence of muscular dystrophy in boys?
    A. The disease is sex-linked and the gene which codes for dystrophin occurs on the Y chromosome.
    B. The disease is sex-linked and the gene which codes for dystrophin occurs on the X chromosome.
    C. Fathers who have the disease pass it on to their sons, but not to their daughters.
    D. Mothers who have the disease pass it on to their sons, but not to their daughters.

150. The functions of dystrophin likely include all but which of the following?
    A. Recognition of protein hormones important to the functioning of the cells
    B. Maintenance of the structural integrity of the plasma membrane
    C. Keeping ion channels within the cells open
    D. Protection of elements within the membrane during contraction of the cells

151. In order for cloning of foreign DNA to take place, bacterial plasmids must:
    A. incorporate the foreign DNA into the DNA in their capsids.
    B. possess several sites at which DNA can be inserted.
    C. be able to resume their usual life cycle after additional sequences of DNA have been incorporated into their genomes.
    D. divide meiotically, so no two daughter cells are exactly alike.

152. Plasmid genomes are circular and a single cleavage converts the DNA into a linear molecule. The two ends can be joined to the ends of a linear foreign DNA to regenerate a circular chimeric plasmid. Which of the following rules would be most important in allowing this process to occur?
    A. DNA replication occurs in a semi-conservative manner.
    B. The genetic code is composed of triplets of bases which correspond to the 20 amino acids used in protein structure.
    C. The stability of the DNA helix is dependent on the number of C-G bonds present.
    D. Phosphodiester bonds must link the plasmid DNA to the foreign DNA.

153. One possible method of treating muscular dystrophy using cloning techniques would be to:

A. splice the nonfunctional genes out of dystrophic muscle cells and clone them in bacterial plasmids.

B. determine the amino acid sequence of dystrophin and introduce the protein into muscle cells artificially.

C. clone the gene responsible for coding dystrophin and insert the normal gene into dystrophic muscle cells.

D. prevent skeletal and cardiac muscle tissue degradation by cloning and inserting the genes for troponin and tropomyosin into dystrophic muscle cells.

154. If the gene which codes for troponin was absent from muscle cells, which of the following processes would NOT be inhibited?

A. The movement of tropomyosin to a new position on the actin molecules

B. The uncovering of the active sites for the attachment of actin to the cross bridges of myosin

C. The hydrolysis of ATP in the myosin head to produce ADP, P_i, and energy

D. The release of Ca^{2+} ions from the sarcoplasmic reticulum

Passage III (Questions 155-160)

Active transport is the energy-consuming transport of molecules against a concentration gradient. Energy is required because the substance must be moved in the opposite direction of its natural tendency to diffuse. Movement is usually unidirectional, unlike diffusion which is reversible.

When movement of ions is considered, two factors will influence the direction in which they diffuse: one is concentration, the other is electrical charge. An ion will usually diffuse from a region of its high concentration to a region of its low concentration. It will also generally be attracted towards a region of opposite charge, and move away from a region of similar charge. Thus ions are said to move down *electrochemical gradients*, which are the combined effects of both electrical and concentration gradients. Strictly speaking, active transport of ions is their movement against an electrochemical gradient powered by an energy source.

Research has shown that the cell surface membranes of most cells possess sodium pumps. Usually, though not always, the sodium pump is coupled with a potassium pump. The combined pump is called the sodium-potassium pump. This pump is an excellent example of active transport.

Table 1: Concentration of Na^+, K^+, and Cl^- inside and outside mammalian motor neurons.

Ion	Concentration (mmol/L H_2O)		Equilibrium potential (mV)
	Inside cell	Outside cell	
Na^+	15.0	150.0	+60
K^+	150.0	5.5	-90
Cl^-	9.0	125.0	-75
Resting membrane potential (V_m) = -70 mV			

155. All of the following explain the ionic concentrations in Table 1 EXCEPT:
  A. Na^+ and Cl^- ions passively diffuse more quickly into the extracellular fluid than K^+ ions.
  B. Na^+ ions are actively pumped out of the intracellular fluid.
  C. the negative charge of the cell contents repels Cl^- ions from the cell.
  D. the cell membrane is more freely permeable to K^+ ions than to Na^+ and Cl^- ions.

156. If cyanide was added to red blood cells, what would be expected to happen to the ionic composition of the cells?
  A. Na^+ ions would be actively pumped into the cell and K^+ ions would be pumped out.
  B. Intracellular Na^+ would increase since the sodium pump would stop functioning.
  C. The potential of the cell membrane would not be reversed so that Cl^- ions would freely enter the cell.
  D. The cell membrane would become freely permeable to Na^+ and Cl^- ions.

157. The temporary increase in the sarcolemma's permeability to Na^+ and K^+ ions that occurs at the motor end plate of a neuromuscular junction is immediately preceded by:
  A. the release of acetylcholine from the motor neuron into the synaptic gap.
  B. the release of adrenaline from the motor neuron into the synaptic gap.
  C. the passage of a nerve impulse along the axon of a motor neuron.
  D. the release of noradrenaline from a sensory neuron into the synaptic gap.

158. The overall reaction which takes place at the sodium pump is given by the equation:

$$3Na^+_{(inside)} + 2K^+_{(outside)} + ATP^{4-} + H_2O \rightarrow$$

$$3Na^+_{(outside)} + 2K^+_{(inside)} + ADP^{3-} + P_i + H^+$$

When a muscle is very active, at the end of glycolysis, pyruvate is converted to lactate by the addition of H^+ ions. During vigorous exercise, how many ions of K^+ could be pumped into a cell per molecule of glucose?

A. 2
B. 4
C. 8
D. 12

159. Active transport assumes particular importance in all but which of the following structures?

A. Cells of the large intestine
B. Alveoli
C. Nerve and muscle cells
D. Loop of Henle

160. At inhibitory synapses, a hyperpolarization of the membrane known as an inhibitory postsynaptic potential is produced rendering V_m more negative. This occurs as a result of:

A. an increase in the postsynaptic membrane's permeability to Na^+ and K^+ ions.
B. an increase in the permeability of the presynaptic membrane to Ca^{2+} ions.
C. the entry of Cl^- ions into the synaptic knob.
D. an increase in the permeability of the postsynaptic membrane to Cl^- ions.

Questions 161-165 are NOT based on a descriptive passage.

161. Consider the following reaction.

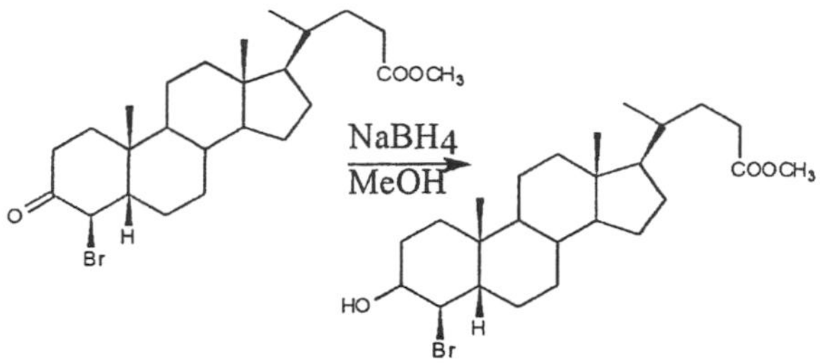
COOCH₃
NaBH4
MeOH
COOCH₃
H
Br
HO
H
Br

The infrared spectrum of the product can be distinguished from that of the starting material by the:

A. disappearance of IR absorption at 3360 cm^{-1}.
B. disappearance of IR absorption at 2820 cm^{-1}.
C. appearance of IR absorption at 3360 cm^{-1}.
D. appearance of IR absorption at 1740 cm^{-1}.

162. The free energy changes for the equilibria cis⇌trans of 1,2-, 1,3-, and 1,4- dimethylcyclohexane are shown below.

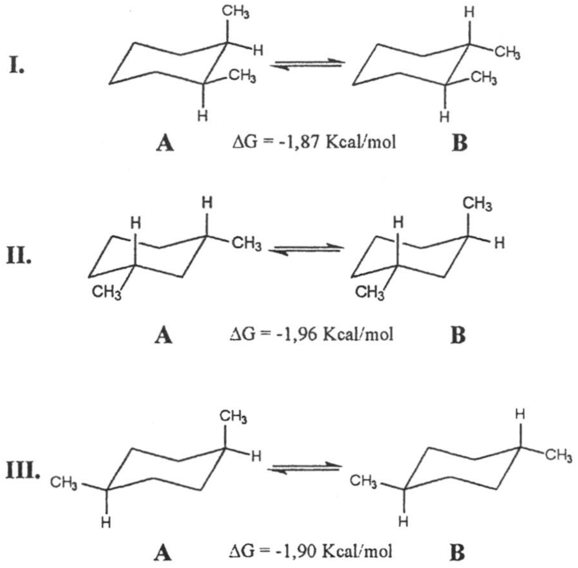
I.
CH₃
H
CH₃
H
H
CH₃
CH₃
H
A
ΔG = -1,87 Kcal/mol
B
II.
H
H
CH₃
CH₃
CH₃
H
H
CH₃
A
ΔG = -1,96 Kcal/mol
B
III.
CH₃
H
CH₃
H
H
CH₃
CH₃
H
A
ΔG = -1,90 Kcal/mol
B

The most stable diastereomer in each case would be:

A. IA, IIB, IIIA
B. IB, IIA, IIIB
C. IA, IIA, IIIA
D. IA, IIB, IIIB

163. Which of the following is required for the human ovum to undergo a second meiotic division?

A. FSH
B. LH
C. Estrogen and progesterone
D. Fertilization

164. All chordates possess a:

A. hollow dorsal nerve cord.
B. vertebral column.
C. closed vascular system.
D. tail in the adult form.

165. When a dilute solution of formaldehyde is dissolved in ^{18}O-labeled water and allowed to equilibrate, ^{18}O incorporation occurs thus indicating the existence of an intermediate product. Which of the following compounds best represents the intermediate product of this ^{18}O exchange?

A.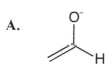

B.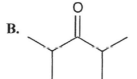

C. HO   OH
      \   /
       C
      / \
     H   H

D. OH⁺
    ‖
    C
   / \
  H   H

Streptococcus mutans is associated with the tooth surface and appears to be the major causative agent of dental caries, or tooth decay. *Streptococcus mutans* produces glucan, a sticky polymer of glucose that acts like a cement and binds the bacterial cells together and to the tooth surface.

Glucan is formed only in the presence of the disaccharide sucrose (the type of sugar found in sweets), through a process catalyzed by an enzyme of the cocci. The enzyme links glucose molecules together to form glucan, while fructose molecules are fermented by the streptococci into lactic acid. Lactic acid can etch the surface of the teeth, enhancing microbial adherence.

Although *S. mutans* initiates dental caries, other bacteria such as *Lactobacillus* and *Actinomyces* species can contribute to caries as secondary invaders. The aggregation of bacteria and organic matter on the surface of the teeth is termed dental plaque. Dental plaque contains a very high number of bacteria, about 10^8 cells per milligram.

In addition to bacteria, certain commensalistic protozoa may inhabit the oral cavity. For example, the flagellated *Trichomonas tenax* may occur in gum margins and in the plaque and cavities of teeth.

166. Once teeth appear, the bacteria comprising the microbial flora of the tissues surrounding the teeth are mainly:
- **A.** gram-negative, aerobes.
- **B.** gram-positive, aerobes.
- **C.** gram-positive, facultative anaerobes.
- **D.** gram-negative, obligate anaerobes.

167. *Streptococcus mutans* and *Lactobacillus* are, respectively:
- **A.** spherical and helical.
- **B.** spherical and cylindrical.
- **C.** cylindrical and helical.
- **D.** helical and cylindrical.

168. The enzyme which catalyzes the formation of glucan is likely located:
- **A.** in the cytosol of the cocci.
- **B.** in lysosomes within the cytoplasm of the cocci.
- **C.** in the nuclei of the cocci.
- **D.** on the cell surface membrane of the cocci.

169. The passage suggests that the enzyme produced by *Streptococcus mutans* initially acts by:
- **A.** catalyzing the formation of glycosidic bonds between glucose molecules.
- **B.** splitting sucrose into fructose and glucose.
- **C.** catalyzing the formation of glycosidic bonds between fructose molecules.
- **D.** catalyzing the fermentation of fructose.

170. The high number of bacteria in dental plaque result from the proliferation of bacteria by all of the following methods, EXCEPT:
- **A.** translocation.
- **B.** transduction.
- **C.** transformation.
- **D.** binary fission.

Passage V (Questions 171-176)

Figure 1 illustrates chemical methods often used by organic chemists for qualitative analysis of water soluble unknowns. Table 1 lists characteristic chemical tests of organic compounds. For instance, Fehling's tests that are positive are indicative of an aldehyde.

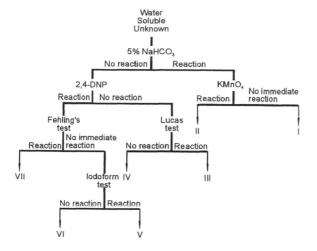

Figure 1

Table 1

Chemical Test	Compounds
Sodium hydroxide	Organic acids: carboxylic acids and phenols
Lucas	Alcohols with 5 or less carbon atoms
Sodium bicarbonate	Carboxylic acids
2,4-Dinitro-phenylhydrazine (DNP)	Aldehydes and ketones
Fehling's solution	Aldehydes
Iodine in sodium hydroxide (Iodoform)	Acetaldehydes and ketones with the CH_3-CO- group Alcohols with the $CH_3CH(OH)$- as a structural feature
Sulfuric acid	Alcohols, ethers, alkenes Soluble Lewis bases

171. Cyclohexanol should fall into which of the following groups?
   A. I
   B. II
   C. III
   D. IV

172. A water soluble unknown is unreactive in the presence of sodium bicarbonate, gives a positive 2,4-DNP test and negative Fehling's and Iodoform tests. In which of the following classes should this compound be classified?
   A. Aldehyde
   B. Ketone
   C. Carboxylic acid
   D. Alcohol

173. When an ether solution of an aldehyde is added to an ether solution of lithium aluminum hydride ($LiAlH_4$), the carbonyl group of the aldehyde will be:
   A. reduced to the corresponding primary alcohol.
   B. hydrated to the corresponding diol.
   C. reduced to the corresponding secondary alcohol.
   D. deoxygenated to the corresponding alkane.

174. Acetone should give positive test results for which of the following chemical tests?
   A. Lucas and sodium bicarbonate
   B. 2,4-DNP and Fehling's
   C. Iodoform and 2,4-DNP
   D. Iodoform and potassium permanganate

175. 3-Pentanone falls into group VI, but acetone falls into group V. This is most likely due to the fact that acetone is:
   A. a cyclic ketone.
   B. an aldehyde.
   C. aromatic.
   D. a methyl ketone.

176. Sodium bicarbonate is a weak base and as such reacts readily with acetic acid. The evolution of bubbles which accompanies this acid-base neutralization reaction is due to the formation of which of the following gases?
   A. $CO(g)$
   B. $CO_2(g)$
   C. $H_2(g)$
   D. $O_2(g)$

Viral hepatitis type B (serum hepatitis) is an infection of humans that primarily damages the liver. The causative agent is a virus called HBV, which is transmitted in much the same way as the HIV virus.

If HBV could be cultivated in the laboratory in unlimited amounts, it could be injected into humans as a vaccine to stimulate immunity against hepatitis type B. Unfortunately, it is not yet possible to grow HBV in laboratory culture. However, the blood of chronically infected people contains numerous particles of a harmless protein component of the virus. This protein, called HBsAg, can be extracted from the blood, purified, and treated chemically to destroy any live virus that might also be present. When HBsAg particles are injected into humans, they stimulate immunity against the complete infectious virus.

Of late, a new source of HBsAg particles have become available. Thanks to genetic engineering, a technique for cloning the gene for HBsAg into cells of the common bread yeast *Saccharomyces cerevisiae* has been developed. The yeast expresses the gene and makes HBsAg particles that can be extracted after the cells are broken. Since yeast cells are easy to propagate, it is now possible to obtain unlimited amounts of HBsAg particles.

177. Before being injected into humans, the HBV virus would first have to:
   A. be cloned in yeast cells to ensure that enough of the virus had been injected to elicit an immune response.
   B. have its protein coat removed.
   C. be purified.
   D. be inactivated.

178. Which of the following physiological processes would be LEAST affected in someone who had viral hepatitis type B?
   A. The production of the fat soluble vitamins A, D, E, and K
   B. The production of fibrinogen and albumin
   C. The breakdown of hemoglobin to amino acids
   D. The conversion of amino acids into carbohydrates

179. HBsAg is likely a component of:
   A. the capsid of the virus.
   B. the nucleic acid core of the virus.
   C. the tail of the virus.
   D. the slimy mucoid-like capsule on the outer surface of the virus.

180. The following graph shows the immune response for an initial injection of HBsAg and a subsequent injection of the HBV virus. Which of the following best explains the differences in the two responses?

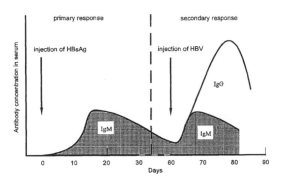

   A. During the initial response, the immune response was carried out primarily by macrophages and B-lymphocytes.
   B. During the secondary response, T-cells possessing membrane receptors, recognized and attacked the viral antigens.
   C. Memory cells produced by T- and B-cells during the first exposure made the second response faster and more intense.
   D. Memory cells produced by macrophages during the first infection recognized the viral antigens more quickly during the second infection, causing antibody production to be increased.

181. Yeast cells used for cloning the gene for HBsAg could be propagated by all but which of the following methods?
   A. Budding
   B. Transduction
   C. Fusion
   D. Meiotic division

Aside from diabetes, thyroid disease is the most common glandular disorder. Over 10 million North Americans are treated for thyroid conditions, often an underactive or overactive gland. Overwhelmingly, women between the ages of 20 and 60 are much more likely than men to succumb to these conditions. The etiology lies in the failure of the immune system to recognize the thyroid gland as part of the body and thus antibodies are sent to attack the gland.

The plasma proteins that bind thyroid hormones are albumin, a prealbumin called thyroxine-binding prealbumin (TBPA), and a globulin with an electrophoretic mobility, thyroxine-binding globulin (TBG). The free thyroid hormones in plasma are in equilibrium with the protein-bound thyroid hormones in the tissues. Free thyroid hormones are added to the circulating pool by the thyroid. It is the free thyroid hormones in plasma that are physiologically active and imbalances in these hormones result in thyroid disease.

In addition, in humans there are four small parathyroid glands that produce the hormone, parathormone, which is a peptide composed of 84 amino acids. Parathormone and the thyroid hormone calcitonin work antagonistically to regulate the plasma calcium and phosphate levels. Overactive parathyroid glands, *hyperparathyroidism*, can lead to an increase in the level of calcium in plasma and tissues.

Table 1: Different plasma proteins and their binding capacity and affinity for thyroxine.

Protein	Plasma Level (mg/dl)	Thyroxine Binding Capacity (μg/dl)	Affinity for thyroxine	Amount of thyroxine bound in normal plasma (μg/dl)
Thyroxine binding globulin (TBG)	1.0	20	High	7
Thyroxine binding prealbumin (TBPA)	30.0	250	Moderate	1
Albumin	...	1000	Low	None
Total protein-bound thyroxine in plasma	...	...	...	8

182. Is it reasonable to conclude that thyroid disease is sex-linked?
A. No, because thyroid disease appears to be caused by a defect of the immune system and not a defective DNA sequence.
B. No, because if the disease was sex-linked, there would be a high incidence in the male, rather than the female, population.
C. Yes, because the high incidence of the disease in women suggests that a gene found on the X chromosome codes for the disease.
D. Yes, because the same factor increases the risk of women getting the disease, regardless of familial background.

183. According to Table 1, it would be expected that:
A. TBG has the highest binding capacity for thyroxine while TBPA has the highest affinity.
B. TBG has the highest binding capacity for thyroxine while albumin has the lowest affinity.
C. albumin has the highest binding capacity for thyroxine while TBPA has the highest affinity.
D. albumin has the highest binding capacity for thyroxine while TBG has the highest affinity.

Question 184 refers to Fig. 1.

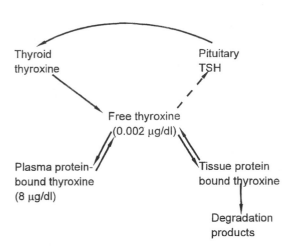

Figure 1

184. According to the equilibrium shown in Fig. 1, an elevation in the concentration of free thyroid hormone in the plasma is followed by:
   A. an increase in tissue protein-bound thyroxine.
   B. an increase in tissue protein-bound thyroxine and plasma protein-bound thyroxine.
   C. an increase in the amount of TSH secreted from the pituitary gland.
   D. an increase in both the amount of TSH secreted from the pituitary gland and the release of thyroxine from the thyroid gland.

185. Symptoms of hypothyroidism and hyperthyroidism, respectively, include:
   A. a fine tremor and diminished concentration.
   B. brittle nails and kidney stones.
   C. rapid heart beat and increased irritability.
   D. lethargy and nervous agitation.

186. Which of the following cell types would be expected to be maximally stimulated in a patient with hyperparathyroidism?
   A. Osteoclasts
   B. Osteoblasts
   C. Fibroblasts
   D. Chondrocytes

187. Parathormone influences calcium homeostasis by reducing tubular reabsorption of PO_4^{3-} in the kidneys. Which of the following, if true, would clarify the adaptive significance of this process?
   A. PO_4^{3-} and Ca^{2+} feedback negatively on each other.
   B. Elevated levels of extracellular PO_4^{3-} result in calcification of bones and tissues.
   C. Increased PO_4^{3-} levels cause an increase in parathormone secretion.
   D. Decreased extracellular PO_4^{3-} levels cause a decrease in calcitonin production.

Questions 188-192 are NOT based on a descriptive passage.

188. Bile, a chemical which emulsifies fat, is produced by the:

A. liver.
B. gallbladder.
C. common bile duct.
D. pancreas.

189. Increased physical activity results in raising the heart rate and blood pressure. The nervous system specifically implicated is:

A. somatic.
B. peripheral.
C. parasympathetic.
D. sympathetic.

190. All of the following are true about a blood pressure of 150/60 EXCEPT:

A. the value usually refers to venous pressure in the arm.
B. 60 refers to the diastolic pressure.
C. the pulse pressure is 90.
D. 150 refers to the pressure resulting from ventricular contraction.

191. Apo-X is a drug which blocks prophase from occurring. When Apo-X is added to a tissue culture, in which phase of the cell cycle would most cells be arrested?

A. Mitosis
B. G_1
C. G_2
D. Synthesis

192. The difference between the bacterium *E. coli* and the fungus *Aspergillus* is:

A. *Aspergillus* contains ribosomes.
B. *E. coli* has a cell wall.
C. *Aspergillus* can undergo anaerobic metabolism.
D. *E. coli* does not have a nucleus.

A chemist studied the mechanisms of the reactions of isopropyl bromide with sodium t-butoxide and with sodium ethoxide.

In Reaction I, the treatment of isopropyl bromide with sodium t-butoxide at 40 °C gave almost exclusively one product. The reaction yielded Compound A which had a molecular formula of C_3H_6. The ^{1}HNMR spectrum of compound A revealed the presence of vinylic protons. The kinetic rate expression indicated second order kinetics for the reaction.

In Reaction II, the treatment of isopropyl bromide with sodium ethoxide (Na^+EtO^-) at 30 °C yielded an ether (Compound B) that had a molecular formula of $C_5H_{12}O$, and Compound A that had a molecular mass of 42 grams. Compound B accounted for only 20% of the total product. The remainder consisted of Compound A.

Compound B was found to be stable to base, dilute acid and most reducing agents. The infrared spectrum of Compound B revealed a strong band at 1100 cm^{-1} and the absence of stretching absorptions at 1730 cm^{-1} was noted.

Compound A was readily oxidized by a neutral solution of cold dilute potassium permanganate. During the oxidation process, the characteristic purple color of the permanganate ion (MnO_4^-) disappeared and was replaced by a brown precipitate indicating the formation of manganese dioxide (MnO_2).

193. Which of the following best describes the reaction mechanisms that led to the formation of products A and B?
   A. B is the S_N2 product and A is derived from an E2 reaction.
   B. A is the S_N2 product and B is derived from an E2 reaction.
   C. B is the S_N1 product and A is derived from an E1 reaction.
   D. B is the S_N1 product and A is derived from an E2 reaction.

194. Compound A belongs to which of the following classes of organic compounds?
   A. Alcohol
   B. Ketone
   C. Alkene
   D. Ester

195. Which of the following most accurately represents the activated complex formed in Reaction II and that subsequently led to Compound A?

A.
$$H-\overset{\overset{\displaystyle CH_3}{|}}{\underset{\underset{\displaystyle CH_3}{|}}{C}} \cdot\cdot\cdot Br$$

B.
$$H-\overset{\overset{\displaystyle CH_3}{|}}{\underset{\underset{\displaystyle CH_3}{|}}{C}} \oplus$$

C.
$$Et-O \overset{\delta^-}{\cdots} H \cdots \overset{\overset{\displaystyle H}{|}}{\underset{\underset{\displaystyle H}{|}}{C}} \overset{\cdots}{\cdots} \overset{\overset{\displaystyle CH_3}{|}}{\underset{\underset{\displaystyle H}{|}}{C}} \overset{\delta^-}{\cdots} Br$$

D.
$$Et-O \overset{\delta^-}{\cdots} \overset{\overset{\displaystyle CH_3}{|}}{\underset{\underset{\displaystyle CH_3}{|}}{C_{\text{\textit{\tiny{H}}}}}} \overset{\delta^-}{\cdots} Br$$

196. Which of the following compounds is an accurate representation of Compound B?
   A. CH_3OCH_3
   B. $C_2H_5OC_2H_5$
   C. $(CH_3)_2CHOCH_2CH_3$
   D. $CH_3CH_2CH_2OCH_2CH_3$

The sequence of events during synaptic transmission at the neuromuscular junction can be summarized as follows.

The depolarization produced by an action potential in the synaptic terminal opens voltage-dependent calcium channels in the terminal membrane. Calcium ions enter the terminal down their concentration and electrical gradients, inducing synaptic vesicles filled with acetylcholine (ACh) to fuse with the plasma membrane facing the muscle cell. The ACh is thereby dumped into the synaptic cleft, and some of it diffuses across the cleft to combine with specific receptors on ACh-activated channels. When ACh is bound, the channel opens and allows sodium and potassium ions to cross the membrane. This depolarizes the muscle membrane and triggers an all-or-none action potential in the muscle cell. The action of ACh is terminated by the enzyme acetylcholinesterase, which splits ACh into acetate and choline.

In order to determine how, and under what conditions, ACh works, the following experiments were done.

Experiment 1
Determining the Effect of the Timing of Calcium Action on Transmitter Release

Calcium ions were removed from the bathing solution of a muscle cell so that release of ACh in response to nerve stimulation was virtually abolished. Calcium ions were then applied to the nerve terminal by ionophoreses, from a micropipette close to the terminal, just before the nerve was stimulated (N), without nerve stimulation, and just after the nerve was stimulated. The results obtained are shown in Fig. 1.

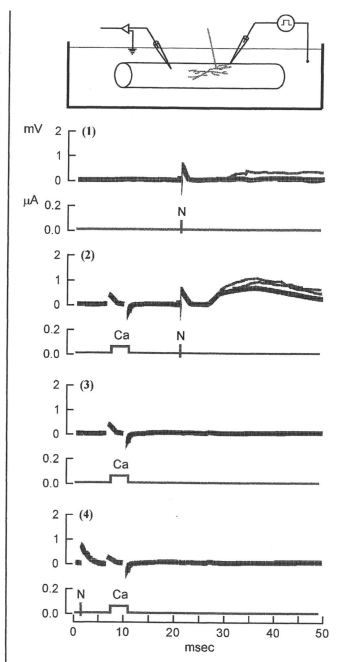

Figure 1

Experiment 2

Determining the Effect of ACh on Neuromuscular Transmission and its Subsequent Action on the Postsynaptic Membrane

Stimulating electrodes were placed on the nerve and a pair of recording electrodes was placed on the muscle. One of the electrodes was placed very close to the end plate region. First curare and then eserine were added to the solution bathing the muscle. The action potentials produced on stimulating the nerve were recorded. The results obtained are shown in Fig. 2.

(A) CONTROL

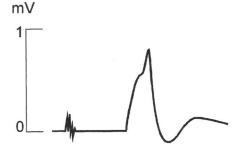

(B) EFFECT OF CURARE

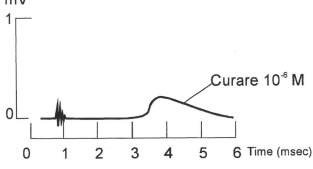

(C) EFFECT OF ESERINE

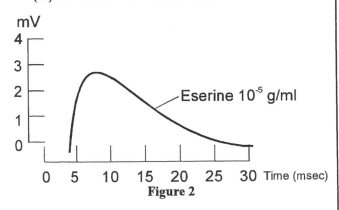

Figure 2

197. At the neuromuscular junction, the receptors on the ACh-activated channels are likely located:
 A. on the tubule of the T system.
 B. in the sarcolemma.
 C. on the muscle surface.
 D. in the synaptic cleft.

198. The depolarization across the muscle membrane triggers an all-or-none action potential in the muscle cell. This suggests that an increase in the amount of transmitter released at the neuromuscular junction would change:
 A. the amplitude of the action potential.
 B. the frequency of the nerve impulses.
 C. the direction of the action potential.
 D. the speed at which nerve impulses travel along the muscle cell.

199. A mutation in the gene which codes for acetylcholinesterase would inhibit all but which of the following processes?
 A. A hyperpolarization in the postsynaptic membrane
 B. A depolarization in the postsynaptic membrane
 C. The passage of a series of nerve impulses along the axon of the postsynaptic neuron
 D. The development of an inhibitory postsynaptic potential

200. According to Fig. 1, which of the following conclusions was confirmed by the experiment?
 A. For transmitter release to occur, calcium ions need only be present after the depolarization of the presynaptic membrane.
 B. The presence of calcium ions is the only variable which affects transmitter release at the synapse.
 C. For transmitter release to occur, calcium ions must be present before and after depolarization of the presynaptic membrane.
 D. For transmitter release to occur, calcium ions must be present before depolarization of the presynaptic membrane.

201. According to Fig. 2, curare and eserine could act by, respectively:
  A. blocking ion channels and binding to the receptors on ACh-activated channels.
  B. blocking ion channels and preventing the hydrolysis of acetylcholinesterase.
  C. initiating the entry of calcium ions into the synaptic knob and initiating the passage of a nerve impulse along the muscle cell.
  D. binding to ACh receptor sites on the postsynaptic membrane and preventing the hydrolysis of acetylcholine.

202. In the control of Fig. 2, the part of the curve between 4 and 5 msec represents:
  A. the absolute refractory period.
  B. the relative refractory period.
  C. the depolarization of the membrane.
  D. saltatory conduction.

Much of the study of evolution of *interspecific* interactions had focused on the results rather than the process of coevolution. In only a few cases has the genetic bases of interspecific interactions been explored. One of the most intriguing results has been the description of "gene-for-gene" systems governing the interaction between certain parasites and their hosts. In several crop plants, dominant alleles at a number of loci have been described that confer resistance to a pathogenic fungus; for each such gene, the fungus appears to have a recessive allele for "virulence" that enables the fungus to attack the otherwise resistant host. Cases of character displacement among competing species are among the best evidence that interspecific interactions can result in genetic change.

Assuming that parasites and their hosts coevolve in an "arms race," we might deduce that the parasite is "ahead" if local populations are more capable of attacking the host population with which they are associated than other populations. Whereas the host may be "ahead" if local populations are more resistant to the local parasite than to other populations of the parasite.

Several studies have been done to evaluate coevolutionary interactions between parasites and hosts, or predators and prey. In one, the fluctuations in populations of houseflies and of a wasp that parasitized them were recorded. The results of the experiment are shown in Fig. 1.

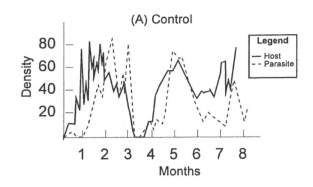

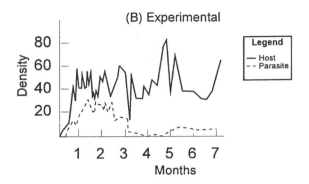

Figure 1

203. A pathogenic fungus is more capable of growth and reproduction on its native population of its sole host, the wild hog peanut, than on plants from other populations of the same species. It is reasonable to conclude that:

   A. the fungus, in this instance, was capable of more rapid adaptation to its host than vice versa.

   B. the fungus, in this instance, was capable of more rapid adaptation to all populations of the host species than vice versa.

   C. the host, in this instance, was capable of more rapid adaptation to the fungus than vice versa.

   D. all populations of the host species were capable of more rapid adaptation to the fungus than vice versa.

204. The passage suggests that one result of interspecific interactions might be:
- **A.** genetic drift within sympatric populations.
- **B.** genetic drift within allopatric populations.
- **C.** genetic mutations within sympatric populations.
- **D.** genetic mutations within allopatric populations.

205. According to Fig. 1, the experiment showed that over time:
- **A.** coevolution caused a decrease in both the host and parasite populations.
- **B.** coevolution caused both a decrease in fluctuation of the host and parasite populations, and a lowered density of the parasite population.
- **C.** coevolution caused a marked increase in the fluctuation of only the host population, and lowered the density of the parasite population.
- **D.** coevolution caused a decrease in the population density of the parasite population but caused a marked increase in the density of the host population.

206. The control in the experiment likely consisted of:
- **A.** members from different populations of the host and parasite species used in the experimental group, that had a short history of exposure to one another.
- **B.** members of the host and parasite species used in the experimental group, that had a long history of exposure to one another.
- **C.** members of the host and parasite species used in the experimental group that had no history of exposure to one another.
- **D.** members from different populations of the host and parasite species used in the experimental group, that had a long history of exposure to one another.

207. Which of the following is the least likely explanation of the results obtained for the control group in Fig. 1?
- **A.** A low parasite population results in a lowered host population by the sheer virulence of the parasite.
- **B.** A low host population can increase a parasite population by eliminating their source for food.
- **C.** A high parasite population destroys the host population resulting in a lowered host population.
- **D.** A high host population creates a breeding ground for parasites thus increasing the parasite population.

208. Penicillin is an antibiotic which destroys bacteria by interfering with cell wall production. Could the development of bacterial resistance to Penicillin be considered similar to coevolution?
- **A.** Yes, a spontaneous mutation is likely to confer resistance to Penicillin.
- **B.** No, an organism can only evolve in response to another organism.
- **C.** Yes, as antibiotics continue to change there will be a selective pressure for bacterial genes which confer resistance.
- **D.** No, bacteria have plasma membranes and can survive without cell walls.

Passage XI (Questions 209-214)

The ninhydrin reaction is a useful analytical detection method for α-amino acids. The reagent ninhydrin produces a characteristic blue color with primary α-amino acids via the following series of reactions (see Fig. 1):

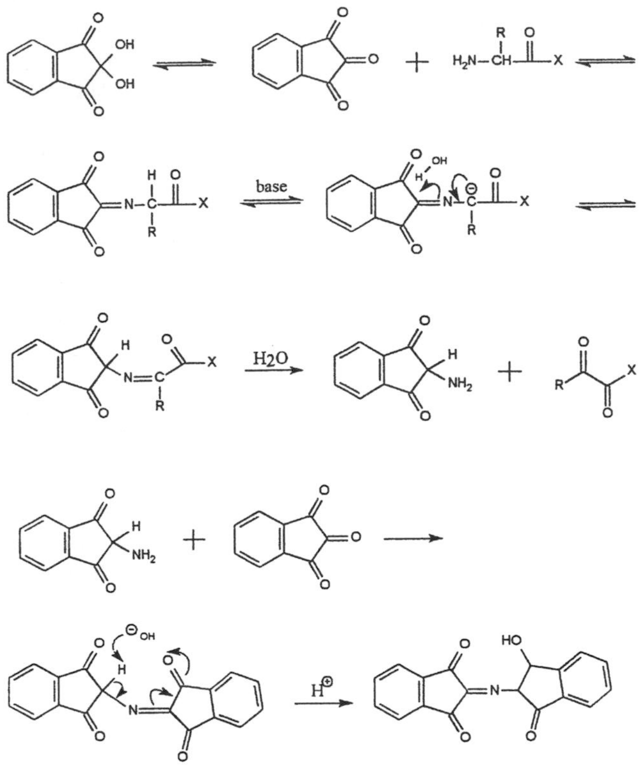

Figure 1

209. In the first reaction of Fig. 1, the inorganic product, which is not written, is:

A. CO_2
B. H_2O
C. HCl
D. H_2O_2

210. Which of the following compounds would be isotopically labeled if $H_2{}^{18}O$ were the only isotype source?

A. 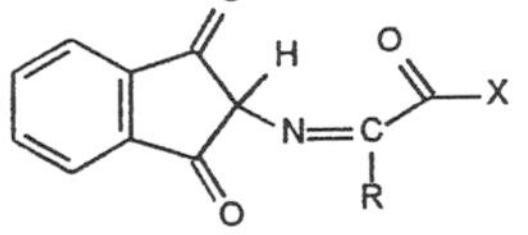

B. 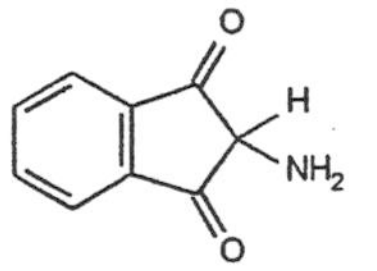

C. 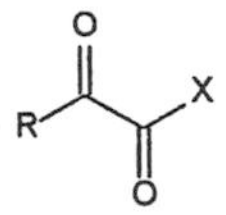

D. 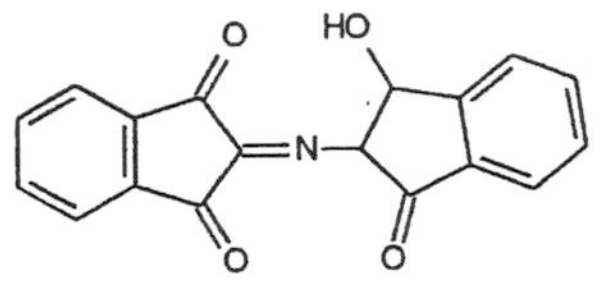

211. Base treatment of an amino acid usually results in the conversion of the acid to a derivative via the amino-carboxylate salt.

$$R-\underset{}{CH}(NH_3^+)-CO_2^- \xrightarrow{B^-} R-CH(NH_2)-CO_2^- + BH$$

The above procedure:

A. decreases the rate of electrophilic reaction of the free amino group.
B. decreases the rate of nucleophilic reaction of the free amino group.
C. enhances the rate of nucleophilic reaction of the free amino group.
D. enhances the rate of electrophilic reaction of the free amino group.

212. A mixture of alanine and benzoyl chloride is treated with dilute aqueous sodium hydroxide to yield compound X. What functional group would be present in compound X?

A. Ester
B. Aldehyde
C. Amide
D. Ether

213. Amino acids can be divided into the following four general categories based on their acid-base charge properties at intracellular pH (~6-7):

Positively charged
Negatively charged
Hydrophobic
Hydrophilic

Consider the following amino acids.

I. 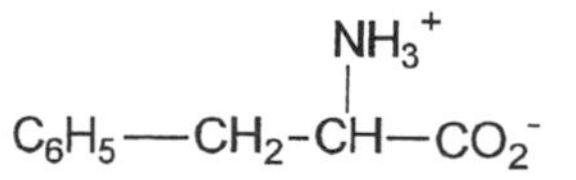 $C_6H_5-CH_2-\underset{\underset{NH_3^+}{|}}{CH}-CO_2^-$

II. 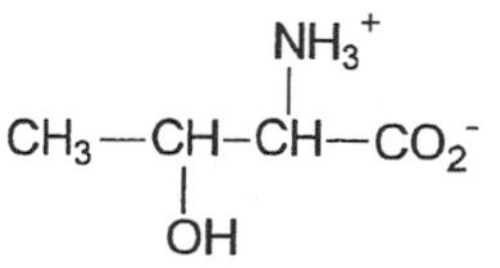 $CH_3-\underset{\underset{OH}{|}}{CH}-\underset{\underset{NH_3^+}{|}}{CH}-CO_2^-$

III. 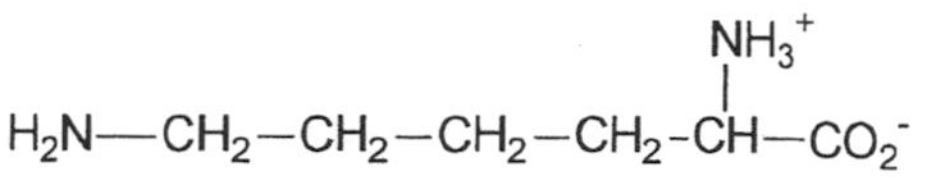 $H_2N-CH_2-CH_2-CH_2-CH_2-\underset{\underset{NH_3^+}{|}}{CH}-CO_2^-$

IV. 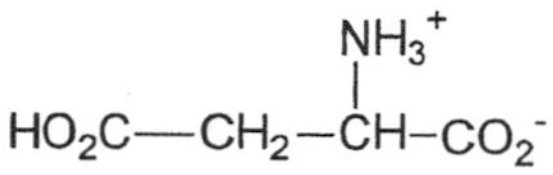 $HO_2C-CH_2-\underset{\underset{NH_3^+}{|}}{CH}-CO_2^-$

Which of the following classification series best represents amino acids I, II, III, and IV, respectively?

A. Hydrophobic, hydrophilic, positively charged, negatively charged
B. Hydrophobic, positively charged, hydrophilic, negatively charged
C. Hydrophilic, negatively charged, hydrophobic, positively charged
D. Positively charged, negatively charged, hydrophilic, hydrophobic

214. The structure of valine is shown below.

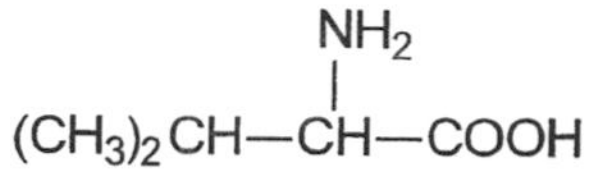

$(CH_3)_2CH-\underset{\underset{NH_2}{|}}{CH}-COOH$

In extremely basic solutions valine possesses 2 basic sites $-CO_2^-$ and $-NH_2$. Monoprotonation of such an alkaline solution would yield which of the following products?

A. 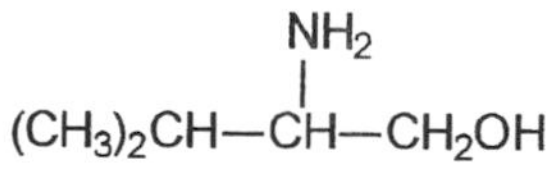 $(CH_3)_2CH-\underset{\underset{NH_2}{|}}{CH}-CH_2OH$

B. 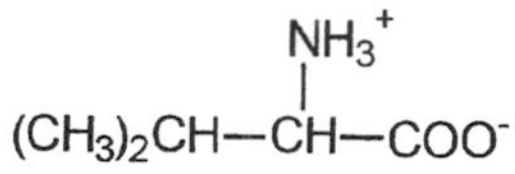 $(CH_3)_2CH-\underset{\underset{NH_3^+}{|}}{CH}-COO^-$

C. 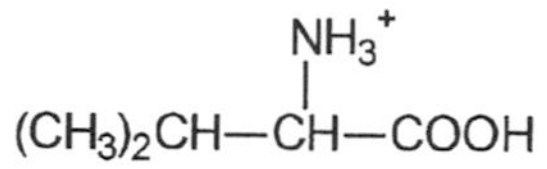 $(CH_3)_2CH-\underset{\underset{NH_3^+}{|}}{CH}-COOH$

D. 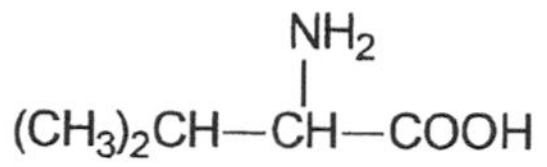 $(CH_3)_2CH-\underset{\underset{NH_2}{|}}{CH}-COOH$

Questions 215-219 are NOT based on a descriptive passage.

215. Von Willebrand's disease is an autosomal dominant bleeding disorder. A man who does not have the disease has two children with a woman who is heterozygous for the condition. If the first child expresses the bleeding disorder, what is the probability that the second child will have the disease?

A. 0.25
B. 0.50
C. 0.75
D. 1.00

216. The structure of β-D-glucose is shown below in two different projection systems. The circled hydroxyl group in Fig. 1 would be located at which position in the modified Fischer projection depicted in Fig. 2?

Figure 1

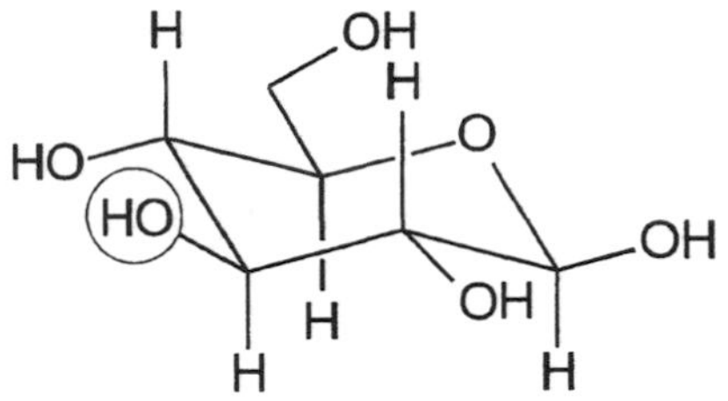

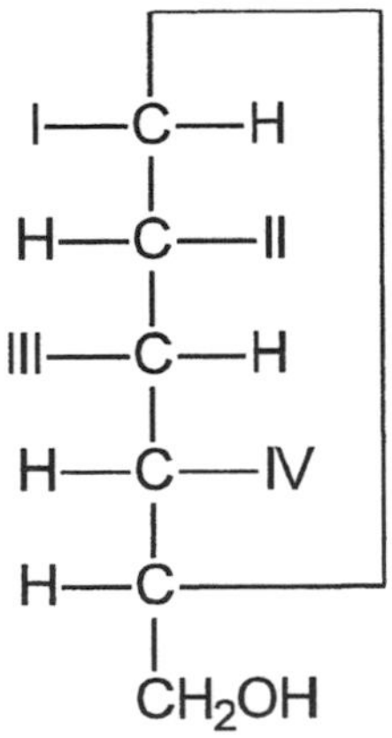

Figure 2

A. I
B. II
C. III
D. IV

217. Which of the following is NOT a product of glycolysis:

A. a net 2 ATP.
B. acetyl-CoA.
C. pyruvate.
D. reducing equivalents.

218. The functional unit of the kidney is the:

A. renal corpuscle.
B. Bowman's capsule.
C. major calyx.
D. nephron.

219. Consider the following conformations of tartaric acid.

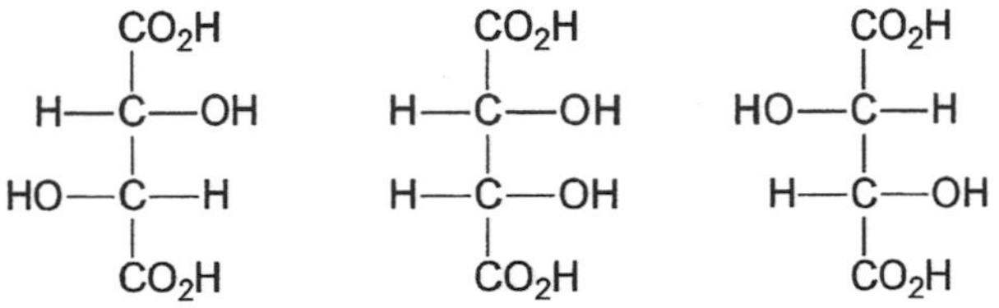

I **II** **III**

A diastereomer which has no enantiomer, thus is achiral, is called a *meso* compound. Which of the above conformations would be classified as *meso*?

A. I only
B. II only
C. I and II only
D. I and III only

END OF BIOLOGICAL SCIENCES. IF TIME REMAINS, YOU MAY GO BACK AND CHECK YOUR WORK IN THIS BOOKLET.

TEST GS-3

Physical Sciences
Questions 1-77
Time : 100 Minutes

OPEN BOOKLET ONLY WHEN TIMER IS READY.

The Gold Standard MCAT* has been designed exclusively to test knowledge and thinking skills. The exam may contain hypothetical statements and/or express controversial ideas. Statements contained herein do not necessarily reflect the policy, position, or view of RuveneCo Publishing.

* MCAT is a registered service mark of the Association of American Medical Colleges, which is not associated with this product.

PHYSICAL SCIENCES

INSTRUCTIONS: Of the 77 questions in the Physical Sciences test, 62 are organized into groups preceded by a passage. After evaluating the passage, select the best answer to each question in the group. Fifteen questions are independent of any descriptive passage or each other. Similarly, select the best answer to these questions. If you are unsure of an answer, eliminate the alternatives that you know to be incorrect and select an answer from the remaining alternatives. To indicate your selection, blacken the corresponding oval on Answer Document 1, GS-3. A periodic table is provided for your use during the test.

PERIODIC TABLE OF THE ELEMENTS

1 H 1.008																	2 He 4.003
3 Li 6.941	4 Be 9.012											5 B 10.81	6 C 12.011	7 N 14.007	8 O 15.999	9 F 18.998	10 Ne 20.179
11 Na 22.990	12 Mg 24.305											13 Al 26.982	14 Si 28.086	15 P 30.974	16 S 32.06	17 Cl 35.453	18 Ar 39.948
19 K 39.098	20 Ca 40.08	21 Sc 44.956	22 Ti 47.90	23 V 50.942	24 Cr 51.996	25 Mn 54.938	26 Fe 55.847	27 Co 58.933	28 Ni 58.70	29 Cu 63.546	30 Zn 65.38	31 Ga 69.72	32 Ge 72.59	33 As 74.922	34 Se 78.96	35 Br 79.904	36 Kr 83.80
37 Rb 85.468	38 Sr 87.62	39 Y 88.906	40 Zr 91.22	41 Nb 92.906	42 Mo 95.94	43 Tc (98)	44 Ru 101.07	45 Rh 102.906	46 Pd 106.4	47 Ag 107.868	48 Cd 112.41	49 In 114.82	50 Sn 118.69	51 Sb 121.75	52 Te 127.60	53 I 126.905	54 Xe 131.30
55 Cs 132.905	56 Ba 137.33	57 *La 138.906	72 Hf 178.49	73 Ta 180.948	74 W 183.85	75 Re 186.207	76 Os 190.2	77 Ir 192.22	78 Pt 195.09	79 Au 196.967	80 Hg 200.59	81 Tl 204.37	82 Pb 207.2	83 Bi 208.980	84 Po (209)	85 At (210)	86 Rn (222)
87 Fr (223)	88 Ra 226.025	89 **Ac 227.028	104 Unq (261)	105 Unp (262)	106 Unh (263)												

*

58 Ce 140.12	59 Pr 140.908	60 Nd 144.24	61 Pm (145)	62 Sm 150.4	63 Eu 151.96	64 Gd 157.25	65 Tb 158.925	66 Dy 162.50	67 Ho 164.930	68 Er 167.26	69 Tm 168.934	70 Yb 173.04	71 Lu 174.967

**

90 Th 232.038	91 Pa 231.036	92 U 238.029	93 Np 237.048	94 Pu (244)	95 Am (243)	96 Cm (247)	97 Bk (247)	98 Cf (251)	99 Es (254)	100 Fm (257)	101 Md (258)	102 No (259)	103 Lr (260)

Various rules of thumb have been proposed by the scientific community to explain the mode of radioactive decay by various radioisotopes. One of the major rules is called the n/p ratio. If all the known isotopes of the elements are plotted on a graph of number of neutrons (n) versus number of protons (p), it is observed that all isotopes lying outside of a "stable" n/p ratio region are radioactive as shown in Figure 1.

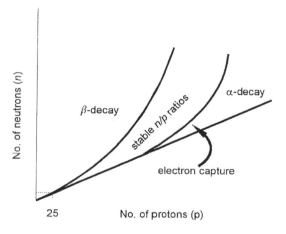

Figure 1

The graph exhibits straight line behavior with unit slope up to p = 25. Above p = 25, those isotopes with an n/p ratio lying below the stable region usually undergo electron capture while those with n/p ratios lying above the stable region usually undergo beta decay. Very heavy isotopes (p>83) are unstable because of their relatively large nuclei and they undergo alpha decay. Gamma ray emission does not involve the release of a particle. It represents a change in an atom from a higher energy level to a lower energy level.

1. How do gamma rays behave in an electric field?
   A. They are not deflected in any direction.
   B. They are deflected toward the positive plate.
   C. They are deflected toward the negative plate.
   D. They oscillate between plates, that is, they are attracted to one plate and then the other.

2. How would the radioisotope of magnesium with atomic mass 27 undergo radioactive decay?
   A. electron capture
   B. alpha decay
   C. beta decay
   D. gamma ray emission

3. The half-life of cobalt-60 is 5.2 years. If a sample's activity is 250 millicuries after 15.6 years, what must its original activity have been?
   A. 500 millicuries
   B. 1000 millicuries
   C. 2000 millicuries
   D. 5000 millicuries

4. In a hypothetical radioactive series, Tl-210 undergoes 3 beta decay processes, 1 alpha decay process and 1 gamma ray emission to yield a stable product. What is the product?
   A. $^{214}_{76}$Os
   B. $^{214}_{84}$Po
   C. $^{206}_{86}$Rn
   D. $^{206}_{82}$Pb

5. $^{230}_{90}$Th undergoes a series of radioactive decay processes, resulting in ^{214}Bi being the final product. What was the sequence of the processes that occurred?
   A. alpha, alpha, alpha, gamma, beta
   B. alpha, alpha, alpha, alpha, beta
   C. alpha, alpha, beta, beta
   D. alpha, beta, beta, beta, gamma

6. Which of the following represents the relative penetrating power of the three types of radioactive emissions in decreasing order?
   A. beta > alpha > gamma
   B. beta > gamma > alpha
   C. gamma > alpha > beta
   D. gamma > beta > alpha

The thermal stability of the salts of the s-block elements is dependent upon three main factors. Firstly, the greater the charge of the ions involved, the stronger the interionic attraction and the more stable the salt. Also, the smaller the ions become in terms of their ionic radii the closer they approach each other in the crystal lattice of their salts and the more stable the salt. Thirdly, if the ions in the lattice are of comparable size, the crystal lattice is arranged in a more uniform fashion and thus possesses greater thermal stability.

There is one other factor that affects thermal stability. The larger the anions in the crystal become, for example CO_3^{2-}, unless the cation is of comparable size, the anions decompose on heating to give smaller anions such as O^{2-}. This point is especially important when considering the thermal stability of the carbonates, nitrates and hydroxides of the s-block elements.

An unknown s-block salt was uncovered at the landing site of a meteor. When converted to its hydroxide, it was found that the K_b of the salt was 1.0×10^{-6}. It did not decompose to the oxide. The metal obtained exhibited the typical properties of most s-block metals:- ductile, malleable, lustre, good electrical and thermal conductivity and a high reactivity. The original salt obtained from the meteor possessed a complex formula and the metal itself had a high molecular weight.

7. Which groups of the periodic table comprise the s-block elements?
   A. Groups I, II and III
   B. Groups I and III
   C. Groups II and III
   D. Groups I and II

8. Given that the CO_3^{2-} anion is approximately the same size as the early Group I cations, what would occur if Na_2CO_3 were heated?
   A. It would decompose to yield Na_2O.
   B. It would decompose to yield Na_2CO_2.
   C. It would decompose to yield NaOH.
   D. No decomposition would occur.

9. Comparing calcium oxide and magnesium oxide, which of the two would be more stable?
   A. Magnesium oxide would be more stable because the magnesium cation is smaller.
   B. Magnesium oxide would be more stable because magnesium has a lower atomic mass than calcium.
   C. Calcium oxide would be more stable because the calcium anion is smaller than the magnesium cation.
   D. Calcium oxide would be more stable because calcium has a greater atomic mass than magnesium.

10. The nitrates of the Group I elements decompose not to the oxide but to the nitrite (NO_2^-) although O^{2-} is smaller than NO_2^-. Why?
    A. Because only doubly charged anions like CO_3^{2-} decompose to the oxide.
    B. Because the double charge on the oxygen would make the salt less stable than a singly charged nitrite anion.
    C. Because the nitrite anion contains two oxygen atoms while the oxide anion contains only one.
    D. Because the nitrite anion is probably about the same size as the Group I cations.

11. When s-block carbonates decompose, a gas is obtained which is heavier than air and does not support a lighted splint. What gas is it?
    A. O_2
    B. CO
    C. CO_2
    D. CO_3

12. What would be the pH of a 1.0 M solution of the unknown salt hydroxide given that the metal is monovalent?
    A. 11
    B. 8.0
    C. 7.5
    D. 13.0

13. Li_2O is often considered to be covalent in nature because of the unusually high electronegativity of lithium. Which of the following would be a plausible Lewis dot structure for the compound?

        A. 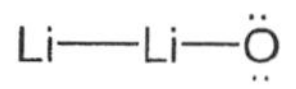   Li—Li—Ö

        B. 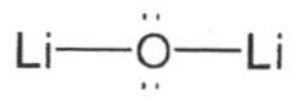   Li—Ö—Li

        C. 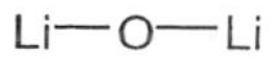   Li—O—Li

        D. 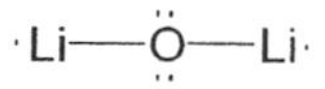   ·Li—Ö—Li·

The Danish physicist Niels Bohr astounded the chemical community when he published his ideas on electron distribution around the nuclei of atoms. What made it even more incredible was that it was the first theory to be based on Planck's revolutionary quantum theory. The theory states that matter cannot absorb energy continuously, but only in small discrete units which he called *quanta*.

Bohr postulated that the electrons are arranged around the atom in regions of space where they had energy corresponding to a whole number of quanta (energy levels). When an electron makes a transition from one energy level to the next, the wavelength of the radiation absorbed or emitted was determined by the energy difference between the two energy levels. The energy levels are numbered starting from the innermost energy level and moving outward.

When the emission spectrum of hydrogen, that is, the wavelengths of electromagnetic radiation emitted during energy level transitions in the molecules, was examined, a number of discrete lines were found, corroborating Planck's theory. These wavelengths corresponded to electron transitions from higher energy levels to lower ones. The Lyman series involves electron transitions to the n=1 energy level and had wavelengths in the ultra-violet region of the electromagnetic (e-m) spectrum. The Balmer series involved transitions to the n=2 energy level and the wavelengths corresponded to the visible range of the e-m spectrum.

The wavelength of radiation emitted in these transitions is given by the following formula:

$$1/\lambda = R_H (1/n_1^2 - 1/n_2^2)$$

where λ = wavelength of radiation emitted in centimeters; n_1 = lower energy level; n_2 = higher energy level; and R_H = Rydberg's constant.

The wavelength of radiation emitted is inversely proportional to the energy difference between the two energy levels. The brightness of each line is related to how many of each type of transition occurred in the sample since transitions between two energy levels in different molecules of the same chemical species emits the same wavelength of radiation.

14. What type of radiation would you expect to be associated with energy transitions down to the n = 3 energy level?
    A. Infrared
    B. Ultraviolet
    C. X-rays
    D. Gamma rays

15. What is the wavelength of the radiation emitted when an electron makes a transition from n = 2 to n =1?
    $$(R_H = 110\ 000)$$

    A. 82 500 cm
    B. 182.82 cm
    C. 6.57×10^{-5} cm
    D. 1.21×10^{-5} cm

16. Which of the following electronic transitions will result in the emission of electromagnetic radiation with the greatest energy?
    A. n = 2 to n = 1
    B. n = 3 to n = 1
    C. n = 3 to n = 2
    D. n = 4 to n = 2

17. The difference between energy levels is directly proportional to which of the following properties of e-m radiation (when it is travelling in a vacuum)?
    A. Amplitude
    B. Frequency
    C. Wavelength
    D. Displacement

18. How would the wavelength of the electromagnetic radiation absorbed change if the number of atoms undergoing the same electronic transition was increased?
    A. There would be no change.
    B. It would be shifted to shorter wavelengths.
    C. It would be shifted to longer wavelengths.
    D. It depends on the magnitude of the increase in the number of atoms.

Passage IV (Questions 19-24)

Due to the fact that many cations form sparingly soluble salts, a method known as *selective precipitation* can be used to separate a mixture of cations. The process involves the addition of a soluble salt containing an anion which forms a sparingly soluble salt with one or more of the cations. If it forms a sparingly soluble salt with only one of the cations in solution, then that cation is effectively separated out of solution.

However, this is not usually the case. More often than not a number of cations in solution will form sparingly soluble salts with the anion. Separation then depends on the magnitude of the K_{sp} value of the sparingly soluble salts that could be formed. The smaller the K_{sp} value for a salt, the earlier it will precipitate out of solution relative to the other salts. Thus the process is similar to a titration: the anion is added gradually in increasing amounts and precipitating each of the salts separately, then the precipitate is removed when all of that particular cation species has been extracted from solution. This is used extensively in the mining industry in the purification of various metal ores and in laboratories in the separation of ions from various bodily fluids.

A mixture of bismuth (Bi^{3+}), silver (Ag^+), zinc (Zn^{2+}) and copper (Cu^{2+}) cations is to be separated using sodium sulfide (Na_2S).

$$K_{sp}(Bi_2S_3) = 1.0 \times 10^{-97}$$
$$K_{sp}(Ag_2S) = 2.0 \times 10^{-49}$$
$$K_{sp}(ZnS) = 1.0 \times 10^{-21}$$
$$K_{sp}(CuS) = 9.0 \times 10^{-36}$$

19. Which cation will precipitate out of solution first on the addition of sodium sulfide?
    A. Bi^{3+}
    B. Ag^+
    C. Zn^{2+}
    D. Cu^{2+}

20. The K_{sp} expression for Bi_2S_3 is:
    A. $[Bi_2^{3+}][S_3^{2+}]$
    B. $[Bi^{3+}][S^{2-}]$
    C. $[Bi^{3+}]^2[S^{2-}]^3$
    D. $[Bi^{3+}]^3[S^{2-}]^2$

21. Cyanide ions (CN^-) could also have been used to precipitate the cations. If after all the cations have been precipitated, the concentration of CN^- is 0.02 M, calculate the pH of the solution given that:

    $$CN^- + H_2O \rightarrow HCN + OH^- \qquad K_b = 1.39 \times 10^{-5}$$

    A. 4.9
    B. 5.4
    C. 7.7
    D. 10 7

22. If in a solution containing only Zn^{2+}, the concentration of zinc ions is 5.0×10^{-3} M, what concentration of S^{2-} is required to just begin the precipitation of zinc sulfide?
    A. 5.0×10^{-24} M
    B. 2.0×10^{-19} M
    C. 3.2×10^{-11} M
    D. 5.0×10^{-3} M

23. An unknown cation X^+ was added to the original solution of cations and was found to precipitate before Ag_2S but after Bi_2S_3. Which of the following gives a plausible value for the solubility product of X_2S?
    A. 3.4×10^{-99}
    B. 1.4×10^{-15}
    C. 8.0×10^{-28}
    D. 4.0×10^{-53}

24. The CuS from the selective precipitation was collected, purified and equal weights of it placed into each of two beakers. Beaker 1 contained distilled water and beaker 2 contained a 0.01 M $Cu(NO_3)_2$ solution. Which of the following statements is true?
    A. More of the CuS will dissolve in beaker 1.
    B. More of the CuS will dissolve in beaker 2.
    C. Equal amounts of CuS will dissolve in both beakers.
    D. No CuS will dissolve in either beaker.

Questions 25-29 are NOT based on a descriptive passage.

25. In the following electrolytic cell, which solution(s) could be used such that the electrode at **A** is the anode?

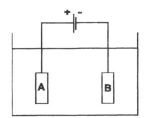

A. Molten NaCl
B. $CuSO_4$
C. $FeBr_2$
D. All of the above

26. A mechanical wave has the following measured values.
amplitude = 0.30 N m^{-2}
speed = 5.0×10^4 m s^{-1}
intensity = 2.0×10^{-4} W m^{-2}
phase angle = $\pi/2$ radians
frequency = 2.5×10^4 Hz

What is the wavelength of this wave?
A. 1.5×10^4 m
B. 2.0×10^4 m
C. 10.0 m
D. 2.0 m

27. Two mechanical waves are made to pass through the same medium with the same frequency. The amplitude of wave X is six units and the amplitude of wave Y is three units. Which of the following pairs of values correctly describes the range of possible amplitudes?
A. 6 units and 9 units
B. 3 units and 18 units
C. 3 units and 9 units
D. 3 units and 6 units

28. A container holds 50 mL of a 0.500 M potassium ion solution. 10 mL of 0.200 M K_2CO_3 is added to the container. What is the concentration of potassium ion after the addition?
A. 0.450 M
B. 0.700 M
C. 0.483 M
D. 0.300 M

29. In a 24 m cylindrical pipeline closed at one end, consecutive resonances occur at two wavelengths. Which pair of values given below corresponds to the possible values of the two wavelengths?

$$L = n\lambda/4 \quad\quad L = \text{length of cylinder}$$
$$n = 1, 3, 5, 7 \ldots$$
$$\lambda = \text{wavelengths}$$

A. 48 m and 12 m
B. 48 m and 19.2 m
C. 12 m and 24 m
D. 32 m and 19.2 m

Passage V (Questions 30-34)

Ordinary chemical reactions consist simply of rearrangements of the electrons in atoms and molecules. In these changes, the atomic nuclei involved are not affected. In the phenomenon of radioactive disintegration, both nuclei and electrons can be involved. A chemical reaction of this kind is referred to as a *nuclear reaction*. One method of producing nuclear alteration involves the bombardment of atomic nuclei with various kinds of high speed particles.

The possibility of artificial transmutation was first suggested when it was discovered that different kinds of atoms are composed of the same fundamental units: protons, electrons and neutrons. Essentially, the problem is in how the number of each of these types of particles could be changed. Rutherford first suggested that alpha particles, which could be easily obtained from radium, could be used. He thought that a few of the particles might make direct hits and either combine with the nuclei or break them up. His theory was proven when he used these particles to transmute ^{14}N to ^{17}O, and the chemical community was shocked. Since then, protons (p), photons (γ-rays in particular), neutrons (n), electrons (e or $_{-1}^{0}e$) and positrons (e^+ or $_{1}^{0}e$) have been used in these types of reactions.

30. What is the nuclear reaction for the transmutation of ^{14}N to ^{17}O ?

A. $_{7}^{14}N + \alpha \rightarrow n + _{8}^{17}O$

B. $_{7}^{14}N + \alpha \rightarrow p + _{8}^{17}O$

C. $_{7}^{14}N + \alpha \rightarrow e + _{8}^{17}O$

D. $_{7}^{14}N + \alpha \rightarrow e^+ + _{8}^{17}O$

31. The larger the bombarding particle and the greater its charge, the more difficult it is to use in artificial transmutation. Which of the following represents the order of particles in terms of increasing ability to be used in these types of reactions given that charge is the more important factor?
A. $n < p < e < \alpha$
B. $n < e < p < \alpha$
C. $\alpha < e < p < n$
D. $\alpha < p < e < n$

32. A radioactive form of phosphorus undergoes β-decay. What would the radioactivity level (R) versus time graph for the decay process look like?

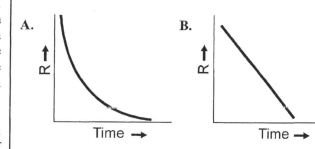

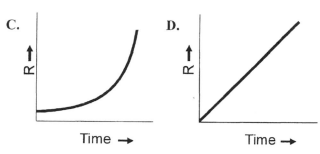

33. How do you suppose a positron will react in an electric field?
A. It would retain its original flight path.
B. It would be attracted to the positive plate.
C. It would be attracted to the negative plate.
D. It would be attracted to the plate with the greater charge density.

34. Given that a particular β particle has a kinetic energy of 2.275×10^{-15} J, what is the velocity of this particle?

Speed of light in free space = 3.0×10^8 m s^{-1}
Mass of an electron = 9.1×10^{-31} kg

A. 1.0×10^8 m s^{-1}
B. 2.5×10^7 m s^{-1}
C. 7.1×10^7 m s^{-1}
D. 1.4×10^7 m s^{-1}

Passage VI (Questions 35-41)

Silver is still one of the most versatile metals known to man, being used in almost everything from electrical wires to jewellery. It is also quite unreactive, and is resistant to attack by common agents such as acid and oxygen. Needless to say, the mining of this precious metal is the mainstay of the economy of many countries. Unfortunately, silver does not occur in its elemental state in nature. It is mined as argentite (Ag_2S containing ore) and horn silver (AgCl containing ore).

The main method used in industry for separating silver from its ores involves *complexation* and the cyanide ligand (CN^-). The cyanide ligand is used to produce the soluble silver cyanide complex according to Reaction I and Reaction II.

$$Ag_2S + 4CN^- \rightarrow 2[Ag(CN)_2]^- + S^{2-} \quad \textbf{Reaction I}$$
$$AgCl + 2CN^- \rightarrow [Ag(CN)_2]^- + Cl^- \quad \textbf{Reaction II}$$

The silver metal in its elemental form is then precipitated by adding zinc dust to the solution as shown in Reaction III.

$$2[Ag(CN)_2]^- + Zn \rightarrow [Zn(CN)_4]^{2-} + 2Ag(s) \quad \textbf{Reaction III}$$

Silver complexes provide one of the most fascinating demonstrations of the relative strengths of different ligands for a particular cation. This is a common occurrence with most complexes of this nature but what makes silver unique is that many of its complexes differ in color. Table 1 is a list of a few of the silver complexes and their colors.

Table 1

Complex	Color
$[Ag(CN)_2]^-$	Clear solution
AgI	Yellow precipitate
$[Ag(EDTA)]^-$	Clear solution
Ag_2S	Black precipitate

One will notice that precipitates are listed in the table. These can be regarded as neutral complexes and as is often the case with neutral complexes, they are quite insoluble and hence precipitate out of solution.

35. The ability of silver ions to form complexes of many different colors identifies it as being a:
   A. univalent metal.
   B. Group IB element.
   C. Period V element.
   D. transition metal.

36. Silverware tarnishes because of a reaction between silver and tiny amounts of a gas in air. What must that gas be?
   A. O_2
   B. N_2
   C. H_2O
   D. H_2S

37. Given that $K_{a1}(H_2S) = 9.1 \times 10^{-8}$ and $K_{a2}(H_2S) = 1.2 \times 10^{-15}$, what would be the effect on Reaction I if protons were added to the reaction mixture at equilibrium?
   A. The equilibrium would shift to the right.
   B. The equilibrium would shift to the left.
   C. There would be no change in the equilibrium position of the reaction.
   D. The change in the equilibrium position cannot be determined from the information given.

38. If Reaction II is at equilibrium, which of the following is true?
   A. The change in entropy is zero.
   B. The change in temperature is zero.
   C. The change in enthalpy is zero.
   D. The change in free energy is zero.

39. 12 grams of silver was extracted from a sample of an ore from which the only source of silver was Ag_2S. How many grams of Ag_2S were in the original sample?
   A. 27.6 grams
   B. 13.8 grams
   C. 8.6 grams
   D. 5.2 grams

40. One of the complexes formed by silver is silver bromide, AgBr. Why would you expect it to be insoluble?
   A. Because it is a neutral complex.
   B. Because Br^- is a large anion.
   C. Because the relative molecular mass of AgBr is large.
   D. Because most bromides are insoluble.

41. From the following data, which of the following ligands would you add to a clear silver complex in solution to determine which of the clear complexes in Table 1 was present?

In order of decreasing affinity for silver ions:
$$EDTA > S^{2-} > CN^- > I^-$$

A. EDTA
B. S^{2-}
C. CN^-
D. I^-

Batman is swinging over the rooftops of Gotham City on his nightly patrol. Suddenly, he sees his old enemy, the Joker, running from a bank firing gunshots behind him. Batman quickly races over and jumps from a four storey building onto a platform below. However, the platform is actually a trap set by his arch nemesis and Batman sticks to the platform when he lands on it. The platform is supported by a sturdy spring with a force constant of $k = 150$ N m^{-1}.

The building was 12 m high and Batman weighs 70 kg. The platform itself weighs 30 kg.

$$(g = 9.8 \text{ m s}^{-2})$$

42. What is the potential energy of Batman at the top of the four storey building?
    A. 0 J
    B. 8232 J
    C. 3528 J
    D. 17640 J

43. What is Batman's velocity just before he strikes the platform? (Assume negligible air resistance)
    A. 15.3 m s^{-1}
    B. 23.4 m s^{-1}
    C. 9.8 m s^{-1}
    D. 32.8 m s^{-1}

44. When the Joker was testing the spring, he applied a 700 N weight to the spring. By approximately how much was the spring compressed from its equilibrium position?
    A. 1.1 m
    B. 2.3 m
    C. 4.7 m
    D. 6.6 m

45. During his tests, the Joker also used a force to compress the spring by 0.5 m. How much elastic potential energy was thus stored in the spring?
    A. 147 J
    B. 18.8 J
    C. 37.5 J
    D. 75 J

46. Although Batman had been foiled, luck was with him that winter night as when the Joker drove away he slid on ice and collided head-on with a stationary truck which weighed 5000 kg. If the Joker's "get away" car weighed 1000 kg and the initial velocity of the Joker's car was 14 m s^{-1}, how fast did the truck initially move if after the collision the velocity of the Joker's car was 2 m s^{-1} in its original direction?
    A. 2.0 m s^{-1}
    B. 2.4 m s^{-1}
    C. 7.0 m s^{-1}
    D. 12.0 m s^{-1}

Passage VIII (Questions 47-51)

Sometimes, one may need to know the number of moles of a substance present. This can be efficiently done by reacting the substance with a reagent which would lead to the production of a gas. Using the ideal gas equation and the stoichiometry of the reaction, one could then determine the number of moles of gas present and hence the number of moles of the substance present.

A good example of this is the determination of the percentage of manganese present in a steel sample. The manganese is extracted from the alloy and converted to the purple manganate (VII) ion (MnO_4^-). This is then made to react with excess hydrochloric acid according to Reaction I.

$$2MnO_4^- + 16H^+ + 10Cl^- \rightarrow 2Mn^{2+} + 5Cl_2(g) + 8H_2O$$
Reaction I

The chlorine gas thus produced is collected in a container and the pressure and volume of the gas is determined. Since the temperature of the system is known, the ideal gas equation can now be used to calculate the number of moles of chlorine gas present. From this value, the number of moles of manganese can then be determined.

47. What type of reaction is Reaction I?
A. Lewis acid - Lewis base
B. Double replacement
C. Oxidation-reduction
D. Dissociation

48. How can the ideal gas equation be rearranged to allow for the determination of n?
A. $n = PV/(RT)$
B. $n = RT/(PV)$
C. $n = PT/(RV)$
D. $n = RV/(PT)$

49. What would be the approximate ratio between the mass of manganese in the steel sample and the mass of chlorine gas produced?
A. 2 : 5
B. 3 : 2
C. 3 : 4
D. 1 : 3

50. Reaction I is endothermic and hence the actual temperature of the reaction vessel may be different from that expected. Given that the initial temperature of the reaction vessel was used in the calculations, how would this affect the predicted value of n?
A. It would be greater than the actual value.
B. It would be less than the actual value.
C. It would be the same as the actual value.
D. This cannot be determined from the information given

51. Pig iron consists of iron with about 5% manganese. Which of the following most accurately describes pig iron?
A. It is a colloid.
B. It is a solid solution.
C. It is a complex molecule.
D. It is an alloy.

Questions 52-56 are NOT based on a descriptive passage.

52. The force between two charged particles is given by n. If the two particles retain their charge, by what distance must they now be separated in order for the force between them to increase to 2n?
A. The distance between them must be increased by a factor of 2.
B. The distance between them must be decreased by a factor of 2.
C. The distance between them must be decreased by a factor of $\sqrt{2}$.
D. The distance between them must be increased by a factor of $\sqrt{2}$.

53. Why does potassium possess a higher first electron affinity than first ionization energy?
A. Its valence shells are only partially filled.
B. The attractive forces between the nucleus and the valence electrons are strong.
C. It possesses very few inner electron shells.
D. Its valence electron shell contains only one electron.

54. A mass of 0.5 kg is attached to a vertically oriented spring with a force constant of 10 N m^{-1}. By approximately how much is the spring stretched? ($g = 10$ m s^{-2})
A. 5.0 m
B. 2.0 m
C. 50 m
D. 0.5 m

55. A sound wave emanating from a stationary observer bounces off an object approaching with velocity *v*. The original wave, relative to the reflected wave, has:
A. a higher wavelength but a lower velocity.
B. a lower wavelength and the same velocity.
C. a higher wavelength and the same velocity.
D. a lower wavelength but a higher velocity.

56. The following reaction was carried out in a closed system:

$$N_2(g) + O_2(g) \rightleftharpoons 2NO(g) \quad \Delta H_{rxn} = \text{-ve value}$$

Which of the following would favor the production of NO?
A. Decreased pressure
B. A catalyst
C. Decreased partial pressure of oxygen
D. Decreased temperature

Passage IX (Questions 57-62)

One of the very innovative methods used to detect radioactive emissions and many other types of particles and energy was devised by Geiger, in conjunction with Muller in the early 1900's. The apparatus works on the principle that many types of small particles and energy (in particular radioactive emissions) convert a gas into a conductor of electricity. The instrument itself consists of a glass tube into which two metal electrodes are sealed: a central cathode and the cylindrical anode lining the glass tube as shown in Figure 1.

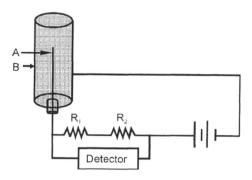

Figure 1

The anode A is a tungsten wire running along the axis of the tube while the cathode B is a thin aluminium cylinder around the circumference of the tube. A potential difference of about 500 V is maintained between the electrodes. The ionizing radiation/particles enters through a mica window and when it interacts with the argon gas present inside the tube (at a pressure of 1300-1600 Pa along with 6% ethanol), the argon atoms are ionized giving rise to cations and free electrons. As the charged particles thus generated are attracted to the electrodes of opposite sign, they are accelerated and ionize other previously neutral argon atoms.

The force exerted on a charged particle in an electric field of strength E is given by $F = q\,E$ where q = charge on the particle in coulombs. The energy of a particle under a potential difference of V volts is given by $E = q\,V$ where E = energy of particle.

Mass of an electron = 9.1×10^{-31} kg
Mass of a proton = 1.7×10^{-27} kg
Mass of a neutron = 1.7×10^{-27} kg
Charge on electron = 1.6×10^{-19} C

57. A certain charged particle experienced an acceleration of 3.2×10^{13} m s^{-2} due to a force of 5.4×10^{-16} N. What was the mass of the particle?
A. 4.7×10^{-28} kg
B. 9.0×10^{-30} kg
C. 9.4×10^{-28} kg
D. 1.7×10^{-29} kg

58. As both the argon cation and electron are accelerated to electrodes of opposite sign, they both have the same initial velocity. Ionization of the gaseous atoms present is dependent only on the velocity of collision. Assuming that they both have the same initial velocity, which of the following statements is true?
A. Both electron and cation will yield the same number of charged particles.
B. The electron will yield more charged particles.
C. The argon cation will yield more charged particles.
D. The answer cannot be determined without knowing the exact value of the initial velocity.

59. What is the energy of an alpha particle (a helium nucleus) under a potential difference of 20 V?
A. 3.5×10^{-18} J
B. 3.2×10^{-18} J
C. 1.3×10^{-18} J
D. 6.4×10^{-18} J

60. If the current that flows into the detector is due only to electron motion and 2.50×10^{19} electrons per second impinge on the positive electrode, what is the value of the current in amperes?
A. 4.00 A
B. 2.00 A
C. 1.00 A
D. 0.20 A

61. A sudden voltage drop across the resistors in Figure 1 appears as a pulse to the detector. If $R_2 = 2R_1$ and R_2 is removed from the circuit, what will the new voltage drop be if the current remains unchanged?
A. 1/2 the original value
B. 1/3 the original value
C. 1/6 the original value
D. The same as the original value

62. Three types of electromagnetic radiation, P, Q and R, were allowed to enter the Geiger counter. Assuming that the current flow is due only to electron motion and that the ionizing power of radiation is directly proportional to its energy, what is the sequence of P, Q and R in order of increasing wavelength (λ)?

Current obtained from P = 1.50 A
Current obtained from Q = 0.75 A
Current obtained from R = 1.00 A

A. $\lambda_P < \lambda_R < \lambda_Q$
B. $\lambda_P < \lambda_Q < \lambda_R$
C. $\lambda_Q < \lambda_R < \lambda_P$
D. $\lambda_Q < \lambda_P < \lambda_R$

Acid-base indicators such as methyl-orange, phenolphthalein and bromothymol blue are substances which change color according to the hydrogen ion concentration of the solution to which they are added.

Most indicators are weak acids (or more rarely weak bases) in which the undissociated and dissociated forms have different, distinct colors. If methyl-orange is used as the example and the undissociated form is written as HMe then the dissociation occurs as shown in Reaction I.

$$HMe \rightleftharpoons H^+ + Me^- \quad \textbf{Reaction I}$$

Red   Colorless   Yellow

The indicator should have a sharp color change coinciding with the equivalence point of the titration. Usually, the color change of the indicator occurs over a range of about two pH units. It should be noted that the eye cannot detect the exact end point of the titration. The pK_a of the indicator should be near the pH of the solution at the equivalence point.

63. By what factor must the hydrogen ion concentration change at the equivalence point for the indicator in solution to change color?
    A. 2
    B. 10
    C. 100
    D. 200

64. Which of the following situations exist at the equivalence point of a titration?
    A. $[H^+] = 10^{-7}$ M
    B. $[H^+] = [OH^-]$
    C. $[OH^-] = 10^{-7}$ M
    D. $[H^+]/[OH^-] = 10^{-14}$

65. A titration between equimolar concentrations of hydrochloric acid and sodium hydroxide has an equivalence point with a pH of 7. Given the following information, which indicator is most suitable for detecting the end point of this titration?

Indicator	K_a
Bromothymol blue	3.16×10^{-7}
Cresol red	7.00×10^{-9}
Bromophenol blue	1.58×10^{-4}
p-Xylenol blue	1.10×10^{-2}

    A. Bromothymol blue
    B. Cresol red
    C. Bromophenol blue
    D. p-Xylenol blue

66. Given that the K_a (methyl-orange) = 4.0×10^{-4}, a solution of pH = 2 containing the indicator would be:
    A. orange.
    B. yellow.
    C. colorless.
    D. red.

67. When indicators are used, what can be done to minimize their interfering with the titration?
    A. Only add a few drops of the indicator.
    B. Add excess of the titrant to negate its effect.
    C. Add excess of the solution to be titrated to negate its effect.
    D. Only use indicators with large K_a values.

Waves can be roughly divided into two categories: those which require media for their propagation (i.e. sound) and those which do not (i.e. electromagnetic radiation). All waves, however, share similar relationships between their physical properties.

A wave travelling through a medium creates a number of high pressure regions (crests) and low pressure regions (troughs) during their propagation. The frequency (f) of a wave is given by the number of crests (or troughs) passing a point in a second. The wavelength of a wave (λ) is the distance between successive crests (or troughs). The amplitude of a wave is given by the maximal displacement of the particles of the medium from their "zero" position. With respect to sound, the frequency of a wave determines what we refer to as pitch, and the amplitude determines what is referred to as loudness or sound intensity.

Sound travels at about 343 m s^{-1} in air, and markedly faster in liquids and solids. The frequency of a particular sound wave remains the same in different media while the other physical properties (velocity and wavelength) are altered.

68. A particular sound wave in air has a pitch of 3500 Hz and a wavelength of 17 m. It then travels through water where it moves four times as quickly as it does in air. What is the ratio of the wavelength of the wave in air to its wavelength in water?
    A. 4 : 1
    B. 1 : 4
    C. 17 : 4
    D. 4 : 17

69. In a liquid, the speed of sound is inversely proportional to the square root of the density of the liquid. If a liquid X has a density equal to twice the density of liquid Y, what is the ratio of the velocity of the wave in X to the velocity of the wave in Y?
    A. $1 : \sqrt{2}$
    B. 1 : 2
    C. 1 : 4
    D. 2 : 1

70. If two sounds measure 93.0 and 90.0 dB, respectively, how many times greater is the sound intensity of the first as compared to that of the second?
    A. 100.0
    B. 20.0
    C. 2.0
    D. 1.0

71. Sonar is one of the applications of sound used extensively in undersea mapping. A transmitter emits a pulse of sound and the time it takes to return is used to determine the depth. If the sound wave takes 20 seconds to return, and sound travels four times as quickly in water as in air, how deep is that region?
    A. 3 430 m
    B. 6 860 m
    C. 13 720 m
    D. 27 440 m

72. A person lying on an air mattress in the ocean rises and falls through one complete cycle every five seconds. The crests of the wave causing the motion are 20.0 m apart. What is the frequency of the wave?
    A. 0.2 Hz
    B. 1 Hz
    C. 4 Hz
    D. 5 Hz

73. When can a real image be formed using a concave (diverging) lens?
A. A real image cannot be obtained.
B. When the object distance is greater than the radius of curvature.
C. When the object distance is less than the radius of curvature but greater than the focal length.
D. When the object distance is less than the focal length.

74. The molarity of a solution is numerically equal to the molality of a solution when which of the following is true?
A. Under any circumstance
B. When the volume of the solvent in cm^{-3} is equal to its mass in grams
C. When the temperature of the solution is 300 K (i.e. room temperature)
D. When the number of moles of solute in solution is less than one

75. The reaction $P + 3Q \rightarrow R$ was studied and the data in Table 1 were collected.

Table 1

Exp.	[P] in M	[Q] in M	Initial rate of reaction
A	0.30	0.90	5.0×10^{-6}
B	0.30	1.80	1.0×10^{-5}
C	0.90	0.90	4.5×10^{-5}

The rate determining step in this reaction probably involves:
A. two molecules of P and two molecules of Q.
B. three molecules of P and one molecule of Q.
C. one molecule of P and three molecules of Q.
D. two molecules of P and one molecule of Q.

76. A uniform plank of length 2 m was suspended on a fulcrum placed 0.50 m from the left end. A mass of 4 kg was placed at a position 0.30 m from the left end of the plank. The system was then in equilibrium. What is the mass of the plank?
A. 0.6 kg
B. 1.0 kg
C. 1.6 kg
D. 2.4 kg

77. Which of the following molecules forms the weakest hydrogen bonds?
A. HF
B. HCl
C. H_2O
D. H_2S

END OF PHYSICAL SCIENCES. IF TIME REMAINS, YOU MAY GO BACK AND CHECK YOUR WORK IN THIS TEST BOOKLET.

THE GOLD STANDARD MCAT*

TEST GS-3

Verbal Reasoning
Questions 78-137
Time : 85 Minutes

OPEN BOOKLET ONLY WHEN TIMER IS READY.

The Gold Standard MCAT* has been designed exclusively to test knowledge and thinking skills. The exam may contain hypothetical statements and/or express controversial ideas. Statements contained herein do not necessarily reflect the policy, position, or view of RuveneCo Publishing.

* MCAT is a registered service mark of the Association of American Medical Colleges, which is not associated with this product.

VERBAL REASONING

INSTRUCTIONS: The Verbal Reasoning test contains nine passages, each of which is followed by several questions. After reading the passage, select the best answer to each question. If you are unsure of the answer, eliminate the alternatives you know to be false then select an answer from the remaining alternatives. Indicate your answer by blackening the corresponding oval on your Answer Document 1, GS-3.

Passage I (Questions 78-84)

"In 1492, Columbus discovered America..." Starting from this disputed fact, each one of us will describe the history of this country in a somewhat different way. Nonetheless, it is reasonable to assume that most of us would include something about what is called the 'democratic process', and how Americans have valued it, or at least have said they valued it. Therein lies a problem: one of the tenets of a democratic society is that men be allowed to think and express themselves freely in any subject... To the extent that our schools are instruments of such a society, they must develop in the young not only an awareness of this freedom, but a will to exercise it, and the intellectual power and perspective to do so effectively. This is necessary so that the society may continue to change and modify itself.

So goes the theory.

In practice, we mostly get a different story. In our society, as in others, we find that there are influential men at the head of important institutions, who cannot afford to be found wrong, who find change inconvenient, and who have financial or political interests they must conserve at any cost. Such men are, therefore, threatened in many respects by the theory of the democratic process... Moreover, we find that there are obscure men who do not head important institutions who are similarly threatened because they have identified themselves with certain ideas and institutions which they wish to keep free from either criticism or change.

Such men as these would prefer that the schools do little or nothing to encourage youth to question any part of the society in which they live... In the early 1960s, Ernest Hemmingway [said], "In order to be a great writer a person must have a built-in, shockproof crap detector." It seems to us, that, in his response, Hemmingway identified an essential survival function of the schools in today's world.

One way of looking at the history of the human group is that it has been a continuing struggle against the veneration of "crap." Our intellectual history is a chronicle of the suffering of men who tried to help their contemporaries see that some part of their fondest beliefs were misconceptions. The mileposts along the road of our intellectual development signal those points at which some person developed a new perspective, or a new metaphor. We have in mind a new education that would set out to cultivate just such people - experts at "crap detecting."

There are many ways of describing this function of the schools, and many men who have. David Reisman calls this the "counter-cyclical approach to education..." Norbert Weiner insisted that the schools must now function as "anti-entropic feedback systems", entropy being the word used to denote a general tendency of all systems to "run down", to reduce to chaos and uselessness. This is a process that can be slowed down and partly controlled... through "maintenance." ...In other words, we must have instruments to tell us when we are running down, when maintenance is required... This is what we mean by "crap detecting."... We are talking about the schools, cultivating in the young that most "subversive" intellectual instrument - the anthropological perspective...

We need hardly ask that achieving such a perspective is extremely difficult, requiring, among other things, considerable courage. We are, after all, talking about achieving a high degree of freedom from the intellectual and social constraints of one's tribe... Our own outlook seems "natural" to us, and we wonder that other men can perversely persist in believing nonsense. Yet, it is undoubtedly true that, for most people, the acceptance of a particular doctrine is largely attributable to the accident of birth... It is the sign of a competent "crap detector" that he is not completely captivated by the arbitrary abstractions of the community in which he happened to grow up.

Adapted from Neil Postman and Charles Weingartner, *Teaching As a Subversive Activity.* © 1969 by Neil Postman and Charles Weingartner.

---

78. Based on the passage, one could reasonably conclude that the authors might encourage debate in the classroom on:

A. the advantages of governmental systems other than the democratic system.

B. how American values could be upheld in a constantly changing world.

C. whether or not Hemmingway was a great writer.

D. whether or not anthropology should really be considered a social science.

79. Based on the passage, which of the following people in American society would likely be most opposed to David Reisman's counter-cyclical approach to education?

A. A politician resolved to facilitating the social and economic development of America

B. An anarchist

C. A young child just entering grade school

D. A high school teacher determined to ingrain into his students those values which he believes has made America the country it is today

80. The "crap" that Hemmingway mentions, likely refers to:

A. the material taught in schools which does not encourage students to exercise their freedom of speech.

B. those ideas which individuals firmly believe, but which are founded on faulty assumptions.

C. the attitudes of people who are opposed to change.

D. the beliefs of individuals from cultures which differ from those of Americans.

81. David Reisman's counter-cyclical approach to education is so named because:

A. it describes a system of education which attempts to question and modify accepted norms of society.

B. it is an approach based on the premise that cycles do not occur in the society in which we live.

C. it is an approach which seeks to accelerate the normal cycle of education, during which information is passed from teacher to student.

D. it facilitates the entropic process acting on the education process.

82. The passage suggests that the "maintenance" instruments described by Weiner likely include:

A. all teachers.

B. those people in society who can recognize when change is needed.

C. those people in society most opposed to change.

D. all students.

83. The passage indicates that the main characteristics of the anthropological perspective is that it:

A. requires students of anthropology to be the main instruments of "maintenance."

B. focuses the attention of individuals on the customs of the many different cultures of the world.

C. facilitates individuals viewing the beliefs of cultures different from their own, as nonsense.

D. demands that individuals view their society objectively, recognizing its limitations.

84. The authors' reference to "...the accident of birth," in the last paragraph suggests that they believe that:

A. the society into which an individual is born has little to do with his ideologies.

B. if an individual was born into another tribe, he would as easily have adopted the beliefs of that tribe.

C. unplanned pregnancies commonly inhibit the adoption of the anthropological perspective by students.

D. all cultures can produce competent "crap detectors."

Critics of the "women's agenda" in both research and policy have complained of its exclusive focus on the experiences of white women. They maintain that as a result of this focus, we know relatively little about the experiences of black women in the labor market compared to those of white women...

Stratification by race and gender shapes the lives of individuals in the United States. Most research treats race and gender stratification as two separate systems. Thus, for women of color, the disadvantage is seen as simply the sum of both systems, with little consideration to whether they experience the system of race stratification differently from men of color. Along a similar vein, scholarship examining gender stratification often fails to consider if women of color experience sexism differently from white women.

Because slavery and a racial caste system form the historical foundation of black women's disadvantages in paid work, their oppression differs from that of white women. As a consequence of their differing histories, black women's current occupational distribution differs markedly from that of white women. Many of the policy initiatives associated with the women's movement and feminist theory have ignored these differences. As a result, black women sometimes perceive feminists' concerns as... ways of redistributing material wealth between white men and white women. One example of a policy initiative supported by many feminists is comparable-worth. Comparable-worth initiatives mandate equal pay for work of equal value in different occupations. However, the occupations that employ the highest concentrations of black women are welfare aide, cook, housekeeper, and private household worker while the occupations that employ the highest percentage of white women are dental hygienist, secretary, and dental assistant. Would the jobs in which black women are concentrated benefit proportionately from comparable-worth? Only by studying the intersection of race and gender in the labor market can we assess the extent to which comparable-worth, or other policies supported by feminists, would benefit black and white women evenly.

More broadly, only by studying intersections of race and gender can we assess the extent to which gender inequality has affected black and white women similarly or the extent to which race inequality has affected men and women similarly. Recently, scholars have asked how these stratification systems intersect. Animating this call is the realization that, even when viewing inequality from the perspective of a group disadvantaged along any one axis, the account given often best fits members of this group who are privileged along the other axis of inequality. This leads discussions of racial inequality to emphasize the plight of black men, while discussions of gender inequality focus on the problems of white women. This phenomenon led Hull, Scott and Smith to entitle their 1982 anthology on black women *All the Women are White, All the Blacks are Men, But Some of Us are Brave.*

Although the writers making this critique have not always chosen statistical language, one implication of their claim is that race and sex should be involved in statistical interaction (with each other or in higher-order interactions that include other variables) in affecting socioeconomic outcomes...

Analyses of gender inequality have often been generalised from data confined to whites. Other analyses have used samples including whites and blacks without separation by race, so that the results are dominated by what holds for whites, because of their much larger numbers. This literature suggests several components of gender inequality in earning, but in many cases we know little about their relative explanatory power for blacks and whites...

Many analyses of racial inequality in earnings have focused exclusively upon men. Past literature suggests several generalizations about racial inequality, but we know little about whether they apply to women or interact with gender.

Adapted from Social Forces, June 1994,72(4), *Effects of Individual, Occupational, and Industrial Characteristics on Earnings.*© The University of North Carolina Press.

85. According to the passage, it is difficult to reach conclusions about the experiences of black women in the labor market because:
   I. most research treats race and gender stratification as two separate systems.
   II. most research focuses exclusively on the experiences of white women.
   III. most research assumes black men and women experience the system of race stratification similarly.

   A. I only
   B. II only
   C. I and II only
   D. I, II and III

86. According to the passage, a black woman's oppression differs from that of a white woman because:
   A. black women perceive feminists' concerns as irrelevant to their experiences.
   B. of their differing histories.
   C. many feminists support the policy of comparable-worth.
   D. many employers are racist.

87. The passage suggests that Hull, Scott and Smith entitled their anthology as they did because:
   A. the plight of black women are rarely the focus of discussions on equality.
   B. the authors of the anthology disliked black women.
   C. comparable-worth initiatives mandate equal pay for work of equal value.
   D. the authors stratified black men and white women in the same manner.

88. On the basis of the author's comments about black women in the labor force, it is reasonable to conclude that the author believes that:
   A. many feminist policies merely involve the redistribution of wealth between white men and white women.
   B. the only way to determine the extent to which black women can benefit from feminist policies is by studying the intersection of race and gender.
   C. black women and white women are presently evenly affected by policies such as comparable-worth.
   D. black men and black women are presently not evenly affected by policies such as comparable-worth.

89. Saying that black women sometimes perceive feminists' concerns as "ways of redistributing material wealth..." (paragraph 3), most nearly means that black women:
   A. are unreasonable.
   B. do not support the feminist movement.
   C. view some feminist policies as irrelevant to their experiences.
   D. experience problems in the labor force that black men do not.

90. Based on the passage, a good study to determine the actual experience of black women in the labor force would be one that:
   A. ascertained what factors explained the gender gap in earnings and whether these factors explained the same portion of this gap among blacks and whites.
   B. ascertained what factors explained the race gap in earnings and whether those factors explained the same portion of this gap among women and men.
   C. ascertained what factors explained the race and gender gaps in earning, independently.
   D. both A and B.

Setaria Beauv. is a genus of about 125 species that includes food crops and a number of important weeds. Some of the weedy *Setaria* species are *S.viridis* (L.) Beauv. (green foxtail), *S.glauca* (Weigel) Hubb. (yellow foxtail), *S.faberii* Herrm. (giant foxtail), *S.verticillata* (L.) Beauv., and *S.geniculata* (Lamarck) Beauv. (knotroot foxtail). *Setaria italica* (L.) Beauv. (foxtail millet), a close relative of *S.viridis,* is an important world grain crop. It has been argued that many temperate weedy foxtails evolved from green foxtail-like ancestors. Green foxtail is primarily self-pollinating, and is morphologically heterogeneous, with many variants. Systematic relationships between these variants are unclear.

Although there have been no explicit phylogenetic analyses of *Setaria,* it has been speculated that Africa is the original home of the genus because 74 out of 125 species occur on that continent. Before being introduced to other continents, green foxtail's natural range was probably Eurasia.

Today, green foxtail is primarily a temperate species but is widely distributed between 45° and 55° N latitudes. It is one of the most widely distributed weedy foxtail species both globally and in the United States. Globally, it ranges from North America, through Central America to parts of South America; from Europe to northern Africa, and from east Asia to south Asia and Australia. It is found in every state in the continental United States and every province in Canada.

Foxtails are of considerable agronomic importance. Their associations with agriculture, as both crops and weeds, date back thousands of years to ancient civilizations. Foxtail millet is one of the oldest cultivated cereals of China, dating back about 6,000 years to the earliest agricultural settlements of the Yang-shao culture phase. Today, this crop is widely grown in Africa, China, India, and scattered areas throughout Eurasia. *Setaria varieties, S.glace,* and *S.fibber* are listed as major weeds worldwide and comprise the second most important weed group in the United States. Foxtail seeds also serve as an important food source for wildlife. Since their introduction to North America, foxtails have expanded in terms of range, population density, and the appearance of new morphological variants. Crop yield losses and herbicide expenditures make control of the foxtails a significant problem in crop production.

Substantial biological diversity, wide geographic distribution, and strong competitiveness in disturbed habitats all mark foxtails as highly successful weeds. There is, however, little understanding of what traits lead to their success as weeds, or the implications and significance of genetic heterogeneity to their adaptation. Answers to these questions require knowledge of both population biology and physiology.

One of the important aspects of population biology is population genetic structure, which forms the basis of plant spatial and temporal organization. Knowledge of population genetic structure has practical implications. It can be used to reconstruct the historical process of migration and colonization, and provide insights into the ecological persistence and evolutionary potential of populations in new habitats, leading to a better understanding of weedy adaptation. Information about the genetic diversity of a species in a particular region can be of value in devising effective biological controls, which match locally adapted weed genotype-predator pairs. In addition, knowledge of population genetic structure could provide clues to the development of a simplified model system to study adaptive functional traits and overcome the limitations inherent in inter- and intraspecific *Setaria* app. heterogeneity.

Developing an understanding of why foxtails are successful weeds is essential for developing future weed management strategies. Current weed management systems rely heavily on herbicides. Problems associated with these chemicals include high annual costs, overdose application as a result of ignorance of weed heterogeneity, selection for herbicide-resistant biotypes, and environmental pollution.

Adapted from the *American Journal of Botany* 82(3); Wang, Wendel and Dekker, 1995.

91. The author supports the argument that "many temperate weedy foxtails evolved from green foxtail-like ancestors" by stating that:
    A. green foxtail is primarily self-pollinating.
    B. green foxtail is morphologically heterogenous.
    C. *Setaria* Beauv. is a genus that includes food crops and a number of important weeds.
    D. *Setaria italica* Beauv. is a close relative of *S. viridis.*

92. Which of the following, if true, would most severely challenge the author's conclusion (paragraph 4) that "foxtails are of considerable agronomic importance"?
A. A domesticated form of foxtail millet is a good food source in India.
B. Foxtails lack biological diversity and are not strongly competitive in disturbed habitats.
C. Foxtail seeds contaminate yields during harvesting.
D. *S. faberii* Herrm. is costing African farmers great losses in yield.

93. According to the passage, it is thought that *Setaria* originated in Africa because:
A. green foxtail's natural range was probably Eurasia.
B. *S. viridis* is primarily a temperate species.
C. many temperate weedy foxtails evolved from green foxtail-like ancestors.
D. the majority of species of *Setaria* occur on the African continent.

94. From the reasoning in the passage, which of the following would be an important property of a successful weed?
A. It is one of the species that make up the genus *Setaria* Beauv.
B. It has substantial biological diversity.
C. It is morphologically heterogenous.
D. It dates back thousands of years to ancient civilization.

95. The passage suggests that North America would be most interested in foxtail population genetic structure:
A. in order to devise effective biological controls to reduce crop loss.
B. because foxtail millet is a food source in North America.
C. foxtail seeds serve as a primary food source for wildlife.
D. foxtail millet provides a food source for China.

96. Based on the passage, which of the following studies would likely be carried out on foxtails by biologists?
A. A study which investigated the geographic patterns of genetic diversity of foxtails at the continental level.
B. A study which assessed the genetic diversity of green foxtails.
C. A study which investigated the traits of foxtails that led to their success as weeds.
D. All of the above

97. The passage implies that green foxtail is one of the most widely distributed species globally:
A. as a result of wind pollination.
B. because it is a close relative of foxtail millet.
C. as a result of its introduction into other continents by external forces.
D. because it is not morphologically heterogenous.

During recent years protest has been vigorous and vehement against the high cost of living. Yet little has been said - publicly at any rate - about the even higher cost of dying. Although that has more than tripled during the last quarter of a century, the general attitude has been that to draw a relationship between funerals and finances is [not] proper.

As a consequence, the cost of death and burial has become one of the most crushing expenses facing American families. In 1935, the average cost of an adult funeral was about $350; by 1960 it had risen to $1100... Statistics give only a poor indication of what this has meant to millions of families, for the expenditure is required not only at a time of great emotional shock, but frequently at a time of great financial dislocation. Most persons, however frugally they may have lived, are dying beyond their means...

Although many unscrupulous morticians have exerted strong pressure to persuade bereaved persons to order elaborate funerals, they have not always needed to exert any pressure at all. For the unusually high sums charged for a funeral are in large measure a reflection of the industry's remarkably successful public relations program - a program that has redefined the ancient concept of respect for the dead to emphasize extravagant display. "It is the task of those in the funeral profession," says the *Psychology of Funeral Service*, an important handbook for morticians, "to educate the public in the right paths."

That "education" has been so effective that the modern American funeral - with its vulgarity, sacrifice of spiritual values to materialistic trappings, and overwhelming abnegation of rational attitudes - has become for many a symbol of cultural sickness... The public relations campaign has managed to make us not only accept extravagant display, but to demand it under the delusion that lavish send-offs are the precise measure of our religion, family love, true-blue Americanism - all of which concepts they violate in a most basic way...

In some cases, of course, persons have willingly gone into debt for an elaborate funeral that has provided them with a means of atonement for their failures in family relationships... This neglect-now, pay-later attitude toward human relationships strikes hard at moral and ethical concepts since it provides easy absolution for all cruelty and coldness, hardness and abuse... one wonders whether the kind of charity that is designed to benefit the giver [rather]

than the receiver can be considered part of the greatest of all virtues...

Not only our attitudes, but most of our laws governing disposal of the dead have also been shaped by undertakers and members of related businesses. Aided by public determination to avoid "unpleasant" talk about death and by the successful lobbying in state capitals, persons in the mortuary and cemetery business are generally free of controls...

Depressing as the situation is, it is certainly not incapable of solution. The idea that the funeral industry is a public utility and as such should be operated by the state or under state regulation has been acknowledged in Europe for years... In the United States, indigents and other public charges are buried at public cost by public agencies; however, great stigma is attached to the idea of a "charity" burial...

In spite of the scope and intensity of the funeral industry's protest, the reform program is growing to such extent that there is genuine hope that the costly and barbaric shows for the dead may be abolished in the interests of the living... The funeral industry has exploited the worst of our motivations and desires: snobbery, vanity, the chance to rid ourselves of feelings of guilt through a payoff.

We are and we have been, in all fairness, our own chief victimizers.

Adapted from Ruth Mulvey Harmer, *The High Cost of Dying.*
© 1963 by The Crowell-Collier Publishing Company.

98. Based on the author's comments in the first paragraph, which of the following would best support the author's claims about the attitude of American's to funeral costs?
   A. Money is no object when one's loved ones are involved.
   B. Funeral costs genuinely reflect the economic state of the families bearing them.
   C. It has been largely shaped by the funeral industry and related businesses.
   D. The right sort of person simply does not consider money at the time of a funeral.

99. According to the passage, the increasing cost of death and burial over the years can be attributed to:
I. unscrupulous morticians.
II. the funeral industry's public relations program.
III. guilt over failures in family relationships.

A. II only
B. I and II only
C. II and III only
D. I, II and III

100. Consider the following: "What father would accept the sacrifice of a child's educational opportunity in the interest of his having a fine funeral?"; which argument presented by the author, does this statement most support?
A. Our laws governing disposal of the dead have also been shaped by undertakers and members of related businesses.
B. Lavish send-offs violate the concepts of religion, family love and true-blue Americanism.
C. The neglect-now, pay-later attitude toward human relationships strikes hard at moral and ethical concepts by easy absolution for cruelty.
D. The modern American funeral has become for many a symbol of cultural sickness.

101. The passage indicates that undertakers have been influential in:
I. creating the laws that govern the disposal of the dead.
II. encouraging the neglect-now, pay-later attitude towards human relationships.
III. shaping the attitude of Americans regarding costs of funerals.

A. II only
B. I and II only
C. I and III only
D. I, II and III

102. Based on the passage, one may conclude that the author believes that the solution to the "high cost of dying" issue in America, involves:
A. educating the public on how to dispose of their loved ones, thus eliminating the need for a funeral industry.
B. appealing to the compassion of the members of the funeral industry and related businesses.
C. reducing the stigma attached to "charity burials," so all funerals would be free.
D. viewing the funeral industry as a public utility, thus allowing funeral cost to be regulated by the state.

103. The author's comments in the passage assert that, on the question of increasing funeral costs over the years:
A. Americans have been completely victimized by undertakers.
B. the blame rests on successful lobbyers.
C. the blame largely rests on the American people.
D. the blame rests on the state for not having completely eliminated the funeral industry years ago.

104. The author claims, but offers no support for the claim that:
A. the cost of death and burial more than tripled in 25 years.
B. the unusually high sums charged for a funeral are in large measure, a reflection of the industry's public relations program.
C. the situation regarding the high cost of dying is not without solutions.
D. persons in the mortuary and cemetery business are generally free of controls.

105. The attitude of the author towards the high cost of dying, could best be described as:
A. disgust.
B. pity.
C. indifference.
D. supportive.

The Roman god Mercury who according to ancient mythology controls the arts of eloquence and communication has also given his name to the most sprightly and changeable of the naturally-occurring elements. It can certainly be said that in the 20th century the god has lived up to his name...

One form the communications revolution has taken this century is the revolution in the manner of physical transportation. The development of the automobile, and the growth in particular of air transport, has given the opportunity and rewards of international travel to wider and wider groups of people. But even more dramatic and far-reaching than the physical transport of people is the revolution in techniques for the communication of information and ideas...

The 16th century saw an earlier revolution in the communication of ideas with the invention of movable type... However, the revolution engendered by print took a long time to develop and had to wait until the 20th century for its full exploitation. The mass reading of newspapers, the growth of advertising, the art of printed persuasion of whole populations, have come into their own only in the last fifty years.

Much of the drive for improving means of communication has been provided by the rewards in terms of efficiency and private profit. Access to effective communications systems amounted to a licence to print money long before the era of commercial television...

The advent of electronics, in particular of the thermionic valve, transformed the science of telecommunication. The thermionic valve was the basis of most electronic circuits until well after the end of World War II, but a further major advance came with the advent of the solid-state device, the transistor. Transistors together with printed circuits have completely transformed the design and production of radio and television sets and indeed most other forms of electronic circuits. The transistor has formed the basis of the growth in the electronics industry since World War II.

The major problem with transatlantic radio transmission has always been atmospheric electrical interference and to avoid this cables have been laid across the Atlantic for transmitting speech across telephone links. Co-axial cables are now used for world telephone transmission... but their cost makes it necessary to search for cheaper means of communication. The most attractive technique is the use of radio waves reflected from or re-transmitted from satellites in space... If a radio relay station is available above the ionosphere, high-frequency speech signals can be re-transmitted over a wide area.

The radio-telescope at Jordell Bank demonstrated these possibilities in 1959 and... subsequently, the American Telegraph and Telephone company launched the Telstar satellite, showing that artificial earth satellites could provide the basis for a practical world-wide communication system...

For twenty-four hour communication, twelve such Telstar satellites continuously circling the earth would by required. Alternatively, a much higher artificial satellite could be used. At about 23 000 miles above the earth's surface a satellite speed is such that it remains stationary with respect to a point on the earth. It can therefore provide communication over a large part of the earth's surface...

The development of mass communication systems such as radio and television has had sweeping social and economic effects. In recent years millions have been able to see, and hear, and read the same message at the same time, whereas before only hundreds could do this... the electronic revolution has turned the world into a "global village." The mass media are expensive to develop and operate so that it has proved necessary to ensure a favourable public response by feeding back into the system the designs and wishes of the masses. The communication media have therefore tended to shift the seat of power from the wishes of a few individuals to the desires of the populace at large. Thus in a limited sense the growth of the global village is placing the determination of the future into the hands of the global villagers themselves.

Adapted from G.B. Niblett, *The Electronics Revolution*, History of the 20th Century, Vol 6(87), © 1969 BPC Publishing Ltd.

106. The author referred to the Roman god of Mercury in order to show that:
   A. people of Italian descent have excellent communication skills.
   B. the element mercury is the foundation of the telecommunications industry.
   C. features of this ancient god serve as a basis for a 20th century revolution.
   D. without the Roman deity advances in communication would not be possible.

107. "The Rothchild's fortune is said to have been based on obtaining before anyone else the result of the battle of Waterloo." This would most strengthen the author's claim that:
   A. the 16th century saw a revolution in the communication of ideas.
   B. the drive for improving communication is provided in part by the rewards of private profit.
   C. a revolution in arms can result in a revolution in ideas.
   D. the English have always been ahead in the field of communications.

108. The passage suggests that movable type was directly responsible for the evolution of all of the following EXCEPT:
   A. the radio.
   B. the newspaper.
   C. magazines.
   D. printed advertising.

109. The America I Satellite, launched in 1995, facilitates communication over a large part of the earth's surface. Based on the passage, the America I Satellite must:
   A. use the thermionic valve as the basis for its communication relays.
   B. be one of twelve similar satellites.
   C. have been launched from the Space Shuttle Explorer.
   D. be about 23 000 miles above the earth's surface to provide dependable service for a large clientele.

110. Which of the following, if true, would LEAST strengthen the claim of the author that mass communication has had sweeping social and economic effects?
   A. Most Americans were deeply affected the day President John F. Kennedy was shot.
   B. National sales of Fox watches increased after its television commercial during the Superbowl.
   C. A small town has banned the advertising of alcohol and now has lowered levels of alcohol abuse.
   D. Violent children enjoy watching violence on television.

111. In the context of the passage, "global villagers" refers to:
   A. the consumers of the communication industry.
   B. the producers of the communication industry.
   C. wealthy individuals who affect communication policies.
   D. computer buffs who use the Internet to access information from around the world.

112. The bulk of the passage is dedicated to showing that:
   A. communication is a key aspect of one's humanity.
   B. electronic technology is the foundation of the modern communications revolution.
   C. World War II helped to improve communications for the "global village."
   D. the development of physical transportation allowed for the evolution of the transportation of ideas.

Passage VI (Questions 113-118)

Recent debates concerning the health care system have been both invigorating and frustrating. On the one hand it was a tremendous display of the power of democracy as debates rang from the coast of California to the shores of Maine, from Pennsylvania Avenue to any avenue in any town in Pennsylvania. It was our national coming-together to take the pulse of our health care system. The pulse was thready, the price was high. Everyone agreed change was necessary. Nothing changed.

Who had not heard of the 30 million Americans who, in their health, were excluded from medical care? But when they fell desperately ill they landed in unfamiliar territory and required the most expensive of all treatment - emergency care. And when they could not afford to remunerate their care-givers, who paid? We all did. Now NASA has nothing over my premiums! There have been cutbacks in benefits, increases in deductibles and so on.

And what of the tens of millions more Americans who were *underinsured*? They were the ones we saw on the evening news who had tilled the soil, paid their premiums, then were bitten with the venom of a chronic disease. Their insurance was not assurance. Their toil could not continue. Her house was sold. He borrowed money from family members and loan sharks. Debt grew, death came; what a way to go. The sailor was stranded in a boat in the open seas and exclaimed: "water everywhere, but none to drink"...

Many felt that getting more individuals and small businesses to coalesce and form associations with massive buying power would reduce costs and increase access for everyone. Some argued vociferously for free choice of one's physician. Yet the system of health care that was growing in popularity since the 1970s had restricted one's choice of physicians - the Health Maintenance Organization (HMO).

The middle name of HMOs is *maintenance*. Thus members, who pay a yearly premium, gain access to regular physical exams. They seek early treatment instead of neglecting their health because of financial considerations. Early diagnosis means treatment at an earlier stage which decreases costs and improves health. Theoretically, HMOs provide a model which could be elaborated during the political debates...

The debate in Washington displayed little concern for compassion, a moderate preoccupation with "containing"

costs, and a supreme infliction with *politicosis*. Politicosis is an illness that even our most excellent health care system cannot cure. Once infected, the unfortunate victim is less likely to weigh the intrinsic value of an opinion as compared to the side of the aisle from which the opinion came.

At first it seemed that all Americans would be insured and health care costs would stabilize or decrease. Then it seemed that 95% would be covered and "We'll work out the costs." Then it seemed 89% would be fully insured. Then nothing changed. Some finger pointing secondary to politicosis ensued. This was followed by a latent period after which the media stopped bringing us stories of the woman who sold her home, or the man who sold his soul.

113. The author suggests that the debates concerning health care were frustrating because:
  A. everyone agreed change was necessary.
  B. there was a national coming-together.
  C. the price of health care was high.
  D. despite the debate, nothing changed.

114. In the context of the passage, the statement "water everywhere, but none to drink" is likely meant to suggest that:
  A. it does not matter how much money a person has, medical care should be universal.
  B. many people become ill for lack of basic necessities like food and water.
  C. surrounded by the most advanced health care system, some die for lack of adequate health care.
  D. many people incurred great debt to pay for health care.

115. According to the passage, the statement concerning those who "tilled the soil" (paragraph 3) is most likely referring to the fact that:
  A. they were all farmers.
  B. they enjoyed planting.
  C. they worked hard.
  D. they were lazy.

116. Which of the following does the author suggest is a disadvantage with regards to HMOs?
    A. The choice of one's doctor is restricted.
    B. They lack interest in maintaining members' health.
    C. HMO's are generally affordable.
    D. Their ability to diagnose disease at an earlier stage.

117. Which of the following findings, if true, would most *weaken* the author's claim that "politicosis" inflicted the health care debate?
    A. Politicians tend to vote along party lines.
    B. During the debate, many bipartisan recommendations were made.
    C. Suggestions that had a high level of support from one party had little support from the other.
    D. Who you favor is more important than what you favor.

118. The overall theme of the passage was that:
    A. the public was excluded from the health care debate.
    B. options should be debated, then an optimal plan enacted.
    C. HMOs should be used as a model for change.
    D. the media's attention for the debate waned.

Admiral Erich Raeder learned many lessons from history, in particular... that if Germany had occupied Norway in 1914, Tirpitz's High Seas Fleet would have been free to operate against Allied trade in the North Atlantic from Norway's northern fiords, instead of being rendered impotent by the blockade maintained by Britain's Grand Fleet from Scapa Flow. Raeder brought this to Hitler's attention as early as October 1939, but not until 1940 did the *Fuehrer* authorize him to plan and organize the necessary operation, which was to be at four days' notice from March 10.

When Germany's radio intelligence indicated that Britain was planning to mine The Leads (the channel inside Norway's numerous offshore islands) in order to stop the flow of high-grade iron ore south from the port to Narvik, Hitler set April 9 as D-day for simultaneous surprise landings in Denmark and Norway. For these, Raeder intended to use almost all his surface Fleet plus a number of troop transports and supply ships, divided into eleven groups. Five of these sailed for ports in Denmark, a country which was unable to offer any resistance. The rest headed for ports in Norway where they were opposed, notably in Oslo fiord where the new 8-inch gun cruiser *Blucher* was torpedoed and sunk by the shore defence.

Ten large destroyers, under Commodore Bonte, carrying 2000 troops of General Dietl's mountain division, were to seize Narvik. These reached Vest Fiord without hindrance on April 8 and at 04:10 next morning steamed into Ofot Fiord. There Bonte detached three ships to deal with supposed forts defending the Ramnes Narrows, and four to occupy the township of Elvegaard in Herjanes Fiord, whilst in his own ship, the *Heidkamp*, he led the *Arnium* and *Thiele* on to Narvik... Before noon General Dietl's division was ashore and in firm control of the port.

By a combination of meticulous planning, surprise, boldness, speed and ruthlessness, German ships and troops thus captured not only defenceless Denmark but Norway's capital and her other principal ports. Allied reaction to these events was in sharp contrast. The British Home Fleet, based on Scapa Flow, was caught off balance in the middle of its operation to mine The Leads. Early on April 7, ten minelaying destroyers were approaching various points on the Norwegian coast. Covering them against German interference was the battle cruiser *Renown*... During this day the British C-in-C, Admiral Sir Charles Forbes, received reports in Scapa Flow that patrol planes of the RAF's Coastal Command had sighted German forces. [The] German purpose seemed to be confirmed early next day, April 8, by a chance encounter between HMS *Glowworm* and the 8-inch cruiser *Hipper*. Before she was sunk by gunfire, this British destroyer not only radioed an enemy report but managed to ram her powerful opponent, whom Forbes promptly ordered Whitworth to intercept. The latter found instead, the next morning, the *Gneisenau* and *Scharnhorst* which were covering the German invasion of Norway against interference by the British fleet. Supposing in the dim light of dawn that the *Renown* was accompanied by the *Repulse*, Admiral Lutjens decided against risking his country's two capital ships and fled to the north-east.

By this time, Forbes had received reports of several of the German landings and understood Germany's real purpose, against which he redeployed his ships. Specifically, he ordered B.A. Warburton-Lee, into Narvik "to make sure that no enemy troops land."

...On the way Warburton-Lee reflected that his intelligence was so sketchy that he would be wise to stop at the entrance to the fiord and seek news from the pilot station. There, he received news which entirely altered the picture. But this did not deter him from prompt action. He turned southwestward to steam down Vest Fiord until dark so as to mislead any enemy who might see him - such as the U51 which duly led Bonte into a false sense of security.

Adapted from G. Bennett, *Narvik: Norway Won and Lost*, No.27('75), International History Magazine.

119. According to the passage, the implied historical and strategic importance of occupying Norway is:
    A. to use the country as a northern base of operations and a source of raw materials.
    B. because of a deep hatred between Germans and Norwegians.
    C. to use as a foothold to launch an attack against Denmark.
    D. to prevent the English from attacking Norway before the Germans get there.

120. The word *fiord* is probably derived from Norwegian meaning:
    A. war.
    B. the open sea.
    C. inlet of sea bordered by land.
    D. sprawling populous city.

121. The *Arnium* and the *Thiele* referred to in paragraph 3 are likely ships in the:
    A. Norwegian Fleet.
    B. English Fleet.
    C. German Fleet.
    D. fleet which had been defending Narvik for years.

122. In the last paragraph, the news which entirely altered the picture for Warburton-Lee was:
    A. the German cruiser *Blucher* was torpedoed and sunk.
    B. Hitler had set April 9 as D-day.
    C. six German destroyers had already occupied the fiord.
    D. Germany did not want to repeat its mistakes from 1914.

123. The U51 referred to in the last paragraph is likely:
    A. an English U-boat.
    B. a German vessel which has potential for unleashing a significant destructive force.
    C. a German port set up in 1939.
    D. a German ship similar to others in the Fleet.

124. Regardless of the outcome of the decision by Warburton-Lee to turn towards the fiord despite being outnumbered by an opposing force, his country would likely see him as a:
    A. prudent military strategist.
    B. fool.
    C. soldier simply following instructions.
    D. hero.

In the early 19th century the idea that women should have equal rights with men was practically unheard of. Mary Wollstonecraft published her *Vindication of the Rights of Women* in 1872; for her pains she was called "a hyena in petticoats."

There were so many things that women lacked besides votes... But equality in these special areas need not have ended women's general status of inferiority. If "the Cause" was to triumph, it needed an issue which all women could accept as their own. The struggle for the vote met this need. Some women who looked far ahead could reckon that, with the vote, they could set many other things right...

In the battles which extended the right to vote to the poorer classes of the male population in the 19th century, the lead was taken by men who already had the vote. On the whole the women had to fight for themselves. And many preferred it that way... Women stood by one another in the struggle and found an unexpected comradeship in it...

Slavery was brought to an end after the Civil War and an amendment to the Constitution laid down that nobody was to be denied the right to vote on account of his color. The amendment completely ignored the women... The only step forward for women was in Wyoming: in 1869 women in the territory were given the right to vote, and when it became a state it insisted on retaining this odd provision in its constitution... the Susan Anthony Amendment - named after the leader and organizer of the movement for women's suffrage...

In the United States the straightforward opposition to equality for women was reinforced by the brewers and distillers, who thought women would vote for prohibition, and by the southern states, who were afraid that it might not be practical to stop black women from voting by beating them up in the way black men were beaten up if they tried to vote.

The suffrage movement made a little progress in the United States in the 1890s when three other western states joined Wyoming. In Australia and New Zealand there were much more decisive changes... None of this was likely to affect the situation in powerful stable countries like Great Britain and the United States...

By 1909 women were becoming militant enough to interrupt Liberal speakers on a great many occasions. They went beyond civil disobedience by breaking the Prime Minister's windows... but it was still true that most of the women arrested were trying to demonstrate more or less peacefully around the House of Commons.

Marches and demonstrations were held in the United States, and there was agitation for the vote in individual states as well as pressure for the Susan Anthony Amendment at Washington. The American movement had been making no progress for a dozen years, but when militancy in Great Britain began to capture the headlines, the suffragists revived.

The eighteen months before August 1914 were the wild period of the suffragette movement. In June 1913 Emily Davison threw herself in front of the King's Horse at the Derby... Paintings were slashed, houses set on fire, telegraph wires cut. The militants had gone far beyond civil disobedience into the tactics of guerilla warfare.

In June 1914, Ireland was building up towards civil war... The war came and the position of women seemed to be revolutionized. When men left for the war, women took on all sorts of jobs. They worked in factories making shells, as bus-conductors, and as auxiliaries for the armed forces.

British war propaganda, much of it directed at the United States, stressed the theme that the allies were on the side of democracy. This implied universal suffrage...

Women's war service and the demand for universal suffrage were brought together in the 1918 Act which gave the vote to men at twenty-one and to women at thirty... In 1928 women got the vote at twenty-one.

Adapted from Trevor Lloyd, *The Fighting Sex*, History of the 20th century, no. 13. © 1969 BPC Publishing LTD.

125. The contrast the author draws between the fight for the right of the men of the poorer classes to vote, and the fight for women to vote would be most directly challenged by evidence showing that:
   A. women fought their battle themselves.
   B. influential men, who believed in "the Cause" had much to do with women eventually getting the vote.
   C. as a result of the struggle of the men of the poorer classes, the women had a less difficult struggle.
   D. women were very influential in preventing men of the poorer classes get the vote.

126. The passage suggests that the rate of progress of the suffrage movement in Australia and New Zealand resulted because:
   A. the suffrage movement in those countries used very violent tactics.
   B. those countries had a much higher female population than the United States and Great Britain.
   C. the governments of the United States and Great Britain were considerably more conservative.
   D. those countries were not weak and politically unstable.

127. The Susan Anthony Amendment likely stated that:
   A. women were equal to men and should be treated as such in the job market.
   B. women, like men, should be allowed to vote at twenty-one.
   C. men of the poorer classes should not be denied the right to vote.
   D. nobody should be denied the right to vote on the basis of gender.

128. The arguments presented by the author in the fifth paragraph suggest that:
   A. though men of the poorer classes had earned the right to vote, black men had not.
   B. though black men had earned the right to vote, they were often prevented from exercising that right.
   C. the southern states opposed the female vote because its economy depended heavily on the alcohol industry.
   D. subsequent to the Civil War, racial tensions subsided considerably in the southern states.

129. Prior to 1913, the tactics of the suffragettes in Great Britain could be most likened to:
   A. the non-violent tactics of Martin Luther King.
   B. those of militant guerrillas fighting for change.
   C. those of passive supporters afraid of confrontation.
   D. those of frustrated peaceful demonstrators, tired of being ignored.

130. According to the passage, which of the following events was a major catalyst in revolutionizing the position of most women?
   A. The American Civil War
   B. The Irish Civil War
   C. World War I
   D. The abolition of slavery

Passage IX (Questions 131-137)

Juvenile misconduct - which comprises grave crime as well as pranks and trifles - is by no means a characteristic feature peculiar to our country and our age. It existed at all times. As revealed in historical documents, most nations know it well, regardless of race, religion, or form of government...

While juvenile misbehavior appears to be a perennial problem, society's ways of dealing with it, and - especially - its tolerance towards it, have been undergoing some significant changes... Nowadays "offenses" of unequal weight are frequently adjudicated simply as juvenile delinquency, without naming the particular crime, in almost all the states. Indeed, the definition of juvenile delinquency can cover everything from the most trivial naughty behavior to brutal murder...

Just before the turn of the century, offenses by youngsters began to be shifted from adult criminal courts to juvenile courts. There, supposedly, a paternalistic and benevolent judge decided in a nonpunitive way what should be done with the young offender to make him a good citizen. While the juvenile court had - and still has - its great merits, its role as a non-criminal, benevolent agency has not always been satisfactorily fulfilled for a number of reasons, among them the lack of adequate budget and facilities that would have provided for appropriate treatment for youngsters with personality disorders.

With the advent of juvenile court, a much broader definition of delinquency began to be applied. No longer need a youngster commit a criminal act to be sent to court. He could also be sent under such vague charges as "being incorrigible", or for "smoking tobacco," "using intoxicating liquor," or "truancy." All these charges were applicable only to youngsters.

Moreover, neglected and dependent children - children who had committed no offenses whatsoever - also found themselves being brought before this so-called benevolent court, and often no differentiation in treatment was made between these youngsters and the delinquents...

Earlier, authorities were reluctant to bring a child to criminal court and expose him to incarceration in the company of hardened criminals, brutal corporal punishment, and possibly even capital punishment... Once the juvenile courts began handling children's cases, the public became less hesitant to send youngsters to these courts. The public's attitude was strengthened by the thought that the court acted in the child's so-called "best interests." The result was that the juvenile courts became overburdened with many cases that had little connection to serious delinquent behavior...

Nowadays, teachers, the police, neighbours, and parents often turn to the juvenile court to handle difficult youngsters - an "easy out" which did not exist in former times. Only recently have we come to recognize that this approach is not always beneficial to the children involved... Youngsters are marked for life with a record even though theoretically juvenile delinquents are not "criminals." Ironically, youngsters who are officially declared as delinquents often begin to think of themselves as such and to conduct themselves accordingly.

To be sure, there is enough robbing and mugging in our cities today to cause alarm. Does this mean there is more crime and delinquency today than, say, one hundred years ago? We must remember that the number of crimes increases with the population. But population growth also means growth in the number of marriages, households, automobile users, and so on. These increases do not necessarily indicate a greater *intensity* of criminal behavior.

But, have delinquency figures not grown faster than the population? True enough, if we look only at the past ten years or so. Unfortunately, reliable and useful national crime and delinquency statistics go back only that far. Recent short-range increases in crime and delinquency may be offering a distorted picture of what has been happening over the years... Actually we should expect even more delinquency today because we now categorize so much more misbehavior as delinquency as compared with the earlier period.

Adapted from Albert G. Hess, *Mankind Magazine* 2(5), 1970.

131. In the context of the passage, perennial means:
   A. a life cycle of every 2 years.
   B. durable.
   C. continuing for a long time.
   D. seasonal.

132. The author highlights the fact that, on the question of juvenile misbehavior, over the years:
   A. society has managed to completely rectify the situation.
   B. society has dealt with the problem in different ways.
   C. society's tolerance towards delinquency has decreased.
   D. there is conclusive evidence that delinquency figures have increased more quickly than the population.

133. Based on the passage, prior to the institution of juvenile courts, the attitude of the public towards juvenile delinquents was that:
   A. they should be treated just like adult criminals.
   B. they were unique to American society.
   C. all youngsters who commit crimes should have access to counselling.
   D. more funding was necessary to treat those with personality disorders.

134. The passage suggests that the institution of juvenile courts affected all of the following EXCEPT:
   A. the public's tolerance towards juvenile delinquency.
   B. the rate of juvenile delinquency.
   C. the fate of hapless youngsters in society.
   D. how difficult children were dealt with by their parents.

135. The author's use of the words "so-called" with respect to the best interests of youngsters in juvenile court, suggests that he:
   A. believes that it is an objective that the court is ill-equipped to achieve.
   B. does not believe that young criminals should be dealt with in juvenile courts.
   C. believes that we should say "best interests" even if we do not mean it.
   D. believes that juvenile misconduct has been ongoing for the span of human history.

136. The author asserts that delinquency figures should be higher today because:
   A. juvenile delinquency is a recent development.
   B. criminal activity in general has been on the rise.
   C. the figures now categorize both crime and misbehavior as delinquency.
   D. there has been increased immigration and decreased emigration.

137. Based on the passage, a plausible explanation for why an increase in automobile users might be accompanied by an increase in juvenile delinquency figures is:
   A. statistics on automobile production are very thorough.
   B. teenagers are inclined to steal automobiles.
   C. delinquency involving a bicycle may go unreported, whereas if a car is involved, it would likely be reported.
   D. the two issues are unrelated.

END OF VERBAL REASONING. IF TIME REMAINS, YOU MAY GO BACK AND CHECK YOUR WORK IN THIS TEST BOOKLET.

TEST GS-3

Writing Sample
Questions : 2
Time : 60 Minutes
Two 30 Minute Prompts,
Timed Separately

OPEN BOOKLET ONLY WHEN TIMER IS READY.

The Gold Standard MCAT* has been designed exclusively to test knowledge and thinking skills. The exam may contain hypothetical statements and/or express controversial ideas. Statements contained herein do not necessarily reflect the policy, position, or view of RuveneCo Publishing.

* MCAT is a registered service mark of the Association of American Medical Colleges, which is not associated with this product.

WRITING SAMPLE

INSTRUCTIONS: This test is designed to evaluate your writing skills. There are two writing assignments. You will have 30 minutes to complete each part.

Your answers for the Writing Sample should be written in ANSWER DOCUMENT 2. Your response to Part 1 must be written only on answer sheets marked " 1 ," and your response to Part 2 on answer sheets marked " 2 ." The first 30 minutes may be used to respond to Part 1 only. The second 30 minutes may be used to respond to Part 2 only. If you finish writing before time is up, you may review your work ONLY on the response you have just completed.

Use your time in an efficient manner. Prior to writing your response, read the assignment carefully. The space below each writing assignment may be used to make notes in planning a response.

Since this is a test of your writing skills, you should use complete sentences as well organized as you can make them in the allotted time. Corrections or additions can be made neatly between the lines but there should be no writing in the margins of the answer booklet.

There are three pages in the answer document for each part of the test. Though you are not expected to use each page, do not skip lines.

Use a black pen to write your response.

Illegible essays cannot be scored.

PART I

Consider the following statement:

In matters of conscience the law of majority is unimportant.

Write a unified essay performing the following tasks. Explain the meaning of the statement. Describe a specific situation in which in matters of conscience the law of majority is important. Discuss what you think determines whether in matters of conscience the law of majority is important or unimportant.

DO NOT TURN TO THE NEXT PAGE UNTIL TIME PERMITS.

PART II

Consider the following statement:

What we obtain too easily, we esteem too lightly.

Write a unified essay performing the following tasks. Explain the meaning of the statement. Describe a specific situation in which that which is obtained easily is not esteemed lightly. Discuss what you think determines whether or not that which is obtained easily is esteemed lightly.

END OF WRITING SAMPLE.
DO NOT RETURN TO PART I.

TEST GS-3

Biological Sciences
Questions 143-219
Time : 100 Minutes

OPEN BOOKLET ONLY WHEN TIMER IS READY.

The Gold Standard MCAT* has been designed exclusively to test knowledge and thinking skills. The exam may contain hypothetical statements and/or express controversial ideas. Statements contained herein do not necessarily reflect the policy, position, or view of RuveneCo Publishing.

* MCAT is a registered service mark of the Association of American Medical Colleges, which is not associated with this product.

BIOLOGICAL SCIENCES

INSTRUCTIONS: Of the 77 questions in the Biological Sciences test, 62 are organized into groups preceded by a passage. After evaluating the passage, select the best answer to each question in the group. Fifteen questions are independent of any descriptive passage or each other. Similarly, select the best answer to these questions. If you are unsure of an answer, eliminate the alternatives that you know to be incorrect and select an answer from the remaining alternatives. To indicate your selection, blacken the corresponding oval on Answer Document 1, GS-3. A periodic table is provided for your use during the test.

PERIODIC TABLE OF THE ELEMENTS

1 H 1.008																	2 He 4.003
3 Li 6.941	4 Be 9.012											5 B 10.81	6 C 12.011	7 N 14.007	8 O 15.999	9 F 18.998	10 Ne 20.179
11 Na 22.990	12 Mg 24.305											13 Al 26.982	14 Si 28.086	15 P 30.974	16 S 32.06	17 Cl 35.453	18 Ar 39.948
19 K 39.098	20 Ca 40.08	21 Sc 44.956	22 Ti 47.90	23 V 50.942	24 Cr 51.996	25 Mn 54.938	26 Fe 55.847	27 Co 58.933	28 Ni 58.70	29 Cu 63.546	30 Zn 65.38	31 Ga 69.72	32 Ge 72.59	33 As 74.922	34 Se 78.96	35 Br 79.904	36 Kr 83.80
37 Rb 85.468	38 Sr 87.62	39 Y 88.906	40 Zr 91.22	41 Nb 92.906	42 Mo 95.94	43 Tc (98)	44 Ru 101.07	45 Rh 102.906	46 Pd 106.4	47 Ag 107.868	48 Cd 112.41	49 In 114.82	50 Sn 118.69	51 Sb 121.75	52 Te 127.60	53 I 126.905	54 Xe 131.30
55 Cs 132.905	56 Ba 137.33	57 *La 138.906	72 Hf 178.49	73 Ta 180.948	74 W 183.85	75 Re 186.207	76 Os 190.2	77 Ir 192.22	78 Pt 195.09	79 Au 196.967	80 Hg 200.59	81 Tl 204.37	82 Pb 207.2	83 Bi 208.980	84 Po (209)	85 At (210)	86 Rn (222)
87 Fr (223)	88 Ra 226.025	89 **Ac 227.028	104 Unq (261)	105 Unp (262)	106 Unh (263)												

*	58 Ce 140.12	59 Pr 140.908	60 Nd 144.24	61 Pm (145)	62 Sm 150.4	63 Eu 151.96	64 Gd 157.25	65 Tb 158.925	66 Dy 162.50	67 Ho 164.930	68 Er 167.26	69 Tm 168.934	70 Yb 173.04	71 Lu 174.967
**	90 Th 232.038	91 Pa 231.036	92 U 238.029	93 Np 237.048	94 Pu (244)	95 Am (243)	96 Cm (247)	97 Bk (247)	98 Cf (251)	99 Es (254)	100 Fm (257)	101 Md (258)	102 No (259)	103 Lr (260)

The last step in translation involves the cleavage of the ester bond that joins the complete peptide chain to the tRNA corresponding to its C-terminal amino acid. This process of *termination*, in addition to the termination codon, requires release factors (RFs). The freeing of the ribosome from mRNA during this step requires the participation of a protein called ribosome releasing factor (RRF).

Cells usually do not contain tRNAs that can recognize the three termination codons. In *E. coli*, when these codons arrive on the ribosome they are recognized by one of three release factors. RF-1 recognizes UAA and UAG, while RF-2 recognizes UAA and UGA. The third release factor, RF-3, does not itself recognize termination codons but stimulates the activity of the other two factors.

The consequence of release factor recognition of a termination codon is to alter the peptidyl transferase center on the large ribosomal subunit so that it can accept water as the attacking nucleophile rather than requiring the normal substrate, aminoacyl-tRNA.

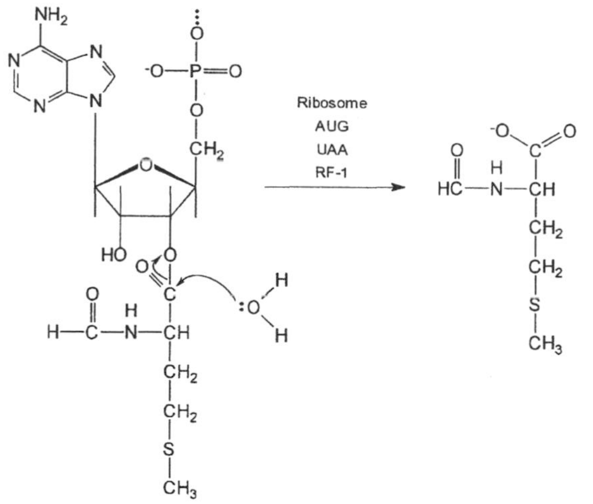

Figure 1

143. Where would the RFs be expected to be found in the cell?
   A. Within the nuclear membrane
   B. Floating in the cytosol
   C. In the matrix of the mitochondria
   D. Within the lumen of the smooth endoplasmic reticulum

144. The alteration to the peptidyl transferase center during the termination reaction serves to convert peptidyl transferase into a(n):
   A. exonuclease.
   B. lyase.
   C. esterase.
   D. ligase.

145. Sparsomycin is an antibiotic that inhibits peptidyl transferase activity. The effect of adding this compound to an *in vitro* reaction in which *E. coli* ribosomes are combined with methionine aminoacyl-tRNA complex, RF-1 and the nucleotide triplets, AUG and UAA, would be to:
   A. inhibit hydrolysis of the amino acid, allowing polypeptide chain extension.
   B. inhibit peptide bond formation causing the amino acid to be released.
   C. induce hydrolysis of the aminoacyl-tRNA complex.
   D. inhibit both hydrolysis of the aminoacyl-tRNA complex and peptide bond formation.

146. If the water in the reaction in Fig. 1 was labelled with ^{18}O, which of the following molecules would contain ^{18}O at the end of the reaction?
   A. The free amino acid
   B. The phosphate group of the tRNA molecule
   C. Oxygen-containing molecules in the cytoplasm
   D. The ribose moiety of the tRNA molecule

147. What sequence of bases would tRNA have, in order to recognize the mRNA codon CAG?
   A. GTC
   B. UAG
   C. CAG
   D. GUC

148. Many codons in the genetic code differ by only one nitrogenous base. The main advantage of this is that:
   A. the code is universal.
   B. DNA replication is simplified.
   C. point mutations are less effective.
   D. the code is non-overlapping.

Passage II (Questions 149-153)

The method of DNA replication proposed by James Watson and Francis Crick is known as semi-conservative replication since each new double helix retains one strand of the original DNA double helix. The evidence for this mechanism was provided by a series of classic experiments carried out by Meselson and Stahl in 1958 which proceeded as follows:

1. Cultures of the bacterium *E. coli*, which has a single circular chromosome, were grown for many generations in a medium containing the heavy isotope of nitrogen ^{15}N.

2. The cells containing the DNA labelled with ^{15}N were transferred to a culture medium containing the normal isotope of nitrogen (^{14}N).

3. After periods of time corresponding to the generation time for *E. coli* (50 min at 3 °C) samples were removed and the DNA extracted.

4. The DNA was then centrifuged at 40 000 times gravity for 20 h in a solution of cesium chloride (CsCl).

During centrifugation the heavy CsCl molecules began to sediment at the bottom of the centrifuge tubes producing an increasing density gradient from the top of the tube to the bottom. The DNA settled out where its density equalled that of the CsCl solution. When examined under ultraviolet light the DNA appeared in the centrifuge tube as a narrow band.

Two other hypotheses were advanced to explain the process of DNA replication. One is known as conservative replication and the other as dispersive replication. These hypotheses are summarized in Fig.1.

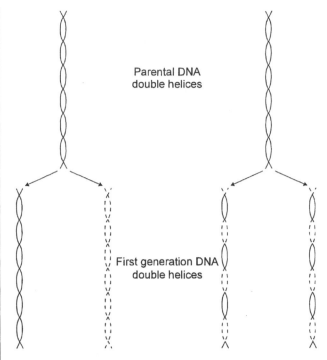

Parental DNA double helices

First generation DNA double helices

Conservative replication   Dispersive replication

Figure 1

149. Based on the passage, which of the following represents the appearance of the tubes after the cells had been allowed to grow in the ^{14}N for two generations?

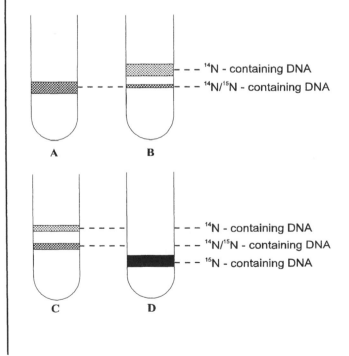

A   B

- - - ^{14}N - containing DNA
- - - $^{14}N/^{15}N$ - containing DNA

C   D

- - - ^{14}N - containing DNA
- - - $^{14}N/^{15}N$ - containing DNA
- - - ^{15}N - containing DNA

150. Had conservative replication been the correct hypothesis, which of the following would represent the appearance of the tubes after the cells had been allowed to grow in the ^{14}N for one generation?

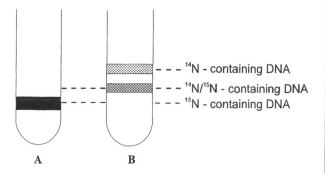

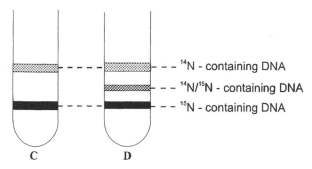

151. Had dispersive replication been the correct hypothesis, which of the following would represent the appearance of the tubes after the cells had been

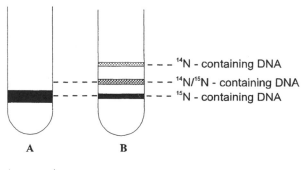

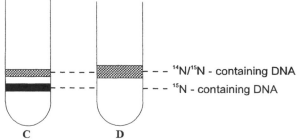

152. Which of the following statements could be held LEAST accountable for DNA maintaining its helical structure?

A. Unwinding the helix would separate the base pairs enough for water molecules to enter between the bases, making the structure unstable.
B. The helix is stabilized by hydrogen bonds between bases.
C. The sugar phosphate backbone is held in place by hydrophilic interactions with the solvent.
D. C-G pairs have 3 hydrogen bonds between them but A-T pairs only have 2.

153. Which of the following enzymes is most important in RNA synthesis during transcription?

A. DNA polymerase
B. RNA replicase
C. RNA polymerase
D. Reverse transcriptase

Passage III (Questions 154-158)

A *monoclonal antibody* is a single pure antibody produced in quantity by a cultured clone of an immune cell called a B lymphocyte. Prior to the development of the monoclonal antibody, the only means of producing large quantities of specific antibodies was immunization of animals with as purified an antigen as possible. But such an antigen still contained many epitopes. Consequently, the antibodies produced by the animals were polyclonal antibodies, with a different antibody produced for each epitope. Now monoclonal antibodies are produced by a single clone of genetically identical cells derived from a single stimulated antibody-producing cell. They can be prepared in large quantities by using special cells called *hybridomas*.

B-lymphocytes that produce antibodies can become cancerous. A myeloma is a cancer, or unchecked proliferation, of an antibody-producing cell. Because a myeloma begins as a single cell, all of its progeny constitute a clone of identical lymphocytes. In 1975, a technique was developed for combining the growth characteristics of myeloma cells and the special characteristics of normal immune spleen cells. In doing so, they developed a "hybrid" cell called a hybridoma, which is a specific antibody-producing factory. In such cells the myeloma portion provides immortality and thus large quantities of monoclonal antibody; the immune lymphocyte portion provides the information for the specificity of the antibody. The technique for making hybridoma cells is as follows:

1. The selected antigen is injected into the spleen of a mouse.

2. The spleen is removed and the antibody-synthesizing cells from the spleen are fused with myeloma cells to make hybridoma cells.

3. Hybridoma cells are grown in a selective culture medium.

4. Individual hybridoma cells are separated into wells and clones are grown.

5. Each clone produced is tested for the desired antibody.

154. What property of spleen cells makes them appropriate for creating hybridomas?
   A. Their ability to produce ATP in large quantities
   B. Their predetermined antibody specificity
   C. Their immortal nature
   D. The rate at which they divide

155. Which of the following biological processes would be inhibited by the removal of an adult human spleen?
   A. The production of erythrocytes
   B. The production of macrophages
   C. The production of T-lymphocytes
   D. The destruction of erythrocytes

156. Based on the passage, does the antigen need to be purified before being injected into the mouse?
   A. No, the separation of the hybridoma cells into wells makes purification unnecessary.
   B. No, only one type of antibody is produced in spleen cells in response to the antigen.
   C. Yes, the injected antigen contains many epitopes.
   D. Yes, an unpurified antigen would kill the mouse.

157. One would expect that the culture medium chosen:
   A. permitted the growth of unfused myeloma and spleen cells as well as hybridoma cells.
   B. permitted the growth of hybridomas, but inhibited the growth of unfused myeloma and spleen cells.
   C. permitted the growth of unfused myeloma and spleen cells, but inhibited the growth of hybridoma cells.
   D. permitted the growth of spleen and hybridoma cells, but inhibited the growth of unfused myeloma cells.

158. What is the major disadvantage of injecting the monoclonal antibody directly into the circulatory system instead of an inactivated form of the antigen?
   A. The myeloma cells increase the risk of tumor development in individuals infected with the antibody
   B. The immune response is faster when the inactivated antigen is injected
   C. The antibodies injected are often recognized as antigens by the immune system, thereby eliciting an immune response
   D. No memory cells are produced when the monoclonal antibody is directly injected into the circulatory system.

159. A compound which has stereocenters yet is achiral, and has no enantiomer, is called a *meso* compound. Which of the following could be classified as a *meso* compound?

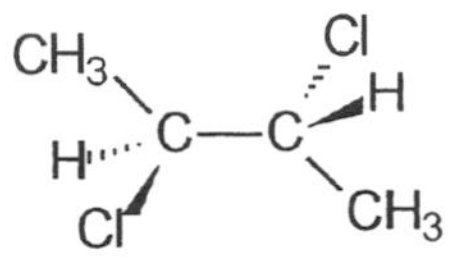

$$CH_3 \quad Cl$$
$$H\cdots C - C \cdots H$$
$$Cl \quad CH_3$$

A.

$$H\cdots C - CH_2CH_3$$
$$I \quad CH_3$$

B.

$$CH_3 \quad H \,Cl$$
$$I\cdots C - C$$
$$H \quad CH_3$$

C.

$$CH_3 \quad Cl\,H$$
$$H\cdots C - C$$
$$Br \quad CH_3$$

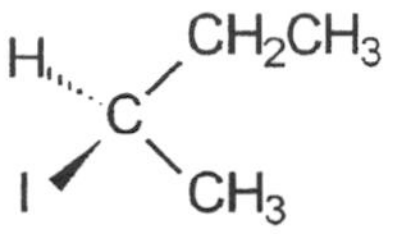

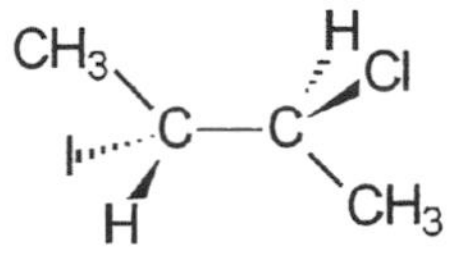

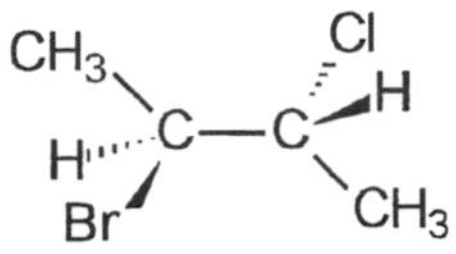

D.

160. The difference between the bacterium *Lactobacillus* and the eukaryote *Trichomonas* is that *Lactobacillus* has no:
   A. ribosomes
   B. cell wall
   C. plasma membrane
   D. lysosomes

161. After fertilization, the zygote will develop into a female if:
   A. the zygote possesses an X chromosome.
   B. the primary oocyte possesses an X chromosome.
   C. the egg possesses an X chromosome.
   D. the sperm possesses an X chromosome.

162. Four isomeric compounds - allyl alcohol, benzoic acid, 2-butanone and butyraldehyde - were identified and stored in separate bottles. By accident, the labels were lost from the sample bottles. The following information was obtained via infrared spectroscopy and was used to identify and relabel the sample bottles.

Infrared absorption peaks (cm^{-1})

Bottle I	Bottle II	Bottle III	Bottle IV
1700 (sharp)	1710	1730 (sharp)	3333 (broad)
	3500-3333 (broad)	2730	1030 (small)

Which of the following most accurately represents the contents of bottles I, II, III, and IV, respectively?
   A. Butyraldehyde, 2-butanone, benzoic acid, allyl alcohol
   B. Benzoic acid, butyraldehyde, allyl alcohol, 2-butanone
   C. 2-Butanone, butyraldehyde, allyl alcohol, benzoic acid
   D. 2-Butanone, benzoic acid, butyraldehyde, allyl alcohol

163. The ^{1}HNMR of compound X is shown in Fig. 1.

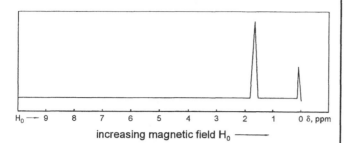

increasing magnetic field H_0 ⟶

Figure 1

Compound X has the molecular formula C_6H_{12} and chemical tests revealed that the compound was an alkene. Which of the following best represents the structure of compound X?

A. CH_3—CH=CH—CH_2—CH_2—CH_3

B.
$$CH_3—\underset{CH_3}{\overset{CH_3}{C}}=\underset{CH_3}{\overset{CH_3}{C}}—CH_3$$

C.
$$\underset{CH_3}{\overset{CH_3}{C}}=\underset{CH_2CH_3}{\overset{H}{C}}$$

D.   (cyclohexene structure)

Conjugated dienes undergo many reactions typical of alkenes such as electrophilic addition. Electrophilic additions invariably produce a mixture of products which result from competing pathways.

For example, 1,3-butadiene reacts with 1 equivalent of Br_2 at 40 °C to give dibromide products A and B, in 20% and 80% yield, respectively. The addition reaction occurs via a resonance stabilized allylic intermediate.

$$CH_2 = CH - CH = CH_2 + Br_2 \rightarrow [intermediate] \rightarrow A + B$$
Reaction I

When the reaction is carried out at -80 °C, the product composition changes to 80% A and 20% B. Product A of the mixture is easily isolated to its pure state by recrystallization at 54 °C.

Both products A and B are stable at -80 °C.

$$A \text{ or } B \xrightarrow{\text{-80°C}} \text{no change}$$

In contrast, upon studying in an ionizing solvent at 40 °C, either product is converted to a mixture identical to that produced by the addition of 1 equivalent of Br_2 to 1,3-butadiene at 40 °C.

$$A \text{ or } B \xrightarrow{\text{40°C}} \underset{(20\%)}{A} + \underset{(80\%)}{B}$$

164. Which of the following pairs most accurately depicts the resonance stabilized intermediate that led to products A and B?

I. $CH_2=CH-\overset{-}{C}HCH_2Br \longleftrightarrow \overset{+}{C}H_2-CH=CHCH_2Br$

II. $CH_2=CH-\overset{+}{C}HCH_2Br \longleftrightarrow \overset{+}{C}H_2-CH=CHCH_2Br$

III. $CH_2=CH-\overset{+}{C}HCH_2Br \longleftrightarrow \overset{-}{C}H-CH=CHCH_2Br$

A. I only
B. II only
C. I and II only
D. II and III only

165. If the bromination of 1,3 butadiene is carried out at -80 °C the major product is Compound A. However, if the reaction is carried out at 40 °C Compound B becomes the major product. Which of the following statements most accurately explains this transformation?
A. A is the thermodynamic product and B is the kinetic product.
B. A is the kinetic product and B is the thermodynamic product.
C. A has a disubstituted double bond and is somewhat less stable than B which has a monosubstituted double bond.
D. A has a monosubstituted double bond and is more stable than B which has a disubstituted double bond.

166. What is the IUPAC name of product A?
A. 3,4-dibromo-1-butene
B. 1,4-dibromo-1-butene
C. 1,4-dibromo-2-butene
D. 3,4-dibromo-2-butene

167. Since products A and B have the same molecular formula ($C_4H_6Br_2$), it is reasonable to assume that products A and B:
A. are enantiomers.
B. form a racemic mixture.
C. are structural isomers.
D. are conjugated dienes.

168. The addition of bromine to cyclohexene will result in which of the following products?

A.

B.

C.

D.

Passage V (Questions 169-173)

The DNA content per haploid genome varies enormously among organisms, even when the species are closely related. Species with high *C values* (a term used to describe DNA content) frequently develop more slowly than those with low C values. The salamander *Plethodon vehiculum*, with a C value almost twice that of *P. cineroeus*, reaches about the same adult size, but with half the number of cells.

It might be supposed that divergence of populations in the number and distribution of repetitive sequences could reduce chromosome pairing in their hybrids and so reduce fertility. Although there is some evidence that pronounced differences in DNA content can interfere with chromosome pairing, the effect is surprisingly slight; hybrids between related species of grasses that differ by as much as 50 percent in DNA content have virtually normal chromosome pairing, chiasma formation, and segregation.

Indeed, there is little evidence that small differences in the number of copies in a gene family have a substantial effect on fitness simply because of total DNA content.

169. The amount of DNA possessed by a haploid organism will LEAST affect which of the following characteristics?
   A. The organism's phenotype
   B. The rate at which meiosis occurs
   C. The length of time between its meiotic divisions
   D. The organism's potential for reproduction

170. If pronounced differences in DNA content did interfere with chromosome pairing, the likely result would be:
   A. genetic drift.
   B. hybrid inviability.
   C. random mating.
   D. disruptive selection.

171. Which of the following processes likely occurs to allow the normal chromosome pairing observed in grass species?
   A. The interstitial repetitive sequences in one homologous chromosome would loop so that pairing could occur.
   B. The unpaired sequences in the homologous chromosome without the interstitial repetitive sequences would duplicate so that pairing could occur.
   C. The homologous chromosome with the interstitial repetitive sequence would undergo a translocation so that pairing could occur.
   D. The homologous chromosome with the interstitial repetitive sequence would undergo a deletion so that pairing could occur.

172. Would the DNA content of the host species or the parasitic species in a parasite-host relationship, be expected, on average, to be lower?
   A. Host, because the host usually reproduces meiotically rather than mitotically.
   B. Host, in order to increase the likelihood of adaptive mutations occurring.
   C. Parasite, because the parasite is usually smaller than the host.
   D. Parasite, because the parasite species usually reproduce more quickly than the host species.

173. The number and distribution of repetitive sequences in a gene family exerts its greatest effect on a species' fitness by:
   A. reducing hybrid viability of the species.
   B. varying the quantities of specific genes produced in the different hybrids of the species.
   C. altering the amount of DNA present in the genome of the species.
   D. reducing the fertility of the species.

Passage VI (Questions 174-180)

E. coli is a bacterial cell which contains a single circular chromosome and three DNA polymerase enzymes - Pol I, Pol II, and Pol III. Replication of DNA in E. coli leads to the formation of a replication eye at which point, the replicating chromosome is referred to as the theta structure.

It is reasonable to conclude that the replication eye contains two partially separated parental DNA strands and two newly synthesized DNA strands. It was not clear for a long time, however, whether or not replication occurred in one direction or both directions about the origin of replication. Eventually, convincing evidence of bidirectional replication was obtained by measuring gene frequencies during replication.

Continuous synthesis on both strands of a replication fork requires synthesis in the 5′ to 3′ direction on one strand and in the 3′ to 5′ direction on the other strand. Since Pol I only adds nucleotides in the 5′ to 3′ direction, it was proposed that Pol I could not be the enzyme responsible for DNA replication in E. coli. In order to prove this and determine the role of Pol I in E. coli, the following experiments were performed.

Experiment 1

The Pol A Mutant of E. coli, which lacks Pol I enzyme activity was grown on agar for several generations and then exposed to ultraviolet light.

Result:

The Pol A Mutants grew in the agar successfully for several generations, but died when they were exposed to ultraviolet light.

Experiment 2

The temperature sensitive type mutants (TS type) of E. coli, which contains a mutant gene that codes for a Pol III enzyme that does not work at high temperatures, were grown on two separate agar dishes. The dishes were incubated at 30 °C and 42 °C, respectively, and left to grow for several generations.

Result:

The TS type E. coli, incubated at 42 °C, did not grow, but the TS type E. coli, incubated at 30 °C, grew successfully for several generations.

174. If replication occurred in a bidirectional manner, the evidence would be that shortly after initiation:
A. each gene in the E. coli genome would be represented only once.
B. each gene in the E. coli genome would be represented twice.
C. DNA duplication would begin on both sides of the origin of replication.
D. gene frequencies should be very high for regions symmetrically disposed about the origin.

175. In Experiment 1, if the researcher wanted to prove that the ultraviolet light had killed the bacteria, she would simultaneously:
A. grow TS type E. coli and expose to ultraviolet light.
B. grow Pol A Mutants and irradiate.
C. grow Pol A Mutants without ultraviolet light.
D. not run an experiment since the conclusion is obvious.

176. The strongest evidence that Pol I was not the main replicating enzyme in E. coli was given by the fact that:
A. Pol A Mutants grew successfully.
B. Pol A Mutants died from exposure to ultraviolet radiation.
C. TS type E. coli grew successfully at 30 °C, but not at 42 °C.
D. the Pol III enzyme does not work at temperatures over 42 °C.

177. The passage suggests that the main reason that TS type E. coli cannot grow above 42 °C, is that:
A. the TS mutant gene causes dehydration of the cell contents at high temperatures.
B. high temperatures cause DNA mutations that cannot be repaired because of the disfunctional Pol III.
C. the TS mutant gene causes the cell to stop producing Pol III at high temperatures.
D. the TS mutant gene causes the tertiary structure of Pol III to be lost at high temperatures.

178. In humans, how is the problem of the unidirectional activity of DNA polymerase overcome during DNA replication?
   A. Only one DNA strand is used as a template for replication.
   B. First one strand is replicated continuously in one direction and then the other strand is replicated continuously in the opposite direction by DNA polymerase.
   C. Only one strand of DNA is continuously replicated, while the other strand is replicated discontinuously by a DNA molecule moving in the opposite direction.
   D. In humans, an enzyme similar to Pol III, and capable of adding nucleotides in both directions, is used during DNA replication.

179. If *E. coli* was allowed to replicate in the presence of ^{3}H-thymidine, during the second round of replication, what would an autoradiograph, which detects irradiation, show if the replication was semi-conservative?
   A. A uniformly unlabeled structure
   B. A uniformly labeled structure
   C. One branch of the growing replication eye would be half as strongly labeled as the remainder of the chromosome
   D. One branch of the growing replication eye would be twice as strongly labeled as the remainder of the chromosome

180. Given that the time for one TS type *E. coli* to divide at 30 °C is approximately 15 minutes, if 10 bacteria should begin dividing in ample culture media, approximately how many would be present 2 hours later?
   A. 500
   B. 1000
   C. 2500
   D. 5000

Fig. 1 illustrates chemical methods often used by organic chemists for qualitative analysis of water insoluble unknowns. Table 1 lists characteristic chemical tests of organic compounds. For instance, sodium bicarbonate tests that are positive are indicative of a carboxylic acid.

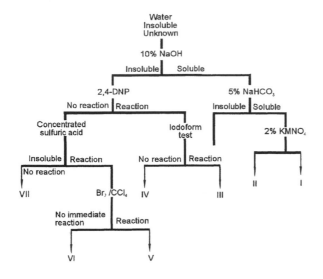

Figure 1

Table 1

Chemical Test	Compounds
Sodium hydroxide	Organic acids: carboxylic acids and phenols
Lucas	Alcohols with 5 or less carbon atoms
Sodium bicarbonate	Carboxylic acids
2,4 Dinitro-phenylhydrazine	Aldehydes and ketones
Iodine in sodium hydroxide (Iodoform)	Acetaldehydes and ketones with the CH_3-CO- group Alcohols with the $CH_3CH(OH)$- as a structural feature
Sulfuric acid	Alcohols, ethers, alkenes Soluble Lewis bases
Bromine	Alkenes

181. Heptane falls into group VII. This is primarily due to the fact that heptane is:
   A. amphiphilic.
   B. hydrophobic.
   C. hydrophilic.
   D. amphoteric.

182. A certain water insoluble unknown is soluble in 10% NaOH, 5% NaHCO₃, and gives a negative test result for the Bayer test. Which of the following is the most probable structure of this unknown?

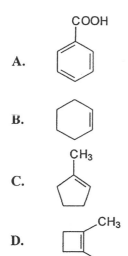

A.

B.

C.

D.

183. The ¹HNMR of compound X was performed with CDCl₃ as a solvent and 8 signals were observed. A second ¹HNMR of compound X was performed after the addition of D₂0 to the ¹HNMR solution, and seven signals were observed. The vanishing of the ¹HNMR signal is an indication that X contains which of the following functional groups?
A. A carboxylic acid
B. An acidic hydrogen
C. An alkene
D. An aldehyde

184. Consider the following aliphatic amines (Et = ethyl).

I.   Et₃N

II. Et₂NCH₂CH₂F

III. Et₂NCH₂CH₂Cl

Which of the following series most accurately represents the basicity of these aliphatic amines in decreasing order?
A. I, II, III
B. II, III, I
C. III, II, I
D. I, III, II

185. A substance X is found to be soluble in sodium bicarbonate and has the molecular formula $C_3H_6O_2$. The IR spectrum has demonstrated a band from 3000 cm⁻¹ to 2500 cm⁻¹ and a sharp absorption peak at 1715 cm⁻¹. Based on the preceding data, compound X is most likely which of the following?

A.

B.

C.

D.

186. All of the following are closely associated with microtubules EXCEPT:
   A. flagella.
   B. cilia.
   C. villi.
   D. centrioles.

187. The structure in the brain responsible for maintaining homeostasis (i.e. body temperature, heart rate, etc.) is the:
   A. pituitary.
   B. thalamus.
   C. hypothalamus.
   D. cerebellum.

188. **Fas/APO-1** is a transmembrane receptor which, when stimulated, may activate intracellular mechanisms leading to cell death. **Fas/APO-1** is likely:
   A. a phospholipid.
   B. a complex carbohydrate.
   C. synthesized in the nucleus.
   D. synthesized by rough endoplasmic reticulum.

189. All of the following are in the correct anatomic order EXCEPT:
   A. trachea → larynx → bronchus.
   B. bronchus → bronchioles → alveolar ducts.
   C. alveolar ducts → alveolar sacs → alveolus.
   D. nose → nasal cavity → nasopharynx.

190. An amino acid in a medium with a pH value above its isoelectric point would have:
   A. a neutral charge.
   B. a net positive charge.
   C. a net negative charge.
   D. either a net positive or net negative charge depending on the pK_a value.

Several models have been developed for relating changes in dissociation constants to changes in the tertiary and quaternary structures of oligomeric proteins. One model suggests that the protein's subunits can exist in either of two distinct conformations, R and T. At equilibrium, there are few R conformation molecules: 10 000 T to 1 R and it is an important feature of the enzyme that this ratio does not change. The substrate is assumed to bind more tightly to the R form than to the T form, which means that binding of the substrate favors the transition from the T conformation to R.

The conformational transitions of the individual subunits are assumed to be tightly linked, so that if one subunit flips from T to R the others must do the same. The binding of the first molecule of substrate thus promotes the binding of the second and if substrate is added continuously, all of the enzyme will be in the R form and act on the substrate. Because the concerted transition of all of the subunits from T to R or back, preserves the overall symmetry of the protein, this model is called the *symmetry model*. The model further predicts that allosteric activating enzymes make the R conformation even more reactive with the substrate while allosteric inhibitors react with the T conformation so that most of the enzyme is held back in the T shape.

191. What assumption is made about the T and R conformations and the substrate?
   A. In the absence of any substrate, the T conformation predominates.
   B. In the absence of any substrate, the R conformation predominates.
   C. In the absence of any substrate, the T and R conformations are in equilibrium.
   D. In the absence of any substrate, the enzyme exists in another conformation, S.

192. The substrate binds more tightly to R because:
   A. T has a higher affinity for the substrate than R.
   B. R has a higher affinity for the substrate than T.
   C. there are 10 000 times more T conformation molecules than R conformation molecules.
   D. the value of the equilibrium constant does not change.

193. A graph representing the addition of substrate to an enzyme over a period of time would be expected to be:
   A. a hyperbole.
   B. a straight line with a positive slope.
   C. a straight line with a negative slope.
   D. sigmoidal.

194. The symmetry model would NOT account for an enzyme:
   A. with many different biologically active conformations.
   B. which engages in positive cooperativity.
   C. with a complex metal cofactor.
   D. which is a catalyst for anabolic reactions.

195. Allosteric enzymes differ from other enzymes in that they:
   A. are not denatured at high temperatures.
   B. are regulated by compounds which are not their substrates and which do not bind to their active sites.
   C. they operate at an optimum pH of about 2.0.
   D. they are not specific to just one substrate.

The Sanger method for sequencing DNA uses newly synthesized DNA that is randomly terminated. The method employs chain-terminating dideoxynucleotide triphosphates (ddXTPs) to produce a continuous series of fragments during catalyzed reactions. The ddXTPs act as terminators because while they can add to a growing chain during polymerization, they cannot be added onto.

When DNA is being sequenced, the appropriate enzymes are added to make a complementary copy of a primed single-stranded DNA fragment. By choosing an appropriate primer, the region of the nucleic acid that is copied can be predetermined. Synthetic reaction mixtures are then set up, each containing one or more radioactive deoxyribonucleoside triphosphates to label the fragments for detection by autoradiography. Each mixture contains a single, limiting amount of dideoxytrinucleoside triphosphate to randomly terminate the synthesized fragments at one of the four nucleotides. The products of four separate reaction mixtures, each containing a different dideoxynucleoside triphosphate, are analyzed.

Following synthesis, the reaction products are separated from the template by denaturation and fractionated by electrophoresis on polyacrylamide gels. After electrophoresis the positions of the fragments on the gel are detected by autoradiography. The sequence is read directly from the autoradiogram, starting with the fastest moving (*smallest*) fragment at the bottom, and then moving up the gel to larger fragments. In order to read the DNA sequence, the individual bands must be followed beginning at the bottom of the gel.

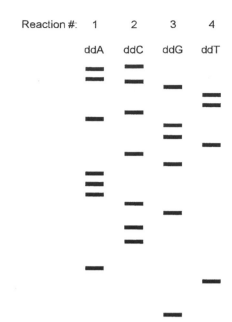

Figure 1: Autoradiogram of a fragmented DNA strand post-synthesis.

196. The passage suggests that dideoxynucleoside triphosphates are able to be used in the Sanger method because they lack a:
    A. hydroxyl group on their phosphoric acid component.
    B. hydroxyl group on C1 of their ribose component.
    C. hydroxyl group on C3 of their ribose component.
    D. hydroxyl group on C5 of their ribose component.

197. Which of the following enzymes would have to be included in the Sanger method in order for it to work?
    A. DNA gyrase
    B. DNA polymerase
    C. Reverse transcriptase
    D. DNA helicase

198. The least likely of the following radioactive deoxynucleoside triphosphates to be used to label the fragments is:

A. dATP

B. dGTP

C. dUTP

D. dCTP

199. According to Fig. 1, the newly synthesized DNA strand began and ended with:

A. an adenine and guanine residue, respectively.

B. a cytosine and guanine residue, respectively.

C. a guanine and cytosine residue, respectively.

D. a cytosine and adenine residue, respectively.

200. According to Fig. 1, the first 8 residues of the DNA template were:

A. GTACCGCA.

B. GAAACGCC.

C. CATGGCGT.

D. CTTTGCGG.

201. One of the latest adaptations of the Sanger method uses four different colored fluorescent derivatives attached to the four different ddXTP terminators. The main advantage of this approach is that:

A. electrophoresis treatment to the denatured DNA would no longer be necessary.

B. the ddXTP terminators would no longer have to be radioactively treated.

C. the technique would be faster and more economical.

D. all four reactions could be carried out simultaneously prior to electrophoresis.

Urine flow through the ureters to the bladder is propelled by contractions of the ureter-wall muscle. The urine is stored in the bladder and intermittently ejected during urination, termed micturition.

The bladder is a balloon-like chamber with walls of muscle collectively termed the detrusor muscle. The contraction of this muscle squeezes the urine in the lumen to produce urination. That part of the detrusor muscle at the base of the bladder, where the urethra begins, functions as a sphincter - the internal urethral sphincter. Beyond the outlet of the urethra is the external urethral sphincter, the contraction of which can prevent urination even when the detrusor muscle contracts strongly.

The basic micturition reflex is a spinal reflex, which can be influenced by descending pathways from the brain. In infants and persons with spinal-cord damage, the contribution of the descending pathways is eliminated. The bladder wall contains stretch receptors whose afferent fibers enter the spinal cord and stimulate the parasympathetic nerves that supply and stimulate the detrusor muscle. As the bladder fills with urine, the pressure within it increases and the stretch receptors are stimulated, thereby reflexively eliciting stimulation of the parasympathetic neurons and contractions of the detrusor muscle. When the bladder reaches a certain volume, the induced contraction of the detrusor muscle becomes strong enough to open the internal urethral sphincter. Simultaneously, the afferent input from the stretch receptors inhibits, within the spinal cord, the motor neurons that tonically stimulate the external urethral sphincter to contract. Both sphincters are now open and the contraction of the detrusor muscle is able to produce urination.

202. The internal and external urethral sphincters consist of:
   A. skeletal and smooth muscle, respectively.
   B. skeletal muscle and connective tissue, respectively.
   C. smooth muscle and skeletal muscle, respectively.
   D. smooth muscle and connective tissue, respectively.

203. On a very hot day, the bladder would likely contain:
   A. a large amount of urine hypertonic to blood plasma.
   B. a large amount of urine hypotonic to blood plasma.
   C. a small amount of urine hypertonic to blood plasma.
   D. a small amount of urine hypotonic to blood plasma.

204. Through the process of micturition, urine is expelled from the bladder into the:
   A. urethra.
   B. ureter.
   C. major calyx.
   D. minor calyx.

205. The following are other physiological systems which depend on stretch receptors EXCEPT:
   A. the circulatory system.
   B. the respiratory system.
   C. the endocrine system.
   D. the digestive system.

206. Damage to which pair of nerves comprising the descending pathways, would likely cause persons with spinal-cord damage to have no control over the micturition process?
   A. Vagus
   B. Abducans
   C. Trigeminal
   D. Hypoglossal

207. The passage indicates that the internal urethral sphincter is:
   A. closed when the detrusor muscle is relaxed.
   B. open when the detrusor muscle is relaxed.
   C. not under the direct control of the detrusor muscle.
   D. innervated directly by motor neurons extending from the descending pathways.

208. The hormone which exerts the most control on the concentration of the urine in the bladder is:
   A. vasopressin.
   B. oxytocin.
   C. thyroxine.
   D. prolactin.

Passage XI (Questions 209-214)

An organic chemistry student was assigned to review two important preparations of alkenes; the dehydration of alcohols and the dehydrohalogenation of alkyl halides.

Experiment I

The treatment of isopropyl iodide with potassium ethoxide in ethanol gave propylene in 94% yield. The reaction revealed first order kinetics in alkyl halide and first order kinetics in base.

Experiment II

1-Bromopentane was treated with potassium hydroxide in ethanol to yield both 1-pentene and ethyl pentyl ether, in 12% and 88% yields, respectively.

Experiment III

Ethyl alcohol was treated with sulfuric acid at 140 °C to produce diethyl ether.

However, when ethyl alcohol was treated with sulfuric acid at an elevated temperature of 170 °C, ethylene was the major product.

209. Which of the following reaction mechanisms best exemplifies the mechanistic process in Experiment I?
A. E1
B. E2
C. S_N1
D. S_N2

210. In a subsequent experiment the student performed the catalytic hydrogenation of propylene by using hydrogen at low temperature in the presence of a platinum catalyst. Which of the following would likely be the major product?

A. $CH_3-CH-CH_3$ with OH

B. $CH_3-CH_2-CH_3$

C. $CH_3-C=CH_2$ with CH_3

D. $CH_3-CH-CH_3$ with CH_3

211. Treatment of ethylene with cold dilute potassium permanganate would yield which of the following compounds?

A.

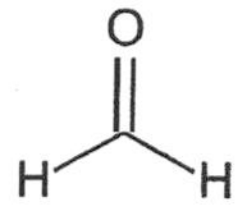

B.

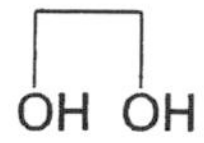

C.

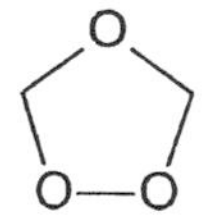

D.

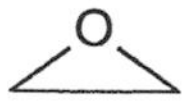

212. In Experiment II, ethyl pentyl ether was the major product. Which of the following assumptions can be made about the mechanism of this reaction?
A. The reaction proceeded by nucleophilic substitution via the S_N2 mechanism.
B. The reaction proceeded by nucleophilic substitution via the S_N1 mechanism.
C. The reaction proceeded by electrophilic substitution via the E1 mechanism.
D. The reaction proceeded by electrophilic substitution via the E2 mechanism.

213. Consider the following reaction:

$$(CH_3)_2\,C = CH_2 + HCl \rightarrow \text{Product}$$

Which of the following compounds best exemplifies the major organic product of the above reaction?

A. $(CH_3)_2\,CHCH_2\,Cl$

B. 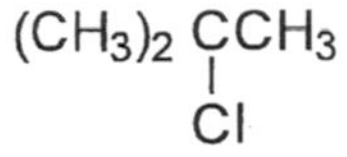 $(CH_3)_2\ \underset{\underset{\displaystyle Cl}{|}}{C}CH_3$

C. $CH_2{=}\underset{\underset{\displaystyle |}{|}}{\overset{\overset{\displaystyle Cl}{|}}{C}}{-}CH_2CH_3$

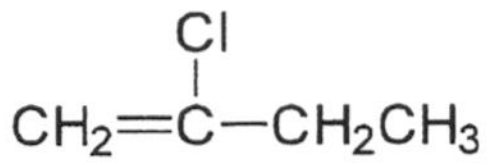

D. 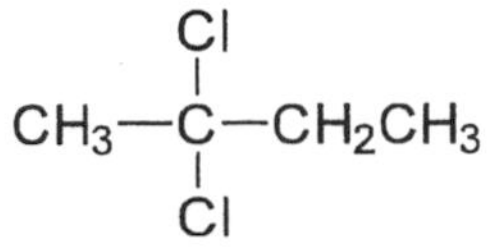 $CH_3{-}\underset{\underset{\displaystyle Cl}{|}}{\overset{\overset{\displaystyle Cl}{|}}{C}}{-}CH_2CH_3$

214. An organic chemist investigated the mode of addition of HBr to terminal olephins via two different mechanisms.

$$CH_3\,CH_2\,CH = CH_2 + HBr \xrightarrow{\text{ionic mechanism}} A \quad \textbf{Reaction I}$$

$$CH_3\,CH_2\,CH = CH_2 + HBr \xrightarrow[\text{mechanism}]{\text{free radical}} B \quad \textbf{Reaction II}$$

Which of the following pairs of compounds represents major products A and B, respectively?

A. 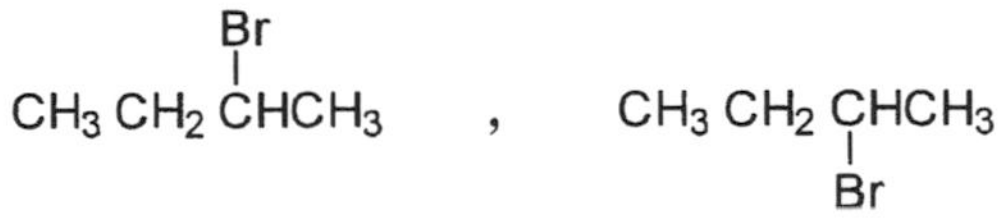 $CH_3\,CH_2\,\underset{\underset{\displaystyle Br}{|}}{C}HCH_3$, $CH_3\,CH_2\,\underset{\underset{\displaystyle Br}{|}}{C}HCH_3$

B. $CH_3\,CH_2\,CH_2\,CH_2\,Br$, $Br\,CH_2\,CH_2\,CH_2\,CH_3$

C. $Br\,CH_2\,CH_2\,CH_2\,Br$, $CH_3\,CH_2\,\underset{\underset{\displaystyle Br}{|}}{C}HCH_3$

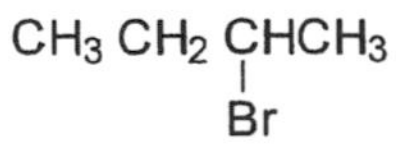

D. 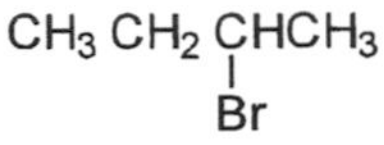 $CH_3\,CH_2\,\underset{\underset{\displaystyle Br}{|}}{C}HCH_3$, $CH_3\,CH_2\,CH_2\,CH_2\,Br$

Questions 215-219 are NOT based on a descriptive passage.

215. If increasing the concentration gradient across the plasma membrane increases the rate of transport until a maximum rate is reached, this would be convincing evidence for:
A. simple diffusion.
B. carrier-mediated transport.
C. osmosis.
D. the Fluid Mosaic model.

216. The structure of lysine is given below.

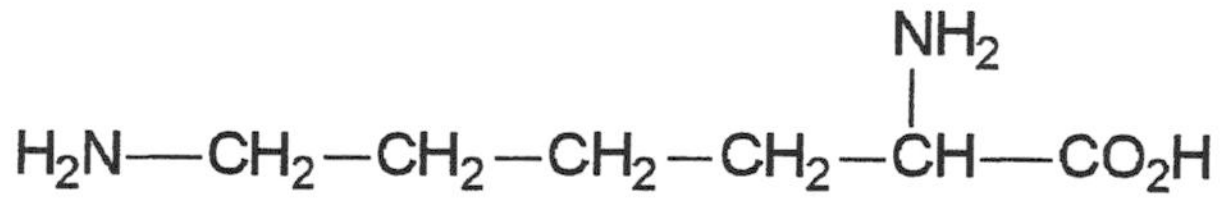
NH2
H2N—CH2—CH2—CH2—CH2—CH—CO2H

If an electrical potential is placed across two electrodes in a lysine solution, lysine will migrate to the cathode or to the anode depending on the pH. It is reasonable to assume that at the isoelectric point:
A. the pH would be above 7 and the net migration of lysine would be toward the cathode.
B. the pH would be above 7 and there would be no net migration of lysine.
C. the pH would be below 7 and the net migration of lysine would be toward the cathode.
D. the pH would be below 7 and there would be no net migration of lysine.

217. A student is synthesizing tripeptides using three different amino acids. How many distinct molecules can she create?
A. 3
B. 4
C. 6
D. 9

218. In the human menstrual cycle, which hormone is preferentially secreted in the follicular phase by the ovary?
A. Estrogen
B. FSH
C. LH
D. Progesterone

219. Cyclohexane derivatives often show significant energy differences between their two chair conformations. In certain instances only one of the two chair conformations is possible and the derivatives are classified as *ring locked.* Which of the following compounds would be classified as ring locked cyclohexane derivatives?

I.

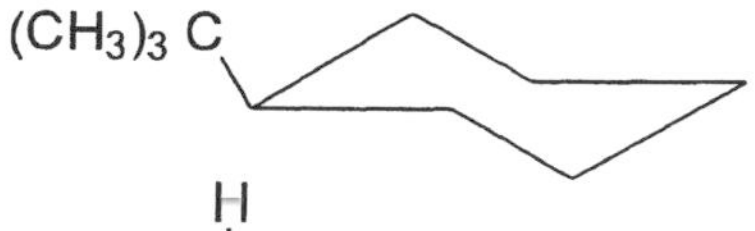
(CH3)3 C

II.

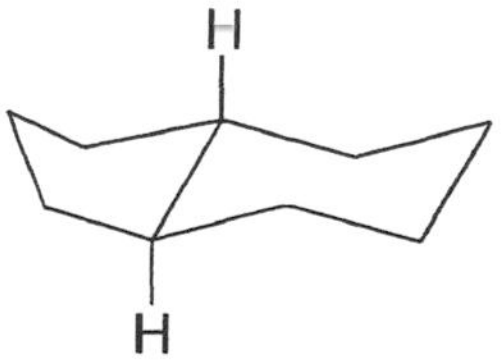
H
H

III.

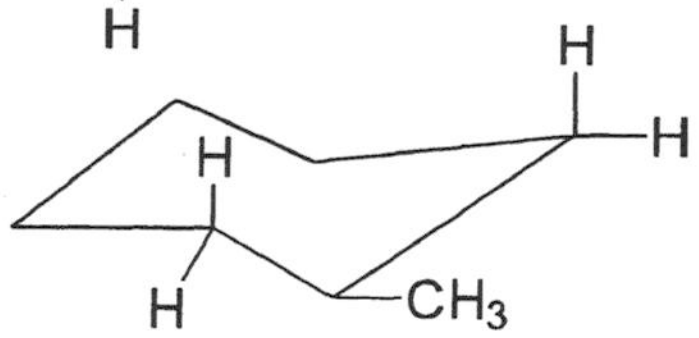
H
H
H
H
CH3

A. I only
B. II only
C. I and II only
D. I, II and III

END OF BIOLOGICAL SCIENCES. IF TIME REMAINS, YOU MAY GO BACK AND CHECK YOUR WORK IN THIS BOOKLET.

Answer Keys & Answer Documents

Answer Document

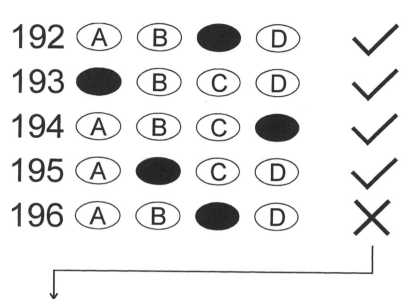

192 Ⓐ Ⓑ ● Ⓓ ✓
193 ● Ⓑ Ⓒ Ⓓ ✓
194 Ⓐ Ⓑ Ⓒ ● ✓
195 Ⓐ ● Ⓒ Ⓓ ✓
196 Ⓐ Ⓑ ● Ⓓ ✗

Answer Key

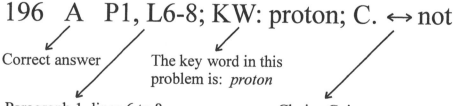

196   A   P1, L6-8; KW: proton; C. ↔ not

Correct answer

The key word in this
problem is: *proton*

Paragraph 1, lines 6 to 8,
is where the answer
can be found

Choice C. is wrong
because of the word "*not*"

TEST GS-1 (PHY = physics section; CHM = chemistry section; BIO = biology section; ORG = organic chemistry section; KW = key word; T = table; E = equation; F = figure; G = graph; L= line(s); P = paragraph; *see* GS Part V, Table 2, for a complete list of symbols and abbreviations)

Item #	Key	INFO			
1	D	PHY 2.3	57	B	PHY 7.2.1; F = mg = kx; k → W
2	C	P3, L5 ; PHY 6.1.3	58	A	EI
3	A	P4, L1: ↑h,↓P	59	D	EI
4	B	PHY 3.3; A + C = B	60	C	PHY 10.1, EI
5	D	PHY 6.1.3; *Continuity then Bernoulli*	61	D	EI
6	D	PHY 6.1.3	62	A	PV/nRT = 1 = const. (ideal)
7	B	CHM 1.6	63	B	#1: F1; CHM 4.1.4/8
8	D	CHM 1.4	64	C	CHM 4.1.2, 4.1.8
9	C	CHM 6.9	65	D	CHM 1.3, 4.1.1/7
10	B	CHM 3.4	66	A	CHM 4.1.2, 4.1.8
11	A	CHM 9.7, 9.8	67	A	CHM 4.1.2
12	B	CHM 9.9	68	B	deduce; P2, L8-13
13	D	CHM 4.1.7	69	D	P2, L7-13
14	B	CHM 6.5, 6.6	70	C	PHY 12.3, 12.4
15	A	PHY 11.4; P2, L3-5; P4, L5	71	A	D.A., PHY 5.7, Ap B.1
16	B	PHY 1.1.1/2	72	C	deduce, PHY 12.3
17	C	PHY 11.4	73	C	CHM 4.2 (3.); ORG 10.1 (P3)
18	B	P4, L5; PHY 11.4	74	A	PHY 9.1.1, 10.1
19	A	PHY 11.4	75	D	CHM 2.3, D. = Helium
20	B	P2; PHY 11.4	76	C	CHM 9.3
21	C	CHM 5.3.2	77	A	CHM 5.1.2
22	B	CHM 5.3.2;B.: *more moles*	78	B	P2, L14-15, 20-23
23	C	P4, L 2-5; T	79	A	P1, L9; P2, L18-19
24	C	P2, L 4-7	80	A	P1, L13-15
25	B	CHM 5.1.1/2	81	B	P3, L1-4
26	B	PHY 3.2, 3.2.1, 3.4	82	C	P4, L5-8
27	A	CHM 3.5T; ORG 1.2	83	B	P5, L6-7
28	B	PHY 9.1.2	84	D	deduce
29	D	PHY 8.3, 8.3.1	85	C	P1, L4-8
30	A	PHY 4.1, 4.1.1	86	A	P4, L5-10; P8, L2
31	D	PHY 4.3/4	87	A	P3, L6-9
32	B	PHY 4.3, 4.4, 4.4.1	88	D	P6, L7-8; P7, L6
33	C	PHY 3.2; F = f < f_{max}; KW: *tries*	89	B	deduce
34	C	PHY 3.2, 3.2.1	90	B	P8, L4-6; P11, L10-13
35	A	PHY 5.4, 1.1.2	91	C	deduce
36	B	CHM 4.3.3	92	A	deduce; P1; P2
37	D	P2, L4-6, deduce	93	C	P3, L1-5
38	A	CHM 8.3, 1.4, ORG 3.2.1	94	D	P4, L9-20
39	A	CHM 9.9	95	C	P4, L15-16; P5, L8-9; P6, L3-4
40	D	CHM 3.5T, ORG 1.2	96	B	deduce; P5
41	C	CHM 2.3 (iv)	97	C	P4, L1-8
42	C	deduce, CHM 7.5	98	A	P2
43	B	PHY 6.1.1	99	D	P4, L3
44	C	CHM 7.5	100	C	P3, L9-10; P3
45	B	D.A.; CHM 8.7	101	D	deduce
46	D	CHM 8.7; deduce	102	A	P1; P2, L1-2
47	A	PHY 6.1.1/2	103	A	P2, L2-10
48	B	CHM 4.3.3	104	A	P5
49	C	CHM 4.2; ORG 11.1.2	105	C	P3, L1-6
50	A	CHM 5.1.1/2; *gluc:*↑particles/gram	106	C	P3, L4-6
51	D	CHM 5.1.2, 4.1.1	107	C	P2, L1-2; P1, L3; P3, L6-7
52	A	PHY 6.1.1, 6.1.2	108	B	P1, L4
53	B	CHM 5.3.1	109	A	P2, L2; C: *traveller*
54	B	CHM 10.1	110	B	P3, L10
55	C	CHM 2.3 (iii)	111	D	P4, L3-4
56	B	PHY 1.6, 2.6, 4.3, 4.4	112	B	P4, L7
			113	D	P3, L8; P5, L8; P6, L2

114	C	P5, L6-7; P6; P8
115	C	P1, L6
116	A	P1, L14-19
117	C	P1, L3-11
118	C	P4, L6-7, L11-12
119	D	P3, L3, L1-8
120	D	P3, L8-10
121	D	P3; P4
122	C	P5, L7-9
123	A	P7, L12-14; P4, L8-11
124	D	P6, L7-10; KW: *counter*
125	B	P2, L8-10
126	D	P7, L4-7, L9-11, L12-14
127	D	P3, L2-3; B. ↔ *only*
128	A	P3, L4-5
129	A	P5; II. ↔ *readying*
130	C	deduce
131	A	P7, L4-7
132	A	deduce
133	A	P2, L2, L9-11; P4, L2
134	C	P4, L6-8; KW: *free*
135	B	P4, L1-2, L8-11; P2, L2-3
136	A	P8, KW: *conflict*
137	B	P1

------------------{Writing Sample}------------------------

143	A	F1; P3, L6; KW: *diastole*
144	A	F1, deduce, B: BIO 7.2
145	C	BIO 7.2; P2, L6-7
146	C	G
147	B	deduce, B: BIO 7.3
148	C	F1
149	B	P1, L2-3; BIO 1.1.1
150	B	P2, L3-5
151	C	deduce; B.↔*not*
152	A	F1; P1, L4-6
153	A	P2, L1-5
154	B	F1, deduce
155	B	P1, L3-6; B: BIO 1.2.1
156	A	P1, L2; BIO 2.2; BIO 4.4/5
157	B	F1 (b)
158	C	F1 (b); cf Q157
159	C	deduce; BIO 1.2.2, 1.3
160	C	ORG 5.2
161	B	BIO 7.3; *vein → lung capillary*
162	A	BIO 14.1
163	C	CHM 9.7/8, 9.10; B: ORG 6.2.1
164	D	ORG 6.2.3/4; cf Q212
165	D	P1, L5-7; BIO 1.1
166	B	BIO 1.2.1
167	C	P1; P2, L1-3
168	B	P3; BIO 5.4.1
169	C	deduce, B: BIO 5.1, 5.1.1/2/3
170	C	P4, L5-8; BIO 5.1
171	D	P1, L6-9; KWs: △, *one*; cf BIO 15.5
172	C	P1, L5-11; ↓O_2 BIO 4.7/8
173	B	F1; BIO 15.3
174	B	F1
175	C	P2, L6-9
176	C	deduce
177	B	ORG 6.2.4
178	C	ORG 14.1

179	D	CHM 2.3 (v), 3.1; Bu⁺: *stable*
180	D	P4; ORG 6.2.3
181	C	ORG 6.2.3; Bu⁺: *stable*
182	B	rate, P4; ORG 6.2.3/4
183	C	CHM 9.5; P2, *spontaneous ∴ exo*
184	B	P1 L10-12; BIO 7.5.1
185	C	P1, L4, L12-16
186	A	P2, L3-4; G
187	B	P1, L12-16; BIO 4.5, *debt: vol. muscle*; BIO 11.2
188	D	deduce
189	B	P1, L12-16; Q188
190	C	BIO 14.5
191	D	BIO 6.1
192	D	BIO 14.7, forewarned!
193	D	BIO 5.2 (i)
194	A	ORG 12.1.2
195	C	P1, L5-6; D.A.
196	A	P2; P3, L4-7; BIO 12.4
197	C	deduce; cf Q196
198	D	P4, L1-4: *post-pulmonary vessel*
199	B	deduce: BIO 12.4
200	B	ORG 10.2, 5.2.2, 12.1.2; CHM 6.3
201	D	F1
202	B	T1, Group III; ORG 8.1
203	D	T1, Group I; BIO 1.1; ORG 12.1.2
204	A	ORG 9.4
205	C	KW: *nature*; ORG 12.3.1
206	C	deduce; P1, L6-10
207	C	BIO 9.3
208	D	BIO 1.1, 1.1.2
209	D	BIO 9.5
210	D	deduce; B: BIO 9.3
211	C	ORG 7.2.2
212	B	ORG 7.1
213	A	F, deduce; B: ORG 4.1
214	B	ORG 7.2.1
215	A	ORG 2.3.2; C: *not chiral*
216	D	BIO 11.3.1; KW: *adult*
217	C	KW: *programmed ∴* DNA; BIO 1.2.2
218	D	BIO 14.3
219	C	ORG 12.3.2

TEST GS-2 (PHY = physics section; CHM = chemistry section; BIO = biology section; ORG = organic chemistry section; KW = key word; T = table; E = equation; F = figure; G = graph; L= line(s); P = paragraph; *see* GS Part V, Table 2, for a complete list of symbols and abbreviations)

Item #	Key	INFO
1	C	PHY 11.3
2	A	PHY 11.5; 2nd I: *virtual*
3	A	PHY 11.5
4	B	PHY 11.5
5	D	PHY 11.5
6	D	PHY 11.5
7	C	CHM 1.3, 1.5
8	C	T1; CHM 6.9.3
9	B	CHM 3.4
10	B	CHM 6.9
11	C	CHM 6.9.3
12	A	CHM 4.2, 4.3.2
13	B	CHM 4.1.7
14	C	PHY 12.1, PoE
15	A	PHY 12.3
16	D	PHY 12.4
17	B	PHY 12.3
18	C	PHY 5.2/3/4/5, 12.3
19	D	PHY 12.3, 12.4
20	B	deduce, EIII, CHM 10.2/4, "GERC"
21	D	CHM 10.1, $(Zn^{2+}/Zn) \neq (Zn/Zn^{2+})$
22	B	CHM 10.1/2
23	B	CHM 10.5
24	B	deduce, CHM 5.3.2
25	D	CHM 5.3.2; KS: $s^3 = \frac{1}{8} \cdot 10^{-15}$
26	A	PHY 10.3.1, Law I
27	B	PHY 7.1.2
28	C	ORG 1.2
29	B	PHY 7.1.3
30	D	PHY 4.1, 4.1.1
31	A	PHY 6.1.1/2; KWs: *max, held*
32	C	PHY 6.1.1/2
33	C	PHY 6.1.1/2
34	C	PHY 6.1.1/2
35	C	PHY 6.1.2; mg did not $\triangle$
36	D	CHM 3.5, P: 3 bonds
37	B	CHM 8.6
38	C	deduce from Q 101.D.
39	A	CHM 1.3, 1.5
40	C	CHM 2.3, 3.2
41	D	CHM 4.1.8
42	A	PHY 9.2.4
43	D	P4, L1-7; T1
44	D	E
45	B	PHY 7.2.1
46	A	E
47	A	PHY 6.1.2
48	C	CHM 4.1.6
49	A	CHM 4.1.8
50	A	deduce; *see* Q113: $\uparrow$T, $\uparrow$M
51	A	CHM 4.1.6/7/8; $\downarrow CO_2(g)$, $\downarrow$P, $\uparrow$M
52	D	CHM 3.1, 5.2
53	D	PHY 7.1.2, 7.1.4
54	A	CHM 10.1
55	A	CHM 2.2, 2.3(iv)
56	D	PHY 4.3, 4.4, 4.4.1, 1.4.1
57	A	CHM 7.5, deduce
58	B	CHM 7.5, deduce
59	D	PHY 6.1.1, deduce
60	B	CHM 8.7
61	A	D.A.
62	D	CHM 2.3
63	B	CHM 10.5
64	C	P2, L3-5; deduce
65	A	CHM 10.1
66	B	CHM 10.1
67	A	CHM 1.6
68	C	PHY 5.4, 3.2.1, 1.1.2
69	C	P2, PHY 1.3/4
70	B	PHY 3.2
71	D	PHY 1.4.1
72	B	PHY 3.2.1; $N = W \cos\alpha$
73	D	CHM 2.3
74	D	PHY 2.6, 1.1.2
75	A	CHM 9.9
76	D	PHY 11.5
77	C	CHM 4.2, ORG 10.1
78	D	P1, L3-6
79	B	P3, L3-6
80	B	P4
81	C	P5, L1-4
82	B	P4, L9-11; P5, L13-16
83	D	P6, L2, L4-6
84	C	P1
85	B	P2, L3-7; P4, L1-5
86	C	P2
87	D	P5, L2-4; P6, L1-2
88	A	P7
89	B	P8, L4-7; P9, L1-3
90	A	P9, L4-8
91	A	P8, L6-8
92	C	P1, L4-6; P2
93	C	P3; KW: *except*
94	A	P6, L1-2; P7
95	C	P4, L3, KW: *gov't*; L7, KW: *even*
96	D	P5, L1-3, L8-9
97	D	P8
98	B	P8, deduce
99	C	P2, L8-11; KW: *best*
100	A	P6
101	B	P6, deduce
102	A	P4; P7, L1-2
103	B	P7, L2-4, L5-8
104	C	P8
105	B	P2, L1-3; P8; C.↔*host*
106	A	P4, L2-3; KW: *susceptible*
107	B	P3
108	A	P5, L3-4
109	C	P4; P6; mom→infant = *horizontal*
110	B	P6, L8
111	D	P7, L5-7; P5, L7-8
112	B	P8, L4-8; C.↔ *inflicted*
113	A	P1, L3-4

114	C	P2
115	C	P3, L2-3, L4-5, L11
116	C	P4; P6; P8
117	C	P4, L8-10
118	D	P6, L3
119	A	P1
120	A	P2, L1-3, L7-9
121	D	P2, L13-18
122	B	P4, L3-5
123	B	P6
124	C	P2, L1-3, L8-9, L16
125	C	P6, L8-9; KW: *wrested*
126	D	P1, L15-16
127	B	P1, L1-2, L19-31; B. = ba
128	C	P2, L4-6
129	C	P2, L13-16
130	B	P3, L2-7, KW: *author*
131	D	P1; P2; C. ↔ *insusceptible*
132	B	P2, L3-5
133	D	P3, L10-12
134	B	P4, L1-2; A. ↔ P3, L13
135	D	P8, L1-8
136	B	P9, L11-14; A.: T/F
137	B	P5, L5-7, deduce
--------------------{Writing Sample}-----------------------		
143	B	BIO 14.5
144	C	BIO 14.5
145	D	BIO 14.2
146	C	P3, L12-13; BIO 3.0
147	A	P3, L12-13; BIO 1.2.2
148	B	BIO 14.5.1
149	B	BIO 15.3; KWs: *best explains*
150	A	P2, L5; BIO 6.3
151	C	P3, L5-7, L9-12
152	D	BIO 1.2.2
153	C	deduce
154	D	BIO 5.2
155	A	T1, deduce; P2, L5-7; B: BIO 5.1.1/2/3
156	B	BIO 4.9; P1, L1-4, P3
157	A	BIO 5.1, 5.1.1/2/3
158	B	C: *anaerobic*; BIO 4.4, CHM 1.5
159	B	BIO 12.3
160	D	T1
161	C	ORG 14.1
162	B	*axial*: ↑ ESR, ORG 3.3, 12.3.2F
163	D	BIO 14.2
164	A	BIO 16.5
165	C	ORG 7.2.2; R^{11} = H
166	C	KW: *facultative*; BIO 2.2
167	B	BIO 2.2; deduce; P2, L3
168	D	C: *glucan = extracellular*; P1, L4-6
169	B	ORG 12.3.2; P2; KW: *initially*
170	A	BIO 2.2, 15.5
171	D	T1, F1, deduce
172	B	T1, F1, deduce
173	A	ORG 7.2.1
174	C	T1, deduce; ORG 7.1
175	D	T1, F1
176	B	BIO 12.4.1 *in reverse*
177	D	P2, L1-3, L7-9; deduce
178	A	P1, L1-2; KW: *production*; BIO 9.4.1
179	A	P2, L6-7; BIO 2.1
180	C	G; BIO 8.2
181	B	BIO 2.3
182	B	P1, L4-6; BIO 15.3
183	D	T1
184	B	F1; CHM 9.9; BIO 6.3.3/6
185	D	BIO 6.3.3
186	A	P3, L5-7; BIO 5.4.4
187	B	deduce; B: BIO 5.4.4, 6.3.3
188	A	BIO 9.4.1
189	D	BIO 6.1.4
190	A	BIO 7.4
191	C	BIO 1.3
192	D	BIO 2.2, 2.3
193	A	ORG 6.2.3/4
194	C	P5; ORG 4.2.2, 6.2.4; B: CHM 6.10
195	C	ORG 6.2.4
196	C	ORG 6.2.3, 10.1
197	B	P2, L7-13; BIO 1.1, 5.2-P4
198	B	BIO 5.1, 5.1.1/2; P2, L11-12
199	B	P2, L13-15; BIO 5.1; deduce
200	D	F1 (2)
201	D	F2, deduce
202	B	F2; BIO 5.1.2
203	A	P2
204	B	P2; BIO 16.3; cf BIO 15.5
205	B	F1 (B), cf (A)
206	C	Ap C
207	A	F1, deduce
208	C	deduce; cf P1/2, BIO16.2; A. ↔ BIO15.5
209	B	F1, deduce
210	C	F1; *Reverse rxn of* ORG 7.2.3
211	C	ORG 11.1.1
212	C	ORG 9.3, 9.1
213	A	ORG 12.1
214	B	ORG 12.1.2
215	B	BIO 15.3, 15.3.1
216	C	ORG 12.3.2
217	B	BIO 4.5
218	D	BIO 10.3
219	B	KWs: *no enantiomer*; ORG 2.2

TEST GS-3 (PHY = physics section; CHM = chemistry section; BIO = biology section; ORG = organic chemistry section; KW = key word; T = table; E = equation; F = figure; G = graph; L= line(s); P = paragraph; *see GS Part V, Table 2, for a complete list of symbols and abbreviations*)

Item #	Key	INFO
1	A	P2, L8; B: PHY 9.1.3, 12.3
2	C	F1; P2; PT
3	C	PHY 12.4
4	D	PHY 12.3/4, PT
5	B	PHY 12.3/4, PT
6	D	PHY 12.3; C: *size/mass*
7	D	CHM 2.3 (ii)
8	D	P2, L1-4
9	A	P1, L4-7; PT; CHM 2.3F
10	D	P2, L1-4
11	C	PoE:PT; Air$\approx N_2 \gg O_2$ (CHM 1.1), $O_2 \rightarrow$ Fire; $CO_3 \neq$ gas (cf. CO_3^{-2})
12	A	CHM 6.6, 6.5
13	B	CHM 3.2
14	A	PHY 9.2.4; P3, L5-12
15	D	E
16	B	E; PHY 9.2.4, 12.5
17	B	PHY 12.5
18	A	P5; PHY 7.1.3F III.B.7.4
19	A	P2, L5-7; CHM 5.3.2
20	C	CHM 5.3.2
21	D	CHM 6.6, 6.6.1
22	B	CHM 5.3.2/3
23	D	P4; P2, L5-7; CHM 5.3.1/2
24	A	CHM 5.3.3
25	D	CHM 10.4; battery $\therefore$ soln irrelevant!
26	D	PHY 7.1.2
27	C	PHY 7.1.3F
28	C	CHM 5.3.1
29	D	E; B: PHY 7.1
30	B	PHY 12.3, 12.4
31	D	PHY 12.3
32	A	PHY 12.4, Ap A.3.2
33	C	PHY 12.3
34	C	PHY 5.3
35	D	New info.
36	D	$Ag/H_2S \rightarrow Ag_2S$ (black); T1
37	B	CHM 5.3.3, 9.9
38	D	CHM 8.10
39	B	CHM 1.3; PT
40	A	P5, L2-4
41	B	T1, deduce
42	B	PHY 5.4
43	A	PHY 5.3/4/5
44	D	PHY 2.1, 7.2.1; mg=(70+30)g= kx
45	B	PHY 5.2
46	B	PHY 4.3, 4.4
47	C	CHM 1.6
48	A	CHM 4.1.6
49	D	CHM 1.3, 1.5; PT
50	B	CHM 4.1.6, 8.2; $\downarrow$T(endo)$\rightarrow \uparrow n_{actual}$
51	D	PoE
52	C	PHY 9.1.2
53	D	CHM 2.3
54	D	PHY 7.2.1
55	C	PHY 8.5, 8.2
56	D	CHM 9.9, 9.8
57	D	PHY 2.2
58	B	PHY 2.1, 2.2
59	D	P3, L3-5; PHY 12.1
60	A	PHY 10.1, D.A.
61	B	PHY 10.1, 10.2, 10.2.1
62	A	PHY 7.1.2, 9.2.4
63	C	CHM 6.5, 6.5.1; P3, L3-4
64	B	CHM 6.9
65	A	CHM 6.9
66	D	R1; P3, L1-4; CHM 6.6.1
67	A	CHM 4.1.2
68	B	PHY 7.1.2, 8.3; P3, L1-5
69	A	deduce; B: PHY 8.2
70	C	PHY 8.3; $\Delta dB = 3$, *solve for* I/I_o.
71	C	PHY 1.3, *use 10 sec. for dist.*
72	A	P2, L3-5; PHY 7.1.2
73	A	PHY 11.5
74	B	CHM 5.3.1
75	D	CHM 9.3, 9.4
76	C	PHY 4.1, 4.1.1
77	D	CHM 4.2, 2.3F, PT
78	A	P1, L9-14
79	D	P3
80	B	P5, L1-5
81	A	P5, L6-10; P6
82	B	P6, L6-11; cf P1 L14-15 & P7 L10-13
83	D	P6, L12-14; P7, L3-5, L10-12
84	B	P7, L8-12; KW: *arbitrary*
85	D	P1, L2-3; P2, L2-3, L5-7
86	B	P3, L1-4
87	A	P4, L11-16
88	B	P3, L21-24
89	C	P3, L1-11
90	D	P3, L21-24; C.$\leftrightarrow$*intersection* $\neq$ *indep.*
91	B	P1, L9-12, KWs: *heterogeneous, many*
92	B	P4, deduce
93	D	P2, L2-4
94	B	P5, L1-3
95	A	P4, L12-16; P6; P7
96	D	P5, L4-5; P6, L9-12,L1-3; KW:*spatial*
97	C	P2; P2, L4-6; P3, L1-3; D.$\leftrightarrow$*not*
98	D	P1, L5-7; A. $\leftrightarrow$ *loved ones?*
99	D	P3, L1-3, L4-6; P5, L1-4
100	B	P4
101	C	P6, L1-3, L5; D.$\leftrightarrow$*willingly* (P5,L1-4)
102	D	P7, L1-5
103	C	P9
104	D	P2, L3-4; P3-4; P7; P6
105	A	deduce
106	C	P1, P2; KWs: *eloquence/communicat.*
107	B	P4; KWs: *fortune/communications/profit*
108	A	P3, L5-6
109	D	P8, L4-7
110	D	deduce; *did TV* Δ *the kids?*

111	A	P9, L10-13; KWs: *masses/populace*
112	B	deduce; P2/3/5/6/7/8
113	D	P1, L9
114	C	P3, deduce; KC: *water ≈ health care*
115	C	deduce
116	A	P4, L4-8; KW: *disadvantage*
117	B	P6, L5-8
118	B	deduce
119	A	P1, L3-5; P2, L4
120	C	P2, L11-13; P3; KWs: *port, shore*
121	C	P2,L1-6;P3,L1-3,L8; *suppos./premat.*
122	C	P3, L9-10; P6, L4
123	B	P6, L7-8 (cf P3); KWs: *false...security*
124	D	deduce
125	B	P3, L4; KWs: *directly challenge*
126	C	P6, L5-6; C: *resistant to* ∆; D.↔*not*
127	D	P4; B.↔*P12*
128	B	P5, L5-7
129	D	P7, L4-6; KW: *most*
130	B	P10; P11
131	C	P1, L3-4; P2, L1
132	C	P2, L2-9; KWs: *highlights/especially*
133	A	P3, L1-3
134	B	P5; P6, L6; P7, L1-3; PoE; KW: *rate*
135	A	P6; P3, L7-12; D.: T/F
136	C	P9, L7-10
137	C	deduce; P8; P9
--------------------{Writing Sample}----------------------		
143	B	BIO 3.0; P1, L3-7
144	C	P1, L1-2; E; ORG 9.4
145	D	P3; E
146	A	ORG 9.4
147	D	BIO 1.2.2, 3.0
148	C	deduce; B: BIO 3.0, 15.5
149	C	deduce; B: BIO 1.2.2, 1.3
150	C	F1; deduce; B: BIO 1.2.2, 1.3
151	D	F1; deduce; B: BIO 1.2.2, 1.3
152	A	PoE
153	C	BIO 3.0
154	B	P2, L7-8, L12-14; D. ↔ P2, L1-3
155	D	BIO 8.3
156	A	P6/7 (#4. and #5.)
157	B	deduce; P2, L20
158	D	deduce; BIO 8.1, 8.2
159	A	KWs: *no enantiomer*; ORG 2.2
160	D	BIO 2.2
161	D	BIO 14.2
162	D	ORG 14.1
163	B	ORG 14.2
164	B	ORG 4.2.1
165	B	CHM 9.6
166	A	ORG 4.2.1;Q164 II, 2° C⁺*more stable*
167	C	ORG 2.1
168	D	ORG 4.2.1; A. ↔ ESR
169	D	PoE
170	B	P2, L1-4; B: BIO 16.3
171	A	deduce
172	D	P1, L3-5; deduce
173	B	deduce
174	C	KW: *bidirectional*
175	C	Ap C

176	A	P4; P5
177	D	P6; ORG 12.2.2
178	C	BIO 1.2.2
179	D	B: BIO 1.2.2; deduce (draw diag.)
180	C	KS: *8 divisions*; 10×2^n, n=8
181	B	F1; T1; ORG 3.1.1
182	A	F1; T1; deduce
183	B	ORG 14.2.1
184	D	ORG 11.1.1
185	C	T1; ORG 8.1
186	C	BIO 1.2
187	C	BIO 6.1
188	D	BIO 1.1, 1.2.1
189	A	BIO 12.2, 12.3
190	C	ORG 12.1.2
191	A	P1, L6-8
192	B	deduce; B: BIO 4.1
193	A	Ap A.3.3; CHM 9.7(F3)
194	A	deduce; B: BIO 4.1
195	B	BIO 4.1, 4.3
196	C	BIO 1.2.2
197	B	BIO 1.2.2; P2, L1-3
198	C	BIO 1.2.2
199	C	F1
200	C	KW: *template*; F1
201	D	deduce
202	C	deduce, BIO 11.2
203	C	deduce; B: BIO 6.3.1
204	A	BIO 10.1
205	C	PoE
206	A	BIO 6.1, 6.1.4; P3, L4-7
207	A	P3, L12-14
208	A	BIO 6.3.1
209	B	ORG 6.24; CHM 9.2
210	B	ORG 4.2.3
211	B	ORG 4.2.2
212	A	ORG 6.2.3
213	B	ORG 4.2.1
214	D	ORG 4.2.1
215	B	BIO 1.1.2
216	B	ORG 12.1.2
217	C	Ap A.1.4; 3! = 6
218	A	BIO 14.3
219	B	deduce; B: ORG 3.3, 12.3.2F

The Gold Standard MCAT
Answer Document 1   Test GS-1

CANDIDATE'S NAME _____

SOCIAL SECURITY NUMBER _____

Mark one and only one answer to each question. Be sure to use a soft lead pencil and completely fill in the space for your intended answer. If you erase, do so completely. Make no stray marks.

Physical Sciences

1 Ⓐ Ⓑ Ⓒ Ⓓ
2 Ⓐ Ⓑ Ⓒ Ⓓ
3 Ⓐ Ⓑ Ⓒ Ⓓ
4 Ⓐ Ⓑ Ⓒ Ⓓ
5 Ⓐ Ⓑ Ⓒ Ⓓ
6 Ⓐ Ⓑ Ⓒ Ⓓ
7 Ⓐ Ⓑ Ⓒ Ⓓ
8 Ⓐ Ⓑ Ⓒ Ⓓ
9 Ⓐ Ⓑ Ⓒ Ⓓ
10 Ⓐ Ⓑ Ⓒ Ⓓ
11 Ⓐ Ⓑ Ⓒ Ⓓ
12 Ⓐ Ⓑ Ⓒ Ⓓ
13 Ⓐ Ⓑ Ⓒ Ⓓ
14 Ⓐ Ⓑ Ⓒ Ⓓ
15 Ⓐ Ⓑ Ⓒ Ⓓ
16 Ⓐ Ⓑ Ⓒ Ⓓ
17 Ⓐ Ⓑ Ⓒ Ⓓ
18 Ⓐ Ⓑ Ⓒ Ⓓ
19 Ⓐ Ⓑ Ⓒ Ⓓ
20 Ⓐ Ⓑ Ⓒ Ⓓ
21 Ⓐ Ⓑ Ⓒ Ⓓ
22 Ⓐ Ⓑ Ⓒ Ⓓ
23 Ⓐ Ⓑ Ⓒ Ⓓ
24 Ⓐ Ⓑ Ⓒ Ⓓ
25 Ⓐ Ⓑ Ⓒ Ⓓ
26 Ⓐ Ⓑ Ⓒ Ⓓ
27 Ⓐ Ⓑ Ⓒ Ⓓ
28 Ⓐ Ⓑ Ⓒ Ⓓ
29 Ⓐ Ⓑ Ⓒ Ⓓ
30 Ⓐ Ⓑ Ⓒ Ⓓ
31 Ⓐ Ⓑ Ⓒ Ⓓ
32 Ⓐ Ⓑ Ⓒ Ⓓ
33 Ⓐ Ⓑ Ⓒ Ⓓ
34 Ⓐ Ⓑ Ⓒ Ⓓ
35 Ⓐ Ⓑ Ⓒ Ⓓ
36 Ⓐ Ⓑ Ⓒ Ⓓ
37 Ⓐ Ⓑ Ⓒ Ⓓ
38 Ⓐ Ⓑ Ⓒ Ⓓ
39 Ⓐ Ⓑ Ⓒ Ⓓ
40 Ⓐ Ⓑ Ⓒ Ⓓ
41 Ⓐ Ⓑ Ⓒ Ⓓ
42 Ⓐ Ⓑ Ⓒ Ⓓ
43 Ⓐ Ⓑ Ⓒ Ⓓ
44 Ⓐ Ⓑ Ⓒ Ⓓ
45 Ⓐ Ⓑ Ⓒ Ⓓ
46 Ⓐ Ⓑ Ⓒ Ⓓ

47 Ⓐ Ⓑ Ⓒ Ⓓ
48 Ⓐ Ⓑ Ⓒ Ⓓ
49 Ⓐ Ⓑ Ⓒ Ⓓ
50 Ⓐ Ⓑ Ⓒ Ⓓ
51 Ⓐ Ⓑ Ⓒ Ⓓ
52 Ⓐ Ⓑ Ⓒ Ⓓ
53 Ⓐ Ⓑ Ⓒ Ⓓ
54 Ⓐ Ⓑ Ⓒ Ⓓ
55 Ⓐ Ⓑ Ⓒ Ⓓ
56 Ⓐ Ⓑ Ⓒ Ⓓ
57 Ⓐ Ⓑ Ⓒ Ⓓ
58 Ⓐ Ⓑ Ⓒ Ⓓ
59 Ⓐ Ⓑ Ⓒ Ⓓ
60 Ⓐ Ⓑ Ⓒ Ⓓ
61 Ⓐ Ⓑ Ⓒ Ⓓ
62 Ⓐ Ⓑ Ⓒ Ⓓ
63 Ⓐ Ⓑ Ⓒ Ⓓ
64 Ⓐ Ⓑ Ⓒ Ⓓ
65 Ⓐ Ⓑ Ⓒ Ⓓ
66 Ⓐ Ⓑ Ⓒ Ⓓ
67 Ⓐ Ⓑ Ⓒ Ⓓ
68 Ⓐ Ⓑ Ⓒ Ⓓ
69 Ⓐ Ⓑ Ⓒ Ⓓ
70 Ⓐ Ⓑ Ⓒ Ⓓ
71 Ⓐ Ⓑ Ⓒ Ⓓ
72 Ⓐ Ⓑ Ⓒ Ⓓ
73 Ⓐ Ⓑ Ⓒ Ⓓ
74 Ⓐ Ⓑ Ⓒ Ⓓ
75 Ⓐ Ⓑ Ⓒ Ⓓ
76 Ⓐ Ⓑ Ⓒ Ⓓ
77 Ⓐ Ⓑ Ⓒ Ⓓ

Verbal Reasoning

78 Ⓐ Ⓑ Ⓒ Ⓓ
79 Ⓐ Ⓑ Ⓒ Ⓓ
80 Ⓐ Ⓑ Ⓒ Ⓓ
81 Ⓐ Ⓑ Ⓒ Ⓓ
82 Ⓐ Ⓑ Ⓒ Ⓓ
83 Ⓐ Ⓑ Ⓒ Ⓓ
84 Ⓐ Ⓑ Ⓒ Ⓓ
85 Ⓐ Ⓑ Ⓒ Ⓓ
86 Ⓐ Ⓑ Ⓒ Ⓓ
87 Ⓐ Ⓑ Ⓒ Ⓓ

88 Ⓐ Ⓑ Ⓒ Ⓓ
89 Ⓐ Ⓑ Ⓒ Ⓓ
90 Ⓐ Ⓑ Ⓒ Ⓓ
91 Ⓐ Ⓑ Ⓒ Ⓓ
92 Ⓐ Ⓑ Ⓒ Ⓓ
93 Ⓐ Ⓑ Ⓒ Ⓓ
94 Ⓐ Ⓑ Ⓒ Ⓓ
95 Ⓐ Ⓑ Ⓒ Ⓓ
96 Ⓐ Ⓑ Ⓒ Ⓓ
97 Ⓐ Ⓑ Ⓒ Ⓓ
98 Ⓐ Ⓑ Ⓒ Ⓓ
99 Ⓐ Ⓑ Ⓒ Ⓓ
100 Ⓐ Ⓑ Ⓒ Ⓓ
101 Ⓐ Ⓑ Ⓒ Ⓓ
102 Ⓐ Ⓑ Ⓒ Ⓓ
103 Ⓐ Ⓑ Ⓒ Ⓓ
104 Ⓐ Ⓑ Ⓒ Ⓓ
105 Ⓐ Ⓑ Ⓒ Ⓓ
106 Ⓐ Ⓑ Ⓒ Ⓓ
107 Ⓐ Ⓑ Ⓒ Ⓓ
108 Ⓐ Ⓑ Ⓒ Ⓓ
109 Ⓐ Ⓑ Ⓒ Ⓓ
110 Ⓐ Ⓑ Ⓒ Ⓓ
111 Ⓐ Ⓑ Ⓒ Ⓓ
112 Ⓐ Ⓑ Ⓒ Ⓓ
113 Ⓐ Ⓑ Ⓒ Ⓓ
114 Ⓐ Ⓑ Ⓒ Ⓓ
115 Ⓐ Ⓑ Ⓒ Ⓓ
116 Ⓐ Ⓑ Ⓒ Ⓓ
117 Ⓐ Ⓑ Ⓒ Ⓓ
118 Ⓐ Ⓑ Ⓒ Ⓓ
119 Ⓐ Ⓑ Ⓒ Ⓓ
120 Ⓐ Ⓑ Ⓒ Ⓓ
121 Ⓐ Ⓑ Ⓒ Ⓓ
122 Ⓐ Ⓑ Ⓒ Ⓓ
123 Ⓐ Ⓑ Ⓒ Ⓓ
124 Ⓐ Ⓑ Ⓒ Ⓓ
125 Ⓐ Ⓑ Ⓒ Ⓓ
126 Ⓐ Ⓑ Ⓒ Ⓓ
127 Ⓐ Ⓑ Ⓒ Ⓓ
128 Ⓐ Ⓑ Ⓒ Ⓓ
129 Ⓐ Ⓑ Ⓒ Ⓓ
130 Ⓐ Ⓑ Ⓒ Ⓓ
131 Ⓐ Ⓑ Ⓒ Ⓓ
132 Ⓐ Ⓑ Ⓒ Ⓓ
133 Ⓐ Ⓑ Ⓒ Ⓓ

134 Ⓐ Ⓑ Ⓒ Ⓓ
135 Ⓐ Ⓑ Ⓒ Ⓓ
136 Ⓐ Ⓑ Ⓒ Ⓓ
137 Ⓐ Ⓑ Ⓒ Ⓓ

Biological Sciences

143 Ⓐ Ⓑ Ⓒ Ⓓ
144 Ⓐ Ⓑ Ⓒ Ⓓ
145 Ⓐ Ⓑ Ⓒ Ⓓ
146 Ⓐ Ⓑ Ⓒ Ⓓ
147 Ⓐ Ⓑ Ⓒ Ⓓ
148 Ⓐ Ⓑ Ⓒ Ⓓ
149 Ⓐ Ⓑ Ⓒ Ⓓ
150 Ⓐ Ⓑ Ⓒ Ⓓ
151 Ⓐ Ⓑ Ⓒ Ⓓ
152 Ⓐ Ⓑ Ⓒ Ⓓ
153 Ⓐ Ⓑ Ⓒ Ⓓ
154 Ⓐ Ⓑ Ⓒ Ⓓ
155 Ⓐ Ⓑ Ⓒ Ⓓ
156 Ⓐ Ⓑ Ⓒ Ⓓ
157 Ⓐ Ⓑ Ⓒ Ⓓ
158 Ⓐ Ⓑ Ⓒ Ⓓ
159 Ⓐ Ⓑ Ⓒ Ⓓ
160 Ⓐ Ⓑ Ⓒ Ⓓ
161 Ⓐ Ⓑ Ⓒ Ⓓ
162 Ⓐ Ⓑ Ⓒ Ⓓ
163 Ⓐ Ⓑ Ⓒ Ⓓ
164 Ⓐ Ⓑ Ⓒ Ⓓ
165 Ⓐ Ⓑ Ⓒ Ⓓ
166 Ⓐ Ⓑ Ⓒ Ⓓ
167 Ⓐ Ⓑ Ⓒ Ⓓ
168 Ⓐ Ⓑ Ⓒ Ⓓ
169 Ⓐ Ⓑ Ⓒ Ⓓ
170 Ⓐ Ⓑ Ⓒ Ⓓ
171 Ⓐ Ⓑ Ⓒ Ⓓ
172 Ⓐ Ⓑ Ⓒ Ⓓ
173 Ⓐ Ⓑ Ⓒ Ⓓ
174 Ⓐ Ⓑ Ⓒ Ⓓ

175 Ⓐ Ⓑ Ⓒ Ⓓ
176 Ⓐ Ⓑ Ⓒ Ⓓ
177 Ⓐ Ⓑ Ⓒ Ⓓ
178 Ⓐ Ⓑ Ⓒ Ⓓ
179 Ⓐ Ⓑ Ⓒ Ⓓ
180 Ⓐ Ⓑ Ⓒ Ⓓ
181 Ⓐ Ⓑ Ⓒ Ⓓ
182 Ⓐ Ⓑ Ⓒ Ⓓ
183 Ⓐ Ⓑ Ⓒ Ⓓ
184 Ⓐ Ⓑ Ⓒ Ⓓ
185 Ⓐ Ⓑ Ⓒ Ⓓ
186 Ⓐ Ⓑ Ⓒ Ⓓ
187 Ⓐ Ⓑ Ⓒ Ⓓ
188 Ⓐ Ⓑ Ⓒ Ⓓ
189 Ⓐ Ⓑ Ⓒ Ⓓ
190 Ⓐ Ⓑ Ⓒ Ⓓ
191 Ⓐ Ⓑ Ⓒ Ⓓ
192 Ⓐ Ⓑ Ⓒ Ⓓ
193 Ⓐ Ⓑ Ⓒ Ⓓ
194 Ⓐ Ⓑ Ⓒ Ⓓ
195 Ⓐ Ⓑ Ⓒ Ⓓ
196 Ⓐ Ⓑ Ⓒ Ⓓ
197 Ⓐ Ⓑ Ⓒ Ⓓ
198 Ⓐ Ⓑ Ⓒ Ⓓ
199 Ⓐ Ⓑ Ⓒ Ⓓ
200 Ⓐ Ⓑ Ⓒ Ⓓ
201 Ⓐ Ⓑ Ⓒ Ⓓ
202 Ⓐ Ⓑ Ⓒ Ⓓ
203 Ⓐ Ⓑ Ⓒ Ⓓ
204 Ⓐ Ⓑ Ⓒ Ⓓ
205 Ⓐ Ⓑ Ⓒ Ⓓ
206 Ⓐ Ⓑ Ⓒ Ⓓ
207 Ⓐ Ⓑ Ⓒ Ⓓ
208 Ⓐ Ⓑ Ⓒ Ⓓ
209 Ⓐ Ⓑ Ⓒ Ⓓ
210 Ⓐ Ⓑ Ⓒ Ⓓ
211 Ⓐ Ⓑ Ⓒ Ⓓ
212 Ⓐ Ⓑ Ⓒ Ⓓ
213 Ⓐ Ⓑ Ⓒ Ⓓ
214 Ⓐ Ⓑ Ⓒ Ⓓ
215 Ⓐ Ⓑ Ⓒ Ⓓ
216 Ⓐ Ⓑ Ⓒ Ⓓ
217 Ⓐ Ⓑ Ⓒ Ⓓ
218 Ⓐ Ⓑ Ⓒ Ⓓ
219 Ⓐ Ⓑ Ⓒ Ⓓ

CANDIDATE'S
SIGNATURE _____
SOCIAL SECURITY NUMBER _____._____

TEST GS-1

Answer Document 2

Writing Sample

1 1 1 1 1

1 1 1 1 1

IF YOU NEED MORE SPACE, CONTINUE ON THE BACK OF THIS PAGE.

1 1 1 1 1

STOP HERE FOR PART 1.

2 2 2 2 2

_____
_____
_____
_____
_____
_____
_____
_____
_____
_____
_____
_____
_____
_____
_____
_____
_____
_____
_____
_____
_____
_____
_____
_____
_____
_____
_____
_____
_____
_____
_____
_____
_____

IF YOU NEED MORE SPACE, CONTINUE ON THE BACK OF THIS PAGE.

2 2 2 2 2

2 **2** **2** **2** **2**

STOP HERE FOR PART 2. DO NOT RETURN TO PART 1.

The Gold Standard MCAT
Answer Document 1   Test GS-2

CANDIDATE'S NAME _____

SOCIAL SECURITY NUMBER _____

Mark one and only one answer to each question. Be sure to use a soft lead pencil and completely fill in the space for your intended answer. If you erase, do so completely. Make no stray marks.

Physical Sciences

1 Ⓐ Ⓑ Ⓒ Ⓓ
2 Ⓐ Ⓑ Ⓒ Ⓓ
3 Ⓐ Ⓑ Ⓒ Ⓓ
4 Ⓐ Ⓑ Ⓒ Ⓓ
5 Ⓐ Ⓑ Ⓒ Ⓓ
6 Ⓐ Ⓑ Ⓒ Ⓓ
7 Ⓐ Ⓑ Ⓒ Ⓓ
8 Ⓐ Ⓑ Ⓒ Ⓓ
9 Ⓐ Ⓑ Ⓒ Ⓓ
10 Ⓐ Ⓑ Ⓒ Ⓓ
11 Ⓐ Ⓑ Ⓒ Ⓓ
12 Ⓐ Ⓑ Ⓒ Ⓓ
13 Ⓐ Ⓑ Ⓒ Ⓓ
14 Ⓐ Ⓑ Ⓒ Ⓓ
15 Ⓐ Ⓑ Ⓒ Ⓓ
16 Ⓐ Ⓑ Ⓒ Ⓓ
17 Ⓐ Ⓑ Ⓒ Ⓓ
18 Ⓐ Ⓑ Ⓒ Ⓓ
19 Ⓐ Ⓑ Ⓒ Ⓓ
20 Ⓐ Ⓑ Ⓒ Ⓓ
21 Ⓐ Ⓑ Ⓒ Ⓓ
22 Ⓐ Ⓑ Ⓒ Ⓓ
23 Ⓐ Ⓑ Ⓒ Ⓓ
24 Ⓐ Ⓑ Ⓒ Ⓓ
25 Ⓐ Ⓑ Ⓒ Ⓓ
26 Ⓐ Ⓑ Ⓒ Ⓓ
27 Ⓐ Ⓑ Ⓒ Ⓓ
28 Ⓐ Ⓑ Ⓒ Ⓓ
29 Ⓐ Ⓑ Ⓒ Ⓓ
30 Ⓐ Ⓑ Ⓒ Ⓓ
31 Ⓐ Ⓑ Ⓒ Ⓓ
32 Ⓐ Ⓑ Ⓒ Ⓓ
33 Ⓐ Ⓑ Ⓒ Ⓓ
34 Ⓐ Ⓑ Ⓒ Ⓓ
35 Ⓐ Ⓑ Ⓒ Ⓓ
36 Ⓐ Ⓑ Ⓒ Ⓓ
37 Ⓐ Ⓑ Ⓒ Ⓓ
38 Ⓐ Ⓑ Ⓒ Ⓓ
39 Ⓐ Ⓑ Ⓒ Ⓓ
40 Ⓐ Ⓑ Ⓒ Ⓓ
41 Ⓐ Ⓑ Ⓒ Ⓓ
42 Ⓐ Ⓑ Ⓒ Ⓓ
43 Ⓐ Ⓑ Ⓒ Ⓓ
44 Ⓐ Ⓑ Ⓒ Ⓓ
45 Ⓐ Ⓑ Ⓒ Ⓓ
46 Ⓐ Ⓑ Ⓒ Ⓓ

47 Ⓐ Ⓑ Ⓒ Ⓓ
48 Ⓐ Ⓑ Ⓒ Ⓓ
49 Ⓐ Ⓑ Ⓒ Ⓓ
50 Ⓐ Ⓑ Ⓒ Ⓓ
51 Ⓐ Ⓑ Ⓒ Ⓓ
52 Ⓐ Ⓑ Ⓒ Ⓓ
53 Ⓐ Ⓑ Ⓒ Ⓓ
54 Ⓐ Ⓑ Ⓒ Ⓓ
55 Ⓐ Ⓑ Ⓒ Ⓓ
56 Ⓐ Ⓑ Ⓒ Ⓓ
57 Ⓐ Ⓑ Ⓒ Ⓓ
58 Ⓐ Ⓑ Ⓒ Ⓓ
59 Ⓐ Ⓑ Ⓒ Ⓓ
60 Ⓐ Ⓑ Ⓒ Ⓓ
61 Ⓐ Ⓑ Ⓒ Ⓓ
62 Ⓐ Ⓑ Ⓒ Ⓓ
63 Ⓐ Ⓑ Ⓒ Ⓓ
64 Ⓐ Ⓑ Ⓒ Ⓓ
65 Ⓐ Ⓑ Ⓒ Ⓓ
66 Ⓐ Ⓑ Ⓒ Ⓓ
67 Ⓐ Ⓑ Ⓒ Ⓓ
68 Ⓐ Ⓑ Ⓒ Ⓓ
69 Ⓐ Ⓑ Ⓒ Ⓓ
70 Ⓐ Ⓑ Ⓒ Ⓓ
71 Ⓐ Ⓑ Ⓒ Ⓓ
72 Ⓐ Ⓑ Ⓒ Ⓓ
73 Ⓐ Ⓑ Ⓒ Ⓓ
74 Ⓐ Ⓑ Ⓒ Ⓓ
75 Ⓐ Ⓑ Ⓒ Ⓓ
76 Ⓐ Ⓑ Ⓒ Ⓓ
77 Ⓐ Ⓑ Ⓒ Ⓓ

Verbal Reasoning

78 Ⓐ Ⓑ Ⓒ Ⓓ
79 Ⓐ Ⓑ Ⓒ Ⓓ
80 Ⓐ Ⓑ Ⓒ Ⓓ
81 Ⓐ Ⓑ Ⓒ Ⓓ
82 Ⓐ Ⓑ Ⓒ Ⓓ
83 Ⓐ Ⓑ Ⓒ Ⓓ
84 Ⓐ Ⓑ Ⓒ Ⓓ
85 Ⓐ Ⓑ Ⓒ Ⓓ
86 Ⓐ Ⓑ Ⓒ Ⓓ
87 Ⓐ Ⓑ Ⓒ Ⓓ

88 Ⓐ Ⓑ Ⓒ Ⓓ
89 Ⓐ Ⓑ Ⓒ Ⓓ
90 Ⓐ Ⓑ Ⓒ Ⓓ
91 Ⓐ Ⓑ Ⓒ Ⓓ
92 Ⓐ Ⓑ Ⓒ Ⓓ
93 Ⓐ Ⓑ Ⓒ Ⓓ
94 Ⓐ Ⓑ Ⓒ Ⓓ
95 Ⓐ Ⓑ Ⓒ Ⓓ
96 Ⓐ Ⓑ Ⓒ Ⓓ
97 Ⓐ Ⓑ Ⓒ Ⓓ
98 Ⓐ Ⓑ Ⓒ Ⓓ
99 Ⓐ Ⓑ Ⓒ Ⓓ
100 Ⓐ Ⓑ Ⓒ Ⓓ
101 Ⓐ Ⓑ Ⓒ Ⓓ
102 Ⓐ Ⓑ Ⓒ Ⓓ
103 Ⓐ Ⓑ Ⓒ Ⓓ
104 Ⓐ Ⓑ Ⓒ Ⓓ
105 Ⓐ Ⓑ Ⓒ Ⓓ
106 Ⓐ Ⓑ Ⓒ Ⓓ
107 Ⓐ Ⓑ Ⓒ Ⓓ
108 Ⓐ Ⓑ Ⓒ Ⓓ
109 Ⓐ Ⓑ Ⓒ Ⓓ
110 Ⓐ Ⓑ Ⓒ Ⓓ
111 Ⓐ Ⓑ Ⓒ Ⓓ
112 Ⓐ Ⓑ Ⓒ Ⓓ
113 Ⓐ Ⓑ Ⓒ Ⓓ
114 Ⓐ Ⓑ Ⓒ Ⓓ
115 Ⓐ Ⓑ Ⓒ Ⓓ
116 Ⓐ Ⓑ Ⓒ Ⓓ
117 Ⓐ Ⓑ Ⓒ Ⓓ
118 Ⓐ Ⓑ Ⓒ Ⓓ
119 Ⓐ Ⓑ Ⓒ Ⓓ
120 Ⓐ Ⓑ Ⓒ Ⓓ
121 Ⓐ Ⓑ Ⓒ Ⓓ
122 Ⓐ Ⓑ Ⓒ Ⓓ
123 Ⓐ Ⓑ Ⓒ Ⓓ
124 Ⓐ Ⓑ Ⓒ Ⓓ
125 Ⓐ Ⓑ Ⓒ Ⓓ
126 Ⓐ Ⓑ Ⓒ Ⓓ
127 Ⓐ Ⓑ Ⓒ Ⓓ
128 Ⓐ Ⓑ Ⓒ Ⓓ
129 Ⓐ Ⓑ Ⓒ Ⓓ
130 Ⓐ Ⓑ Ⓒ Ⓓ
131 Ⓐ Ⓑ Ⓒ Ⓓ
132 Ⓐ Ⓑ Ⓒ Ⓓ
133 Ⓐ Ⓑ Ⓒ Ⓓ

134 Ⓐ Ⓑ Ⓒ Ⓓ
135 Ⓐ Ⓑ Ⓒ Ⓓ
136 Ⓐ Ⓑ Ⓒ Ⓓ
137 Ⓐ Ⓑ Ⓒ Ⓓ

Biological Sciences

143 Ⓐ Ⓑ Ⓒ Ⓓ
144 Ⓐ Ⓑ Ⓒ Ⓓ
145 Ⓐ Ⓑ Ⓒ Ⓓ
146 Ⓐ Ⓑ Ⓒ Ⓓ
147 Ⓐ Ⓑ Ⓒ Ⓓ
148 Ⓐ Ⓑ Ⓒ Ⓓ
149 Ⓐ Ⓑ Ⓒ Ⓓ
150 Ⓐ Ⓑ Ⓒ Ⓓ
151 Ⓐ Ⓑ Ⓒ Ⓓ
152 Ⓐ Ⓑ Ⓒ Ⓓ
153 Ⓐ Ⓑ Ⓒ Ⓓ
154 Ⓐ Ⓑ Ⓒ Ⓓ
155 Ⓐ Ⓑ Ⓒ Ⓓ
156 Ⓐ Ⓑ Ⓒ Ⓓ
157 Ⓐ Ⓑ Ⓒ Ⓓ
158 Ⓐ Ⓑ Ⓒ Ⓓ
159 Ⓐ Ⓑ Ⓒ Ⓓ
160 Ⓐ Ⓑ Ⓒ Ⓓ
161 Ⓐ Ⓑ Ⓒ Ⓓ
162 Ⓐ Ⓑ Ⓒ Ⓓ
163 Ⓐ Ⓑ Ⓒ Ⓓ
164 Ⓐ Ⓑ Ⓒ Ⓓ
165 Ⓐ Ⓑ Ⓒ Ⓓ
166 Ⓐ Ⓑ Ⓒ Ⓓ
167 Ⓐ Ⓑ Ⓒ Ⓓ
168 Ⓐ Ⓑ Ⓒ Ⓓ
169 Ⓐ Ⓑ Ⓒ Ⓓ
170 Ⓐ Ⓑ Ⓒ Ⓓ
171 Ⓐ Ⓑ Ⓒ Ⓓ
172 Ⓐ Ⓑ Ⓒ Ⓓ
173 Ⓐ Ⓑ Ⓒ Ⓓ
174 Ⓐ Ⓑ Ⓒ Ⓓ

175 Ⓐ Ⓑ Ⓒ Ⓓ
176 Ⓐ Ⓑ Ⓒ Ⓓ
177 Ⓐ Ⓑ Ⓒ Ⓓ
178 Ⓐ Ⓑ Ⓒ Ⓓ
179 Ⓐ Ⓑ Ⓒ Ⓓ
180 Ⓐ Ⓑ Ⓒ Ⓓ
181 Ⓐ Ⓑ Ⓒ Ⓓ
182 Ⓐ Ⓑ Ⓒ Ⓓ
183 Ⓐ Ⓑ Ⓒ Ⓓ
184 Ⓐ Ⓑ Ⓒ Ⓓ
185 Ⓐ Ⓑ Ⓒ Ⓓ
186 Ⓐ Ⓑ Ⓒ Ⓓ
187 Ⓐ Ⓑ Ⓒ Ⓓ
188 Ⓐ Ⓑ Ⓒ Ⓓ
189 Ⓐ Ⓑ Ⓒ Ⓓ
190 Ⓐ Ⓑ Ⓒ Ⓓ
191 Ⓐ Ⓑ Ⓒ Ⓓ
192 Ⓐ Ⓑ Ⓒ Ⓓ
193 Ⓐ Ⓑ Ⓒ Ⓓ
194 Ⓐ Ⓑ Ⓒ Ⓓ
195 Ⓐ Ⓑ Ⓒ Ⓓ
196 Ⓐ Ⓑ Ⓒ Ⓓ
197 Ⓐ Ⓑ Ⓒ Ⓓ
198 Ⓐ Ⓑ Ⓒ Ⓓ
199 Ⓐ Ⓑ Ⓒ Ⓓ
200 Ⓐ Ⓑ Ⓒ Ⓓ
201 Ⓐ Ⓑ Ⓒ Ⓓ
202 Ⓐ Ⓑ Ⓒ Ⓓ
203 Ⓐ Ⓑ Ⓒ Ⓓ
204 Ⓐ Ⓑ Ⓒ Ⓓ
205 Ⓐ Ⓑ Ⓒ Ⓓ
206 Ⓐ Ⓑ Ⓒ Ⓓ
207 Ⓐ Ⓑ Ⓒ Ⓓ
208 Ⓐ Ⓑ Ⓒ Ⓓ
209 Ⓐ Ⓑ Ⓒ Ⓓ
210 Ⓐ Ⓑ Ⓒ Ⓓ
211 Ⓐ Ⓑ Ⓒ Ⓓ
212 Ⓐ Ⓑ Ⓒ Ⓓ
213 Ⓐ Ⓑ Ⓒ Ⓓ
214 Ⓐ Ⓑ Ⓒ Ⓓ
215 Ⓐ Ⓑ Ⓒ Ⓓ
216 Ⓐ Ⓑ Ⓒ Ⓓ
217 Ⓐ Ⓑ Ⓒ Ⓓ
218 Ⓐ Ⓑ Ⓒ Ⓓ
219 Ⓐ Ⓑ Ⓒ Ⓓ

TEST GS-2

Answer Document 2

Writing Sample

1 1 1 1 1

1 1 1 1 1

_____

_____

_____

_____

_____

_____

_____

_____

_____

_____

_____

_____

_____

_____

_____

_____

_____

_____

_____

_____

_____

_____

_____

_____

_____

_____

_____

_____

IF YOU NEED MORE SPACE, CONTINUE ON THE BACK OF THIS PAGE.

1 1 1 1 1

STOP HERE FOR PART 1.

2 2 2 2 2

IF YOU NEED MORE SPACE, CONTINUE ON THE BACK OF THIS PAGE.

2 2 2 2 2

STOP HERE FOR PART 2. DO NOT RETURN TO PART 1.

The Gold Standard MCAT
Answer Document 1   Test GS-3

CANDIDATE'S NAME _____

SOCIAL SECURITY NUMBER _____

Mark one and only one answer to each question. Be sure to use a soft lead pencil and completely fill in the space for your intended answer. If you erase, do so completely. Make no stray marks.

Physical Sciences

1 Ⓐ Ⓑ Ⓒ Ⓓ	47 Ⓐ Ⓑ Ⓒ Ⓓ	88 Ⓐ Ⓑ Ⓒ Ⓓ	134 Ⓐ Ⓑ Ⓒ Ⓓ	175 Ⓐ Ⓑ Ⓒ Ⓓ
2 Ⓐ Ⓑ Ⓒ Ⓓ	48 Ⓐ Ⓑ Ⓒ Ⓓ	89 Ⓐ Ⓑ Ⓒ Ⓓ	135 Ⓐ Ⓑ Ⓒ Ⓓ	176 Ⓐ Ⓑ Ⓒ Ⓓ
3 Ⓐ Ⓑ Ⓒ Ⓓ	49 Ⓐ Ⓑ Ⓒ Ⓓ	90 Ⓐ Ⓑ Ⓒ Ⓓ	136 Ⓐ Ⓑ Ⓒ Ⓓ	177 Ⓐ Ⓑ Ⓒ Ⓓ
4 Ⓐ Ⓑ Ⓒ Ⓓ	50 Ⓐ Ⓑ Ⓒ Ⓓ	91 Ⓐ Ⓑ Ⓒ Ⓓ	137 Ⓐ Ⓑ Ⓒ Ⓓ	178 Ⓐ Ⓑ Ⓒ Ⓓ
5 Ⓐ Ⓑ Ⓒ Ⓓ	51 Ⓐ Ⓑ Ⓒ Ⓓ	92 Ⓐ Ⓑ Ⓒ Ⓓ		179 Ⓐ Ⓑ Ⓒ Ⓓ
6 Ⓐ Ⓑ Ⓒ Ⓓ	52 Ⓐ Ⓑ Ⓒ Ⓓ	93 Ⓐ Ⓑ Ⓒ Ⓓ		180 Ⓐ Ⓑ Ⓒ Ⓓ
7 Ⓐ Ⓑ Ⓒ Ⓓ	53 Ⓐ Ⓑ Ⓒ Ⓓ	94 Ⓐ Ⓑ Ⓒ Ⓓ		181 Ⓐ Ⓑ Ⓒ Ⓓ
8 Ⓐ Ⓑ Ⓒ Ⓓ	54 Ⓐ Ⓑ Ⓒ Ⓓ	95 Ⓐ Ⓑ Ⓒ Ⓓ		182 Ⓐ Ⓑ Ⓒ Ⓓ
9 Ⓐ Ⓑ Ⓒ Ⓓ	55 Ⓐ Ⓑ Ⓒ Ⓓ	96 Ⓐ Ⓑ Ⓒ Ⓓ		183 Ⓐ Ⓑ Ⓒ Ⓓ
10 Ⓐ Ⓑ Ⓒ Ⓓ	56 Ⓐ Ⓑ Ⓒ Ⓓ	97 Ⓐ Ⓑ Ⓒ Ⓓ		184 Ⓐ Ⓑ Ⓒ Ⓓ
11 Ⓐ Ⓑ Ⓒ Ⓓ	57 Ⓐ Ⓑ Ⓒ Ⓓ	98 Ⓐ Ⓑ Ⓒ Ⓓ		185 Ⓐ Ⓑ Ⓒ Ⓓ
12 Ⓐ Ⓑ Ⓒ Ⓓ	58 Ⓐ Ⓑ Ⓒ Ⓓ	99 Ⓐ Ⓑ Ⓒ Ⓓ	**Biological Sciences**	186 Ⓐ Ⓑ Ⓒ Ⓓ
13 Ⓐ Ⓑ Ⓒ Ⓓ	59 Ⓐ Ⓑ Ⓒ Ⓓ	100 Ⓐ Ⓑ Ⓒ Ⓓ		187 Ⓐ Ⓑ Ⓒ Ⓓ
14 Ⓐ Ⓑ Ⓒ Ⓓ	60 Ⓐ Ⓑ Ⓒ Ⓓ	101 Ⓐ Ⓑ Ⓒ Ⓓ		188 Ⓐ Ⓑ Ⓒ Ⓓ
15 Ⓐ Ⓑ Ⓒ Ⓓ	61 Ⓐ Ⓑ Ⓒ Ⓓ	102 Ⓐ Ⓑ Ⓒ Ⓓ	143 Ⓐ Ⓑ Ⓒ Ⓓ	189 Ⓐ Ⓑ Ⓒ Ⓓ
16 Ⓐ Ⓑ Ⓒ Ⓓ	62 Ⓐ Ⓑ Ⓒ Ⓓ	103 Ⓐ Ⓑ Ⓒ Ⓓ	144 Ⓐ Ⓑ Ⓒ Ⓓ	190 Ⓐ Ⓑ Ⓒ Ⓓ
17 Ⓐ Ⓑ Ⓒ Ⓓ	63 Ⓐ Ⓑ Ⓒ Ⓓ	104 Ⓐ Ⓑ Ⓒ Ⓓ	145 Ⓐ Ⓑ Ⓒ Ⓓ	191 Ⓐ Ⓑ Ⓒ Ⓓ
18 Ⓐ Ⓑ Ⓒ Ⓓ	64 Ⓐ Ⓑ Ⓒ Ⓓ	105 Ⓐ Ⓑ Ⓒ Ⓓ	146 Ⓐ Ⓑ Ⓒ Ⓓ	192 Ⓐ Ⓑ Ⓒ Ⓓ
19 Ⓐ Ⓑ Ⓒ Ⓓ	65 Ⓐ Ⓑ Ⓒ Ⓓ	106 Ⓐ Ⓑ Ⓒ Ⓓ	147 Ⓐ Ⓑ Ⓒ Ⓓ	193 Ⓐ Ⓑ Ⓒ Ⓓ
20 Ⓐ Ⓑ Ⓒ Ⓓ	66 Ⓐ Ⓑ Ⓒ Ⓓ	107 Ⓐ Ⓑ Ⓒ Ⓓ	148 Ⓐ Ⓑ Ⓒ Ⓓ	194 Ⓐ Ⓑ Ⓒ Ⓓ
21 Ⓐ Ⓑ Ⓒ Ⓓ	67 Ⓐ Ⓑ Ⓒ Ⓓ	108 Ⓐ Ⓑ Ⓒ Ⓓ	149 Ⓐ Ⓑ Ⓒ Ⓓ	195 Ⓐ Ⓑ Ⓒ Ⓓ
22 Ⓐ Ⓑ Ⓒ Ⓓ	68 Ⓐ Ⓑ Ⓒ Ⓓ	109 Ⓐ Ⓑ Ⓒ Ⓓ	150 Ⓐ Ⓑ Ⓒ Ⓓ	196 Ⓐ Ⓑ Ⓒ Ⓓ
23 Ⓐ Ⓑ Ⓒ Ⓓ	69 Ⓐ Ⓑ Ⓒ Ⓓ	110 Ⓐ Ⓑ Ⓒ Ⓓ	151 Ⓐ Ⓑ Ⓒ Ⓓ	197 Ⓐ Ⓑ Ⓒ Ⓓ
24 Ⓐ Ⓑ Ⓒ Ⓓ	70 Ⓐ Ⓑ Ⓒ Ⓓ	111 Ⓐ Ⓑ Ⓒ Ⓓ	152 Ⓐ Ⓑ Ⓒ Ⓓ	198 Ⓐ Ⓑ Ⓒ Ⓓ
25 Ⓐ Ⓑ Ⓒ Ⓓ	71 Ⓐ Ⓑ Ⓒ Ⓓ	112 Ⓐ Ⓑ Ⓒ Ⓓ	153 Ⓐ Ⓑ Ⓒ Ⓓ	199 Ⓐ Ⓑ Ⓒ Ⓓ
26 Ⓐ Ⓑ Ⓒ Ⓓ	72 Ⓐ Ⓑ Ⓒ Ⓓ	113 Ⓐ Ⓑ Ⓒ Ⓓ	154 Ⓐ Ⓑ Ⓒ Ⓓ	200 Ⓐ Ⓑ Ⓒ Ⓓ
27 Ⓐ Ⓑ Ⓒ Ⓓ	73 Ⓐ Ⓑ Ⓒ Ⓓ	114 Ⓐ Ⓑ Ⓒ Ⓓ	155 Ⓐ Ⓑ Ⓒ Ⓓ	201 Ⓐ Ⓑ Ⓒ Ⓓ
28 Ⓐ Ⓑ Ⓒ Ⓓ	74 Ⓐ Ⓑ Ⓒ Ⓓ	115 Ⓐ Ⓑ Ⓒ Ⓓ	156 Ⓐ Ⓑ Ⓒ Ⓓ	202 Ⓐ Ⓑ Ⓒ Ⓓ
29 Ⓐ Ⓑ Ⓒ Ⓓ	75 Ⓐ Ⓑ Ⓒ Ⓓ	116 Ⓐ Ⓑ Ⓒ Ⓓ	157 Ⓐ Ⓑ Ⓒ Ⓓ	203 Ⓐ Ⓑ Ⓒ Ⓓ
30 Ⓐ Ⓑ Ⓒ Ⓓ	76 Ⓐ Ⓑ Ⓒ Ⓓ	117 Ⓐ Ⓑ Ⓒ Ⓓ	158 Ⓐ Ⓑ Ⓒ Ⓓ	204 Ⓐ Ⓑ Ⓒ Ⓓ
31 Ⓐ Ⓑ Ⓒ Ⓓ	77 Ⓐ Ⓑ Ⓒ Ⓓ	118 Ⓐ Ⓑ Ⓒ Ⓓ	159 Ⓐ Ⓑ Ⓒ Ⓓ	205 Ⓐ Ⓑ Ⓒ Ⓓ
32 Ⓐ Ⓑ Ⓒ Ⓓ		119 Ⓐ Ⓑ Ⓒ Ⓓ	160 Ⓐ Ⓑ Ⓒ Ⓓ	206 Ⓐ Ⓑ Ⓒ Ⓓ
33 Ⓐ Ⓑ Ⓒ Ⓓ		120 Ⓐ Ⓑ Ⓒ Ⓓ	161 Ⓐ Ⓑ Ⓒ Ⓓ	207 Ⓐ Ⓑ Ⓒ Ⓓ
34 Ⓐ Ⓑ Ⓒ Ⓓ		121 Ⓐ Ⓑ Ⓒ Ⓓ	162 Ⓐ Ⓑ Ⓒ Ⓓ	208 Ⓐ Ⓑ Ⓒ Ⓓ
35 Ⓐ Ⓑ Ⓒ Ⓓ	**Verbal Reasoning**	122 Ⓐ Ⓑ Ⓒ Ⓓ	163 Ⓐ Ⓑ Ⓒ Ⓓ	209 Ⓐ Ⓑ Ⓒ Ⓓ
36 Ⓐ Ⓑ Ⓒ Ⓓ		123 Ⓐ Ⓑ Ⓒ Ⓓ	164 Ⓐ Ⓑ Ⓒ Ⓓ	210 Ⓐ Ⓑ Ⓒ Ⓓ
37 Ⓐ Ⓑ Ⓒ Ⓓ	78 Ⓐ Ⓑ Ⓒ Ⓓ	124 Ⓐ Ⓑ Ⓒ Ⓓ	165 Ⓐ Ⓑ Ⓒ Ⓓ	211 Ⓐ Ⓑ Ⓒ Ⓓ
38 Ⓐ Ⓑ Ⓒ Ⓓ	79 Ⓐ Ⓑ Ⓒ Ⓓ	125 Ⓐ Ⓑ Ⓒ Ⓓ	166 Ⓐ Ⓑ Ⓒ Ⓓ	212 Ⓐ Ⓑ Ⓒ Ⓓ
39 Ⓐ Ⓑ Ⓒ Ⓓ	80 Ⓐ Ⓑ Ⓒ Ⓓ	126 Ⓐ Ⓑ Ⓒ Ⓓ	167 Ⓐ Ⓑ Ⓒ Ⓓ	213 Ⓐ Ⓑ Ⓒ Ⓓ
40 Ⓐ Ⓑ Ⓒ Ⓓ	81 Ⓐ Ⓑ Ⓒ Ⓓ	127 Ⓐ Ⓑ Ⓒ Ⓓ	168 Ⓐ Ⓑ Ⓒ Ⓓ	214 Ⓐ Ⓑ Ⓒ Ⓓ
41 Ⓐ Ⓑ Ⓒ Ⓓ	82 Ⓐ Ⓑ Ⓒ Ⓓ	128 Ⓐ Ⓑ Ⓒ Ⓓ	169 Ⓐ Ⓑ Ⓒ Ⓓ	215 Ⓐ Ⓑ Ⓒ Ⓓ
42 Ⓐ Ⓑ Ⓒ Ⓓ	83 Ⓐ Ⓑ Ⓒ Ⓓ	129 Ⓐ Ⓑ Ⓒ Ⓓ	170 Ⓐ Ⓑ Ⓒ Ⓓ	216 Ⓐ Ⓑ Ⓒ Ⓓ
43 Ⓐ Ⓑ Ⓒ Ⓓ	84 Ⓐ Ⓑ Ⓒ Ⓓ	130 Ⓐ Ⓑ Ⓒ Ⓓ	171 Ⓐ Ⓑ Ⓒ Ⓓ	217 Ⓐ Ⓑ Ⓒ Ⓓ
44 Ⓐ Ⓑ Ⓒ Ⓓ	85 Ⓐ Ⓑ Ⓒ Ⓓ	131 Ⓐ Ⓑ Ⓒ Ⓓ	172 Ⓐ Ⓑ Ⓒ Ⓓ	218 Ⓐ Ⓑ Ⓒ Ⓓ
45 Ⓐ Ⓑ Ⓒ Ⓓ	86 Ⓐ Ⓑ Ⓒ Ⓓ	132 Ⓐ Ⓑ Ⓒ Ⓓ	173 Ⓐ Ⓑ Ⓒ Ⓓ	219 Ⓐ Ⓑ Ⓒ Ⓓ
46 Ⓐ Ⓑ Ⓒ Ⓓ	87 Ⓐ Ⓑ Ⓒ Ⓓ	133 Ⓐ Ⓑ Ⓒ Ⓓ	174 Ⓐ Ⓑ Ⓒ Ⓓ	

TEST GS-3

Answer Document 2

Writing Sample

1 1 1 1 1

IF YOU NEED MORE SPACE, CONTINUE ON THE NEXT PAGE.

1 1 1 1 1

IF YOU NEED MORE SPACE, CONTINUE ON THE BACK OF THIS PAGE.

1 1 1 1 1

_____

_____

_____

_____

_____

_____

_____

_____

_____

_____

_____

_____

_____

_____

_____

_____

_____

_____

_____

_____

_____

_____

_____

_____

STOP HERE FOR PART 1.

2 2 2 2 2

IF YOU NEED MORE SPACE, CONTINUE ON THE BACK OF THIS PAGE.

2 2 2 2 2

IF YOU NEED MORE SPACE, CONTINUE ON THE NEXT PAGE.

2 2 2 2 2

STOP HERE FOR PART 2. DO NOT RETURN TO PART 1.

Understanding

GS-1

Physical Sciences

Q 1 D   PHY 2.3

Let's use the process of elimination. **A.** is untrue as the fast moving air causes a lower pressure in the region above the wing (*see* Q2). **B.** has no relation to the question. **C.** is false because such a difference in pressure *between* the wings would lead to serious imbalances during flight. **D.** is correct and is the only answer which refers to two forces acting in opposite directions on the same object.

Q 2 C   P3, L5; PHY 6.1.3

A. and **B.** are false as stated in the passage (paragraph 3, line 5). Next, let's look at a bit of math: given "$xy + z$ = constant," means that if z increases, then xy must decrease for the equation to remain constant; if z remains the same but x doubles, then y must be halved for the equation to remain constant; etc. Let's look at the equation you're given: *Bernoulli's equation*:

$$P + \tfrac{1}{2}\rho v^2 + \rho gh = \text{const.}$$

We are told (P3, L5) that air (= *a fluid*) flows more rapidly (= *greater velocity*, v) above the wing than below the wing. Thus if the velocity 'v' is *less* <u>below</u> the wing, according to Bernoulli's equation, the pressure 'P' must be *higher* <u>below</u> the wing in order to keep the equation constant. {*A Phun with Physics Phact: wings are shaped as they are* (P3) *in order to allow pressure to increase under the wing which provides the force of 'lift' for the airplane and allows it to fly!*}

Q 3 A   P4, L1

Once again our friend Bernoulli has the answer. This time the velocity is constant but the height 'h' is changing. By looking at Bernoulli's equation it is clear that if the height 'h' increases then pressure 'P' must decrease - and *vice versa* (answer choice **A.**) - in order for the equation to remain constant. {*Superkeeners may try to argue that according to Newton's Law of Gravity, the force of gravity which affects 'g' should decrease as the plane moves farther from Earth, i.e. at higher altitudes. This argument is true but not relevant because moving from a low altitude to a higher one (which is measured from the plane to the <u>surface</u> of the Earth) is affected by magnitudes more than gravity over the same change in height (recall that the distance 'r' in Newton's Law of Gravity is measured from the plane to the <u>center</u> of the Earth!*)}

Q 4 B   PHY 3.3; *A + C = B*

The acceleration of an object which is moving in a circle (*centripetal acceleration*) acts toward the center of the circle when the object is at *constant speed* (that is, along answer choice **C.**). However, since the speed of the plane is <u>decreasing</u>, it experiences a <u>deceleration</u> (= *negative* acceleration) which acts along the tangent to the circle <u>opposite</u> to the direction of its velocity (that is, along answer choice **A.**). The resultant acceleration vector can be obtained by finding the vector sum of **A.** and **C.**, and this gives vector **B.** {*Had the speed been <u>increasing</u>, we would add **C.** plus a vector to be drawn in the direction of the velocity at point 'P' (i.e. opposite to **A.**); the sum vector would be in the general direction of **D.** See PHY Chap. 1 for vectors*}

Q 5 D   **PHY 6.1.3;** *Continuity, then Bernoulli*
From the continuity equation (Av = const.), the velocity of the fluid must be at its smallest value when the cross-sectional area of the region is the greatest. From Bernoulli's equation (which is valid because the flow is laminar, not turbulent), the region with the highest pressure is also the one with the smallest velocity (*see* Q2).

Q 6 D   **PHY 6.1.3**
It's this simple:

$$Flow = R = (volume)/(time) = Av = \textbf{CONSTANT !}$$

Thus the flow must be constant throughout (laminar).

Q 7 B   **CHM 1.6**
Let's look at H_2SO_3. The oxidation number of H is +1 and that of oxygen is -2. Therefore, not including S, the total oxidation state is $(+1 \times \underline{2}) + (-2 \times \underline{3}) = -4$. Since the molecule has no overall charge, the oxidation state of S added to -4 must be equal to zero; thus S = +4.

Q 8 D   **CHM 1.4**
The relative atomic mass of O is ≈ 16; that of H is 1.0; and that of S is ≈ 32. Thus the relative molecular mass of H_2SO_3 is $(2 \times 1.0) + 32 + (16 \times 3) = 82$. The mass of the molecular oxygen $(16 \times 3 = \underline{48})$ is more than half of 82. There is only one answer choice (**D.**) which is greater than 0.5! Alternatively, you can do it the old fashioned way: 48/82 etc. etc.

Q 9 C   **CHM 6.9**
The first end point in Fig. 1 uses a volume of NaOH of 30 mL and results in a pH of 3.6. The indicator used must change color in a range which *includes* the expected end point (= 3.6).

Q 10 B   **CHM 3.4**
By definition, a Lewis acid is a chemical species which accepts an electron pair (CHM 3.4). Answer choice **A.** is the Bronsted-Lowry definition of an acid (CHM 6.1).

Q 11 A   **CHM 9.7, 9.8**
Catalysts only affect the *rate* at which equilibrium is achieved, *not* the equilibrium position itself.

Q 12 B   **CHM 9.9**
Reaction I is <u>exothermic</u> (ΔH *is negative* ∴ *heat is released*). The reaction could be written as:

$$2SO_2(g) + O_2(g) \rightleftharpoons 2SO_3(g) + Heat$$

Adding heat (*increasing the temperature*) adds to the right hand side of the equilibrium forcing a shift to the left in order to compensate. The reverse occurs by *decreasing* the temperature thus creating a shift to the right which would produce more $SO_3(g)$ and more heat is *released*. {*Note: an increase in pressure would also lead to a right shift; see* Le Chatelier's Principle, CHM 9.9}.

Q 13 D   CHM 4.1.7

The sum of the mole fractions of each species present must be unity (= 1). Therefore, the partial pressure of O_2 is 1 - (1/6 + 1/2) = 1/3. The partial pressure of a species is given by the product of its mole fraction and the total pressure of the system. Therefore, the answer is given by 1/3 × 1 atm = 0.33 atm, approximately.

Q 14 B   CHM 6.5, 6.6

Since we are *told* to consider the first ionization of H_2SO_3 as if from a strong acid (Reaction II), we assume that the first proton completely dissociates. However, the second proton ionizes as if from a *very* weak acid (Reaction III). After all, a $K_a \approx 10^{-6}$ means that the product of the reactants is about 1 000 000 (*one million!*) times greater than the product of the products (*which includes the second proton; for* K_a *see* CHM 6.1). The preceding fact combined with the imprecision of the available multiple choice answers means that our answer can be estimated by assuming that H_2SO_3 acts as a strong monoprotic acid like HCl.

Therefore, one proton completely dissociates while the second proton's concentration is relatively negligible; thus $[H^+]$ = 0.01 mol dm^{-3} (1 dm^{-3}= 1 L^{-1}, App. B.2). The pH is equal to the negative logarithm of $[H^+]$ = -log (0.01) = -log (10^{-2}) = 2.

Q 15 A   PHY 11.4; P2, L3-5; P4, L5

The passage states that the refractive index is equal to the ratio of the velocities of light in a vacuum and in the medium (P2, L3-5).

$$n_{medium} = v_{medium}/ c$$

Since the value for n_{medium} is 1.00 when the medium is air (P4, L5), the velocity of light in air (v_{medium}) must be approximately that of light in a vacuum (that is, "c").

Q 16 B   PHY 1.1.1/2

If you know your trigonometry, this problem becomes a joke ☺ (PHY 1.1.1/2). Using the rules for right-angled triangles, tan θ_2 = 1000/1700 = 1/1.7. From knowledge, tan 30° = 1/($\sqrt{3}$), which is approximately equal to 1/1.7. Therefore, θ_2 is approximately 30°.{*Mathfax:* $\sqrt{2} \approx 1.4$}

Q 17 C   PHY 11.4

Time for equationrama !

$$v_1/v_2 = n_2/n_1 \therefore v_1 n_1 = v_2 n_2 = constant$$

Thus

$$v_{red} n_{red} = v_{violet} n_{violet} = constant \therefore \text{ given } \downarrow v_{violet} \text{ then } \uparrow n_{violet}$$

Q 18 B   P4, L5; PHY 11.4

Using the derivation of Snell's law which refers to the critical angle, $\sin \theta_c = n_2/n_1 = n_{air}/n_{water}$ (P4, L5), where "θ_c" is the unknown critical angle. Thus $\sin \theta_c = 1.00/1.33 \approx 1/(4/3) = 3/4 = 0.75$. {*Notice the importance of simple algebra, manipulating fractions, speed, etc.*}

Q 19 A   PHY 11.4

First: $\sin \theta_c = n_2/n_1 = n_{air}/n_{water}$

Now: $\sin \theta_{c2} = (n_{air} + x)/n_{water}$

Thus we increased the numerator by some value "x" which means $\sin \theta_{c2} > \sin \theta_c$, which also means $\theta_{c2} > \theta_c$.

Q 20 B   P2; PHY 11.4

From the passage, both <u>velocity</u> and <u>wavelength</u> (*different colors*) change (P2; *recall velocity and wavelength are directly proportional*, PHY 7.1.2). One should also know that the <u>intensity</u> (= *the rate of energy propagation through space*, PHY 8.3) of a light ray decreases when it passes through a medium other than air (*its velocity decreases in the medium and this leads to an overall loss of energy*).

Q 21 C   CHM 5.3.2

Since $MgCO_3 \rightleftharpoons Mg^{2+} + CO_3^{2-}$, $K_{sp} = [Mg^{2+}][CO_3^{2-}] = s \times s = s^2$, where s is the solubility. From the table provided, $s = 1.30 \times 10^{-3}$ mol L^{-1}. Thus $K_{sp} = [Mg^{2+}][CO_3^{2-}] = s^2 = (1.30 \times 10^{-3})^2 = 1.69 \times 10^{-6} \approx 1.7 \times 10^{-6}$. {*Mathfax:* $(13)^2 = 169 \therefore (1.3)^2 = 1.69$; *also, to increase speed you should at least be able to recognize the squares of numbers between 1-15, i.e.* $(12)^2 = 144$; *rules of exponents:* App A.4.1}

Q 22 B   CHM 5.3.2; B.: *more moles*

Consider these two equations:

    (i) $CaSO_4$ $\rightleftharpoons$ $Ca^{2+} + SO_4^{2-}$

    (ii) $Ca(OH)_2$ $\rightleftharpoons$ $Ca^{2+} + 2OH^-$

If $[Ca^{2+}] = s$ = solubility of salt, then:

    For (i) : $s^2 = K_{sp}$, therefore s = square root of K_{sp}

    For (ii): $(2s)^2 \times s = K_{sp}$, therefore s = cube root of $(1/4 \times K_{sp})$

Since K_{sp} is always *less* than 1 for sparingly soluble salts (i.e. *see the table provided in the problem*), the value for s obtained in (ii) *necessarily* is greater than that obtained in (i). {*For fun (!), work out values for 's' in (i) and (ii) using any value for* K_{sp} *less than 1*}

Q 23 C   P4, L 2-5; T

$SrCO_3$ is actually less soluble than the salt below it (*see the table in the passage*) despite the fact that Ba is situated lower down Group II in the periodic table. Thus the explanation given in the last paragraph has to be considered to explain the *stability* or extremely *low solubility* of $SrCO_3$.

Q 24 C   P2, L 4-7

The answer is clearly explained in the middle of the second paragraph.

Q 25 B   CHM 5.1.1/2

A non-volatile solute causes a lowering of the vapor pressure of the solvent and hence an elevation of the boiling point. The preceding is a *colligative property*.

Q 26 B   PHY 3.2, 3.2.1, 3.4

Since the 200 N block is <u>not in motion</u>, the value of the **frictional force** is *equal* and opposite in direction to the **applied force**, that is, 10 N.

Q 27 A   CHM 3.5T; ORG 1.2

As in ethene and SO_2, the sp^2 hybridized atom has a trigonal planar orientation.

Q 28 B   PHY 9.1.2

From the equation $F = kq_1q_2/r^2$, if the distance r is doubled then $(2r)^2 = 4r^2$, which means $4 \times r^2$ in the *denominator*. Thus the original force is quartered (= *decreased by a factor of* 4).

Q 29 D   PHY 8.3, 8.3.1

Let the number of decibels of sound Y be $dB_Y = 10 \log (I/I_o)$. If the intensity 'I' of sound X increases by a factor of 1000 then:
$$dB_X = 10 \log (1000 \times I/I_o) = 10 \log (10)^3 + 10 \log (I/I_o) = 30 + dB_Y .$$

{*For rules of logarithms see* CHM 6.5.1}

Q 30 A   PHY 4.1, 4.1.1

A simple torque force problem: let the fulcrum (= *the center of gravity of the bar*) be the pivot point (*draw a vector diagram i.e* PHY 4.1.1):
$$\Sigma L = CCW - CW = (100 \text{ kg} \times g \times 0.5 \text{ m}) - (75 \text{ kg} \times g \times x) = 0$$
Thus $(100 \text{ kg} \times g \times 0.5 \text{ m}) = (75 \text{ kg} \times g \times x)$
g cancels, manipulate to get: x = 50/75 = 2/3 m = 0.67 m (*CW is to the <u>right</u> of the fulcrum*).

Q 31 D   **PHY 4.3/4**

The external force acting on the cars is tiny compared to the large forces of the colliding vehicles (i.e. *friction is negligible*), so momentum is conserved (PHY 4.3). The total kinetic energy before collision is not equal to the total kinetic energy after the collision, thus it is not conserved and the collision is not completely elastic. It must be remembered that during a collision energy may change form (i.e. kinetic, heat, sound, etc.), but *total* energy must be conserved.

Q 32 B   **PHY 4.3, 4.4, 4.4.1**

Using the principle of Conservation of Momentum:

Momentum before collision = Momentum after collision

$(1200 \text{ kg} \times 7.5 \text{ m s}^{-1}) + (8000 \text{ kg} \times 3.0 \text{ m s}^{-1}) = (1200 \text{ kg} \times 3.0 \text{ m s}^{-1}) + (8000 \text{ kg} \times x \text{ m s}^{-1})$

Divide through by 400: $(3)(7.5) + (20)(3) = (3)(3) + 20x$

Isolate x: $(7.5 + 20 - 3)3/20 = x$

Thus $x = (24.5)(3/20) = 73.5/20 = 3 \; 13.5/20 \approx 3 \; 7/10 = 3.7 \text{ m s}^{-1}$.

{*Recall: momentum is a <u>vector</u>; in this problem the sign for the velocities are always positive because we are told that the vehicles are always moving in the same (i.e. northerly) direction*}

Q 33 C   **PHY 3.2; F = f < f$_{max}$; KW:** *tries*

This question is fun! We begin with the fact that the maximum frictional force that can be exerted occurs when the car is just about to move, and is equal to the product of the coefficient of friction (*static*) and the normal force on the car. Since the car is not moving perpendicular to the surface, using Newton's Second Law (F = ma), since the acceleration 'a' when the car is *about* to move is zero, the normal force is equal to the weight of the car (i.e. $\Sigma F = N - Mg = ma = 0$; thus N = Mg).

Therefore, the maximum frictional force $= 1/3 \times 1200 \text{ kg} \times 10 \text{ m s}^{-2} = 4000 \text{ N}$, approximately since we estimated 'g'. Since the force the car exerts (300 N) is less than the *maximum* frictional force on the car (4000 N), the car is *not* in motion. For an object not in motion, the sum of forces must be equal to zero (Newton # II !). Because the exerted force is 300 N, the *actual* frictional force must be 300 N in the *opposite* direction (cf. Q26).

Q 34 C   **PHY 3.2, 3.2.1**

The normal force on an object always acts perpendicular to the **surface**, in this case, the road. Friction depends on the normal force (*see* Q33). Since only a component of the weight of the car acts perpendicular to the hill, the value of the normal force <u>decreases</u>. Since the coefficient of friction remains the same, the value of the maximum frictional force <u>decreases</u>. {*Once an object is on an incline: N < weight of the object as determined by the cosine of the angle of the incline; this is worked out in* PHY 3.2.1}

Q 35 A   **PHY 5.4, 1.1.2**

Too easy! The potential energy (P.E.) = mass (m) × gravitational acceleration (g) × **perpendicular** height (h). "h" is given by $40\sin 30° = (40)(1/2) = 20$ m. The weight "m × g" is given already as 12 000 N. Thus $(20)(12\ 000) = 240\ 000$ J.

Q 36 B   CHM 4.3.3

Answer choice **B.** is a typical phase diagram for a substance. The exceptions to this rule include substances which exhibit larger intermolecular forces than usual, for example *hydrogen bonding*. These include water and ammonia, which would yield a phase diagram such as that in answer choice **A.** {*See the last paragraph of* CHM 4.3.3}

Q 37 D   P2, L 4-6, deduce

From the second paragraph, it is seen that the layers in graphite can move relative to one another. Hence, it can be used as a lubricant. No evidence is provided for any of the other properties as they relate to the layered structure of graphite.

Q 38 A   CHM 8.3, 1.4, ORG 3.2.1

From Table I we are *not* given $\Delta H_{formation}$; rather, we are provided with a new parameter which the table describes as the enthalpy of combustion ΔH_c of carbon. The end product of combustion (the oxide) of carbon is carbon dioxide. Now we can use Hess's Law knowing that the ΔH_c for $C_{graphite}= -393.3$ kJ mol^{-1} and for $C_{diamond}= -395.1$ kJ mol^{-1}. We can summarize the process as follows:

$$
\begin{aligned}
C_{graphite} &\rightarrow CO_2 & \Delta H_c &= -393.3 \text{ kJ mol}^{-1} \\
\underline{CO_2 \rightarrow C_{diamond}} & & \underline{\Delta H_c = 395.1 \text{ kJ mol}^{-1}} \\
C_{graphite} &\rightarrow C_{diamond} & \Delta H_c &= 1.8 \text{ kJ mol}^{-1}
\end{aligned}
$$

{*Notice the change in direction of the equation for* $C_{diamond}$ *was necessary in order to cancel the* CO_2; *thus the sign for* ΔH_c *was changed from negative to positive*}

Q 39 A   CHM 9.9

Since the density of diamond is greater than that of graphite (*see* Table I), the same number of carbon atoms occupy less volume in diamond than in graphite (density = mass/volume). An increase in pressure leads to a decrease in volume, therefore diamond formation will be facilitated (Le Chatelier's Principle). Although these rules usually apply to gases, extremely high pressures make the process possible with solids.

Q 40 D   CHM 3.5T, ORG 1.2

The rule is that an atom which exhibits tetrahedral geometry is sp^3 hybridized.

Q 41 C   CHM 2.3 (iv)

The smaller the atomic radii of the two atoms, the shorter the bond length. Bond **strength** is inversely related to bond **length**. Carbon has the *smaller* atomic radius thus it has the *greater* bond strength. {*This force of attraction is analogous to Coulomb's Law*, PHY 9.1.2, *where the positive nucleus is attracted to the bond which contains negative electrons*}

Q 42 C   deduce, CHM 7.5
Dark colors absorb light (*radiant energy*) to a greater extent than lighter colors.

Q 43 B   PHY 6.1.1
The passage explains how the solar collector can harness energy from the sun first by heating water. Liquids expand on heating and thus occupy a greater volume. Since density = mass/volume, the density of the liquid decreases when it is heated. Thus the heated water leaving the collector in draining pipes is less dense than the water being supplied to the collector. Of course, 1 L of the less dense water would yield a lower weight.

Q 44 C   CHM 7.5
Radiation is the only heat transfer process which can occur in a vacuum (outer space is essentially a vacuum in this instance).

Q 45 B   D.A.; CHM 8.7
Dimensional analysis is cool because it means you don't need to memorize an equation (!), you just have to define the terms and follow the units . . .
Area of collector = 20 m × 20 m = 400 m^2
Incident solar energy = 1600 W m^{-2} = 1600 J s^{-1} m^{-2}
Therefore, energy received per second by collector = 1600 J s^{-1} m^{-2} × 400 m^2 = 640 000 J s^{-1}
Rate of flow of water = 4 L s^{-1} = 4000 cm^3 s^{-1} {*see* Appendix B.2}
Mass of water going through collector in one second = 4000 cm^3 × 1 g cm^{-3} = 4000 g
From Q = mcΔt: 640 000 J = 4000 g × 4.2 J g^{-1}°C^{-1} × Δt
Thus   Δt = 38.1 °C
{*The answer could be quickly estimated by approximating 'c' as 4 and dividing through by 16 000; the answer obtained would be 40°C which is sufficiently accurate for this problem*}

Q 46 D   CHM 8.7; deduce
The <u>specific heat capacity</u> is the energy required to raise the temperature of a unit of mass of a substance by one degree. The smaller the specific heat capacity, the *less energy is required* to raise the temperature of that substance by a certain amount.

Q 47 A   PHY 6.1.1/2
Less dense solids or liquids float on *denser* liquids.

Q 48 B   CHM 4.3.3
The negative slope of the solid-liquid equilibrium curve in the phase diagram depicts that increasing the pressure causes a decrease in the melting point.

Q 49 C   CHM 4.2; ORG 11.1.2
Ammonia, like water, is a polar molecule. Ammonia possesses a partially negative nitrogen atom and a partially positive hydrogen atom (*see* ORG 11.1.2). Thus ammonia exhibits <u>hydrogen bonding</u>, which is the basis for the negative slope of the solid-liquid equilibrium curve in the phase diagram for water.

Q 50 A   CHM 5.1.1/2; *gluc*: increased particles/gram
This question tests your understanding of *colligative properties*. From the equation $T_b = K_B m$, where K_B is constant, "m" or the molality is the factor to be considered. Recall that m = (Number of moles solute)/(1000 g solvent) and number of moles = (Mass of substance present)/(Relative molecular mass). Since glucose has a smaller relative molecular mass than sucrose, there will be a greater number of moles of glucose present when equal masses of the two substances are used. Therefore, the molality of glucose is greater and hence the boiling point elevation is greater.

Q 51 D   CHM 5.1.2, 4.1.1
From the equation $T_f = K_f m$, $T_f = (2.0\,°C\,mol^{-1})(0.5\ molal + 0.5\ molal) = 2.0\,°C$. Therefore, the freezing point of this solution is $0\,°C - 2\,°C = -2\,°C = (273 - 2)\ K = 271\ K$.
{*Recall: acetic acid is a weak acid thus relatively very little dissociates*; CHM 6.1, 6.6}

Q 52 A   PHY 6.1.1, 6.1.2
The percentage of height of ice **below** the surface of mercury is = density of ice/density of mercury = $0.98\ g\ cm^{-3}/13.60\ g\ cm^{-3} = 1/14$ approximately = 7%. Therefore, the percentage of height of ice **above** the surface of mercury is = 100% - 7% = 93%.

Q 53 B   CHM 5.3.1
Let's begin with the total number of moles of Mg^{2+} present in the final solution: 0.05 moles/L × 0.02 L = 0.001 moles of Mg^{2+}. Next, let's look at the number of moles of Mg^{2+} obtained from $MgCl_2$: 0.005 moles/L × 0.005 L = 0.000025 moles of Mg^{2+}. Now we know the number of moles of Mg^{2+} we need supplied from $Mg_3(PO_4)_2$: (0.001 - 0.000025) moles = 0.000975 moles. Thus from the 15 mL of $Mg_3(PO_4)_2$ we need 0.000975 moles of Mg^{2+}. But each mole of $Mg_3(PO_4)_2$ contains **3** moles of Mg^{2+}! Therefore, the concentration of $Mg_3(PO_4)_2 = [(0.000975\ moles)/(0.015\ L)] \times 1/3 = 0.022\ mol\ L^{-1} = 2.2 \times 10^{-2}\ M$.
{*Note: the math is much faster if you notice that the answer to the second step is negligible thus you can skip the third step and the final calculation is easier*}

Q 54 B   CHM 10.1

The reduced species of the electrochemical equilibrium with the most negative $E°$ value is the strongest reducing agent (CHM 10.1). Memory aside (!), it is of value to note that a reducing agent reduces the other substance, thus <u>a reducing agent is oxidized</u>. Note that only answer choices **B.** and **C.** are oxidized (= *lose electrons*). When you write the two relevant equations as oxidations, instead of reductions like the table provided, you will note that only answer choice **B.** has a positive $E°$ value indicating the spontaneous nature of the reaction. The table provided demonstrates <u>half-reactions</u> written as <u>reduction potentials</u>. In order to write the oxidation, simply reverse the reaction and change the sign of $E°$:

Oxidation: $Cr^{2+} \rightleftharpoons Cr^{3+} + e^-$ $E° = 0.410$

Q 55 C   CHM 2.3(iii)

As one moves across the periodic table, the atomic radius decreases as a result of the increasing effective nuclear charge (*without an increase in the number of atomic orbitals*). In other words, the nucleus becomes more and more positive from left to right on the periodic table resulting in the drawing of negatively charged orbital electrons nearer and nearer to the nucleus. As a result, atoms will accept electrons more readily as we go across the periodic table and the electron affinity becomes more negative (*less positive*).

Q 56 B   PHY 1.6, 2.6, 4.3, 4.4

There are two parts to this problem. We begin by calculating the impact velocity of the 0.2 kg ball using the equation for speed V at any time t (i.e. PHY 1.6, 2.6): $V = V_o + at$, where V_o is the original speed. Since the ball starts at rest we get:
$$V = 0 \text{ m s}^{-1} + (5 \text{ m s}^{-2})(5 \text{ s}) = 25 \text{ m s}^{-1}$$

Using the principle of Conservation of Momentum and momentum = mass × velocity, we get:
Total momentum before collision = total momentum after collision
$$(0.2 \text{ kg})(25 \text{ m s}^{-1}) + (0.5 \text{ kg})(0 \text{ m s}^{-1}) = (0.2 \text{ kg})(0 \text{ m s}^{-1}) + (0.5 \text{ kg})(x \text{ m s}^{-1})$$
Isolate x: $x = 10.0 \text{ m s}^{-1}$

Q 57 B   PHY 7.2.1; F = mg = kx; k leading to W

At equilibrium the force of the weight ($W = mg$) will be equal to the spring force ($F_s = -kx$), thus: $kx = mg$, $k = mg/x = (1 \text{ kg} \times 10 \text{ m s}^{-2})/(0.5 \text{ m}) = 20 \text{ kg s}^{-2}$
Work done (*spring*) = $1/2 \ kx^2 = 1/2 \ (20)(0.5)^2 = 1/2 \ (20)(1/4) = (20)/(8) = 5/2 = 2.5$ J.

{*Note F = mg, g is estimated as 10 m s^{-2}*}

Q 58 A   E1

Simply plug the values into the equation; be careful about blood flow = (V/t) [= 80 cm^3 s^{-1}; P1, L11].

Q 59 D   **E1**

The radius is raised to the highest power in the equation (4). Therefore, a change in this value by any amount will be more pronounced than a similar change in another variable.

Q 60 C   **PHY 10.1, E1**

Manipulate Equation I to get: $\Delta P = (8Ln)/(\pi R^4) \times (V/t)$, which we are told is similar to $V = IR$, Ohm's Law. Therefore, if P is similar to the voltage and the flow V/t is similar to resistance, we are left with the term $(8Ln)/(\pi R^4)$ which must be similar to current.

Q 61 D   **E1**

If the radius is halved then R^4 changes to $(1/2 \times R)^4 = 1/16 \times R^4$. In order to balance this change by changing only one variable (i.e. *pressure*; see E1), pressure has to be increased by a factor of 16.

Q 62 A   **PV/nRT = 1 = const. (ideal)**

For an ideal gas, since $PV = nRT$ (CHM 4.1.6) then $PV/nRT = 1 = \underline{constant}$ for all measured values of the variables.

Q 63 B   **#1: F1; CHM 4.1.4/8**

Having deduced what a graph would look like for an ideal gas, examine carefully the positive slope of H_2 in the figure in Passage X. Notice how the curve shows values which are always *greater than* ideality (the constant PV/nRT). Ideally we would expect, if all else remains constant, if you double the pressure (i.e. from 50 atm to 100 atm), then according to 'PV = nRT' the volume would be halved (i.e. from 1 dm^3 to 500 cm^3). However, since we are evaluating a curve (H_2) whose values for PV/nRT are always *higher* than expected, then for a given pressure at constant temperature, the volume would necessarily be higher than expected (i.e. V > 500 cm^3).{*Recall: 1 dm^3 = 1 L = 1000 mL = 1000 cm^3*, App. B.1/2; *Plow and Thigh*, CHM 4.1.8}

Q 64 C   **CHM 4.1.2, 4.1.8**

The Kinetic Theory of Gases acknowledges that the particles in a gas possess kinetic energy, thus mass (*although they have negligible volume*).

Q 65 D   **CHM 1.3, 4.1.1/7**

We are told that the salt Na_2SO_4 is a "drying agent" thus we can assume it absorbs only water.
Number of moles of water absorbed = (Mass of water)/(relative molecular mass H_2O)
= 35.0 g / 18.0 g mol^{-1} = 36 g / 18.0 g mol^{-1} approximately = 2 moles
Given: 1 mole of a gas at room temperature and pressure = 24 dm^3 mol^{-1}
Therefore, volume occupied by 2 moles H_2O = 24 dm^3 mol^{-1} × 2 mol = 48 dm^3
Therefore, volume occupied by N_2 = Total volume of gas - volume of H_2O

$= 200 \text{ dm}^3 - 48 \text{ dm}^3 = 152 \text{ dm}^3$

Mole fraction of N_2 = (Volume occupied by N_2)/(Total volume of gas)

$= 152 \text{ dm}^3 / 200 \text{ dm}^3 = 19/25$

Partial pressure of N_2 = Mole fraction of N_2 × Total pressure

$= 19/25 × 1.00 \text{ atm} = 0.76 \text{ atm} = 0.8 \text{ atm}$ to one significant figure

Q 66 A   CHM 4.1.2, 4.1.8

A gas most closely approaches ideality at very low pressures (*thus making the relative volume that the gas particles occupy and the attractive forces between them negligible*) and at high temperatures (*so that the energy loss in inelastic collisions is negligible*).{*Plow and Thigh !*}

Q 67 A   CHM 4.1.2

If a gas is ideal, its particles have absolutely no attractive forces between them. Therefore, it should remain as a gas at all temperatures since liquefaction and solidification are based on mutual electrostatic forces of attraction between particles.

Q 68 B   deduce; P2, L8-13

The critical mass or size (P2, L8-10) would be achieved leading to a nuclear explosion via a nuclear chain reaction.

Q 69 D   P2, L7-13

The best answer is that the chain reaction depends on the *size* of the uranium sample, being of the *critical size*, which facilitates at least one neutron produced from a uranium-235 fission splitting another uranium-235 nucleus (that is, the chain reaction).

Q 70 C   PHY 12.3, 12.4

The sum of the atomic numbers (*bottom figures or subscripts*) and mass numbers (*top figures or superscripts*) must be the same on both sides of the arrow since matter cannot be destroyed or created (*at least not in MCAT Physics!*). From this, it is seen that "X" must be (essentially) massless and without charge. Gamma rays fit this description.

Q 71 A   D.A., PHY 5.7, Ap B.1

This problem is strictly a matter of dimensional analysis (*see* Part II, 2.3, #16 in The Gold Standard text).

1 Megawatt $= 10^3 \text{ kW} = 10^6 \text{ W}$

Therefore, power in watts = (Total number of watt-years)/(Number of years)

$= 2 × 10^6 \text{ watt-years}/6 \text{ years} = 0.33 × 10^6 \text{ W} = 3.3 × 10^5 \text{ W}$

Q 72 C   deduce, PHY 12.3

Gamma rays are the most energetic and have no mass, and hence they are the most penetrating kind of radioactive emission; consequently, gamma rays require the most pronounced safety precautions.

Q 73 C   CHM 4.2(3.); ORG 10.1(P3)

Answer choice **C.** is not necessary for the formation of a hydrogen bond. A classic example is that of ethers (ORG 10.1, P3). Ethers are water soluble because the oxygen in ether, which is covalently bonded to two carbons, can hydrogen bond with the hydrogen in H_2O.

Q 74 A   PHY 9.1.1, 10.1

Using $Q = It$

$$Q = (2.0 \text{ A})(1.5 \text{ min} \times 60 \text{ s min}^{-1}) = 180 \text{ C}$$

Therefore, the total charge Q is 180 C. The charge on an electron is 1.6×10^{-19} C per electron. Thus the number of electrons $n = Q/e$:

$n = 180 \text{ C}/(1.6 \times 10^{-19} \text{ C per electron}) = (180/1.6) \times 10^{19} = (1800/16) \times 10^{19}$

$n = (450/4) \times 10^{19} = 110 \times 10^{19}$ approximately $= 1.1 \times 10^{21}$ electrons

Q 75 D   CHM 2.3, D. = Helium

Helium (electronic configuration $= 1\underline{s}^2$) is unique since it is an s-block element and is a noble gas (Group VIII). All other s-block elements are in groups I and II, including answer choice **A.** (calcium), answer choice **B.** (magnesium), and answer choice **C.** (beryllium).

Q 76 C   CHM 9.3

By looking at Table 1, we can see that when the concentration of X is quadrupled (factor of 4^1) while [Y] is unchanged (Exp. 1 and 3), the rate is increased by a factor of $4 = 4^1$. Thus the order of the reaction with respect to X is 1. When the concentration of Y is doubled (factor of 2^1) while [X] remains the same (Exp. 1 and 2), the rate of reaction is quadrupled (factor of $4 = 2^2$). Thus, the order of reaction with respect to Y is 2. The rate equation is Rate = $[X][Y]^2$. {*Notice that the stoichiometric coefficients are not relevant*}

Q 77 A   CHM 5.1.2

Sucrose would be degraded to smaller molecules by the enzyme. Thus the number of molecules in solution would increase, leading to an increase in the number of moles of molecules. The molality of the solution would then increase [Molality = (Number of moles of solute) / (1000 g solvent)]. From $T_f = K'_f m$, the freezing point **depression** would increase and hence the freezing point would decrease. {*This problem is a classical example of a colligative property which depends on the underline{number} not the underline{type} of molecule or particle present*}

Understanding

GS-1

Verbal Reasoning

Explanation: the basis for the answers for Verbal Reasoning is the passage. Most answers are found directly in the passage which we have cross-referenced for you by paragraph and line in The Gold Standard Answer Key. Therefore, explanations for Verbal Reasoning are only given for selected questions which are either more challenging or reveal some teaching point. It is recommended that you review Part II, Chapter 3 in The Gold Standard text.

Q 81 B   P3, L1-4
When the question states "X is *like* Y. . . ," this is called a *simile*. Thus we must look for traits that are present in *both* X and Y. Answer choices **A.** and **D.** may be present in either a budding artist or an embryo but not necessarily both! Answer choice **C.** is false because an embryo is hardly influenced by cultural forces. Answer choice **B.** is correct because the simile begins with: "Just as an embryo retraces much of its *evolutionary past*, so the artist reinvents the first stages of art." That which is similar between the evolutionary past of an embryo and the development of a budding artist has nothing to do with culture but everything to do with answer choice **B.** This question is tricky for some students because the passage goes on to discuss the cultural aspect of the artist's development (P3, L3-6). As long as you remain focused on the question - *looking for that which is similar between X and Y* - then you can't be tricked!

Q 84 D   deduce
"The main idea of the passage" is a classic MCAT statement. You can bet that the answer choices will include more than one true statement from the passage even though only one answer will represent the actual *main* idea. How do we determine what a main idea is? It is the *theme* of the passage, a dominant concern or characteristic which can be ascribed to the passage. The main idea is *not* simply a topic which happened to be mentioned in a line or paragraph.

Answer choice **A.** is false since not only does the passage *not* focus on psychiatrists, there is no mention of art being "little understood by psychiatrists"; rather, in one paragraph (P4) there is mention of one psychiatrist who did not do "justice to artistic creativity." Answer choice **B.** is false despite the fact that it sounds appealing (!) and you may find some support for this response in the last paragraph; the fact is, sufficient support cannot be given for this response as being the *main* concern or characteristic of the passage.

Answer choice **C.** is false since its focus is "since the beginning of man" which may be alluded to sparsely in the passage but the history of art was clearly *not* the focus of the passage. Answer choice **D.** is true because paragraphs 1, 4 and 5 are all written to show that art *is* "one of the greatest forms of expression" **and** the largest paragraph (P2) focused on demonstrating that art "separates us from all other creatures across an evolutionary gap that is unbridgeable" (= *"available exclusively to humans"*).

Q 89 B   deduce
You must fully understand the main idea of the phenomenon described in the question before attempting to choose an answer. The 'phenomenon' referred to is that of four dimensions creating a "hypercube" which can exist without being detectable through usual human methods. The application of this concept to the study of the paranormal is similar: that psychic signals can exist without being physically detected, answer choice **B.** The central idea in this case is the basis for the speculation that psychic theorists might make. Answer choices **A.** and **C.** take an aspect of the concept described in the question that was not essential to the central idea and use this aspect to create a view of the paranormal. While this view might be taken, the

phenomenon in the question does not provide the basis for it.   In answer choice **D.**, the statement does not draw simply from the information given in the question, but on a further conclusion by the theorist that the concept described is wrong. The speculation is not based on the phenomenon described but on the beliefs of the theorist about the phenomenon.

Q 91 C   deduce

You first need to identify the theme of the passage. The passage starts out by acknowledging that too many cases of paranormal activity have occurred to explain them all away by coincidence (P1). However, while various means of explaining psychic phenomena have been proposed, there is no physical evidence to support any of these theories (P3; P8; P11, L10-13). The answer must be consistent with the ideas put forth in the passage. Answer choice **A.** has no basis in the passage. The passage in no way explores the issue of people who seek attention through lying about paranormal experiences. Answer choice **B.** states that the people actually have a special ability and even goes so far as to explain how this ability works. This information is stated as though it were a fact and this suggests some form of proof or evidence for the existence of this type of activity. Throughout the entire passage, the message is that these are proposed but unproven ideas. Therefore, they cannot be attributed to people as though they have been proven to exist. Answer choice **D.** is flawed in the same way as answer choice **B.** in that it states a method by which psychic signals may travel as though it is a proven fact. The passage stresses that there is no physical evidence, so these answer choices are not consistent with that theme.   Answer choice **C.** is consistent with the passage because it reaffirms the main ideas discussed in the passage.

Q 92 A   deduce; P1; P2

It is obvious that the U.S. government viewed overpopulation as a problem and that they actively tried to promote this view through the public schools. However, the passage also states that no law had committed the United States to this policy (P4, L3-4), eliminating answer choice **D.** The U.S. government could not have been indifferent to population growth, as stated in answer choice **C.**, because they actively promoted one side of the issue. Answer choice **B.** is incorrect because the passage states that at the same time as the campaign against population growth was going on, experts had yet to agree about whether a problem of overpopulation even existed, and some evidence was surfacing that population growth could be beneficial (P4, L4-8). The government had not based its actions on a determination of the actual effects of population growth, because if it had, its message would have been quite different. Answer choice **A.** is the only statement that is consistent with the information in the passage.

Q 96 B   deduce; P5

The statement "If not on the side of angels" is not meant to be taken literally. It is used to demonstrate a point. Angels are used as a symbol in this case. Angels for many people signify an embodiment of all that is good and moral, just as the devil is viewed as an embodiment of evil. By saying that Ehrlich was not on the side of angels, the author is suggesting that Ehrlich was not doing the right thing or was misguided in some way. Answer choices **A.** and **D.** take the view that the author was referring to angels quite literally which is not consistent with the rest of the passage. The statement is not used in the passage to introduce religion into the discussion, as the issue is never explored further. This eliminates answer choice **C.** Answer choice **B.** is correct because if Ehrlich was not on the side of angels (e.g. goodness, morality), he must have been on the wrong side of the issue.

Q 97 C   P4, L1-8

Two points to remember about this question: (i) in general, we are looking for the *best* answer; (ii) in this case, we are looking for the reason that the author is *most* disappointed in the government. There is no clear statement about that which has rendered the author most disappointed. Thus we must analyze the passage for suggestions of how the author might feel given the way she has written the article.

There is no evidence in the passage that answer choice **A.** is correct. However, answer choices **B.**, **C.** and **D.** seem like valid reasons why the author would be disappointed in the government. Now we must seek the *best* answer. This is easy because one of the answer choices is *overriding*; that is, one answer explains the others, thus one answer is most important. The passage suggests that the government disregarded available evidence supporting population growth (P4, L1-8; **C.**), then the <u>fall-out</u> from this primary error is that the government became committed to supporting programs which were aimed at reducing population growth *including* those programs geared to teaching children.

Q 101 D   deduce

Reading the end of the passage, you find the author saying that the attitude that population growth is bad for the country has become part of the way that vast numbers of people think (P6, L1-5). The author believes that the idea has simply been accepted without justification or further examination (P6, L6-7). Any attempt to examine the situation does not do so objectively, but starts by stating the current belief and works from there (P6, L8-10). From reading the passage, it is obvious that the author feels that the campaign against population growth was misguided and without sound basis (cf. Q96). For the author to feel anything but disheartened, there would have to be evidence that people are discovering or at least attempting to discover for themselves how out of tune with reality their beliefs about overpopulation really are. This is not the case, as shown in the author's closing remarks. People are not attempting to seek the truth as the author believes it to be, so answer choice **D.** is correct in saying that the author is disheartened (= *discouraged*).

Q 109 A   P2, L2; C: *traveller*

In paragraph two of the passage, we learn of Antipater of Sidon who listed six of the seven wonders of the ancient world. The passage suggests that the ancient wonders stretch into three continents (P3, L8; P5, L8; P6, L2). Thus Antipater must have been in a position in which he travelled or continually met travellers. Certainly, a general in a powerful army (i.e. *at war with or conquering other nations*) would fulfil both criteria.

Q 117 C   P1, L3-11

This question presents a simile (*see* Q81). Answer choice **B.** is not pertinent and **D.** uses the word "deobjectifies" which, when referring to the "camera" analogy as used in the passage, is exactly false! Answer choice **A.** is enticing only if one does not read the signals from the first paragraph of the passage. The emphasis when speaking of the "first image," science, is objectivity and neutrality. Thus the analogy of a camera is used effectively. In the context of the passage, answer choice **C.** mentions only the *similarities* between a camera and science as an objective field.

Q 121 D   P3; P4

Strategy: this passage and the questions that follow can be easy if you take the extra few seconds to annotate. For example, the passage states that the atmosphere *loses* carbon dioxide because of photosynthesis (P3, L3-4). Write "↓ CO_2" next to answer choice **A.** The passage states that in periods of oil formation the **earth retains** carbon dioxide (P3, L7-9). In other words, the atmosphere does not gain and in the long term *loses* carbon dioxide to the earth. Write "↓ CO_2" next to answer choice **B.** The passage states that great volumes of carbon dioxide is *lost* from the atmosphere when there are dolomite deposits (P4, L2-5). Write "↓ CO_2" next to answer choice **C.** And finally, the passage suggests that carbon dioxide may be *added* to the atmosphere from the interior of the earth by volcanoes. Write "↑ CO_2" next to answer choice **D.** Thus it is answer choice **D.** which changes the carbon dioxide balance in a different direction from the other answer choices. Annotating makes the answer very clear.

Q 124 D   P6, L7-10; KW: *counter*

Strategy: a quick reading of the answer choices reveals an important signal: answer choices **A.** and **D.** are in direct opposition. When two answers contradict each other, often but not always, one of the two answer choices is the correct answer to the question. In this case, the author describes the effect of the sun's radiation (P6, L3-7) in order to *counter* the theory that a colder climate is accompanied by increased precipitation (P6, L1-3; answer choice **D.**) and to *conclude* that colder climates result in decreased precipitation (*less snow*; P6, L7-10).

Q 129 A   P5; II. is false because of the word *readying*

This question is somewhat subtle. The passage clearly names books which have triggered the American Revolution and the Civil War (P5, L6-9). Thus you can put a tick (√) indicating 'correct' next to the response **I.** Now let's analyze the response **II.** which is essentially asking the following: was a book influential in *readying* England for vast expansion? The passage clearly notes that England *was* ready for vast expansion at the time *Wealth of Nations* was being written (P5, L3-5). The implication is that the latter influenced *how* the expansion occurred but the book clearly came during or after England's readiness for the said expansion. And finally, response **III.** is essentially asking the following: was a book influential in fuelling Hitler's rise to power? In the passage, there is no mention of any book with reference to Hitler. Thus you could put an "X" indicating false next to responses **II.** and **III.** providing you with answer choice **A.** as your final answer.

Q 130 C   deduce

Strategy: <u>beware of "true but unrelated" statements.</u> For example, the question refers to books which have there full impact years after the initial publication *within the context of the passage*. The author continually mentions books which have had enormous cultural, economic and political impact (P3; P5; P6). Answer choices **A.**, **B.** and **D.** may contain true statements but they are unrelated to the question in the context of the passage. On the other hand, answer choice **C.** presents a book with clear cultural, economic and political impact, all of which was felt years after its initial publication.

Q 132 A   deduce

Strategy: <u>beware of "politically incorrect statements"</u>! More often than not, statements like answer choice **B.** are false. Answer choice **D.** is false because the author actually demonstrates the opposite by continually providing specific dates, times and numbers. There is no strong evidence for answer choice **C.** However, almost every paragraph in the passage either alludes to human suffering from war or explicitly describes it. Thus answer choice **A.**, which happens to sound "politically correct," is the correct answer. {*Note the similarities in Q137*}

Q 136 A   P8, KW: *conflict*

This is another question where "to annotate is great"! Let's begin at the bottom. Response **III.** is essentially asking: did the author explore the *conflict* between lives preserved <u>versus</u> lives sacrificed? Paragraph 5 of the passage explores the preceding conflict thus you can put a tick next to response **III.** Paragraphs 2 and 3 explicitly explore the *conflict* between Imperialist Japan <u>versus</u> images of suffering Japanese. Consequently, you can put a tick next to response **II.** By now the process of elimination has begun to reveal the answer. But let's ask the question: did the author explore the *conflict* between modern Japan <u>versus</u> American culture? No, quite the opposite is revealed! The last paragraph of the passage (P8) shows that different elements of American culture are very popular in modern Japan (*suggesting harmony, not conflict*).

Understanding

GS-1

Biological Sciences

<u>Explanation: the basis for the biology and organic chemistry questions within Biological Sciences is very different. Thus we have chosen to provide the answers in different formats. Most biology answers are found directly in the passage which we have cross-referenced for you by paragraph, line and/or figure or diagram (when applicable). Therefore, explanations for biology are given in a similar format to the one used for Physical Sciences. On the other hand, MCAT organic chemistry questions usually rely on the ability to decipher the important information from the given passage and an understanding of the basics including mechanisms. Thus all organic chemistry questions and answers are explored in detail, beginning with a review of the passage itself.</u>

☞ You will often find that the Biology passages deal with advanced level topics or experiments. The key is not to become deterred by fancy words; rather, know what you know and concentrate on quickly understanding any graph or table presented. Do not try to understand details from the passage. Instead, read quickly and then focus on the questions.

Q 143 A   F1;P3, L6; KW: *diastole*
This question requires you to incorporate information from the figure with information given in the passage. Following vertically down from position P in Figure 1, note that it occurs during a period of diastole. In P3, L6 the passage gives information concerning the actions of the heart during diastole which would lead to answer choice **A.** Alternatively, the answer can be deduced through information in the passage and figure. In P1, L6-7 diastole is described as a period of ventricular relaxation, ruling out answer choice **B.** Position P in Figure 1 occurs during a period of diastole and it occurs at a point about halfway through that period, ruling out answer choices **C.** and **D.**

Q 144 A   F1, deduce, B: BIO 7.2
This entire passage relies little on your previous knowledge or understanding of cardiovascular physiology; rather, emphasis is on your ability to read a graph and, at times, correlate the information with the passage. This question indicates that we should be looking at the graph representing "Heart sounds" in Figure 1. The graph for heart sounds can be described thus: a horizontal line is followed by a narrow burst of spikes or activity; prior to the spikes is the label "1st" implying that the spikes represent the 1st heart sound. The first heart sound begins immediately after the first long vertical line. By following this vertical line downwards, we can note any other events which may initiate or occur at the time as the first heart sound: beginning near the bottom of Figure 1, note that the first heart sound occurs (i) in phase 2 of the cardiac cycle; (ii) at the beginning of ventricular SYSTOLE; (iii) during a period that the aortic and pulmonary valves are not opened (i.e. closed); and (iv) the first heart sound begins exactly when the position of the AV valves *just become closed*. Therefore, strictly according to the figure, during ventricular systole the AV valves suddenly close just as the first heart sound is created. Thus answer choice **A.** is the only plausible answer.

Q 145 C   BIO 7.2; P2, L6-7
Thicker walls in a particular part of the heart would indicate that it is more muscular, and therefore is more efficient or forceful during its contraction. This immediately rules out answer choices **B.** and **D.**, as they suggest that the thicker walled chamber would be less efficient or forceful. It should be known from the biology review (BIO 7.2) that the ventricles are more muscular (thicker-walled), but in the event that this is not initially known, information regarding the function of both the atria and the ventricles from the passage may help lead to this conclusion. First, systole, the period of contraction, refers to the period of contraction of the ventricles not the atria (P1, L5). This would indicate that the contraction of the ventricles might be more relevant in some way. Second, during diastole, atrial contraction occurs after

most of the ventricle is already filled (P3, L6-7) and serves to push the small amount of blood necessary to complete the filling into the ventricles. Since the atrial contraction does not need to move a large amount of blood (the ventricle is already mostly full), it does not need to be as muscular.

Q 146 C   G

This question is easily answered by reading the graph. Compared to the curve labelled 'control', the curve labelled 'sympathetic stimulation' is always at a higher stroke volume for a given end-diastolic volume. However, by looking at stroke volume values for both curves at any end-diastolic volume value (i.e. 200), it is clear that the stroke volume for sympathetic stimulation is always less than twice the control (i.e. 160 vs. 100), thus eliminating answer choice **A.** Thus we are left with answer choice **C.**

Q 147 B   deduce, B: BIO 7.3

It is commonly known that as a rule, the size of a muscle is proportional to its strength. The heart, which is a muscle, contains a chamber which must pump blood into the aorta to perfuse the grand majority of the body's tissues. Clearly, this chamber (= *the left ventricle*) must contain thicker muscle (= *stronger*) than a chamber that pumps blood only to the lungs (= *the right ventricle through the pulmonary artery*). The stronger chamber pumps blood with a greater force which means a higher pressure (*recall from physics: P = F/A;* PHY 6.1.2).

Q 148 C   F1

Close analysis of Figure 1 (*compare to* Q 144) reveals that during the period that the aortic and pulmonary valves are OPEN, the curve for left ventricular volume drops (= *decreases*) but does not rise (= *increase*).

Q 149 B   P1, L2-3; BIO 1.1.1

The passage states that sweat is less concentrated (with electrolytes) than blood plasma. The question asks how electrolytes would be transported *from* blood plasma (high concentration) *to* sweat (low concentration). Osmosis is the mechanism by which water, not electrolytes, is transported across membranes. Active transport is used to move molecules *against* their concentration gradient. Simple diffusion is the movement of molecules in the direction in which they naturally tend to move: from areas of high concentration to areas of low concentration, as in this case.

Q 150 B   P2, L3-5

The effect of two changes to the temperature of the body on sweating is being questioned here. One change, exposing the skin to heat, affects the outer parts of the body. The other, drinking iced water, affects the inner core of the body. The passage clearly states that sweating only occurs as a result of a rise in core body temperature (P2, L3-5). Therefore, heating the skin will not affect sweating. Since we now know that it is the iced water which will affect sweating it is a question of exactly what effect the iced water will have. A rise in core body temperature causes an increase in sweating, so it stands to reason that a decrease in core body temperature (caused by the iced water) will cause a decrease in sweating.

Q 151 C   deduce; B. is false because of the word *not*
This question, which is not well phrased, can be translated thus: you have been told that the temperature is constant (= 45 °C) and from Figure 1 you can see that the evaporation rate remains relatively constant for the first 20 minutes, why is this so? To begin with, what happens *after* 20 minutes? Points (a), (b) and (c) represent the moments when water is swallowed. Prior to these points we have a person at constant temperature, in a particular environment, with a constant rate of evaporation. The rate of evaporation is constant because the subject was provided time to enter a dynamic equilibrium or equilibrate with his environment. This time is necessary in order to understand what effects swallowing iced water will have on the equilibrium which was established in the first 20 minutes (= *baseline*).

Q 152 A   F1; P1, L4-6
By examining the figure, a direct relationship between hypothalamic temperature and rate of sweating (energy lost by evaporation) is shown. When one curve increases, the other increases and when one decreases, the other decreases. This leaves options **A.** and **B.** The passage states that the hypothalamus has a role in thermoregulation, which includes sweating (P1, L4-6). Thus it can easily be concluded that the rate of sweating is controlled by the hypothalamus and not vice versa.

Q 153 A   P2, L1-5
Since sweating occurs only as a result of changes in the core body temperature (P2, L4-5), drinking iced water will have an effect on sweating (*see* Q150). It decreases core body temperature, which will result in decreased sweating. Sweating causes heat to be lost from the body as latent heat of evaporation (P2, L1-2). When sweating is decreased less heat is lost through the skin, so skin temperature will increase. Alternatively, the other answer choices can be eliminated. Option **B.** does not answer the question. It gives an explanation as to why the skin temperature rose, but not why it rose after drinking iced water. Option **C.** hints at homeostasis, but the skin itself is never described in the passage as having a direct role in this function. Option **D.** states an observation, not an explanation.

Q 154 B   F1, deduce
The word *petite* is taken from the French word for *small*. The real question is: what's so small about the petite mutants? To begin with, we are told that their mitochondria have mutated such that this mutant yeast is an obligate anaerobe (= *an organism that survives in the absence of*

oxygen thus produces energy via anaerobic respiration only; P1, L2-3; BIO 2.2). Normally mitochondria produce energy via aerobic respiration which is much more energy efficient than the anaerobic pathway (BIO 4.4/5). Thus the mutants have, relative to the normal yeast cells, less energy from metabolism to reproduce, grow, etc. Consequently, we would expect a group (= *colony*) of petite mutants to be smaller than a group of normal yeast cells (= answer choice **B.**). Answer choice **D.** is physically impossible since daughter cells have nuclei and a nucleus is much larger than a mitochondrion (BIO 1.1F).

Q 155 B   P1, L3-6; B: BIO 1.2.1

The mutation in the wild-type mutant is such that the organism can still function. However, some part of a protein or enzyme must be affected in order to make the yeast an obligate anaerobe. Also, the mutation involves only the mitochondria, which have their own DNA. Therefore, the mutation which causes this phenotype would be located in the mitochondrial DNA, and would be such that no drastic changes would occur (as would be likely in a translocation). Options **A.** and **D.** can be ruled out because the passage states that the mutation is inherited in a nonchromosomal fashion (P1, L4).

Q 156 A   P1, L2; BIO 2.2; BIO 4.4/5

The mutant is identified by the fact that it is an obligate anaerobe, suggesting that normal phenotypes are likely facultative anaerobes. Thus the difference between the two will be related to this difference in mode of respiration. In the obligate anaerobe the anaerobic pathway is the only pathway that can be used. The anaerobic pathway leads to less ATP production per glucose molecule than the aerobic pathway. Facultative anaerobes can use either aerobic or anaerobic pathways depending upon the prevailing conditions. This means that the facultative anaerobe has the potential to produce more ATP than the obligate anaerobe, and this is the essential difference.

Q 157 B   F1 (b)

The processes of meiosis and mitosis with respect to the inheritance of the "petite" mutation are both drawn out in Figure 1. The end result of meiosis is four cells with both mutant and normal mitochondria present. The end result of mitosis can include cells which contain only the mutant mitochondria [i.e. complete inheritance of the "petite" mutation; notice the third cell from the left in the bottom of Figure 1 (b)]. Option **C.** can be ruled out because no division takes place in between the meiotic and mitotic divisions and therefore complete inheritance of any trait cannot occur. Option **D.** is incorrect because the passage states that the "petite" mitochondrial phenotype is inherited in a nonchromosomal fashion, and metaphase is a stage in chromosomal cell division.

Q 158 C   F1 (b); cf. Q 157

A respiratory deficiency would be present in cells that contain only the "petite" mitochondria. From the figure, all daughter cells of meiosis will contain a mix of both normal and mutant mitochondria, ruling out option **B.** The diploid zygote would combine two of these kinds of daughter cells, leaving a zygote also containing a mix of normal and mutant mitochondria. This rules out option **A.** Option **D.** is clearly incorrect as it states that the parent cell contains normal mitochondria. Only the daughter cells of mitosis as shown in Figure 1 could contain only the mutant mitochondria (*see* Q157).

Q 159 C   deduce; BIO 1.2.2, 1.3

The question is asking which component of the cell is involved in cell division. From the biology review it should be known that lysosomes are involved in digestive processes, the Golgi apparatus is involved in modification and packaging of proteins, and that tRNA is involved in protein synthesis. The only option left is DNA, which must have a function in directing cell division.

Q 160 C   ORG 5.2

This question is answered by ORG 5.2. For your interest, you may recall that a Lewis acid *accepts electrons* (CHM 3.4). In this way, the catalyst ferric bromide makes the reactant bromine quite positive. Bromine does not like to be positive!!!!!{*see* CHM 2.3 *and* PT} Now Br really, really, really wants electrons (= powerful electrophile). That's why it can add to the electron dense benzene ring.

Q 161 B   BIO 7.3; *vein → lung cap.*

This question can be translated thus: if something enters a vein in your arm, where is the *first* capillary bed which will be encountered? The following is simply part of the basic cardiovascular anatomy you need to know: vein in arm (= *upper body*) → larger veins → *superior* vena cava → right atrium of the heart → right ventricle of the heart → pulmonary artery → smaller arteries in the lung → arterioles in the lung → **capillary beds in the lung** → venules in the lung → veins in the lung → pulmonary veins → left atrium of the heart → left ventricle of the heart → aorta → many different arteries → many different arterioles → many different **capillary beds of the body system** including those that supply the heart muscle, the arms, the kidneys, the brain, the liver, etc. → venules → veins, and the story repeats itself.

Q 162 A   BIO 14.1

The structures and processes of the male reproductive system should be understood from the biology review.

Q 163 C   CHM 9.7/8/10; B: ORG 6.2.1

Q163 tests your understanding of a catalyst: they speed up the rate of a reaction, they decrease the activation energy, they do not affect K_{eq}, they are not used up in a reaction, and finally, to make a reaction more inclined to occur, ΔG, which is a measure of spontaneity, <u>decreases</u> (CHM 9.5, 9.7, 9.8, 8.10). If you're interested in dehydration of alcohols (!) see ORG 6.2.1.

Q 164 D   ORG 6.2.3/4; cf. Q212

This question will be fully explored in the answer for <u>Q 212</u> using LDA as an example.

Q 165 D   P1, L5-7; BIO 1.1

The passage gives various functions of glycoproteins. The question asks which of the cellular components has characteristics that would suit the special functions of a glycoprotein. A phospholipid bilayer is a membrane, and one of the functions of the oligosaccharide attached to a protein is to anchor the protein to a membrane.

Q 166 B   BIO 1.2.1

To answer this question basic knowledge of the function of various cell components is necessary.

Q 167 C   P1; P2, L1-3

The passage states that the glycoprotein is formed by attaching carbohydrate groups through covalent bonds. Therefore, to interfere with this formation, an agent that destroys these covalent bonds is needed.

Q 168 B   P3, BIO 5.4.1

From the passage it is found that collagen involves a disaccharide linked to hydroxylysine. If all hydroxylysine residues are replaced by asparagine, the function of collagen is sure to be affected. It is necessary to know from the biology review that collagen is an important component of the loose connective tissue in order to correctly answer the question (BIO 5.4.1). It is possible, however, to narrow down the options. One function of the oligosaccharide part of the glycoprotein is to aid in recognition (P1, L6-7). Since only the protein part of the glycoprotein is changed, protein recognition should remain possible. This rules out option **D.**

Q 169 C   deduce, B: BIO 5.1. 5.1.1/2

Given that glycolipids are a critical component in membranes, including myelin sheaths (P4), and all four answer choices involve cellular events which involve the plasma membrane, the real question becomes: which of the following processes relies *least* on the glycolipid part of the plasma membrane. The initial generation of a nerve impulse depends on the activity of membrane channels which are <u>proteins</u> (BIO 1.1/2/3, 5.1.3).

Q 170 C   P4, L5-8; BIO 5.1
The passage states that glycolipids are found in abundance on the surface of nerve cells, as part of the myelin sheath. To answer the question, knowledge about the structure of neurons is required (BIO 5.1). Fibers lying in grooves on the surface of the neurolemma of glial cells are unmyelinated. Nodes of Ranvier are unmyelinated spaces *between* myelin sheaths. Cell bodies of neurons are not covered by a myelin sheath. Schwann cells themselves make up the myelin sheath and will thus be most affected by any irregularity in glycolipid production.

Q 171 D   P1, L6-9; KWs: *change, one*; cf. BIO 15.5
The key to this question is to realize that the passage describes the mutation resulting in the <u>change</u> of <u>one</u> amino acid of the 146 amino acids (P1, L6-9). The passage does NOT state that the number of amino acids was *reduced* to 145 (answer choice **B.** is false), nor that *two* amino acids changed (answer choice **A.** is false), nor that the number of amino acids *increased* to 147 (answer choice **C.** is false). Only a <u>substitution</u> of one amino acid for another results in the *change* of *one* amino acid of 146 without altering the length of the polypeptide.

Q 172 C   P1, L5-11; ↓O_2 BIO 4.7/8
Sickle cell anemia lowers the oxygen-carrying capacity of red blood cells. This means that less oxygen is reaching the cells for use in cellular respiration. Fermentation of pyruvate to lactate and ATP will occur in the absence of oxygen, which is not the case here. Glycolysis occurs whether oxygen is present or not, so this process will also be unaffected. Option **D.** states that carbon dioxide is produced through the processes of the Electron Transport Chain, which is incorrect. We are left with option **C.** which makes sense because oxygen is needed to form carbon dioxide and water, and is also used in *oxidative* phosphorylation.

Q 173 B   F1; BIO 15.3
This question tests your understanding of Mendelian genetics (BIO 15.3) and your ability to understand Figure 1. Let "S" = the sickle-cell allele, let "s" = absence of the sickle-cell allele; each individual has two alleles, thus "SS" = homozygous resulting in sickle-cell anemia, "ss" = homozygous for normal red blood cells, "Ss" = heterozygous meaning sickle-cell trait (P1, L11-12; F1). Now we turn our attention to Figure 1. Carefully read the explanation which follows the diagram. Thus the heterozygous male is the square at the top left corner of Figure 1. If this were a homozygous normal male (ss, *as the question proposes*) mating with the homozygous normal female in the diagram (ss), the result is ss × ss. Using a Punnett square, it becomes clear that all possible offspring (= *second generation*) will also be ss. Thus in the second generation, we have an ss male mating with an Ss female (i.e. ss × Ss). The Punnett

square reveals that the offspring (= *third generation*) will be 2/4 or 1/2 normal (ss) and 2/4 or 1/2 sickle-cell trait (Ss), thus the ratio is 1:1.

	S	s
s	Ss	ss
s	Ss	ss

Q 174 B   F1
Carefully read the explanation which follows Figure 1. Now you can count only 1 circle which is "filled" (= *shaded*), indicating a female who is homozygous for sickle cell anemia. Now by looking at the column directly underneath the filled circle, we see <u>one</u> line which corresponds to 13 kb on the y-axis (*no deeper understanding required!*).

Q 175 C   P2, L6-9
The passage suggests that detection of polymorphisms (through restriction fragment length polymorphism) could be useful in pre- or postnatal diagnosis. It would follow that if the polymorphism can be detected in the child, then the same polymorphism could be detected in one or both of the parents. In this way parents may be advised of their chances of producing a child who will display the particular trait that is associated with the polymorphism before they try to conceive (e.g. genetic counselling). The other applications listed as answer choices may be useful in characterizing particular groups of people, but the practical implications are not explored by the passage.

Q 176 C   deduce
This question is challenging. Answer choice **A.** is false because for survival, eukaryotes usually require oxygen, carbohydrates, etc., but *not* a specific amino acid in a specific polypeptide; even if it were the case that the organism needed the replaced amino acid to survive, it could certainly find that amino acid in other cellular proteins. Answer choice **B.** is false because the explanation is improbable (BIO 15.5) and the passage does not even hint of linked genes. Answer choice **D.** is false because the word "patients" implies people with the disease yet the question only refers to people with the trait (cf. P4/F1). Then we are left with the plausible explanation in answer choice **C.** which suggests that the organism cannot procreate in an environment where 40% of the hemoglobin is abnormal (P1, L11-14).

GS-1, Passage VI, Questions 177-183

Since this is our first organic chemistry passage together we'll discuss it in detail. Afterwards, you'll begin to notice the trends then we'll speed up a bit more.

▸ Principle #1: Organic Chemistry is simple.

▸ Principle #2: It's OK to learn new words (i.e. *solvolysis*) during the exam!

Let's solve the problem. Read the first paragraph. Now you should want to know what tert-butyl bromide looks like. Draw it below. {*If you can't, see* ORG 3.1 *for tert-butyl and simply attach "Br" to the free bond*}

▸ Principle #3: Think about the preceding molecule. Begin by assessing electronics: bromine is a halogen to the right of carbon on the periodic table thus it is more electronegative (inscribe δ^- next to Br). Since Br is drawing electrons away from the central carbon which it is attached to, that carbon becomes partially positive, δ^+. {*see* ORG 1.5; CHM 2.3}

▸ Principle #4: Recognize. Notice how bulky the molecule is. Compare the molecule with less hindered ones with the same number of carbons, i.e. sec-butyl which has a secondary carbon or n-butyl (*normal* butyl) which has a primary carbon. Steric hindrance {*see* ORG 6.2.3/4} means that the partially positive carbon has so many attached groups around it that if you were a nucleophile, with your negative or partially negative charge, you would have a difficult time gaining access to that carbon which attracts you. If you can't reach the carbon *nucleus* then you can't engage in *nucleo*philic substitution.

Remember, you're still a nucleophile. You want something positive but you can't get to the carbocation. However, you have your pick of hydrogens! {*H is slightly more electropositive compared to carbon see* ORG 1.5; CHM 2.3} Removing or *eliminating* H from t-butyl is the start of an *elimination* reaction. Note, for this reaction to occur, we would need a hydrogen-hungry strong nucleophile like OH⁻ or $C_2H_5O^-$ (*ethoxide*, which was added to Reaction I in the passage).

☞ KEY CONCEPT: If we started with a primary compound (i.e. n-butyl bromide) and added a nucleophile (you!), the nucleophile has easy access, and is attracted, to the partially positive carbon. Thus the nucleophile adds to the central carbon and bumps off the leaving group (Br) = *nucleophilic substitution, second order* = S_N2. "Second order" emphasizes that the rate-determining step depends on the concentration of <u>two</u> compounds - the nucleophile and n-butyl bromide (ORG 6.2.3).

However, <u>this problem</u> begins with a <u>tertiary</u> <u>hindered</u> compound which, as we described, may undergo *elimination*, and for the same reason as previous, it is also *second order* = **E2** (ORG

6.2.4). Once a hydrogen is eliminated by the nucleophile, we are left with the very unstable but intermediate primary carbanion whose electrons are quickly put to use by forming a double bond and bumping off Br^-. Thus the product is $(CH_3)_2C=CH_2$. It's name is 2-methyl-1-propene. It contains hydrogens that are arranged similar to those of the vinyl group (ORG 4.1). Draw the E2 mechanism and the product below (ORG 6.2.4).

Is there a second possible mechanism? That question is both excellent and rhetorical! Here is an expression to memorize: *tertiary carbocations are relatively stable*. Why? Here is another expression to memorize: *alkyl groups are somewhat electron donating*. In other words, if you were a primary carbocation, you would be pretty unstable! You would try to hold on to a formal positive charge without any help - too difficult. However, if you were a tertiary carbocation surrounded by three alkyl groups - each of which will tend to reduce the burning positive charge on the central carbon with cool electrons!

Because of the stability of tertiary compounds, the second mechanism has one*** compound in its rate-determining step: t-butyl bromide in solution can simply dissociate into Br^- and the stable t-butyl$^+$. Draw this reaction.

Now a nucleophile would be happy to *quickly* mate with the positive carbocation (*nucleophilic substitution, first*** order* = S_N1). If the nucleophile is hydroxide, or water (**Q 178**), then the product would be the tertiary alcohol tert-butanol $(CH_3)_3C$-OH {*note* -OH *substituted* -Br}. If the nucleophile is ethoxide, or ethanol, then the product would be the ether $(CH_3)_3C$-OCH_2CH_3. {*The preceding product can be named t-butyl ethyl ether, or, ethoxy t-butane; see ORG 10.1*}

Now let's read the second paragraph in the problem! By analyzing the possible mechanisms we now can say with confidence that Compound A must be the S_N1 product ethoxy t-butane $[C_6H_{14}O = (CH_3)_3C$-$OCH_2CH_3]$. Compound B, with its vinylic protons, must be the E2 product 2-methyl-1-propene $[C_4H_8 = (CH_3)_2C=CH_2]$. The latter is the answer to **Q 177**.

The third paragraph tells us what we already know! This includes: (i) there are two possible mechanisms each of which are identified with different rate constants k_1 and k_2; (ii) since the rate is given by:

$$\text{rate} = k_1 [\text{t-BuBr}] + k_2 [\text{t-BuBr}][C_2H_5O^-]$$

Thus the first reaction mechanism (k_1) is first order (S_N1) while the second (k_2) must be second order (**E2**). {*the order of the reaction = the sum of exponents, see CHM 9.2*}

Back to the passage! After some irrelevant info, we come to the final two paragraphs concerning Reaction II. Once again, we already KNOW ALL THIS STUFF!!! To begin with, the ethanol in the solvent system created the compounds A and B according to the S_N1 and E2 mechanisms we've discussed. Then Compound C is produced by the reaction of t-BuBr and the water in the solvent system producing tert-butanol $(CH_3)_3C\text{-}OH$ (S_N1 which we looked at a few paragraphs ago...). Thus the passage gives us the correct molecular formula, $C_4H_{10}O$, and the correct IR absorbance for an alcohol (= hydroxyl group, **Q 178**) which *we*'ve memorized from ORG 14.1 !

On to **Q 179**: for the purposes of the MCAT, the key rule of thumb is that increasing strength of the conjugate acid (*see* CHM 2.3 (v) *and* PT *for trends in electronegativity which affects a compounds ability to ionize*) means better leaving group (*see* ORG 6.2.4, *last paragraph*).

Q 180 can be answered by looking at the rate expression or by working out the S_N1 mechanism as we did. Note that E2 is not an answer choice. But if it were, it still would <u>not</u> be the best answer! "Pure ethanol" = no ethoxide = no hydrogen-hungry strong nucleophile = E2 is about as probable as adoring your in-laws. It's not impossible, but it's not likely either.

Q 181 reminds us that the S_N1 mechanism occurred in *both* reactions I and II. In other words, t-Bu$^+$ is the stable tertiary <u>carbocation</u> intermediate prior to the nucleophilic reaction with ethanol/ethoxide (Reaction I) or water (Reaction II). {*see* ORG 6.2.3}.

Q 182 has been answered many different ways already: A=S_N1, B=E2, and C=S_N1.

Q 183 points to the second paragraph of the passage which suggests that the reaction occurred spontaneously, which means $\Delta G < 0$ (see CHM 8.10), which also means that the great likelihood is that $\Delta H < 0$. The latter is called an *exothermic* reaction (CHM 8.2). Since energy is released, the reactants must have a higher energy and the products must have a lower energy (sample curves: CHM 9.5). The only possible answers are **A.** and **C.** However, the intermediate in **A.** has a low energy which indicates stability implying that any further reaction is not likely to be spontaneous (from the mechanisms we did we know this to be false, untrue and unpleasant to hear). Answer choice **C.** suggests a higher energy intermediate which would be happy to engage in a further reaction to create a low energy, very stable final product.

Q 184 B   P1, L10-12; BIO 7.5.1
The passage states that "the net effect of GBP is to <u>shift</u> the oxygen-binding curve . . ." (P1, L10-11), thus the curve may move in one direction or the other but the passage does not say that the *shape* of the curve is altered. Therefore, to answer this question, we only need to

identify a curve with the same shape as the oxygen-binding curve (= *oxygen dissociation curve*) which is sigmoidal (BIO 7.5.1).

Q 185 C   P1, L4, L12-16
The effect of GBP is to cause a greater release of oxygen at areas of lower oxygen tension, without affecting the ability of hemoglobin to pick up oxygen at high pressures (i.e. in the lungs). To release oxygen to the cells, the affinity of hemoglobin for oxygen must be low, but only at those points at which oxygen is needed (where oxygen concentration is low; B: BIO 7.5.1).

Q 186 A   P2, L3-4; G
According to the passage, myoglobin will only start to release oxygen at pressures below 20 mmHg. To answer the question you must find the curve on the graph which shows the percent saturation of oxygen to be very high at oxygen partial pressures greater than 20 mmHg with a distinct lowering of the percent saturation occurring at pressures lower than 20 mmHg.

Q 187 B   P1, L12-16; BIO 4.5, *debt: vol. muscle*; BIO 11.2
The passage suggests that when exposed to body tissues other than lung, in other words parts of the body with relatively low oxygen concentrations, both myoglobin (P2, L2-6) and hemoglobin with GBP (P1, L12-16) begin to release oxygen at a tremendous rate. The question can be translated thus: which of the following tissues can deplete its oxygen reserves quickest and thus would benefit most from a molecule which is used to delivering oxygen to oxygen-starved tissue? Oxygen debt can be most pronounced in skeletal muscle. Voluntary or *skeletal* muscle can deplete its oxygen stores so quickly that it switches to anaerobic respiration thus incurring an oxygen debt (BIO 4.5). The oxygen tension (= *partial pressure* = *concentration*) in this tissue is extremely low and will therefore benefit most from an influx of oxygen. {*Note that myoglobin like myosin implies muscle*}

Q 188 D   deduce
This question reveals an interesting physiology lesson. Here is a statement you can easily deduce or should be memorized (!): *an exercising muscle is acidic, hot and has a high partial pressure of carbon dioxide; an exercising muscle requires increased quantities of oxygen* (= answer choice **D.**).

For your interest, we will examine the details: an exercising muscle is acidic because of (i) the accumulation of lactic *acid* (BIO 4.5) and (ii) the high partial pressure of carbon dioxide which results in an increase carbonic *acid* (BIO 12.4.1). An exercising muscle is hot because of the increased metabolic rate and blood flow. Carbon dioxide is in high concentration in an exercising muscle since it is a product of aerobic respiration (BIO 4.4).

If you were to draw a sigmoidal shaped oxygen-binding curve to the right of answer choice **B.** in Q186, you will notice that for a given partial pressure of oxygen, the curve shows a greater tendency to unload oxygen (= *a lower oxygen saturation*). Thus the exercising muscle gets increasing oxygen delivery as the curve shifts to the right.

Q 189 B   P1, L12-16; Q188

This question boils down to the following: as described in the answer for Q188, if the tissue is acidic then it needs increased oxygen delivery to those tissues. Only answer choice **B.** delivers oxygen to the tissues.

Q 190 C   BIO 14.5

The stages of embryogenesis must be known from the biology review to answer this question.

Q 191 D   BIO 6.1

Only two of the answer choices should seem possible: the ganglion and the nucleus. A ganglion is a cluster of nerve cell bodies in the *peripheral* nervous system, while a nucleus is a cluster of nerve cell bodies in the *central* nervous system.

Q 192 D   BIO 14.7

You can only understand fetal circulation (BIO 14.7) if you understand normal adult circulation (BIO 7.2/3). The *ductus arteriosus* connects the pulmonary artery to the aorta. If the ductus arteriosus remains open or *patent* after birth, some of the deoxygenated blood from the pulmonary artery will flow through the ductus into the aorta which contains fresh oxygenated blood from the newborn's lungs. Thus the mixing causes a <u>decrease</u> in oxygen and an <u>increase</u> in carbon dioxide partial pressures in the aorta. The aorta leads the blood into systemic arteries and circulation.

Q 193 D   BIO 5.2 (i)

The process of muscle contraction must be well understood to answer this question. Option **C.** contains a correct statement, however it does not answer the question as it is not related to muscle contraction.

Q 194 A   ORG 12.1.2

You should be familiar with the concept of isoelectric point from the organic chemistry review.

Q 195 C   P1, L5-6; D.A.
Minute ventilation = tidal volume × respiratory rate
Minute ventilation = 500 ml/breath × 12 breaths/minute × (1 L)/(1000 ml) = 6.0 L/minute
{*D.A. = dimensional analysis*, Part II 2.3 #16 in The Gold Standard text}

Q 196 A   P2; P3, L4-7; BIO 12.4
By various mechanisms (BIO 12.4), inspiration increases the size of your chest, or more precisely, your thoracic cavity. The increased amount of air in the chest in combination with the chest's desire to return to its initial position (= *recoil*) leads to an increased pressure in the lungs (= *transpulmonary*). Airway radius is inversely proportional to airway resistance (P2).

Q 197 C   deduce; cf. Q196
We are told that there exists fibers which *pull* on the airways and become *stretched* during inspiration. The preceding implies that the radius of the airway is increased by the stretching of the fibers. Thus both transpulmonary pressure (Q196) and lateral traction result in an increase in airway radius.

Q 198 D   P4, L1-4; deduce: *post-pulmonary vessel*
This is a classic MCAT/Sesame Street type of question: "one of these things is not like the other . . ." The vena cava, the pulmonary artery and the femoral ***vein*** all carry deoxygenated blood to the lungs. Among our choices, only the aorta carries blood *away* from the lungs. Thus the aorta would be a perfect place to have receptors which would indicate whether the carbon dioxide exchange in the lung required an increase or decrease in respiratory rate (P4) in order to improve the quality of the blood supply to the rest of the body's organs.

Q 199 B   deduce: BIO 12.4
Clearly if food is stuck, for example, in the trachea then inspiration may pull the food into the lung (= *not good!*), but <u>expiration</u> could expel the food from the body (= *much better!*). The events in expiration normally include <u>decreasing</u> the size of the thoracic cavity and relaxation or <u>raising</u> of the diaphragm (BIO 12.4). The fact that the Heimlich Maneuver includes an upward abdominal *thrust* means that it is a <u>forcible</u> maneuver which suddenly increases the size and pressure in the thoracic cavity thus dislodging the food.

GS-1, Passage IX, Questions 200-204

Now that we know each other, we don't have to go into too much detail! The passage is self-explanatory so let's look at the questions. . .

Q 200 shows how irrelevant a passage can be! This question is testing your ability to combine a few important ideas: (i) substituents affect the acidity of phenols (ORG 10.2); (ii) halides (i.e. Br) are weakly deactivating groups but they are O-P Directors (ORG 5.2.2); (iii) activating groups (O-P Directors *except* halides) decrease the acidity of the phenol (ORG 10.2); (iv) in summary, where EDG = electron donating group and EWG = electron withdrawing group, we get:

EDG	**EWG**	**EWG: Halogens**
activates the ring	*deactivates the ring*	*weakly deactivating*
O/P Directing	Meta Directing	O/P Directing
i.e. alkyl groups	i.e. nitro ($-NO_2$)	i.e. bromine
acid weakening	acid strengthening	acid strengthening
↑ pK_a	↓ pK_a	↓ pK_a

☞ The Reasoning: Electron withdrawing groups can stabilize the *negative* charge on oxygen which encourages oxygen to lose a proton (i.e. *become more acidic*). When a compound becomes more acidic, K_a *increases* (CHM 6.3) thus pK_a *decreases* because $pK_a = -\log K_a$.

Q 201 tests your ability to read the diagram. For each compound, there are only two choices: Sol. (*soluble*) or Insol. (*insoluble*). By following the diagram, step by step, only one compound can be <u>insoluble</u> in water, NaOH, HCl, and H_2SO_4: compound IX. Why not compound III? Because it is <u>soluble</u> in NaOH !

Q 202 is seeking to remind you that benzoic acid is a carboxylic acid with 7 carbon atoms (*see* ORG 8.1). By quickly examining Table 1 in the passage, you may agree that Group III includes benzoic acid. And finally, looking at Group III in Figure 1 makes the answer reveal itself!

Q 203 sends us back to Figure 1. Group I is soluble in water which is defined as *hydrophillic* (BIO 1.1). The only possible answers are **A.** and **D.** The former is not the better answer since it only mentions the <u>basic</u> feature of amino acids. But of course amino acids, even small ones, contain both basic and acidic groups = *amphoteric* (ORG 12.1.2).

Q 204 can be solved by drawing a quick diagram of the acid-catalyzed ester hydrolysis reaction (see the third reaction in ORG 9.4). For your own interest consider drawing the whole mechanism (in the exam it should quickly fly across your cerebral cortex).

The story goes something like this: The catalyst (H^+), being the most charged substance is implicated first. Thus the electrons from the electronegative oxygen (O^*) are attracted to the proton (H^+) and bonds. Now oxygen (O^*) has the positive charge. Electronegative oxygen does not like to carry positive charges! Thus with haste it draws electrons to itself from a covalent bond (i.e. its bond to the central carbon). Thus HO*R' is the leaving group and now the central carbon carries the positive charge. Now the juicy lone pair of electrons on the oxygen in H_2O is quickly attracted (= *nucleophile*) and then bonds to the carbocation. The extra hydrogen in water is kicked out as a proton (regenerating our catalyst) producing a carboxylic acid.

Back to the question: if water is exchanged for an alcohol, the only thing that changes is the last step in the story. Now the alcohol is the nucleophile. Instead of producing a carboxylic acid, we produce another ester.

Q 205 C   KW: *nature*; ORG 12.3.1

The question asks which characteristic of carbohydrates does not add to their diversity *in nature*. Naturally occurring carbohydrates exhibit both linear and ring form. They can form tautomers (B: ORG 7.1), and may also differ in the structure of the linkages between monosaccharides. However in nature, nearly all carbohydrates exhibit the D form of the two possible optical isomers at the highest numbered chiral carbon. This limits the effect that optical isomerism will have on the diversity of carbohydrates.

Q 206 C   deduce; P1, L6-10

Cellulose is passed through the mouth, stomach and small intestine unchanged. It is only because of bacteria in the large intestine that cellulose gets broken down at all. This would indicate that humans do not possess enzymes to break down this particular polysaccharide (cf. P2).

Q 207 C   BIO 9.3

The components of gastric juice in the stomach should be known from the biology review. One of these, pepsinogen, converts to its active form in low pH to become pepsin. Pepsin acts to break down proteins in the stomach. However, the great majority of digestion is completed in the small intestine.

Q 208 D   BIO 1.1, 1.1.2

Membranes are usually semipermeable. Small neutral molecules can pass relatively freely by diffusion. Monosaccharides, however, are large *polar* molecules thus require some assistance in crossing the hydrophobic interior of plasma membranes. Exocytosis and endocytosis are found most commonly in the context of releasing proteins or ingesting large particles (i.e. viruses, bacteria). Therefore, carrier mediated transport is most likely.

Q 209 D   BIO 9.5

From the biology review it should be clear that bile salts do not *absorb* fat, they *emulsify* fat. This immediately rules out options **A.** and **B.** Most products of digestion are absorbed and processed in the liver, but fat products are an exception. Fats are absorbed into the lymphatic system via lacteals, giving answer **D.**

Q 210 D   deduce; B: BIO 9.3

The question is asking why an enzyme exists in the stomach which is present in an inactive form until conditions exist in which it is converted into its active form (e.g. a zymogen). You should be able to recognize that the question is referring to pepsinogen and should be familiar with its function. Nothing exists in the stomach which would break down pepsin should it remain in its active form. As well, pepsinogen converts to its active form, pepsin, in the presence of low pH. It would not make sense that the active enzyme would neutralize the acid, as this would cause the enzyme to be converted back to its inactive form. The inactive form offers no enhancement of activity, but suggests some form of protection, either for the enzyme itself or for surrounding cells. Option **D.** makes sense because if the enzyme remained active even when not needed, perhaps it could continue to function on molecules it was not meant to break down.

GS-1, Passage XI, Questions 211-214

No, you are not expected to know the mechanisms of synthesis of the millions of biochemicals in nature! Yes, you are supposed to remain cool under pressure. No, you are not expected to be intimidated by the mere SIZE of a molecule! And yes, you should know your mechanisms well enough such that if different molecules are presented to you, you can key in on the functional groups you know to be reactive.

Q 211 provides us with only one answer which could possibly have the correct geometry! Nonetheless, let's work through the mechanism (cf. ORG 7.2.2).

The story goes something like this: The catalyst (H^+), being the most charged substance is implicated first. Thus the electrons from the electronegative oxygen (O in the carbonyl, C=O) are attracted to the proton (H^+) and bonds. To remain neutral oxygen loses its pi bond with carbon, leaving only a single bond and secondary carbocation. The δ^- charge on the oxygen from the *diol* (= a compound with 2 alcohol - OH - groups) attacks the positively charged carbocation. The extra hydrogen on the oxygen which now attaches to carbon is kicked out as a proton (regenerating our catalyst). Now we have our "*hemi-ketal*": the ketone has been converted into a hydroxyl group and the diol (*minus one hydrogen*).

Next, the proton strikes again! It can be attracted to the hydroxyl group which falls off as water (*a great leaving group*), thus we have a secondary carbocation, again. Now we have a partial negative charge (the oxygen of the free arm of the diol) and a positive charge (the carbocation) in close proximity in the same molecule! In a very fast *intra*molecular reaction, the nucleophile meets the carbon nucleus and regenerates the proton catalyst. The product is answer choice **C.**, a ketal.

Q 212 presents two important points: (i) it describes a compound called LDA as *hindered* (= bulky) and (ii) its conjugate acid has a pK_a of about 40. Of course, pK_a equals $-\log K_a$ and K_a is the acid dissociation constant (Chapter 6, CHM). A K_a which is extremely low ($\approx 10^{-40}$), indicating that the conjugate acid is verrrrry weak, would give a pK_a of about 40. All to say, weak conjugate acid = strong base ! Translation of Q212: *what does a strong bulky base like to do?*

Before we answer, what does a strong *small* base like to do in organic chemistry? They tend to engage in nucleophilic substitution reactions (i.e. OH⁻, CN⁻). A big bulky base usually has difficulty accessing carbon for a nucleophilic reaction. Instead, it takes the easy way out: it plucks protons off a molecule like oranges off a tree!

Of course some H^+'s are easier to remove than others. This depends on the stability of the suggested product. For example, removing a H^+ from the methoxy substituent would create a primary carbanion (verrrry unstable) with no real stable options to get rid of the negative charge.

On the other hand, examine the carbon in the ring which is attached to the methyl group. If you remove the only hydrogen attached to that 'ringed' carbon (= *α-hydrogen which is happy to be plucked, see* ORG 7.1), you get a <u>tertiary</u> carbanion. Furthermore, you get a logical ensuing reaction: the negative charge is quickly attracted to the carbonyl carbon which is δ^+ thus forming a double bond. Simultaneously, the pi electrons from the carbonyl group are kicked up to the oxygen creating an enolate anion (*almost identical to <u>keto-enol</u> tautomerism*, ORG 7.1).

Q 213 relies on the powers of ☺bservation. The question leads us to looking at step I in the mechanism provided. The products are labelled **A** and **B**. A stern glance will reveal the only difference between the two products: the location of the double bond in the cyclohexene derivative. The next step is to recall that a vinyl group is simply a carbon double bonded to a carbon with hydrogens as substituents (ORG 4.1). At the double bond in question, Product A has *no* hydrogens attached to the carbon double bond, while Product B has two hydrogens (*if you are having trouble counting hydrogens, see* ORG 3.1). The difference can be picked up by proton NMR which reveals the number and *types* of protons (ORG 14.2).

Q 214 B   ORG 7.2.1
This question is quick and easy! By looking at Step IX we notice $NaBH_4$, a very important reducing agent (ORG 7.2.1). Thus the carbonyl group becomes an alcohol group (*hydroxy*) in a <u>reduction reaction</u>.

Q 215 A   ORG 2.3.2; C: *not chiral*
This question shows the structure of 1,1-dichloroethane. The molecule's central carbon has two identical substituents (Cl). Thus it is <u>not</u> chiral (*a chiral carbon has four different substituents,* ORG 2.2). Only chiral substances can rotate plane polarized light (ORG 2.3.2).

Q 216 D   BIO 11.3.1; KW: *adult*
Cartilage can exist in all of the listed tissues. However, the question asks about cartilage in *adult* tissues. In children who are still growing, a disc of cartilage exists between the epiphysis and diaphysis of long bones, but in adults, this cartilage has been replaced by bone. The other tissues listed will remain as cartilage even in adults.

Q 217 C   KW: *programmed* ∴ DNA; BIO 1.2.2
The question refers to programmed cell death which indicates that it is a planned event that will be carried out by cell components based on some sort of instruction or signal. Proteins or other cell components may play a role in the actual killing of the cell, but the signal to do so must come from the DNA. Nucleotides are the subunits which polymerize to produce DNA.

Q 218 D   BIO 14.3
You must be familiar with the graph of the menstrual cycle in order to know which curve is referring to which hormone. There are four hormones involved: luteinizing hormone (LH), follicle stimulating hormone (FSH), estrogen and progesterone. If the menstrual cycle is understood well, you should immediately know that both estrogen and progesterone are secreted by the corpus luteum which came from the ovary. Alternatively, if the pituitary hormones are known, it is easy to eliminate LH and FSH because they are secreted by the anterior pituitary.

Q 219 C   ORG 12.3.2
This question tests your memory of the direction of bonds. If you spend some time reading ORG 12.3.2 and really following the representations in Figure IV.B.12.1, then this question should be easy. The structure of glucose shows six carbons (*this should be consistent with your knowledge of the molecule!*). Only answer choices **A.** and **C.** have six carbons. The structure given never has 2 hydroxy groups attached to the same carbon. That eliminates **A.** as an option.

THE GOLD STANDARD

Understanding

GS-2

Physical Sciences

Q 1 C   PHY 11.3

In order for the eyepiece to magnify the first image formed by the objective, this image has to be real. If it were virtual, no light rays would emerge from it and therefore it could not be magnified by the eyepiece.

Q 2 A   PHY 11.5; 2ⁿᵈ i: *virtual*

The only way an image can be formed on the same side of a converging lens as the original object (*or the first, real image which serves as an object for the eyepiece*) is for that object or real image to be at a distance from the lens which is less than the focal length of the lens. This can be verified using the lens maker's equation. Note that the final enlarged image will be virtual.

Q 3 A   PHY 11.5

In order for magnification by the eyepiece to occur on the same side of the lens as the object (*or first, real image which serves as an object for the eyepiece*), the first image must be formed at a distance from the eyepiece which is less than F_e (i.e. Q2). However, as the first image distance from the eyepiece becomes smaller than F_e, the smaller the second (*virtual*) image formed becomes (verified by the lens equation). Since the closer the two lenses are, the closer their focal lengths are, the closer the first image forms relative to the eyepiece.

Q 4 B   PHY 11.5

I, II and III are facts about optics.

Q 5 D   PHY 11.5

The total magnification of the object is equal to the product of the magnification contributed by each lens. Therefore, total magnification = $15 \times 40 = 600$. From magnification = (image height)/(object height), we get $600 = 25/x$, thus $x = 25/600 = 1/24 = 1/25$ approximately = 0.04 mm.

Q 6 D   PHY 11.5

Using diopters = 1/(focal length in **meters**)
Number of diopters = $1/(0.50 \times 10^{-2}$ m$) = [10^2/0.5] = 10^2/(1/2) = 2 \times 10^2 = 200$

Q 7 C   CHM 1.3, 1.5

Reaction I shows us that the stoichiometric ratio between Cl_2 and HCl is 1:2.
Using Number of moles Cl_2 = (Mass used)/(relative molecular mass Cl_2)
Number of moles Cl_2 = 10 g/[(35.5 × 2) g mol^{-1}] = 10 g/(71.0 g mol^{-1})
From the ratio above, number of moles HCl produced = 2 × number of moles Cl_2
Number of moles HCl = 2 × 10 g/(71.0 g mol^{-1})
Using Number of grams HCl = Number of moles HCl × Relative molecular mass of HCl

Number of grams HCl = 2 × 10 g/(71.0 g mol^{-1}) × (1 + 35.5 g mol^{-1}) ≈ 2 × 10 g × 1/2
= 10 g

Q 8 C   T1; CHM 6.9.3
HCl is an acid, so one would expect the pH of the reaction mixture to **decrease** (that is, become more acidic) as increasing volumes of HCl are added. Thus only **C.** and **D.** are possible answers. Answer choice **D.** is wrong because there should be two "plateaus" (*that is, where the slope of a curve approximates 0 in that region*) in this type of graph, there are just regions where the slope approaches infinity (*that is, the slope is almost vertical which is not logical for a titration curve; furthermore, consider the data in Table 1 for pH = 8.8*).

Q 9 B   CHM 3.4
The lone pair of electrons on the nitrogen atom allows it to **donate** a pair of electrons which is the definition of a Lewis acid.

Q 10 B   CHM 6.9
The range of the indicator should include the range where the graph depicts an almost vertical slope, that is, it should include the *equivalence point* in the middle of that region. This is approximately 4.6 in this instance (*see Q8 C. and Table 1*).

Q 11 C   CHM 6.9.3
Once the $C_6H_5NH_2$ is depleted (*producing $C_6H_5NH_3^+$*), additional protons from the HCl can no longer be neutralized. Thus the [H$^+$] increases dramatically, leading to a **decrease** in pH.

Q 12 A   CHM 4.2, 4.3.2
The hydrogen bonding present requires energy to be broken before the HCl can enter the gaseous phase, thereby making HCl more difficult to boil (i.e. *the boiling point is elevated*). Neither Cl_2 nor H_2 engage in H-bonding.

Q 13 B   CHM 4.1.7
Using Partial pressure = Mole fraction × Total pressure
For Cl_2:   35 atm = x × 100 atm
Thus   x = 35 atm/100 atm = 7/20
Also, the mole fraction of HCl is given as 0.40.
Using the fact that the sum of the mole fractions of all species is one,
For H_2: Mole fraction = 1 - (0.4 + 7/20) = 1 - (4/10 + 7/20)
Mole fraction = 1 - (8/20 + 7/20) = 1 - (15/20) = 1 - (3/4) = 1/4
Partial pressure H_2 = Mole fraction H_2 × Total pressure
Partial pressure H_2 = 1/4 × 100 atm = 25 atm

{Though the above is pretty(!), there is a much faster way: since the total pressure is 100 atm, the mole fraction of 0.40 for HCl represents 40 atm; we are given 35 atm for Cl_2, thus 100 - (40 + 35) = 25 atm}

Q 14 C   PHY 12.1, PoE

Since a neutron has no charge, it would not be impeded in its motion by the positively charged nucleus, unlike the similarly charged proton. {*Note: answer choices **A.** and **B.** are false; answer choice **D.** is true for both a neutron and a proton and is thus an inappropriate answer*}

Q 15 A   PHY 12.3

An alpha particle is defined as a (*doubly positively charged*) helium nucleus.

Q 16 D   PHY 12.4

Using Fraction of activity remaining = (Final activity)/(Initial activity)
Fraction of activity remaining = 10.8 dpm g^{-1}/43.0 dpm g^{-1} = 1/4, approximately
Using Fraction of activity remaining = $(1/2)^{\text{number of half-lives}}$
$1/4 = (1/2)^x$, thus x = 2

Q 17 B   PHY 12.3

Since the radioactive emission angled up toward the positive plate, it must be oppositely charged, that is, negatively charged. The only negatively charged species in the answer choices is the beta particle which is, by definition, an electron. Note that gamma rays are not deflected in electromagnetic fields.

Q 18 C   PHY 5.2/3/4/5, 12.3

The neutron is a mass in motion and as a result possesses <u>kinetic energy</u>. The final product is one with a greater atomic <u>mass</u> than uranium.

Q 19 D   PHY 12.3, 12.4

Equation I: $^{238}_{92}U \rightarrow {^x_y}Z + 3{^4_2}He + 2{^0_{-1}}e^- + 3$ (gamma rays)
Since the sum of the atomic numbers and mass numbers on either side of the equation must be equal:
$238 = x + (3 \times 4) + (2 \times 0) + (3 \times 0)$
$x = 226$
$92 = y + (3 \times 2) + (2 \times -1) + (3 \times 0)$
$y = 88$
Thus, from the answer choices, Z = Ra; note that gamma rays are a form of electromagnetic radiation (PHY 9.2.4) and thus have no charge and no mass.

Q 20 B   deduce, E III, CHM 10.2/4, "GERC"

Since the hydroxide is being formed as a result of a **reduction** (Equation II), that terminal is referred to as the <u>cathode</u>. Since the bicarbonate (HCO_3^-) *neutralizes* the product of the cathode (Equation III), it can be referred to as an <u>inhibitor</u> since OH^- contributes to the rusting process. {P2, P3; "GERC"= Gain Electrons Reduction at the Cathode}

Q 21 D   CHM 10.1, (Zn^{2+}/Zn) ≠ (Zn/Zn^{2+})

The electrochemical reaction for the standard reduction potential $E^\circ(X^{n+}/X)$ of a metal "X" is: $X^{n+} + ne^- \rightleftharpoons X$. The more negative the E° value, the greater the tendency for the equilibrium to shift to the <u>left</u>, that is, toward the production of cations. In order to minimize the reaction with Fe (*rusting*) and maximize the reaction with Zn (*galvanizing*), we want the following: since the cation of Zn is supposed to react more readily with the hydroxide ions (P4) than with iron (Fe), it would be facilitated if it ionized more readily than the iron, that is, if its <u>standard reduction potential was more negative</u> than that of iron.

Q 22 B   CHM 10.1/2

Written as standard reduction potentials, we get:

$O_2 + 2H_2O + 4e^- \rightleftharpoons 4OH^-$ $E^\circ = +0.401$ V   Cathode (*gain of electrons*)

$2Fe^{2+} + 4e^- \rightleftharpoons 2Fe$ $E^\circ = -0.440$ V   Anode (*loss of electrons, see* **Equation I**)

$E^\circ_{reaction} = E^\circ_{reduction} - E^\circ_{oxidation}$

$E^\circ_{reaction} = +0.401 - (-0.440) = +0.841$ V

Q 23 B   CHM 10.5.1

Using Quantity of electricity (Q) = Current(I) × Time(t)

Q = 0.2 A × (80 min × 60 s min^{-1}) = 960 C

Number of faradays required to add **2 moles of electrons** to one mole of Fe^{2+} (*to obtain one mole of Fe, see* **Equation I**) = 2 × F = 2 × 96000 C.

Using Number of moles Fe obtained = Q/(Number of Faradays required to produce 1 mole Fe)

Number of moles Fe = 960 C/(2 × 96000 C) = 1/(100 × 2) = 1/200 mol

Using Number of grams Fe = Number of moles Fe × Relative atomic mass Fe

Number of grams Fe = 1/200 mol × 55.8 g mol^{-1}

Number of grams Fe = (1/200 × 56) g approximately = 7/25 g = 28/100 g = 0.28 g in one hour

{*Nice math!*}

Q 24 B   deduce, CHM 5.3.2

Electrolytes, by their very nature and definition, are charge carriers when in the molten state or in solution. Since the electrons must move from the center of the drop to the exterior (P2, L4-6), facilitating this process would increase the rate of the rusting.

Q 25 D CHM 5.3.2; KS: $s^3 = 1/8 \times 10^{-15}$

Equation: $FeX_2 \rightleftharpoons Fe^{2+} + 2X^-$

Solubility s can be calculated using the above equation and $K_{sp} = [Fe^{2+}][X^-]^2$:

$K_{sp} = (s)(2s)^2 = 4s^3$

Thus $s^3 = (K_{sp}/4) = (5.0 \times 10^{-16})/4 = (1.25 \times 10^{-16}) = 0.125 \times 10^{-15} = 1/8 \times 10^{-15}$

$s = [\text{cube root } (1/8)] \times [\text{cube root } (10^{-15})] = 1/2 \times 10^{-5} = 5.0 \times 10^{-6}$ mol L^{-1}

Q 26 A PHY 10.3.1, Law I

Kirchoff's Law I: *the sum of current at a junction is equal to zero.* Let all current arriving at the junction be positive while all current leaving the junction is negative:

$Q + T - S - U \pm R = 0$

$7 A + 8 A - 4 A - 11 A \pm R = 0$

$15 A - 15 A \pm R = 0$ A, thus R = 0.

Q 27 B PHY 7.1.2

Using velocity = frequency × wavelength:

7.5×10^3 m s^{-1} = x × 1.5 m

Thus x = $(7.5 \times 10^3$ m s$^{-1})/(1.5$ m$) = 5.0 \times 10^3$ s$^{-1} = 5.0 \times 10^3$ Hz

Q 28 C ORG 1.2

The atom has 2 equal sp orbitals and 2 p orbitals perpendicular to the sp orbitals. As seen in *acetylene* (HCCH), the orbital geometry would be linear.

Q 29 B PHY 7.1.3

When maximum destructive interference occurs, amplitude = 8 - 4 = 4 units; when maximum constructive interference occurs, amplitude = 8 + 4 = 12 units, thus the range is between 4 and 12.

Q 30 D PHY 4.1, 4.1.1

A diagram and the principle that for a system in equilibrium (*that is, with no net forces acting on the system*), the sum of the moments acting in opposite directions are equal (= *rotational equilibrium*) are used.

Using Moment of force = force × distance from axis of rotation (= *pivot point*)

50 kg × g × 0.60 m = x kg × g × 0.30 m, thus mass x = 100 kg

The weight x = 100 kg × 10 m s^{-2} approximately = 1000 N (gravitational acceleration g = 9.8 m s^{-2} = 10 m s^{-2}, approximately)

Q 31 A PHY 6.1.1/2; KWs: *max, held*

Using volume of cube = (length of side)^3

Therefore: Volume of the block (P2, *square block*) = $(4.0 \text{ m})^3$ = 64 m^3 = *volume of fluid displaced* since the entire block must be *held* under the surface of the water in order for there to be <u>maximum</u> buoyant force.
Using density = (Mass)/(Volume)
Mass of fluid displaced = Density of fluid × Volume of fluid
Mass of fluid displaced = $(1.00 \times 10^3 \text{ kg m}^{-3}) \times (64 \text{ m}^3)$ = 6.4×10^4 kg
Using Weight of fluid displaced = Mass of fluid displaced × gravitational acceleration
Weight of fluid displaced = $(6.4 \times 10^4 \text{ kg}) \times (10 \text{ m s}^{-2})$ approximately = 6.4×10^5 N
{*Recall Archimedes' Principle: the buoyant force equals the weight of the fluid displaced*}

Q 32 C   PHY 6.1.1/2
Using **Specific Gravity** or Fraction of block in water = (Density of block)/(Density of water)
Fraction of block in water = $(500 \text{ kg m}^{-3})/(1.0 \times 10^3 \text{ kg m}^{-3})$ = 1/2
Therefore, fraction of block out of water = 1 - 1/2 = 1/2
If 1/2 of the block is above the water, then 1/2 of its volume is out of the water and hence 1/2 its height is out of the water. Thus the height of the block out of water = 1/2 × 4.0 m = 2.0 m

Q 33 C   PHY 6.1.1/2
From the equation in the answer for Q32, if the density of the block increases, the fraction of the block in the water increases and therefore the fraction of the block out of the water decreases. Thus, the height of the block out of the water decreases.

Q 34 C   PHY 6.1.1/2
Tricky! You must recognize that the half immersed block would sink as long as its density is greater than that of the original wood block which floats half immersed (*see* Q32). Thus the second block may: (i) have a specific gravity between 0.5 and 1.0 (which means the block's density would be *less* than that of water); or (ii) it could have a density *equal* to that of water; or (iii) it could have a density *greater* than that of water: either way, it would sink from a position of being held half immersed [*thus answer choice* **B.** *is not the best answer because of the preceding points (i) and (ii)*]. When the block sinks, it will *certainly* displace more water than it did initially; therefore, the buoyant force <u>increases</u> to its maximum.{*cf. Archimedes Principle, Q31*}

Q 35 C   PHY 6.1.2; mg did not change
The object displaces an amount of water equal to its <u>weight</u> when it is floating. Thus, if the object were to change state, since its **mass** remains constant, the level of the water would remain constant.

Q 36 D   CHM 3.5, P: 3 bonds

Phosphorus is in Group V. It can therefore either have a valency of 3 *or* 5 (*you can memorize this or determine it through VSEPR modelling*). Answer choice **D.**, which has *three* bonds to each phosphorous, is the only answer which fulfils this requirement.

Q 37 B   CHM 8.6

Equation: Red phosphorus → White Phosphorus $\Delta H_{reaction}$ = x kJ mol^{-1}

$\Delta H_{formation}$: -2900 kJ mol^{-1}(red), -3020 kJ mol^{-1}(white)

$\Delta H_{reaction}$ = $\Delta H_{products}$ - $\Delta H_{reactants}$ = -3020 kJ mol^{-1} - (-2900 kJ mol^{-1}) = -120 kJ mol^{-1}

Q 38 C   deduce from Q 101.D.

Each face of the molecule is a triangle, each "side" consisting of the same type of bond(s). Therefore, the triangle would be expected to resemble an equilateral triangle, where each angle is 60°.

Q 39 A   CHM 1.3, 1.5

Using Number of moles = (Mass)/(Relative molecular mass)

For PCl_3: Number of moles = (68.75 g)/[(31.0 + 35.5 × 3) g mol^{-1}] = 68.75/137.5 = 1/2

Equation: P_4 (s) + $6Cl_2$ → $4PCl_3$

Thus, Number of moles of P_4 = 1/4 × Number of moles PCl_3 = 1/4 × 1/2 mole = 1/8 mole

Using 1 mole of particles = 6.0 × 10^{23} particles (*Avogadro's # = 6.023 × 10^{23} particles/mole*)

1/8 mole P_4 = 1/8 × 6.0 × 10^{23} = 3/4 × 10^{23} = 0.75 × 10^{23} P_4 molecules

Q 40 C   CHM 2.3, 3.2

Phosphorus is in Group V and therefore requires three more electrons to approach the more stable noble gas electronic configuration. If these are shared with another phosphorus atom, three covalent bonds exist between the two atoms. Multiple bonds usually contain one sigma bond, the other bonds being pi bonds. Each atom will also possess a lone pair of electrons. {*Notice this is the same as for N_2 as nitrogen is in the same group as phosphorus in the periodic table; when you see something you are unfamiliar with, always look for similarities with something you know well*}

Answer choice **A.** is incorrect because if phosphorus loses three electrons, it will have a total of 12 electrons, which does not correspond to a stable noble gas-like configuration.

Q 41 D   CHM 4.1.8

The molecular mass of the real gas P_4 is 124 g/mol (i.e. 4 × 31.0 g/mol). The question is really asking: what is the difference between a real gas and an ideal gas if the molecular weight is the same?

An increase in density depends on an increase in the mutual forces of attraction between particles, causing the volume occupied by the same mass of those particles to decrease [density

= (mass)/(volume)]. Ideal gases possess no intermolecular forces so its density should be less than that of any real gas.

Q 42 A   PHY 9.2.4

The electromagnetic spectrum from longer to shorter wavelength goes as follows: radiowaves, microwaves, infrared, visible, ultraviolet, X-rays, gamma rays.

Q 43 D   P4, L 1-7; T1

Since both sulphur and carbon have the same electronegativity, there is an even charge distribution and as a result, no permanent dipole. Since there is no dipole, there is no absorption of infrared (P4, L1-4).

Q 44 D   E

Let M = original effective mass of system = $(m_1 + m_2)/(m_1 m_2)$
Using frequency = $(1/2\pi) \times \sqrt{(k/M)}$
Original frequency = $(1/2\pi) \times \sqrt{(k/M)}$
Let M' = new effective mass of system = $(2m_1 + 2m_2)/(2m_1 \times 2m_2) = 2(m_1 + m_2)/4m_1 m_2$
$M' = (m_1 + m_2)/(2m_1 m_2) = 1/2M$
Thus New frequency = $(1/2\pi) \times \sqrt{(k/M')} = (1/2\pi) \times \sqrt{[k/(1/2M)]}$
New frequency = $\sqrt{(2)} \times (1/2\pi) \times \sqrt{(k/M)} = \sqrt{(2)} \times$ Original frequency

Q 45 B   PHY 7.2.1

From Hooke's Law

Q 46 A   E

$M = (2 + 2)/(2 \times 2) = 4/4 = 1$
Using Frequency = $(1/2\pi) \times \sqrt{(k/M)}$
Frequency = $(1/2\pi) \times \sqrt{(4/1)} = (1/2\pi) \times 2$
Frequency = $1/\pi$ Hz

Q 47 A   PHY 6.1.2

Since the height of water on the left side of the manometer is lower, the pressure inside the vessel must be greater than atmospheric pressure. In other words, you can imagine that if pressure builds up within the container (*see the drawing in the passage*), the additional pressure would "push" on the fluid in the U-tube. Recall that the *difference* in pressure $\Delta P = \rho gh$. Thus:
Pressure in vessel = ρgh + atmospheric pressure
Pressure = (1000 kg m^{-3} × 9.8 m s^{-2} × 0.50 m) + atmospheric pressure
Pressure = 4900 kg m^{-1} s^{-2} + atmospheric pressure = 4900 N m^{-2} + atmospheric pressure

Q 48 C   CHM 4.1.6

Using the ideal gas equation and Number of moles (n) = [Mass (w)]/[(Relative molecular mass (M)]

PV = nRT = (wRT)/M, thus M = (wRT)/(PV).

Q 49 A   CHM 4.1.8

Unlike an ideal gas, carbon dioxide possesses intermolecular attractive forces; therefore, the ideal gas equation will not hold exactly. {*Recall (ORG 1.5) CO_2 has δ^- oxygens and a δ^+ carbon which creates a force of attraction of opposite charges between <u>different</u> CO_2 molecules*}

Q 50 A   deduce, ↑T, ↑M

We are told that the initial temperature is lower than the final temperature. Since the initial temperature is used in the equation M = (wRT)/(PV)[*see* Q48, CHM 4.1.6], the predicted M would be less than the <u>recorded</u> value which occurs with the <u>actual</u>, higher temperature.

Q 51 A   CHM 4.1.6/7/8; ↓$CO_2(g)$, ↓P, ↑M

Because CO_2 dissolves in water, the amount of gas obtained would be less than expected. Thus, the pressure of the gas would be less than expected and from the equation M = (wRT)/(PV), the value for M would be larger than expected.

Q 52 D   CHM 3.1, 5.2

Magnesium phosphate is a salt, which can ionize, and has the empirical formula $Mg_3(PO_4)_2$. Thus for each mole of $Mg_3(PO_4)_2$, three moles of magnesium cations will be obtained. Therefore, the concentration of magnesium ions will be three times that of the magnesium phosphate.

$$Mg_3(PO_4)_2 \rightleftharpoons 3Mg^{2+} + 2PO_4^{3-}$$

Q 53 D   PHY 7.1.2, 7.1.4

Resonance involves a system vibrating at its natural or intrinsic frequency, and under these conditions, the system vibrates at maximum amplitude. Energy and power are both proportional to the square of the amplitude, so they will also be at their maximum values.

Q 54 A   CHM 10.1

The more positive the E° value, the greater the tendency for that half-reaction to proceed to the right. Since the E° value for the Ce^{4+}/Ce^{3+} equilibrium system is more positive than that for the HNO_2/NO equilibrium system, the latter will be shifted to the left, that is, NO will be oxidized (= *lose electrons; recall LEO is a GERC!*; CHM 10.2).

Q 55 A   **CHM 2.2, 2.3 (iv)**
A half-filled electron shell contains subshells each of which possesses one unpaired electron. All unpaired electrons have parallel spins and this half-filled system confers extra stability to the atom. Thus more energy than would be expected (*from a consideration of the ionization energies of other elements in the same period*) is required to remove a valent electron from the neutral atom.

Q 56 D   **PHY 4.3, 4.4, 4.4.1, 1.4.1**
Using momentum = mass × velocity and the Principle of Conservation of Momentum
Total momentum before collision = total momentum after collision
$(1 \text{ kg} \times 12 \text{ m s}^{-1}) + (2 \text{ kg} \times 0 \text{ m s}^{-1}) = [(1 \text{ kg} + 2 \text{ kg}) \times x \text{ m s}^{-1}]$
$12 \text{ kg m s}^{-1} = (3 \times x) \text{ kg m s}^{-1}$
$x = 4 \text{ m s}^{-1}$
Using $V = V_o + at$, where the final velocity V is 0, the initial velocity of the balls V_o is $x = 4$, and the time t to reach the final velocity is 10 seconds:
$0 \text{ m s}^{-1} = 4 \text{ m s}^{-1} + (a \times 10 \text{ s})$
$10 \times a = -4$
Thus $a = -4/10 \text{ m s}^{-2} = -0.4 \text{ m s}^{-2}$
Therefore, **deceleration** $= 0.4 \text{ m s}^{-2}$

Q 57 A   **CHM 7.5, deduce**
Light colors tend to reflect incident electromagnetic radiation including infrared rays, the main type of electromagnetic radiation associated with heat. The answer is easily deduced since there is only one answer which refers to the *reflective* property of the metal foil (P2, L7).

Q 58 B   **CHM 7.5, deduce**
Air is a poor *conductor* of heat. Both radiation and convection typically need air, or some other fluid, as a medium to transmit energy/heat.

Q 59 D   **PHY 6.1.1, deduce**
Cold air is denser, not actually heavier since the same particles are involved, and the particles of cold air associate more closely with each other because they possess less kinetic energy than warm air particles (*kinetic energy is proportional to temperature*).

Q 60 B   **CHM 8.7**
The specific heat capacity of a substance is the energy required to raise the temperature of unit mass of a substance by one degree. Therefore, the smaller this value, the greater the temperature change on the addition or subtraction of a certain quantity of energy. Therefore, the temperature of the oil will increase by the greatest value, then the ethanol, then the water ($c_{oil} < c_{ethanol} < c_{water}$). Alternatively, using the equation $Q = mc\,\Delta T$, where Q and m are constant, clearly an increase in c results in a lowering of the temperature change.

Q 61 A   D.A.

This problem is solved by giving <u>special attention to units</u> (i.e. 1 W = 1 J per s):

Rate of incident solar energy = 70 000 m^2 × 120 $J\ s^{-1}\ m^{-2}$ = 8 400 000 $J\ s^{-1}$

From Quantity of heat (Q) = Mass (m) × Specific heat capacity (c) × temperature change (T)

Thus <u>in one second</u>: Q = 8 400 000 J = m × (4.2 $J\ g^{-1}\ °C^{-1}$) × (10 °C)

42 × m = 8 400 000; thus m = 200 000 g = 200 kg

Using Density = (Mass)/(Volume)

Volume = (Mass)/(Density) = 200 kg/1000 $kg\ m^{-3}$ = 0.2 m^3 = 0.2 m^3 × 1000 dm^3/m^3

Volume = 200 dm^3 = 200 L <u>in one second</u>

Q 62 D   CHM 2.3

A half-filled orbital has extra stability associated with it since all the electrons are unpaired and have parallel spins. Thus it is more difficult to remove an electron from this system and hence it requires more energy.

Q 63 B   T1; CHM 10.5

From Table 1 we can see that each mole of sulfate ions requires *two* moles of electrons for reduction to one mole of sulfur dioxide, but each mole of chromium (III) cations requires *three* moles of electrons for reduction to one mole of chromium metal. Hence, the ratio of the number of moles of electrons available to produce the chromium metal will be 2:3 producing 0.67 moles of the metal.

Q 64 C   P2, L 3-5; deduce

Answer choice **C.** is the only absolute requirement for ligand association with a transition metal. Though the ligand must possess a lone pair of *electrons* to associate with the *positive* charged metal cations, no formal charge is necessary. {*Incidental: a coordinate covalent bond is where the contribution of electrons in a covalent bond comes from <u>one</u> atom i.e. NH_3 (lone pair e^- on N) + H^+ (no e^- to share) → NH_4^+ (1 coord. cov. bond); in a normal covalent bond, each atom contributes an electron to the bond,* CHM 3.2}

Q 65 A   CHM 10.1

The key to the problem is the following: *a reaction will tend to be spontaneous if the final (overall) $E°$ for the reaction is <u>positive</u>.* For the reduction of Fe^{3+} to occur, the $E°$ of the other half-reaction used must be <u>more</u> negative or <u>less</u> positive than that of the Fe^{3+}/Fe^{2+} equilibrium system so that the equilibrium will shift to the right, that is, reduction of Fe^{3+} with an overall positive $E°$ for the reaction. Only two half reactions do *not* fulfil the preceding requirement: VO_2^+/VO^{2+} and $Cr_2O_7^{2-}/Cr^{3+}$.

Q 66 B   CHM 10.1

The direction of the reactions are chosen such that a positive $E°$ occurs for the overall reaction (i.e. Q65).

$$VO_2^+ + 2H^+ + e^- \rightleftharpoons H_2O + VO^{2+} \qquad E^\circ = +1.00 \text{ V}$$
$$- \qquad VO^{2+} + 2H^+ + e^- \rightleftharpoons H_2O + V^{3+} \qquad -(E^\circ = +0.34 \text{ V})$$

$$VO_2^+ + V^{3+} \rightleftharpoons 2VO^{2+} \qquad E^\circ = +0.66 \text{ V}$$

Q 67 A   CHM 1.6

The oxidation state of oxygen is usually -2. Therefore, the total oxidation state due to oxygen = 7 × -2 = -14. The overall charge on the molecule is -2. There are 2 Cr atoms per $Cr_2O_7^{2-}$ molecule, thus:

2 × oxidation state of Cr + (-14) = -2

2 × oxidation state of Cr = 12

Oxidation state of Cr = 12/2 = 6

Q 68 C   PHY 5.4, 3.2.1, 1.1.2

After you draw a line diagram, the calculations are quite straightforward:

From Potential Energy = Mass (m) × gravitational acceleration (g) × **Vertical** height (h)

Potential Energy = (5 000 kg + 1 000 kg) × 9.8 m s^{-2} × (5 m × sin 30°)

Potential Energy = (6 000 × 10 × 5 × 1/2) J approximately = 150 000 J = 1.5×10^5 J

Q 69 C   P2, PHY 1.3/4

Uniform acceleration is depicted as a straight line with a *positive* gradient (= *slope*) on a velocity-time graph. Of course, uniform velocity, since the velocity *does not change*, is depicted as a straight horizontal line. Uniform deceleration (= *negative acceleration*) is depicted as a straight line with a *negative* gradient on a v-t graph.

Q 70 B   PHY 3.2

Using Maximum frictional force f_{MAX} = Coefficient of friction × Normal force

Using Newton's Second Law (F = ma) in the vertical plane, the normal force is equal to the weight of the truck as there is no acceleration (or motion) in this plane

f_{MAX} = 1/3 × (5 000 kg + 1 000 kg) × 9.8 m s^{-2} = 1/3 × 6 000 kg × 10 m s^{-2} approximately = 20 000 N.

Q 71 D   PHY 1.4.1

Using V = V_0 + at, the original velocity V_0, time t, and acceleration a = 6 m s^{-2}:

V = 14 m s^{-1} + (6 m s^{-2} × 5 s) = 44 m s^{-1}

Now let's determine deceleration using V = V_0 + at

0 m s^{-1} = 44 m s^{-1} + (a × 8 s) {*Note that the final velocity for the acceleration becomes the original velocity for the deceleration; cf Q69 C.*}

a = -5.5 m s^{-2}; therefore, **deceleration** = 5.5 m s^{-2}

Ratio of acceleration to deceleration = 6 : 5.5 = 12 : 11

Q 72 B   **PHY 3.2.1; N = W** *cos (α)*

When the angle decreases, the component of the weight of the truck which is related to the normal force [mg × cos (angle)] increases. Hence the normal force increases. {*Notice that the value of the function cosine <u>increases</u> as its angle decreases; also notice that when there is no angle (= 0º), the value of cosine is 1 (= maximal) indicating that N is at its maximal value for this problem: N = mg*}

Q 73 D   **CHM 2.3**

Because the attractive forces between the nuclei and the valence electrons are strong, there is less tendency for electrons to be lost and hence a greater tendency for an electron to be gained in order to attain the more stable noble gas configuration.

Q 74 D   **PHY 2.6, 1.1.2**

The horizontal component of the velocity = V × cos (angle) = 30 × cos 45° = 30 × (square root 2)/2.

The vertical component of the velocity = V × sin (angle) = 30 × sin 45° = 30 × (square root 2)/2.

Q 75 A   **CHM 9.9**

Less particles are on the left side of the equation (9 moles versus 10). Therefore, the increase in pressure favors a shift in the equilibrium position to the left as the reactants occupy less volume (*Le Chatelier's principle*).

Q 76 D   **PHY 11.5**

The object is placed at a distance equal to half the radius of curvature, that is, at the focal length. Therefore, no image will be formed (*verified using the lens equation, $1/f = 1/i + 1/o$, where o = f*).

Q 77 C   **CHM 4.2, ORG 10.1**

Ethers possess a highly electronegative atom (*oxygen*), but no hydrogen atom is directly bonded to an oxygen or any other electronegative atom. As a result, another molecule with an electropositive hydrogen (i.e. water) can form hydrogen bonds with the oxygen atom of an ether, but the ether's hydrogen atoms will not be involved in hydrogen bonding.

THE GOLD STANDARD

Understanding

GS-2

Verbal Reasoning

Explanation: the basis for the answers for Verbal Reasoning is the passage. Most answers are found directly in passage which we have cross-referenced for you by paragraph and line in The Gold Standard Answer Key. Therefore, explanations for Verbal Reasoning are only given for selected questions which are either more challenging or reveal some teaching point. It is recommended that you review Part II, Chapter 3 in The Gold Standard text.

Q 82 B   P4, L9-11; P5, L13-17

A mother who discourages independent thinking and encourages conformity is more likely strict, which leads to less differentiation (P4, L9-11), than permissive. Agriculturalists, for example, also have less differentiation and higher field dependence (P6) which translate into relatively poor performance in RFT and EFT tests (P5). Answer choice **D.** is false though the passage suggests that agriculturalists tend to do poorly on the RFT and EFT tests, *nowhere is the opposite suggested*. In other words, test performance only reveals how dependent or independent on environmental cues the child might be, but it does not indicate whether or not the child will most likely be a hunter or a farmer!

Q 98 B   P8, deduce

The "adversary function" of the press is mentioned in the discussion of the media's new role of scrutinizing public officials, statements and issues (P8). The question asks which event might have been influenced by this new role. Answer choice **A.** clearly could not have occurred as a result of the media's close examination of public officials, as it involves the media's exploration of other forms of media. Answer choice **C.** is a case of an editor <u>agreeing</u> with the President. The event was not adversarial since a member of the media (the editor) was actually in agreement with the President. Answer choice **D.** shows how the media can bring relevant issues into the spotlight so that something may be done, but no careful inspection is involved nor mention of adversarial reporting. Only answer choice **B.** involves a close examination of a public (consistent with P8, L7-9) official (the researching and publishing of evidence linking the senator to organized crime) which leads to a certain event occurring (the senator retires).

Q 101 B   P6; deduce

The question asks for a negative effect of killing large numbers of *Culex* mosquitoes through the use of synthetic egg-laying pheromone (e.g. the tests in Kenya, P6). The effects mentioned in answer choices **C.** and **D.** are in no way explored or implicated in the paragraph discussing the tests done in Kenya (P6). In general, the massive destruction of any species is not desirable and holds many negative consequences. However, *Culex* mosquitoes carry various forms of harmful diseases (P6, L6-8), so in this case the decrease in number of *Culex* mosquitoes is not a negative effect, in fact it is the intended effect. This eliminates answer choice **A.** However, the same insecticide by which large numbers of *Culex* mosquitoes are destroyed could also affect populations of other insects. If these insects do not pose the same risk as the disease-carrying *Culex* mosquitoes, their destruction might very well have negative consequences.

Q 137 B   P5, L5-8, deduce

The fact that the people saw a huge silver disk and concluded that it was a fulfilment of a "prophecy of the Virgin Mary" does not support the statement in answer choice **A.** because no judgement (i.e. that they are occultists, that they cannot accept modern society) about the people who saw the disk is made in the account of the event. Answer choice **C.** is not supported by the account of the incident in 1917 because no information is given about what the people in Fatima may have believed about existence. Even if the account included that the people of Fatima fervently believed that there was more to life than they could know, this does not support the statement given because it would be an observation about these fifty thousand people, and not all people in general over time. Answer choice **D.** contains a statement about people in antiquity, which from the passage can be inferred to be hundreds of years ago (P8, L8-13) and, actually, refers to the period *before* the Middle Ages (= c. 470-1450 A.D.). The date given in the account in the question, 1917, is far too recent for this account to be used as supporting evidence for the statement given. The only reasonable option is answer choice **B.** The people in Fatima saw a silver disk. However, their interpretation of this event, that it was a fulfilment of prophecy, was much different from the interpretations of the "Ufologists."

Understanding

GS-2

Biological Sciences

Explanation: the basis of the biology and organic chemistry questions within Biological Sciences is very different. Thus we have chosen to provide the answers in different formats. Most biology answers are found directly in the passage which we have cross-referenced for you by paragraph, line and/or figure or diagram (when applicable). Therefore, explanations for biology are given in a similar format to the one used for Physical Sciences. On the other hand, MCAT organic chemistry questions usually rely on the ability to decipher the important information from the given passage and an understanding of the basics including mechanisms. Thus all organic chemistry questions and answers are explored in detail, beginning with a review of the passage itself.

☞ You will often find that the Biology passages deal with advanced level topics or experiments. The key is not to become deterred by fancy words; rather, know what you know and concentrate on quickly understanding any graph or table presented. Do not try to understand details from the passage. Instead, read quickly and then focus on the questions.

Q 143 B   BIO 14.5
You must be familiar with the stages of embryogenesis to answer this question.

Q 144 C   BIO 14.5
You must be familiar with the stages of embryogenesis to answer this question.

Q 145 D   BIO 14.2
You must be familiar with gametogenesis in males to answer this question.

Q 146 C   P3, L11-13; BIO 3.0
The passage states that non-genetic material in the germ plasm is responsible for germ cell formation. This rules out nuclear DNA as an option. Mitochondria (*energy*) and microtubules (*structural*) are unlikely answers as they have very limited roles to actively change their outside environment. RNA and protein molecules can actively change the environment around them by aiding in the production of proteins, through functioning as enzymes (catalysing reactions), as structural proteins, etc. Thus they are the most likely to induce germ cell function.

Q 147 A   P3, L12-13; BIO 1.2.2
The conclusion drawn from the experiment is that non-genetic material induces germ cell formation. You must identify the experimental results that would suggest that this conclusion is incorrect and that genetic material actually *does* have a role in germ cell formation. Option **B.** is simply the same experiment as that in the passage but with the germ plasm injected at a different site. The results are the same, so it does not contradict the conclusion made in the passage. Option **C.** states that breaking down proteins (*proteases*) interferes with the induction of germ cell formation. This does not contradict the conclusion made since proteins are not genetic material. Option **D.** shows that the interference in germ cell formation in the irradiated fly was not due to genetic mutations, which further supports the conclusion given in the passage. Option **A.** indicates that the only thing present in the germ plasm appears to be genetic material (nucleotides). Since it was the germ plasm that induced germ cell formation in the experiment, genetic material is implicated. This is the only evidence that contradicts the conclusion made in the passage.

Q 148 B   BIO 14.5.1
The point at which a blastomere is committed to becoming a germ cell is different from the point at which the germ cell actually starts to function as a germ cell (i.e. producing cell-specific proteins). Determination is the point at which a cell is committed to becoming a particular type of cell, although it may not display any specific characteristics that would yet identify it as a specific type of cell. After determination, a cell will differentiate into a particular type of cell, and the fully differentiated cell is called *specialized*. Determination is the crucial point at which the fate of the blastomere is decided.

Q 149 B   BIO 15.3; KWs: *best explains*
Muscular dystrophy occurs due to the absence or malfunction of dystrophin (P2). If muscular dystrophy occurs much more commonly in males (P1), the trait is likely sex-linked. The gene coding for dystrophin cannot be on the Y chromosome otherwise *no* females would have genes coding for dystrophin. The only method in which a father could pass the disease to his sons but no daughters is through the Y chromosome, which again, would mean that females do not have the gene. There is no method of inheritance by which mothers can pass a trait exclusively to male offspring. This leaves only option **B.** which accurately explains the higher incidence of the disease in males since males receive only one copy of the X chromosome. If this one copy contains the disease-causing allele, there exists no homologous pair that may contain a normal allele to mask the effects of the mutant allele. Females have two X chromosomes, thus significantly reducing their chances of having the disease as they must receive two mutant alleles in order to display characteristics of the disease.

Q 150 A   P2, L5; BIO 6.3
The passage clearly states that the protein dystrophin is located on the *inner* surface of the plasma membrane (P2, L5). All that is required for this question is that you recall that protein hormones (answer choice **A.**) do *not* diffuse across the plasma membrane (BIO 6.3) and thus have their effect on the *outer* surface of the membrane (cf. *steroid hormones*). This recognition is then transduced into an intracellular message using intermediates like intrinsic proteins which span the membrane and cyclic AMP.

Q 151 C   P3, L5-7, L9-12
To clone a piece of DNA, large quantities of DNA must be produced (P3). The method by which this is done is through the use of bacterial plasmids. The foreign DNA is inserted into plasmid DNA (not capsid, as in option **A.**; *see* BIO 2.1). The bacterial plasmid is replicated through the normal life cycle of bacteria, which is short enough to allow rapid replication of the foreign sequence. For cloning to take place sites must exist where foreign DNA can be inserted. However, inserting the DNA is of no use unless the bacteria can complete its usual life cycle after being altered in such a way.

Q 152 D   BIO 1.2.2
Let's translate the question into more basic language: if you have a DNA molecule (*plasmid*) and you want to add another DNA molecule (*foreign DNA*), how can this be done? The answer is that a DNA molecule is <u>elongated</u> via phosphodiester bonds (answer choice **D.**; BIO 1.2.2; ORG 12.5). DNA *replication* is a completely different mechanism as it refers to the duplication of DNA strands *within* a DNA molecule which is related to appropriate base pairing (cf. answer choice **C.**) and occurs in a semi-conservative manner (answer choice **A.**). Answer choice **B.** is irrelevant.

Q 153 C   deduce
Answer choice **A.** is false because we are looking for a *functional* gene for dystrophin! Answer choice **B.** is false since it does not refer to any cloning techniques as requested in the question. Answer choice **D.** is false since it is known that dystrophin (P2) and not troponin or tropomyosin is responsible for muscular dystrophy. Answer choice **C.** presents a possible method to treat the disease by: (a) using a cloning technique and (b) inserting the needed gene into diseased cells which would then make them capable of producing dystrophin. {*Incidental: this type of research is currently being done on humans using special viruses to insert the missing gene into the cells of the patient*}

Q 154 D   BIO 5.2
You must understand the structures and processes involved in muscle contraction to answer this question.

Q 155 A   deduce; T1; P2, L3-7; B: BIO 5.1.1/2/3
Answer choice **A.** is a false statement making it the correct answer! Table 1 shows us that the inside of the membrane is negatively charged (V_m = -70 mV; cf. BIO 5.1.1), yet there are 10 times the number of sodium cations *outside* the membrane as compared to inside. The passage suggests that there should be a strong gradient for positively charged sodium to diffuse into the *intracellular* fluid (P2, L3-7; *opposite charges attract*). Also, since Table 1 shows that the ionic concentration of sodium outside the cell is so much greater than inside, then this would be another reason that sodium should diffuse into the cell. Thus the only way for sodium to be driven against its charge <u>and</u> concentration (= *electrochemical*) gradient is by **active transport** not diffusion (P2; BIO 1.1.2).

Q 156 B   BIO 4.9; P1, L1-4, P3
The sodium-potassium pump uses energy to transport these molecules against their concentration gradients. Cyanide is an inhibitor of an essential enzyme of the electron transport chain (BIO 4.9), which is a major source of ATP (*energy*) for the cell (BIO 4.4). If cyanide is added to the cells, considerably less energy will be produced, and the sodium potassium pump will be unable to function.

Q 157 A   BIO 5.1, 5.1.1/2/3

To answer this question you must know that acetylcholine is an excitatory neurotransmitter that is important in motor neurons. Acetylcholine must cause an action potential in the following cell to continue the signal to the appropriate muscle. Action potentials start with the membrane becoming temporarily more permeable to sodium ions, causing depolarization of the membrane. Therefore, the post-synaptic membrane (*motor end plate*; BIO 5.1F) will become more permeable to the positive ions immediately following acetylcholine being released from the pre-synaptic membrane and reaching receptors on the post-synaptic membrane by diffusion.

Q 158 B   C: *anaerobic*; BIO 4.4, CHM 1.5

Since the exercise is "vigorous," mostly anaerobic conditions prevail (BIO 4.5). Therefore, two molecules of glucose produce four molecules of ATP (BIO 4.4). Now you can multiply the given equation (Q158) through by four.

Q 159 B   BIO 12.3

Active transport moves molecules against a gradient and requires energy (P1; B: BIO 1.1.2). Blood returning to the lungs from the rest of the body is deoxygenated and comes into contact with a high concentration of O_2 in the lungs. Clearly O_2 does not need to be actively transported and, rather, will readily diffuse. The alveoli of the lungs require such fast and efficient transport of O_2 into the body and CO_2 out of the body that only the rapid process of diffusion will do.

Q 160 D   T1

Let's begin by translating the question: *how do we make the membrane potential (V_m) more negative?* The easy way to answer is simply by looking at the equilibrium potentials of the ions in Table 1. Only chloride and potassium have equilibrium potentials more negative than V_m. If the permeability of either of the two ions could be increased then V_m would become more negative (i.e. the value would become closer to that of the ion whose permeability increased). Thus answer choice **D.** is the only possible answer. In reality the membrane is always *very* permeable to potassium and that is an important reason resting V_m is negative (BIO 5.1.1). Thus increasing the already very high potassium permeability is not an important factor in membrane hyperpolarization. Imagine what would happen if the permeability to sodium suddenly increased: V_m would tend towards the equilibrium potential of sodium which is positive (= *depolarization*; BIO 5.1.2/3).

Q 161 actually asks two straightforward questions: (i) what is the difference between the initial molecule and the final one? A: in the bottom left hand corner of the molecule, the carbonyl group is converted to a hydroxyl group; and (ii) have you memorized the IR absorption of a carbonyl group and a hydroxyl group?! A: ☹ or ☺ ! The IR absorption range for the carbonyl group is 1630-1780 and hydroxyl is 3200-3650 (ORG 14.1). Taking question (i) into consideration, we would expect a *disappearance* in the 1630-1780 range and an *appearance* in the 3200-3650 range.

⊠ Incidental #1: $NaBH_4$ is the mild reducing agent which reduces ketones and aldehydes to alcohols (i.e. Q 161; ORG 7.2.1, cf 8.2).

⊠ Incidental #2: 'MeOH' is shorthand for methanol (EtOH = ethanol).

Q 162 tests two concepts.

☞ Just like atoms or molecules, groups attached to a ring have electrons in their outermost shells. Like charges repel. Thus *electron shell repulsion* means substituents want to be maximally apart.

☞ There are two positions for substituents of a ring: *axial* and *equatorial*. Equatorial substituents are maximally apart (ORG 3.3; ORG 12.3.2, Fig IV.B.12.1).

Q 163 D   BIO 14.2
You must understand the process of gametogenesis in females to answer this question.

Q 164 A   BIO 16.5
You must be familiar with characteristics of the phylum Chordate and the subphylum Vertebrate. While vertebrates share many characteristics of chordates, they are somewhat more complex in that they have vertebral columns and closed vascular systems. Chordates have a tail at some point in development, but not necessarily in the adult form. The only option that applies only to chordates is the hollow dorsal nerve cord.

Q 165 begins with your ability to write the molecular structure for formaldehyde (*a carbonyl group with two hydrogens attached to carbon*; ORG 7.1). Next, let's treat formaldehyde with water. Draw the mechanism below.

The δ^- oxygen in water is attracted to the δ^+ carbonyl carbon. The pi bond breaks and the free electrons go to oxygen. The attached water molecule now has three bonds (two H's and one carbon) and thus is positively charged. Electronegative oxygen is not happy! Oxygen pulls electrons to itself from its bond to H, thereby kicking off the proton H^+. The proton is attracted to the oxygen with the free electron pair. Our product is a *diol* (= *2 alcohol groups*). Note that the mechanism is the same as for hemiacetal formation (ORG 7.2.2), where R=H, R'=H, and R'''=H.

Q 166 C   KW: *facultative*; **BIO 2.2**
To begin with, the issue of gram positive or gram negative is irrelevant and should not distract you. This question actually reduces to the following simple concepts: your mouth is sometimes open (*exposed to oxygen*) and sometimes closed (*little or no oxygen*). Thus in order to survive in your mouth, a bacterium would need to be able to produce energy in the presence or absence of oxygen (= *facultative anaerobe*; BIO 2.2).

Q 167 B   BIO 2.2; deduce; P2, L3
The suffix 'coccus' refers to the shape and means sphere. The suffix 'bacillus' also refers to the shape and means cylindrical (BIO 2.2). {P.S.: *never let the mere size of a word or molecule intimidate you!*}

Q 168 D   C: *glucan = extracellular*; **P1, L4-6**
From the description in the passage it is clear that glucan is formed outside of the bacteria. It adheres to the teeth and is present between bacteria. Therefore, the enzyme which catalyzes the formation of glucan must be located on an external surface of the bacteria.

Q 169 B   ORG 12.3.2; P2; KW: *initially*
From the second paragraph it is found that glucan is formed only in the presence of sucrose, which is a disaccharide made up of fructose and glucose. The enzyme acts on glucose molecules to form glucan and fructose molecules to form lactic acid. However, the question asks how the enzyme acts *initially*. To get the glucose and fructose which the enzyme will ultimately change, the enzyme first needs to split its starting product, sucrose, into those constituent sugars.

Q 170 A   BIO 2.2, 15.5
Answer choices **B.**, **C.** and **D.** are processes by which bacteria multiply or by which they change their genetic makeup thereby enhancing their chances of survival (which contributes to their proliferation). Answer choice **A.** sounds very similar to these bacterial processes, but is not associated with an increase in viability or with multiplication.

GS-2, Passage V, Questions 171-176

Q 171 refers to cyclohexanol which is a cyclic alcohol with six carbons (ORG 6.2.4). Now we look at Figure 1 to see where the four possible answers are. Note that in order for I or II to be possible, there would have had to be a reaction with the 5% sodium bicarbonate. However, Table 1 shows that a sodium bicarbonate test is positive with carboxylic acids (*which is not cyclohexanol!*).

Now let's compare III and IV in Figure 1. The only difference between the two is their response to the Lucas test. From Table 1 the Lucas test is positive with alcohols with *five or less* carbons (*which is not cyclohexanol!*). The only possible answer is IV which is **D.**

Q 172 simplifies to the following: they tell us only one test is positive - the 2,4-DNP test. By looking at Table 1, we see that aldehydes and ketones are the only two possibilities. But how can we differentiate the two? Easy! Also in Table 1, we see that Fehling's is positive with aldehydes. Since Fehling's is negative in our problem, then the answer must be ketones

Q 173 reminds you of one of the very important reducing agents, LiAlH$_4$, which can reduce aldehydes and ketones to their corresponding alcohols (ORG 7.2.1). However, an aldehyde has only <u>one</u> R group as a substituent but a ketone has <u>two</u> R groups (ORG 7.1). Thus an aldehyde is reduced to a <u>primary</u> alcohol and a ketone is reduced to a <u>secondary</u> alcohol.

Q 174 simply tests your recognition of acet*one* as a ket*one* and whose molecular formula is CH$_3$-CO-CH$_3$ (ORG 7.1). Next, a quick glance at Table 1 reveals ketones besides 2,4-DNP and CH$_3$-CO- besides Iodoform.

Q 175 *is* **Q 174** in wolf's clothing! The relevant difference between the two ketones is the CH$_3$-CO- R (*methyl ketone*) group on acetone producing the positive Iodoform test (*which is the difference between groups IV and V*).

Q 176 is asking you to spell out the reaction. Recall Na$^+$ is a spectator ion (ORG 1.6) and acetic *acid* is simply a proton donor (CHM 6.1). Thus the reaction simplifies to the following:

$$HCO_3^- + H^+ \rightleftharpoons H_2CO_3 \rightleftharpoons H_2O + CO_2$$

The preceding is the reverse of the reaction in BIO 12.4.1.

Q 177 D   P2, L 1-3, L7-9, deduce
In order to be effective, the vaccine must elicit an immune response without giving the person the full-blown disease. Before injecting the virus it must be cloned, but it cannot simply be injected in its natural harmful form. Also, the protein coat is how the immune system will initially identify the virus in order to produce antibodies against it. For this reason, the protein coat should not be destroyed. The most important thing is to ensure that the virus will be unable to cause harm (inactivated), yet will still elicit the appropriate immune response.

Q 178 A P1, L1-2; KW: *production*; BIO 9.4.1

The liver is affected in people with viral hepatitis type B. You must understand the functions of the liver to answer this question. The liver produces bile which emulsifies fat. This aids in the *absorption* of vitamins A, D, E and K (they are fat soluble) and the liver may even store some of these vitamins. However, the liver has no role in *producing* these vitamins.

Q 179 A P2, L6-7, BIO 2.1

You should know the basic structure of a virus (BIO 2.1). HBsAg is a protein (P2, L6-7). A virus is very simple in structure and the protein outer coating is called the *capsid*. Viruses do not have 'slimy mucoid-like' capsules around them like some bacteria.

Q 180 C G; BIO 8.2

Basic knowledge of the immune response would be helpful here; nonetheless, certain options can be ruled out. The question has asked for an explanation of why the first immune response differs from the second. An appropriate answer should include some information about both responses to show the difference. Options **A.** and **B.** contain one statement concerning only one of the two immune responses. This is not useful in explaining why the two are different. You should also know that macrophages do not produce memory cells, and this rules out option **D.** By carefully examining the graph it is clear that the antibody concentration in serum is higher (*more intense*) and faster in the secondary response. This is consistent with option **C.** and information from the biology review (BIO 8.2).

Q 181 B BIO 2.3

You must understand the basic processes involved in the reproduction of fungi to answer this question.

Q 182 B P1, L4-6; BIO 15.3

You should be familiar with the reasoning behind sex-linked diseases. The disease in question cannot be sex-linked because it occurs more often in women. If the gene for this disease were located on sex chromosomes, the male would get the disease more often (BIO 15.3).

Q 183 D T1

This question is very straightforward. You simply need to read the table and find the highest values for the two columns, then see which protein had that value.

Q 184 B F1; CHM 9.9; BIO 6.3.3/6

According to Figure 1, free thyroxine (thyroid hormone) is involved in an equilibrium reaction with both tissue protein-bound thyroxine and plasma protein-bound thyroxine. By Le

Chatelier's principle, a change in the system (increasing free thyroxine) will cause the system to evolve in such a way as to minimize the change. So adding more free thyroid hormone will cause both equilibria to shift to the product side, producing more tissue and plasma protein-bound thyroxine.

Q 185 D   BIO 6.3.3

The prefix 'hypo' tends to refer to things that are low or slowed down in some way (lethargy). The prefix 'hyper' tends to refer to things that are elevated or overactive (i.e. your kid brother!).

Q 186 A   P3, L5-7; BIO 5.4.4, 6.3.3

Hyperparathyroidism refers to an overactive parathyroid gland. The passage states that this condition leads to an increase in the level of calcium in plasma and tissues (P3, L5-7). This calcium comes from the breaking down of bone by *osteoclasts*, which are stimulated by parathyroid hormone.

Q 187 B   deduce; B: BIO 5.4.4, 6.3.3

If it is true that elevated levels of extracellular phosphate results in the calcification of bones and tissues (answer choice **B.**), then circulating calcium must be *lowered* in order to participate in the calcification process. However, parathormone *increases* circulating calcium. Thus in would be logical that parathormone finds ways to reduce extracellular phosphate in order to avoid the calcification process.

Q 188 A   BIO 9.4.1

This is very simple question. You should know that the liver produces bile and the gallbladder stores it.

Q 189 D   BIO 6.1.4

The sympathetic nervous system is involved in 'fight or flight' reactions. These reactions include many of the same effects that are caused by increasing physical activity.

Q 190 A   BIO 7.4

Blood pressure is not measured in the veins, it is measured in the brachial artery.

Q 191 C   BIO 1.3

The order of events in the cell cycle is: G_1, S (*synthesis*), G_2, Prophase, Metaphase, Anaphase, Telophase. If a drug prevents prophase from occurring, most cells will be arrested at the stage immediately prior to prophase, G_2.

Q 192 D   BIO 2.2, 2.3

The question is asking for a difference between a bacterium and a fungus. Options **A.**, **B.** and **C.** may very well be correct attributes of the organism stated, but for it to be the correct answer it must be a characteristic that the other organism does not also possess. Bacteria are prokaryotes and therefore do not have a nucleus. Fungi, on the other hand, are eukaryotes and therefore contain a nucleus, so this is the difference between the two organisms. Note that both fungi and bacteria have cell walls, ribosomes and can undergo anaerobic metabolism (BIO 2.2, 2.3).

GS-2, Passage VIII, Questions 193-196

This is a fun passage! {☺ !} Begin by drawing the molecular structures of isopropyl bromide, Na$^+$ tert-butoxide, and Na$^+$ ethoxide (*if you have problems review* ORG 3.1 *and* 6.1; *isopropyl bromide = 2-bromopropane*):

The ethoxide molecule, being relatively small and negatively charged, will (*but not exclusively*) be attracted to the δ^+ central carbon in isopropyl bromide. Thus ethoxide is the nucleophile and Br is the leaving group = S$_N$2. The product would be ethyl isopropyl ether. {*mechanism*: ORG 6.2.3; *to name ethers*: ORG 10.1} Draw this S$_N$2 mechanism:

However, with the big bulky base, Na$^+$ tert-butoxide, it would have difficulty accessing the central carbon in isopropyl bromide. Instead, it takes the easy way out: it plucks protons off a molecule like oranges off a tree! {I think I've said that before!} This leaves the unstable primary carbanion intermediate whose electrons are quickly attracted to the neighboring δ^+ carbon thus bumping out Br = E2 mechanism. Thus the product is propene (ORG 6.2.4; *yes, Na$^+$ ethoxide often engages in E2 reactions!! However, the difference between the two oxides in this problem is size which affects the probability of the occurrence of a given reaction*). Draw the E2 mechanism for the production of propene:

In the second paragraph in the passage, we learn what we have already worked out! Compound A is propene, C_3H_6, the reaction occurs by second order kinetics (=E2), and it has vinylic protons (ORG 4.1). In the third paragraph we also learn that its molecular mass is 42 grams.

Paragraph 3 introduces Compound B which we already worked out as $C_5H_{12}O$, ethyl isopropyl ether.

Paragraphs 4 and 5 are irrelevant! However, to learn more about ethers see ORG 10.1. For info about alkene oxidation with $KMnO_4$ see ORG 4.2.2.

Q 193 has been answered in the preceding paragraphs (Compound A = E2, B = S_N2).

Q 194 has been worked out to reveal Compound A as prop*ene*, an alk*ene*.

Q 195 relies on your understanding of the key events in the E2 mechanism as illustrated in ORG 6.2.4. The dotted lines are meant to represent *partial* bonds. Thus we're looking for an option that shows the attraction of the electrons from a negatively charged group (i.e. ethoxide) to a proton; as the <u>positive</u> proton is being *eliminated* (<u>E</u>2) the <u>negative</u> electrons on the primary carbon are being attracted to the neighboring δ^+ carbon with the good leaving group which is electronegative. Answer choice **C.** fills our requirements! Answer choice **D.** represents the S_N2 mechanism.

Q 196 was determined to be $C_5H_{12}O$, ethyl isopropyl ether.

Q 197 B   P2, L7-13; BIO 1.1, 5.2-P4
The synaptic terminal faces the muscle and the acetylcholine released must reach receptors on the muscle (P2). These receptors should logically be located on the surface of the muscle with which the neurotransmitter will first come into contact (*motor end plate*, BIO 5.1F). However, it should be known from the biology review that muscle fibers are covered by a plasma membrane, or sarcolemma (BIO 5.2). This will be the first surface the neurotransmitter comes into contact with, so it should contain receptors (BIO 1.1).

Q 198 B   BIO 5.1, 5.1.1/2; P2, L11-12
We are told that the muscle cell engages in an "all-or-none" action potential. In other words, either the action potential occurs (100%) or it does not occur (0%), but there is nothing in between. Another way of considering the concept "all-or-none" is graphically. Figure 2 (A) is the control in Experiment 2 which is the classic action potential curve (BIO 5.1.2) which occurs under <u>natural</u> conditions. Thus in nature, either the curve occurs essentially as drawn or it does not (i.e. no action potential), but the action potential curve does *not* occur in a graded fashion (*all-or-none*). Thus answer choice **A.** is false.

Q 199 B   **P2, L13-15; BIO 5.1; deduce**

Acetylcholine (ACh) can depolarize the postsynaptic membrane (P2; BIO 5.1). Acetylcholinesterase terminates the action of ACh. Thus if acetylcholinesterase no longer had its normal activity (i.e. because of a mutation) then ACh could continue to depolarize the postsynaptic membrane uninhibited.

Q 200 D   **F1 (2); B: BIO 5.1**

Read the information below "Experiment 1" which describes the four trials in Figure 1. In the first trial marked (1) in Fig. 1, we have two tracings. The top tracing is in the units mV or milli*volts*, which must refer to V_m, the membrane potential from the presynaptic and postsynaptic cells. The way you can determine this information is by examining the line drawing at the top of Figure 1: notice how the second electrode, which is symbolized as if it is recording information, has its tip placed at the junction between the neuron (*presynaptic*) and the muscle cell (*postsynaptic*), thus both voltages can be recorded. {*The preceding junction is called the motor end plate*; BIO 5.1F}

The second tracing is in the units µA or micro*amps*, which must refer to the *current* used to stimulate the nerve (N = nerve stimulation, Ca = calcium). Thus Fig. 1 (1) shows us that after the nerve is stimulated in the absence of calcium, there is little or no increase in voltage (= *depolarization; follow the tracings to the right of the point of stimulation*) of the muscle cell. Fig. 1 (2) shows us that if we give calcium prior to nerve stimulation, we get a clear and significant depolarization of the muscle cell. Fig. 1 (3) shows us that if we give calcium alone, there is no depolarization. And finally, Fig. 1 (4) shows us that if we give calcium *after* the nerve is stimulated (N), there is *no* resulting depolarization of the muscle cell.

Q 201 D   **F2, deduce**

By looking at Figure 2 we can see three graphs. The first (A) is the "control" which is actually a classic tracing of an action potential (BIO 5.1.2). The next curve (B) demonstrates that adding curare drastically reduces the depolarization. The final curve (C) demonstrates that the addition of eserine greatly increases the depolarization [*notice that the x and y-axis for (C) is several times greater than (A) or (B)*]. Thus curare (B), which reduces depolarization, may block (*bind*) acetylcholine (ACh) receptors on the muscle cell (= *postsynaptic membrane*) preventing ACh from engaging in depolarization. And eserine (C), which increases depolarization, may prevent the hydrolysis of acetylcholine thus prolonging and increasing its depolarization capability. {*Compare eserine's action to Q199*}

Q 202 B   **F2; BIO 5.1.2**

You need to examine the figure carefully to determine that between four and five msec the membrane potential is in the process of returning to its resting potential [note that (A) and (B) are drawn to the same scale]. The lowest point in the curve has just been passed at four msec. The period between the highest point of the curve and the lowest point corresponds to the absolute refractory period in which another action potential cannot be generated. In the process of returning from the lowest point to the resting potential, action potentials may be generated but with difficulty. This corresponds to the relative refractory period.

Q 203 A   P2

The fungus is better adapted to live on one population of the host species than another. In this case the fungus displays more rapid adaptation than the host since the fungus is better able to live on this host than others. The fungus did not display more rapid adaptation with respect to all host populations, as its ability to grow and reproduce on other populations of hosts is limited.

Q 204 B   P2; BIO 16.3; cf BIO 15.5

The passage discusses evolution within two different species. Within a species, the passage distinguishes between "local" populations and "other" populations which suggests that the populations live apart (= *allopatric*; BIO 16.3). Since the local population evolves differently (i.e. *"more capable of attacking the host . . ."*), genetic drift may be implicated. Recall that genetic mutations are usually either negative or neutral with regard to the organism's survival (BIO 15.5).

Q 205 B   F1 (B), cf (A)

By looking at the experimental results (B) in Figure 1 you can see that over time the parasite population noticeably declines. The fluctuation (frequency of oscillation of the curve) of both populations is also somewhat reduced compared to the control (A).

Q 206 C   Ap C

The passage suggests (= *hypothesis*) that evolution occurs between two different species, a parasite and a host, which have had prolonged exposure to each other [= *experimental group*; Fig.1 (B)]. To prove that the preceding is true and significant, the result must first be compared to a control which is not exposed to the "treatment" (i.e. *members of the parasite and host species which have no prior exposure to each other*). In this manner, we can attribute the *difference* in the two graphs to the only factor which changed - the exposure to each other which is the basis for coevolution.

Q 207 A   F1, deduce

You need to identify what the trend is in the graph for the control group in order to identify possible explanations for these events. As the host population increases [Fig. 1 (A)], the parasite population also increases until a point at which the host population declines, probably as a result of too many parasites. The parasite population quickly drops off in response to this decline (i.e. too few hosts to infect). The host population starts to increase again, followed shortly after by the parasite population. Options **C.** and **D.** are adequate explanations of the events occurring in the populations. Option **B.** is less likely, as eliminating the parasite's source of food is not likely to increase that population. However, a decrease in the host population is followed shortly after by an increase in parasite population and in this way option **B.** provides an unlikely explanation of events that actually do occur. Option **A.** is illogical as the virulence of the parasites when the population is low is unlikely to have a large enough effect to decrease the host population significantly. Also, this option explains an event which does not occur on the graph. In no place does the parasite population lower first, followed by a lowering of the host population.

Q 208 C   deduce; cf P1/2, BIO 16.2; A.↔ BIO 15.5

Knowledge of bacteria or even current affairs should tell you that it is definitely possible for a bacterium to develop resistance to a drug. Those bacteria which happen to be able to survive in the presence of the drug (because of mutations or other reasons) will be the ones that will reproduce, likely passing this resistance on to the new bacteria (selective pressure) which are similar to the mechanisms described in the passage for coevolution.

GS-2, Passage XI, Questions 209-214

Recall Principle #1: Organic Chemistry is simple! Do not waste precious exam time working out details which are not relevant to your success! Thus the initial paragraph of the problem is read, then a quick, fleeting (!) glimpse at the reaction, then we get to the point: *the questions*!

Q 209 can only go wrong if you're "thinking too much"!! On the most basic level, in the first reaction we saw a large ugly molecule on the left side of the equation and a *similarly* ugly molecule on the right side. The difference being 2 H's and 1 O. Mmmmm, 2 H's and 1 O, H_2O, water! Superkeeners will complain about the imprecise way the reaction is written: *where did the second molecule come from?* When you're offered a gift, don't reject it because it's not exactly the way you wanted it to be!

Q 210 is trying to test your *understanding* of a mechanism. This is done by labelling oxygen in some way and seeing if you can work out where *that* oxygen, in water, ends up in the product. First we need to determine which reaction involves water as a reactant. A quick look at Figure 1 reveals H_2O on the third line. Of course, oxygen in H_2O is δ^- (CHM 2.3, PT) and thus will be attracted to a δ^+ atom. The carbon double bonded to the nitrogen must be δ^+. Furthermore, since nitrogen is δ^- and the hydrogens in H_2O are δ^+ then their mating is also inevitable. In summary, the hydrogens in H_2O help form the amino group $-NH_2$ while the oxygen in H_2O, which we are tracing, helps form the second carbonyl group, C=$\underline{O}$, in the illustrated product (line 3, Figure 1). The reverse reaction is represented in ORG 7.2.3; tracing oxygen in a reaction is shown for esters in ORG 9.4.

Q 211 tests your recognition of the δ⁻ nitrogen in the amino group as a *nucleophile* (= *nucleus-loving, AKA positive charge-loving!*). Now only answer choices **B.** and **C.** are possible. Recall that nitrogen's lone pair electrons are essential to carrying out a nucleophilic reaction. In the reaction provided in the question, we go from a nitrogen with four bonds (= *no lone pair available*) to one with three bonds thus the addition of a base freed up the lone pair which can now engage in a nucleophilic reaction. Furthermore, the free amino group prior to the addition of a base was positively charged thereby being a distinctly terrible nucleophile!! {*ORG Chapter 11: Amines*}

Q 212 begins with the issue of nomenclature. Alanine should be recognized as an amino acid. Draw the *general* structure of an amino acid below (ORG 12.1 *or see* Q211).

Benz*oyl chloride* should be recognized as an acid halide. Draw the general structure of an acid chloride below (ORG 9.1; *note that 'Benz' refers to benzyl, as in the benzene ring* [ORG Chap. 5], *which is stable to nucleophilic reactions so we need not account for its presence!*).

Now if you were able to get Q211 correct then Q212 is just a follow-up. The *amino* acid contains a δ⁻ nitrogen in the *amino* group which is a nucleophile. The nucleophile is attracted to the δ⁺ carbon of the carbonyl group in benzoyl chloride. The weakest bond breaks (*the π bond within the double bond*, ORG 1.3.1), and the electron pair lands on the electronegative oxygen. Now carbon is surrounded by *three* electronegative atoms making carbon verrrrry δ⁺! This is an unstable situation!

Thus the negatively charged free electrons on oxygen quickly mate with the verrrrry δ⁺ carbon. However, since carbon can only be bonded four times, one of its substituents has to go! Since chloride is an excellent leaving group (*see the last paragraphs of* ORG 6.2.4), we are left with an *amide* (ORG 9.3). Draw the mechanism below.

Why was the medium "dilute aqueous sodium hydroxide"? Once again we turn our attention back to Q211. Base treatment of an amino acid increases the rate of a nucleophilic reaction of the free amino group.

Would the "dilute aqueous sodium hydroxide" create other products in the reaction? Because it is *dilute* we would expect very little contamination or by-products. But just for fun, let's treat both our reactants with *concentrated* aqueous sodium hydroxide.

Now NaOH in water (= *aqueous*) means Na^+ and OH^- (CHM 5.2), which simply means the nucleophile OH^- since Na^+ is a spectator ion (ORG 1.6). Note that both compounds have a carbonyl group which are internationally popular in attracting nucleophiles! Treat your preceding reactants with OH^-. The nucleophile is quickly attracted to the δ^+ carbon of the carbonyl group (i.e. ORG 8.1). The weakest bond breaks (*the π bond within the double bond*, ORG 1.3.1), and the electron pair lands on the electronegative oxygen. Now carbon is surrounded by *three* electronegative atoms making carbon verrrrry δ^+! This is an unstable situation! {*does this sound familiar?!*}

Thus the negatively charged free electrons on oxygen quickly mate with the verrrrry δ^+ carbon. However, since carbon can only be bonded four times, one of its substituents has to go! In the case of the amino acid, the hydroxyl group leaves simply re-establishing the <u>carboxylic acid</u>. In the case of the acid chloride, chloride is an excellent leaving group (*see the last paragraphs of* ORG 6.2.4), thereby creating a <u>carboxylic acid</u>.

Q 213 reminds you of Principle #4: isn't it remarkable how many questions in a row that you can answer without reading the passage?

This question can be answered very quickly with some strategy and some basic info about amino acids (ORG 12.1, 12.1.1/2). Amino acid **I.** has the side group C_6H_5- which is the benzene ring (ORG 5.1) which is neither *ionic* nor *polar* and is thus <u>hydrophobic</u>. Amino acid **II.** has the side group -OH which *is* polar and thus <u>hydrophilic</u>. Therefore, without going any further, the answer must be **A.**

For interest, we note that amino acid **III.** has the amino side group which is protonated at neutral pH (= *positively charged*; ORG 12.1.2). Amino acid **IV.** has the carboxylic *acid* side group which *loses a proton* at neutral pH (= *negatively charged*).

Q 214 is really asking: what is the better base (*proton acceptor*) an amino group $-NH_2$ or the carboxylate anion $-CO_2^-$, which is an anion because carboxyl is an <u>ACID</u> (*carboxylic acid*). Mmmmm, I'd go with the amino group also! (ORG 12.1.2)

Q 215 B   BIO 15.3, 15.3.1
We are told that Von Willebrand's is an autosomal dominant disease. Let V be the allele for the disease while v is the absence of the allele for the disease. Thus the father is vv and the mother who is heterozygous is Vv. The Punnett square (BIO 15.3) reveals the following:

	V	**v**
v	Vv	vv
v	Vv	vv

Thus the frequency of Vv is 0.50 (= 2/4) and that of vv is also 0.50 (= 2/4). Since the gene is dominant all heterozygotes (Vv) will have the disease. The chance that the next child expresses the disease is not dependent on what happened to the parent's previous children (BIO 15.3.1).

Q 216 C   ORG 12.3.2

This can be solved quickly: focus on the -CH$_2$OH substituent in Figure 1. The shortest route between it and the circled hydroxyl contains *three* carbons. Now look at the -CH$_2$OH substituent in the modified Fischer projection (Fig. 2) of β-D-glucose. We should be able to count three carbons along the shortest route between it and I, II, III, or IV. The answer must be III. {ORG 12.3.2, Fig IV.B.12.1}

Q 217 B   BIO 4.5

Glycolysis is the process by which glucose is broken down into two molecules of pyruvate. At this point the lysis of glucose (glyco-lysis) is finished. The following step of converting the pyruvate molecules into acetyl-CoA is not a part of glycolysis.

Q 218 D   BIO 10.3

The nephron is the functional unit of the kidney and contains Bowman's capsule and the renal corpuscle.

Q 219 B   KWs: *no enantiomer*; ORG 2.2

This question tests your ability to identify a molecule which has no enantiomer. In other words, a molecule whose mirror image *can* be superimposed on itself (ORG 2.2). Examine molecule I. Note that its mirror image is molecule III. If you just picked up molecule III and tried to put it on top of molecule I, it doesn't work (*the hydroxyl groups never cover each other*). Even if you rotate molecule III around 180°, you still cannot superimpose it on molecule I. Molecules I and II are enantiomers of each other!

Examine molecule II. Draw its mirror image. Note that when you turn the mirror image 180°, you end up with the same molecule. Thus it has no enantiomer and may be referred to as a *meso* compound.

Understanding

GS-3

Physical Sciences

<u>**Q 1 A**</u>   **P2, L8; B: PHY 9.1.3, 12.3**

Since gamma rays are uncharged electromagnetic rays, they are not deflected in magnetic or electric fields under normal conditions.

<u>**Q 2 C**</u>   **F1; P2, L1-5; PT; B: PHY 12.2**

From the graph and the fact that the n/p (= *# neutrons/ # protons*) ratio for magnesium is 27/12, which is greater than 1 (= *unit slope*; P2, L1-5).

<u>**Q 3 C**</u>   **PHY 12.4**

Using Number of half-lives elapsed = (Elapsed time)/(Length of half-life)
Number of half-lives = 15.6 years/5.2 years = 3
Using Fraction of initial activity remaining = $(1/2)^{\text{number of half-lives elapsed}}$
Fraction of initial activity remaining = $(1/2)^3 = 1/8$
Since Activity after 15.6 years = 250 millicuries
Initial activity = 8×250 millicuries = 2000 millicuries

<u>**Q 4 D**</u>   **PHY 12.4, PT**

$$^{210}_{81}\text{Th} \rightarrow {}^{x}_{y}Z + 3\,^{0}_{-1}e^- + {}^{4}_{2}\text{He}^{2+} + \text{gamma ray}$$

Since the sum of the atomic numbers and mass numbers on either side of the equation must be equal (matter cannot be created or destroyed), we get:
$210 = x + (3 \times 0) + 4 + 0$; x = 206
$81 = y + (3 \times -1) + 2 + 0$; y = 82
You can stop at this point or examine the periodic table for the name of the correct element (answer choice **D.**). Note that the atomic number and mass number of gamma rays are both zero.

<u>**Q 5 B**</u>   **PHY 12.4, PT**

$^{230}_{90}\text{Th} \rightarrow {}^{214}_{83}\text{Bi} + x\,^{0}_{-1}e^- + y\,^{4}_{2}\text{He}^{2+} + z$ (*gamma ray*)
Since the sum of the atomic numbers and mass numbers on either side of the equation must be equal (matter cannot be created or destroyed), we get:
$90 = 83 - x + 2y$ Equation (i)
$230 = 214 + 4y$; y = 4 (i.e. *4 alpha decay reactions*)
Substituting for y in Equation (i)
$90 = 83 - x + 8$; x = 1 (i.e. *1 beta decay reaction*)
The order of the reactions is irrelevant (i.e. alpha, beta, ..). Since gamma rays have no atomic number or mass number, the value of z does not affect this particular calculation.

<u>**Q 6 D**</u>   **PHY 12.3, 4.2; deduce**

Alpha radiation consists of the largest particles (*helium nuclei* with a mass number of 4 thus the greatest inertia, PHY 4.2) and are the slowest (about 1/3 times the speed of light). Beta radiation consists of smaller (*electrons*, 1/1370 times lighter than a proton), faster particles (about 4/5 times the speed of light). Gamma radiation consists of the smallest particles (*photons*, no mass) which travel at the greatest speed (at the speed of light).

Q 7 D   CHM 2.3 (ii)

The s-block elements are those whose s-orbital is the valent orbital.

Q 8 D   P2, L1-4

Given in the second paragraph of the passage and knowing that sodium (Na) is a group I cation (CHM 2.3).

Q 9 A   P1, L4-7; PT; CHM 2.3F

Given in the first paragraph of the passage.

Q 10 D   P1, L7-10; P2, L1-4

Given in the first and second paragraphs of the passage. Note that answer choice **B.** is false because of P1, L2-4.

Q 11 C   PoE: PT, Air ≈ N_2, O_2 leading to Fire, CO_3 ≠ gas (cf. CO_3^{2-})

Let's use the process of elimination. Answer choice **A.** is false because it would support a lighted splint (*translation: fire burns in the presence of oxygen!*). Answer choice **B.** (molecular weight or MW = 28 g/mol) is somewhat lighter that air which is mostly nitrogen (78%, MW = 28 g/mol) with oxygen (21%, MW = 32 g/mol). Answer choice **D.** is really an anion (*carbonate*) not a gas (P2). Thus we are left with carbon dioxide (MW = 44 g/mol) which is heavier than air and does not support a lighted splint.

Q 12 A   CHM 6.6, 6.5

Using $K_b = ([X^+][OH^-])/[XOH]$; X is most probably a Group I metal since no decomposition occurred (P3, L3-4), implying that the anion (OH^-) and cation (X^+) are of comparable size (P2, L1-4).

Assuming that $[X^+] = [OH^-]$ approximately

$K_b = [OH^-]^2/[XOH]$, where XOH ≈ 1.0 M at equilibrium, thus:

$1.0 \times 10^{-6} = [OH^-]^2/1$

$[OH^-]^2 = 1.0 \times 10^{-6}$

$[OH^-] = 1.0 \times 10^{-3}$ mol dm^{-3}

$pOH = -\log[OH^-] = -\log(1.0 \times 10^{-3}) = -(-3) = 3$

Using pH + pOH = 14, we get:

pH = 14 - pOH = 14 - 3 = 11

Q 13 B   CHM 2.3

Lithium only has one valent electron (Group I, PT; CHM 2.3). Therefore, one would expect only one covalent bond per lithium atom with no extra valent electrons on the lithium (that is, no lone pairs nor single electrons).

Q 14 A   PHY 9.2.4; P3, L5-12

The trend according to the passage is that the lower in energy the radiation emitted, the greater the principal quantum number of the orbital the electron goes down to. Therefore, the radiation emitted in this problem (*transitions down to* n = 3) should possess less energy than visible light (*transitions down to* n = 2; PHY 9.2.4).

Q 15 D   E

Using the equation given:

$1/(\lambda) = 110\ 000 \times (1/1^2 - 1/2^2) = 110\ 000 \times (1 - 1/4)$

$1/(\lambda) = 110\ 000 \times \times 3/4 = 3 \times 27\ 500 = 72\ 500 = 7.25 \times 10^4\ m^{-1}$

$\lambda = 1/(7.25 \times 10^4) = (1/7.25) \times 10^{-4}$

$\lambda = 1/8 \times \times 10^{-4}$ approximately $= 0.125 \times 10^{-4} = 1.25 \times 10^{-5}\ m$

Q 16 B   E; PHY 12.5; 9.2.4

The determining factor will be the size of the $1/n_1^2 - 1/n_2^2$ term from the given equation. The larger the term is, the larger the value of $1/(\lambda)$ and since the energy difference is inversely proportional to λ (P5, L1-3), the greater the energy, the smaller the value of λ. Thus we want the $1/n_1^2 - 1/n_2^2$ term to be as high as possible. Quickly plugging in values reveals answer choice **B.** as true.

Q 17 B   PHY 9.2.4, 12.5, 7.1.2

$E = hf$

Q 18 A   P5, PHY 7.1.3F

The wavelength of the radiation is dependent on the energy difference between the two orbitals, not on the number of atoms participating. However, the brightness (= *amplitude*) of the lines depends on the number of the relevant transitions occurring (P5).

Q 19 A   CHM 5.3.1, 5.3.2; P2, L 5-7

The stoichiometry of the salt often affects the solubility of the salt, so the least soluble salt is not necessarily the one with the smallest solubility constant. Simply for interest (!), let's derive the general formula:

Equation: $A_xB_y = xA^{y+} + yB^{x-}$

Considering 1 L of solution p moles of A_xB_y will yield a maximum of $(x \times p)$ moles A^{y+} and $(y \times p)$ moles of B^{x-}.

$K_{sp} = [A^{y+}]^x[B^{x-}]^y = (xp)^x \times (yp)^y$

p = solubility of salt = [(x + y) root of $(K_{sp}/(x^x \times y^y))$]
Therefore, Solubility of $Bi_2S_3 = 10^{-20}$ approximately
Solubility of $Ag_2S = 10^{-16}$ approximately
Solubility of $ZnS = 10^{-10.5}$ approximately
Solubility of $CuS = 3.0 \times 10^{-18}$; thus Bi_2S_3 has the lowest solubility which means that in solution Bi^{3+} would be the first cation to precipitate.

ALTERNATIVELY, the same results could be obtained in the traditional fashion where s = solubility and K_{sp} is given in the passage:
$K_{sp}(Bi_2S_3) = (2s)^2(3s)^3 = 108s^5 = 10^{-97}$
$K_{sp}(Ag_2S) = (2s)^2 (s) = 4s^3 = 2 \times 10^{-49}$
$K_{sp}(ZnS) = (s)(s) = s^2 = 10^{-21}$
$K_{sp}(CuS) = (s)(s) = s^2 = 9.0 \times 10^{-36}$

Q 20 C   CHM 5.3.2
$Bi_2S_3 \rightleftharpoons 2Bi^{3+} + 3S^{2-}$
$K_{sp} = [Bi^{3+}]^2[S^{2-}]^3$, *see* CHM 5.3.2
{Compare with the calculation of solubility in Q19}

Q 21 D   CHM 6.6, 6.6.1
Using $K_b = [HCN][OH^-]/[CN^-]$
Assuming that $[HCN] = [OH^-]$ approximately
$K_b = [OH^-]^2/[CN^-]$
$[OH^-]^2 = K_b \times [CN^-] = 1.39 \times 10^{-5} \times 0.02 = 1.39 \times 10^{-5} \times 2 \times 10^{-2} = 2.78 \times 10^{-7}$
$[OH^-] = \sqrt{(2.78 \times 10^{-7})} = \sqrt{(27.8 \times 10^{-8})}$
$[OH^-] = (\sqrt{27.8}) \times 10^{-4} = (\sqrt{25}) \times 10^{-4}$ approximately $= 5 \times 10^{-4}$
Using $pOH = -\log[OH^-]$
$pOH = -\log(5 \times 10^{-4}) = -\log(5) + [-\log(10^{-4})] = -\log(5) + 4$
{To see how a log can be estimated within reasonable error, see the end of CHM 6.6.1}
$pOH = 3.5$ approximately
Using $pH + pOH = 14$
$pH = 14 - pOH = 14 - 3.5$ approximately $= 10.5$

Q 22 B   CHM 5.3.2/3
Equation $ZnS \rightleftharpoons Zn^{2+} + S^{2-}$
Using $K_{sp} = [Zn^{2+}][S^{2-}]$
$1.0 \times 10^{-21} = (5.00 \times 10^{-3})[S^{2-}]$
$[S^{2-}] = (1.0 \times 10^{-21})/(5.00 \times 10^{-3}) = 1/5 \times 10^{-18} = 0.2 \times 10^{-18} = 2.0 \times 10^{-19}$

Q 23 D   P4; P2, L5-7; CHM 5.3.1, 5.3.2

The solubility product should be between that of Ag_2S (= 2.0×10^{-49}) and Bi_2S_3 (= 10^{-97}) making answer choice **D.** the only possibility. Just for interest (!!), let's see if the **solubility** is also between the values for the two salts. Since the X^+ cation is singly charged:

Equation: $X_2S \rightleftharpoons 2X^+ + S^{2-}$

From the answer to Q19

Solubility = cube root of $K_{sp}/4$ = cube root $4.00 \times 10^{-53}/4 = 10^{-17.7}$ approximately

Compare to the solubilities of Ag_2S and Bi_2S_3 (Q19).

Q 24 A   CHM 5.3.3

Due to the common ion effect, the CuS will dissolve to a lesser extent in the presence of copper (II) ions (or sulfide ions).

Q 25 D   CHM 10.4; battery therefore soln irrelevant!

A is the <u>positively charged electrode</u> i.e. <u>anode</u> in the diagram so the electrolyte used is irrelevant.

Q 26 D   PHY 7.1.2

Using velocity = frequency × wavelength

5.0×10^4 m s^{-1} = 2.5×10^4 Hz × λ

$\lambda = (5.0 \times 10^4)/(2.5 \times 10^4)$ m = 2.0 m

Q 27 C   PHY 7.1.3F

If destructive interference occurs (*minimum value*), amplitude = 6 - 3 = 3 units.

If constructive interference occurs (*maximum value*), amplitude = 6 + 3 = 9 units.

Q 28 C   CHM 5.3.1

Using Number of moles in solution = (Concentration × volume used)/1000mL

50 mL of 0.500 M K^+ solution = (0.500 M × 50 mL)/1000 mL= 0.025 moles K^+

10 mL 0f 0.200 M K_2CO_3 solution = [(0.200 M × 10 mL)/1000 mL] × 2 moles K^+ since there are 2 moles of K^+ for each mole of K_2CO_3 = 0.004 moles K^+

Total number of moles K^+ present = 0.025 + 0.004 = 0.029 moles

Total volume of solution = 50 mL + 10 mL = 60 mL

Using Concentration = (Number of moles × 1000 mL)/(volume of solution)

Concentration = (0.029 × 1000)/(60) M = 29/60 M = 2.9/6 M = 0.483 M

Q 29 D   E; B: PHY 7.1

From L = (n × λ)/4, λ = 4L/n

First wavelength = (4 × 24)/1 = 96

Second wavelength = (4 × 24)/3 = 32

Third wavelength = (4 × 24)/5 = 19.2

Fourth wavelength = $(4 \times 24)/7 = 13.7$ approximately
Fifth wavelength = $(4 \times 24)/9 = 10.7$ approximately

Q 30 B   PHY 12.3, 12.4

$^{14}_{7}N + alpha \rightarrow {}^{x}_{y}Z + {}^{17}_{8}O$
$^{14}_{7}N + {}^{4}_{2}He^{2+} \rightarrow {}^{x}_{y}Z + {}^{17}_{8}O$

Since the atomic numbers and mass numbers for the equation must be the same on both sides of the equation (matter is neither created or destroyed), thus:
$14 + 4 = x + 17$; $x = 1$
$7 + 2 = y + 8$; $y = 1$
Therefore, $Z = H$ (= p, a proton)

Q 31 D   PHY 12.3

The alpha particle is the largest <u>and</u> it is doubly charged (= *a helium nucleus*) thus it is the worst candidate for "artificial transmutation". Protons and electrons have the same magnitude of charge (± 1), but a proton is much larger than an electron. And finally, since a neutron has no charge, on such a basis alone, it becomes the best particle for the described reaction.

Q 32 A   PHY 12.4, Ap A.3.2

This is the shape of the graph for all natural radioactive decay processes (and all first order reactions).

Q 33 C   PHY 12.3

It would be attracted to the plate of opposite charge, negative, since a positron is positively charged.

Q 34 C   PHY 5.3

Using Kinetic Energy = $1/2 \times mass \times (velocity)^2$
2.275×10^{-15} J $= 1/2 \times (9.1 \times 10^{-31}) \times v^2$
$v^2 = (2.275 \times 10^{-15} \times 2)/(9.1 \times 10^{-31})$
$v^2 = (4.55 \times 10^{-15})/(9.1 \times 10^{-31}) = 1/2 \times 10^{-15}/10^{-31} = 0.5 \times 10^{16} = 5 \times 10^{15}$
$v = \sqrt{(5 \times 10^{15})} = \sqrt{(50 \times 10^{14})} = \sqrt{(50)} \times 10^7 \approx \sqrt{(49)} \times 10^7$
$v = 7 \times 10^7$ m s^{-1} approximately

Q 35 D   New info

Colored complexes are a well-known characteristic of most transition metals.

Q 36 D $Ag/H_2S \rightarrow Ag_2S$ (black); T1

Tarnished silver is black and from the passage (Table 1), Ag_2S is a black solid. Now we just need to find an answer choice which contains sulfur. H_2S is a gas found in small amounts in air and would react with silver to yield the sulfide.

Q 37 B   CHM 5.3.3, 9.9

Because the acidity constants are small, the undissociated form of the acid tends to predominate in solution, that is, the equilibria $H_2S \rightleftharpoons HS^- + H^+$ ($K_{a1} \approx 10^{-7}$) and $HS^- \rightleftharpoons H^+ + S^{2-}$ ($K_{a2} \approx 10^{-15}$) both are heavily shifted to the left. According to Le Chatelier's principle, this would lead to Reaction I shifting to the right to counteract the effects of H_2S, if it were added. A shift to the left would occur to counteract the addition of protons (H^+) and/or HS^-.

Q 38 D   CHM 8.10

Answer choice **D.** is true for all equilibria.

Q 39 B   CHM 1.3; PT

Using Number of moles = (Mass)/(Relative atomic mass)
Number of moles Ag extracted = 12 g/107.9 g mol^{-1} = 12/108 mol approx = 1/9 mol approx
Equation $2Ag^+ + S^{2-} \rightarrow Ag_2S$, for each mole of silver extracted, ½ mole of silver sulfide is required.
Therefore, number of moles Ag_2S obtained = 1/2 × 1/9 = 1/18 mol
Using Mass = Number of moles × Relative molecular mass
Mass of Ag_2S in original sample = 1/18 × [(107.9 × 2) + 32.1] g = 1/18 × 247.9 g
= 1/18 × 247.5 g approx. = 1/2 × 27.5 g approx. = 13.75 g = 13.8 g

Q 40 A   P5, L2-4

As stated in the passage.

Q 41 B   T1, deduce

When sulfur is added, if $[Ag(CN)_2]^-$ is present, sulfur has the higher affinity for Ag thus a black precipitate will form (= Ag_2S, see Table 1). If $[Ag(EDTA)]^-$ is present, the clear solution will persist because EDTA has a greater affinity for Ag as compared to sulfur. All of the other methods will result in the same solution or precipitate for each of the two complexes.

Q 42 B   PHY 5.4

From Potential energy = Mass (m) × gravitational acceleration (g) × vertical height (h)
Potential energy = 70 kg × 9.8 m s^{-2} × 12 m = 8 232 J

Q 43 A   PHY 5.3/4/5

Using the Principle of conservation of energy and Kinetic Energy = 1/2 × Mass × (velocity)^2

8 232 J = 1/2 × 70 kg × v² {see Q42}
v² = 235.2 = 225 approximately
v = √225 = 15 m s⁻¹

Q 44 D   PHY 2.1, 7.2.1; mg = (70 + 30)g = kx
Using Force = kx (Hooke's Law)
The force is the Joker's applied force: 700 N *and* the weight of the platform: 30 kg × 9.8 m s⁻²
= the spring constant: 150 N m⁻¹ × (x)
Estimate gravity as 10 m s⁻² and we get:
x = (700 + 300)/150 = 1000/150
x = 6.7 m

Q 45 B   PHY 5.2
Using: Potential energy = 1/2kx² (*spring*)
= 1/2 × 150 kg s⁻² × (0.5)² = 75 × (1/2)² = 75 × 1/4 = 18.75 = 18.8 J

Q 46 B   PHY 4.3, 4.4
Using the Principle of conservation of momentum and Momentum = Mass × Velocity:
Total momentum before collision = Total momentum after collision
(1 000 kg × 14 m s⁻¹) + (5 000 kg × 0 m s⁻¹) = (1 000 kg × 2 m s⁻¹) + (5 000 kg × x m s⁻¹)
x = (14 000 - 2 000)/(5 000) = 12/5 = 2 2/5 = 2.4 m s⁻¹

Q 47 C   CHM 1.6
The oxidation state of oxygen is -2; therefore, the total oxidation state of the oxygens in MnO₄⁻
= -2 × 4 = -8. Since the net charge on the ion is -1,
Oxidation state of Mn + (-8) = -1, thus Mn = -1 + 8 = +7
Since the oxidation state of Mn in Mn²⁺ is +2, there has been a decrease in the oxidation state,
that is, a reduction has occurred. {GERC = *gain electrons reduction* . . .CHM 10.2}
The oxidation state of Cl in Cl⁻ is -1 and is 0 in Cl₂ (*the oxidation state of an element in
naturally occurring form* = 0) so an increase in the oxidation state, that is, an oxidation has
occurred. {LEO = *loss of electrons is oxidation* . . .}

Q 48 A   CHM 4.1.6
From the ideal gas equation PV = nRT, n = (PV)/RT

Q 49 D   CHM 1.3, 1.5; PT
From the Reaction I, mole ratio between Mn and Cl₂ = 2 : 5
Relative atomic mass of Mn = 55 approximately (*see the periodic table*)
Relative molecular mass of Cl₂ = 35.5 × 2 = 71.0
Therefore, the mass ratio between Mn and Cl₂ = (2 × 55) : (5 × 71.0)

= 110 : 355 = 11 : 35.5 = 1 : 3 approximately

Q 50 B   CHM 4.1.6, 8.2; decrease T(endo) → increase in n_{actual}

Since the reaction is endothermic, the final temperature of the reaction vessel would be lower than the initial temperature. From the equation obtained in the answer for question 48, if the temperature used in the calculation is greater than the actual temperature, the value of n predicted will be less than the actual value.

Q 51 D   PoE

A solid mixture of two or more metals is referred to as an *alloy*.

Q 52 C   PHY 9.1.2

Using Coulomb's equation : $F = kq_1q_2/r^2$
At original distance, $f = kq_1q_2/r^2$
$r = \sqrt{(kq_1q_2/f)}$
At new distance x, $2f = kq_1q_2/x^2$
$x = \sqrt{(kq_1q_2/2f)}$
$x = (1/\sqrt{2}) \times \sqrt{(kq_1q_2/f)} = (1/\sqrt{2}) \times r = r/\sqrt{2}$

Q 53 D   CHM 2.3

Since potassium only has one electron in its outer shell, it is easily removed (i.e. low first ionization potential/energy), thus leaving potassium with the more stable noble gas-like configuration (i.e. Ar). On the other hand, adding an electron to neutral potassium would require much energy (i.e. high first electron affinity) which would leave potassium with two valence electrons which would not be stable.

☞ Noble gases are the most stable elements in the periodic table.

Q 54 D   PHY 7.2.1

Using Force = kx (Hooke's Law), where the force is the weight mg:
$0.5 \text{ kg} \times 9.8 \text{ m s}^{-2} = 10 \text{ kg s}^{-2} \times x$
x = 0.5 m approximately

Q 55 C   PHY 8.5, 8.2

From the equation $f_o = f_s(V \pm v_o)/(V \pm v_s)$
Since the distance between object and observer is decreasing, use $+v_o$ and $-v_s$, and given $v_o = 0$, we get:
$f_o = f_s(V)/(V - v_s) > f_s$, thus $f_o > f_s$
{The preceding is true because the term $(V)/(V - v_s)$ is necessarily greater than 1 (*plug in any real, which means positive, imaginary values*), thus f_o must be greater than f_s}

Therefore, the observed frequency is greater which means that the wavelength is lower from the observers point of view (from velocity = frequency × wavelength). Thus the wavelength from the source (= the original wavelength) is higher. As long as the environment (i.e. temperature) is relatively constant, the velocity of sound is constant (PHY 7.1.2, 8.2, 8.5).

Q 56 D   CHM 9.9, 9.8
Using Le Chatelier's principle, the reaction will shift in the direction to counteract the stress put on the equilibrium system. Since ΔH is negative (*exothermic*), the reaction can be written thus:

$$N_2 + O_2 \rightleftharpoons 2NO + heat$$

Thus an increase in temperature or heat applies stress to the right, shifting the equilibrium to the left. Conversely, a decrease in temperature or heat shifts the equilibrium to the right (answer choice **D.**). Since the number of moles on both sides of the equilibrium is the same (i.e. 2), a change in pressure does not alter the equilibrium. An *increase* in the partial pressure (*concentration*) of O_2 would shift the equilibrium to the right. A catalyst speeds up the rate of a reaction but does not affect K_{eq}.

Q 57 D   PHY 2.2
Using Newton's Second Law (F = ma)
5.4×10^{-16} N = m $\times 3.2 \times 10^{13}$ m s^{-2}
m = $(5.4 \times 10^{-16})/(3.2 \times 10^{13})$ = 5.4/3.2 $\times 10^{-16}/10^{13}$
m = 5.4/3.2 $\times 10^{-29}$ = 1.7×10^{-29} kg, approximately

Q 58 B   PHY 2.1, 2.2
Both species experience the same force, the *initial* velocity is the same. Therefore, from Newton's Second Law (F = ma), the electron which has the smaller mass will experience a larger acceleration and as a result will have a greater velocity. The greater the velocity of the collision, the more charged particles will be formed.

Q 59 D   P3, L 3-5; PHY 12.1, 12.3
The charge on the helium nucleus is caused by the loss of two electrons (He^{2+}), each having the same charge. Since it must have an equal but opposite charge to the sum of the charges of the two electrons, its charge = $+1.6 \times 10^{-19} \times 2 = 3.2 \times 10^{-19}$ C.
From E = qV (last paragraph)
E = 3.2×10^{-19} C $\times$ 20 V = 64×10^{-19} J = 6.4×10^{-18} J

Q 60 A   PHY 10.1, D.A.
Using Q = It = ne
I(1 s) = $(2.50 \times 10^{19})(1.6 \times 10^{-19})$ = 2.5 × 1.6 = 4.0 A

ALTERNATIVELY, use dimensional analysis:
2.50×10^{19} electrons/second $\times 1.6 \times 10^{-19}$ coulombs/electron $= 4.0$ C/s $= 4.0$ A

Q 61 B   PHY 10.1, 10.2, 10.2.1

Using Ohm's Law : $V = IR$, and $R_{Total} = R_1 + R_2$ (*in series*):
Total resistance before $= 3R_1$; $V_{before} = 3IR$
Total resistance after $= 3R_1 - 2R_1 = R_1$; $V_{after} = IR = 1/3 \times V_{before}$

Q 62 A   PHY 7.1.2, 9.2.4

Energy of electromagnetic radiation is directly proportional to frequency which is inversely proportional to wavelength ($E = hf$; $v = \lambda f$). Therefore, since $E_P > E_R > E_Q$, then wavelength P < wavelength R < wavelength Q.

Q 63 C   CHM 6.5, 6.5.1; P3, L3-4

Two pH units (P3, L3-4) are equivalent to a 100 fold $[H^+]$ difference as shown below.
pH $= -\log(x) = \pm 2$
$x = 10^{\pm 2} = 100$ or $1/100$

Q 64 B   CHM 6.9

Answer choices **A.** and **C.** are characteristics of a neutral solution, which may not necessarily exist at the equivalence point of a titration.

Q 65 A   CHM 6.9

The pK_a of the indicator ($= -\log K_a$) should be near the equivalence point of the titration (P3, L5-7; pH ≈ 7). Only one indicator has a K_a with a factor of 10^{-7} [recall: $-\log (10^{-7}) = 7$].

Q 66 D   R1; P3, L1-4; CHM 6.6.1

Since the pH is less than the pK_a of the indicator, the undissociated form predominates.
pH $= 2$; $pK_a = -\log K_a = -\log (4 \times 10^{-4}) = 4 - \log(4) > 2$
{*for the math see* CHM 6.5.1, *and the end of* CHM 6.6.1}
Since the pH of the solution is less than the pK_a of the indicator, $\downarrow$pH means $\uparrow[H^+]$, looking at Reaction I and remembering Le Chatelier's Principle, if the stress is on the right side of the equilibrium (i.e. $\uparrow[H^+]$), the reaction shifts to the left which gives the red color (i.e. $\uparrow[HMe]$).

Q 67 A   CHM 4.1.2

By only using a few drops of indicator, the number of protons (i.e. Reaction I) that the indicator interacts with is kept to a minimum.

Q 68 B   PHY 7.1.2, 8.3; P3, L1-5
Using velocity = frequency × wavelength
Since the frequency of the wave remains constant (P3, L1-5), if the velocity is quadrupled, the wavelength must also be quadrupled in the process.

Q 69 A   deduce; B: PHY 8.2
From the question, velocity (v) is inversely proportional to the square root of the density of the medium (ρ). Let $\mathbf{v} \sim \mathbf{1}/(\sqrt{\rho})$, where " $\sim$ " *means* proportional to; if density increases by a factor of 2, density (ρ_X) = $2\rho_Y$
Knowing that $v_Y \sim 1/(\sqrt{\rho_Y})$, we get:
New velocity (v_X) = $1/\sqrt{(2\rho_Y)}$ = $1/(\sqrt{2}) \times 1/(\sqrt{\rho_Y})$ = $1/(\sqrt{2}) \times v_Y$
Thus $(v_X)/(v_Y)$ = $1/\sqrt{2}$

Q 70 C   PHY 8.3; change in dB = 3, *solve for* I/I_0
The difference between the two sounds is 3.0 dB.
Using Number of dB = $10\log(I/I_o)$
$$3.0 = 10\log(I/I_o)$$
$$3/10 = \log(I/I_o)$$
$$I/I_o = 10^{3/10}$$
This value is less than 10 (= 10^1), but greater than 1 (= 10^0), which reveals only one possible answer.

Q 71 C   PHY 1.3, *use 10 sec. for dist.*
Speed of sound in water = (343×4) m s^{-1}
Time taken to return = 20 s
Therefore, time taken to reach = 1/2 × time taken to return = 10 s
Depth of region = (343×4) m s^{-1} × 10 s = 13 720 m

Q 72 A   P2, L3-5; PHY 7.1.2
One cycle = 5 s ; Period = 5 s
Using frequency = 1/(Period)
frequency = 1/(5 s) = 0.2 Hz

Q 73 A   PHY 11.5
This can be verified using the lens maker's equation, paying close attention to the signs of the values used (focal length is negative for a diverging lens).

Q 74 B   CHM 5.3.1
Molarity = Number of moles per liter [= mol/(1000cm^3)]
Molality = Number of moles per 1000 g of solvent [= mol/(1000 g)]

Then, if $1000 \text{ cm}^3 = 1000 \text{ g}$,
Molarity = Molality

Q 75 D   CHM 9.3, 9.4

When [P] is increased by a factor of 3 (Exp A and C, [Q] *is constant*), the initial rate of reaction is increased by a factor of 9 (= 3^2). Thus the order of reaction with respect to P is 2. When [Q] is increased by a factor of 2 (Exp A and B, [P] *is constant*), the initial rate of reaction is also increased by a factor of 2 (= 2^1). Therefore, the order of reaction with respect to Q is 1. The order of reaction with respect to a certain component tells you how many molecules of that component are involved in the rate determining step of the reaction which may not be equivalent to the stoichiometric coefficients.

Q 76 C   PHY 4.1, 4.1.1

Since the bar is uniform, its center of gravity is at the center of the bar. Using the fact that for a system in equilibrium, the sum of the moments in opposite directions are equal (= *rotational equilibrium*) and: Moment = Force × perpendicular distance from the axis of rotation, we get:
$4 \text{ kg} \times 9.8 \text{ m s}^{-2} \times 0.20 \text{ m} = x \text{ kg} \times 9.8 \text{m s}^{-2} \times 0.50 \text{ m}$ {9.8m s^{-2} cancels}
$x = 0.80/0.50 = 1.60/1.0 = 1.6$

Q 77 D   CHM 4.2, 2.3F, PT

Among the answer choices, S is the least electronegative of the different atoms bonded to hydrogen. This can be deduced from the periodic table: it is below oxygen in Group VI, in a lower period than fluorine, and before chlorine in its period, each of which makes it less electronegative than the other atoms. The <u>relatively</u> low electronegativity translates in a lower force of attraction between the δ^- sulfur and neighboring δ^+ hydrogens (*see* H-bonding, CHM 4.2, #3).

Understanding

GS-3

Verbal Reasoning

Explanation: the basis for the answers for Verbal Reasoning is the passage. Most answers are found directly in passage which we have cross-referenced for you by paragraph and line in The Gold Standard Answer Key. Therefore, explanations for Verbal Reasoning are only given for selected questions which are either more challenging or reveal some teaching point. It is recommended that you review Part II, Chapter 3 in The Gold Standard text.

Q 92 B   P4, deduce
You must determine what is meant by "agronomic importance" and then choose an answer which demonstrates that foxtails do not have this. From the author's discussion concerning foxtail's agronomic importance (P4), it can be inferred that foxtails are agronomically important because they have various functions (i.e. food, important weeds), are widely distributed with a long history, and they pose problems in crop production. It seems that agronomic importance refers to the depth of the foxtail's involvement or association with the economics of agriculture. Answer choices **A.**, **C.**, and **D.** all affirm the fact that foxtails are agronomically important because they state situations that are described in the passage as being examples of the foxtail's agronomic importance. Answer choice **B.** is the only one that demonstrates that foxtails might not be agronomically important.

Q 100 B   P4
The statement is a rhetorical question through which the writer is suggesting that it is not respectable for a father to sacrifice a child's education in order to fund an elaborate funeral. All four answer choices include statements which the author has made; however, only one answer choice is *most* supported by the given statement. Answer choice **B.** is the best among other possible answers because it refers directly to "having a fine funeral"(= "lavish send-offs"). Also, there is reference to the idea that the father should really put his funds to use for his son's education rather than his own funeral ("family love and true-blue Americanism").

Q 104 D   P2, L3-4; P3; P4; P6; P7
Answer choice **A.** is supported by the figures in P2, L3-4. Answer choice **B.** is amply supported by paragraphs 3 and 4. Answer choice **C.** is supported by the possible solution provided in P7. The statement in answer choice **D.** is made in P6 but not supported. For example, in what way are they generally free of controls? What evidence is there that they have any different controls than other businesses? Etc.

Q 105 A   deduce
The attitude of the author towards the high cost of dying can be inferred from the strong words used to describe the situation throughout the passage. The author refers to morticians who encourage expensive funerals as "unscrupulous" (P3, L1). The commonly held belief that the extravagance of the funeral is somehow a measure of the dead person's worth is described as a "delusion" (P4, L7). The author calls the situation "depressing" (P7, L1). The use of these words makes it clear that the author is neither supportive nor indifferent to the high cost of dying. If the author's attitude was one of pity there would be more exploration of the struggles of families to finance the funerals. It is quite obvious that the author regards the high cost of dying as deplorable or disgusting.

Q 110 D   deduce; *did TV change the children?*
Answer choices **A.**, **B.** and **C.** present situations in which mass communication *affected* people in different ways leading to social and economic consequences. However, answer choice **D.**

states that "violent children enjoy watching violence on television." Does the preceding mean that television, which *is* a form of mass communication, has affected or influenced the violent children leading to some social consequence? No, we do not know since the children were violent to begin with, thus there is no evidence in this problem that television *changed* the children. However, if the statement was "children who watch violence on television become violent," then the assertion would lend evidence to one of television's social effects.

Q 112 B   deduce; P2/3/5/6/7/8

The objective in this question is to determine what most of the passage is attempting to demonstrate to the reader. Answer choice **A.** is only explored peripherally at the end of the passage (P9, L10-15), so it clearly cannot be the answer. Answer choice **C.** mentions World War II and the "global village," both discussed only briefly and not in relation to one another in the passage. Answer choice **D.** focuses on an aspect that the passage discusses (P2), but the exploration of this aspect does not extend into most of the passage. The passage cites several examples of new technologies being used to improve communications, which supports answer choice **B.** The inventions of moveable type (P3), electronics (P5), telephone transmissions (P6), satellites (P7) and radio and television (P9) and their effects on global communications are discussed, making up a large portion of the passage.

Q 114 C   P3, deduce; KC: *water ≈ health care*

The statement "water everywhere, but none to drink" is not meant to be taken literally, as in answer choice **B.** Obviously in the United States, most people are not going without food and water; furthermore, this literal perspective is not explored by the passage. The statement provided really suggests that even in an abundance of something vital, people are still going without. Answer choice **A.** is incorrect as the statement includes those with little money (e.g. *not* an abundance) who should have access to health care. Answer choice **D.** states that people incurred great debt to pay for health services, however, in this statement no one is going without something (i.e. answer choice **D.** is a true statement but unrelated to the question). Answer choice **C.** fits the statement given in the question in that it suggests an abundance of something vital, health care, which some people cannot access.

Q 115 C   deduce

The author uses the words "tilled the soil" to demonstrate that the people referred to were working. Notice that after they had developed a chronic disease, they could no longer work ("Their toil could not continue"; P3, L3-5). The statement provided certainly does not mean that the people were all farmers, or even that they actually planted anything. The author is referring to people who were unable to cover their health expenses because their insurance did not provide adequate coverage. This situation could obviously not occur exclusively to farmers or to those who enjoyed planting! However, these people all had insurance, so it is possible that this situation happened only to those who worked hard to pay for that insurance.

Q 118 B   deduce

You need to decide what is the overall theme of the passage. Answer choice **A.** states that the public was excluded from the health care debate. However, in the passage people from all over the United States were debating the future of health care (P1, L4-6) and no exclusion is mentioned. Health Maintenance Organizations (HMOs) are discussed in the passage, but this is by no means the main theme. Though some positive points are presented, HMOs are criticized as restricting the patient's choice of physician (P4, L5-7) and cited as a basis on which to improve (P5, L6-8). The focus of the passage is not on exactly what particular changes to make, as answer choice **C.** suggests. Answer choice **D.** suggests that the main idea of the passage is something which is not even mentioned until the last sentence (P7, L6-8). This is obviously incorrect. Answer choice **B.** is consistent with the author's main ideas. The author makes it clear that change is necessary, and that there are options which need to be discussed. It is also clear that further than just discussing the issue, as has occurred in the past, the passage suggests that a plan (P1, P5, P6, P7) needs to be enacted.

Q 124 D   deduce

Warburton-Lee was ordered to go into Narvik to make sure that no enemy troops landed there (P5, L4-5). However, before arriving Warburton-Lee received information that led him to change his course of action from that which he was ordered to do. For this reason, Warburton-Lee would not be regarded as a soldier simply following instructions, as in answer choice **C.** Warburton-Lee's new course of action was not a result of carefully thought-out plans, it was simply a result of re-evaluating his situation with respect to new information. Furthermore, to be prudent (answer choice **A.**) would be to *avoid* confronting or being seen by the enemy. The intention of Warburton-Lee when he chose his new course of action was to mislead enemy troops as to the future actions of the British troops (P6, L6-7). In this sense, Warburton-Lee was successful (P6, L8) and would therefore not be regarded as a fool, but rather he would be regarded as a hero (answer choice **D.**).

Q 137 C   deduce; P8; P9

There is no evidence in the passage to support answer choices **A.**, **B.** and **D.** However, paragraphs 8 and 9 bring out some important points: (i) the number of auto users has increased; (ii) delinquency figures are higher now than in an earlier period; and (iii) the author believes that increases in the number of crimes does not necessarily indicate a greater intensity of criminal behavior. Thus it can be reasonably inferred from the passage that some crimes (i.e. stealing a bicycle) may have gone unreported in the past because the value was much less than other crimes (i.e. stealing a car) which are now: (a) more common (more users) and (b) would consistently be reported as a crime. Despite this, the frequency or intensity of "stealing" may have remained the same, yet the figures (*reported*) increased.

Understanding

GS-3

Biological Sciences

Explanation: the basis of the biology and organic chemistry questions within Biological Sciences is very different. Thus we have chosen to provide the answers in different formats. Most biology answers are found directly in the passage which we have cross-referenced for you by paragraph, line and/or figure or diagram (when applicable). Therefore, explanations for biology are given in a similar format to the one used for Physical Sciences. On the other hand, MCAT organic chemistry questions usually rely on the ability to decipher the important information from the given passage and an understanding of the basics including mechanisms. Thus all organic chemistry questions and answers are explored in detail, beginning with a review of the passage itself.

☞ You will often find that the Biology passages deal with advanced level topics or experiments. The key is not to become deterred by fancy words; rather, know what you know and concentrate on quickly understanding any graph or table presented. Do not try to understand details from the passage. Instead, read quickly and then focus on the questions.

Q 143 B   BIO 3.0; P1, L3-7

Releasing factors need to be located near ribosomes engaging in protein synthesis (P1). You should know that such ribosomes are located in the cytosol (answer choice **B.**) or associated with *rough* endoplasmic reticulum, not within the nucleus, nor *smooth* endoplasmic reticulum (BIO 1.2.1), nor mitochondria.

Q 144 C   P1, L1-2; E; ORG 9.4

The name of an enzyme is usually related to its function. In termination, cleavage of an *ester* bond is required (P1, L1-2). Therefore, *ester*ase is the most appropriate name.

Q 145 D   P3; E; B: ORG 12.2.1

Peptidyl transferase is involved in making the peptide bonds in the forming amino acid (P3). In termination, the activity of peptidyl transferase is altered by releasing factors so that a molecule of water may be added (= *hydrolysis*; ORG 12.2.1) instead of another aminoacyl tRNA (P3; E; cf. Q144). So, if peptidyl transferase activity is inhibited, both of these processes are inhibited.

Q 146 A   ORG 9.4

Attack of the carbon shown in Figure 1 by water will cause the oxygen that is already attached to the sugar to leave the amino acid (see arrow in Figure 1). The oxygen of the water will become part of the amino acid as it loses its hydrogens (ORG 9.4→8.1→12.2.1).

Q 147 D   BIO 1.2.2, 3.0

You must know that A pairs with T and C pairs with G (BIO 1.2.2). However, the question is asking about RNA, not DNA. In RNA, T is replaced by U. Therefore, the complementary sequence of CAG is GUC.

Q 148 C   deduce; B: BIO 3.0, 15.5

The question is asking what advantage is conferred by having many codons with very similar sequences. The choices provided may be true statements about the genetic code, but only one is an advantage that arises because of this feature. Point mutations, which affect a single nitrogenous base, are not as detrimental to the genetic code since a change in one base may not affect the amino acid for which the new codon will code.

Q 149 C   deduce; B: BIO 1.2.2, 1.3

This problem begins with you understanding that nitrogen is an integral part of the subunits (*nucleotides*: BIO 1.2.2) which polymerize to form DNA. After the part of the experiment labelled **1.**, essentially all bacterial DNA will contain the isotope of nitrogen ^{15}N. Thus the original molecules contain only ^{15}N. By semi-conservative replication in the presence of only ^{14}N (part **2.** and **3.** in the experiment), the first new molecules will each contain one strand of ^{15}N (= the parent or template) and one strand of ^{14}N (= the new or daughter strand). In the second replication, the $^{15}N/^{14}N$ molecule created in the first replication will be separated and used as a template. One strand of ^{15}N will be used as a template for a new $^{15}N/^{14}N$ molecule and one strand of ^{14}N will be used as a template for a new molecule that will contain only ^{14}N. This will produce equal amounts of the $^{15}N/^{14}N$ and the ^{14}N molecules in the second generation.

Q 150 C   F1; deduce; B: BIO 1.2.2, 1.3

If conservative replication had occurred the initial strand which contained only ^{15}N (*see* Q149) would not separate to form templates for two new strands (*conservative* = to resist or oppose change). The replication would produce no DNA molecules containing a mix of the old strand (^{15}N) and the new strand (^{14}N) [*see* Figure 1]. After one generation there would be the original old strand with ^{15}N and an equal number of new daughter strands with ^{14}N.

Q 151 D   F1; deduce; B: BIO 1.2.2, 1.3

Dispersive replication takes the original molecule and produces two new molecules which are both mixtures of the old and new strands (*see* Figure 1). Therefore, the centrifuge of a mixture which had replicated in this manner would show only a large band of $^{15}N/^{14}N$ molecules.

Q 152 A   PoE; B: BIO 1.2.2

Option **D.** is an accurate description of how the nitrogenous bases bind together to form the helical structure. Option **C.** is also a feature of the molecule which aids in maintaining the shape. The hydrophobic bases are kept in the center of the helix while the hydrophillic backbone interacts with the outside environment. Option **B.** is similar to option **D.** in that it describes the bonds which give the helical molecule its strength. Option **A.** is a description of a negative consequence of DNA not holding its helical structure. It is not a process or interaction by which DNA maintains its shape.

Q 153 C   BIO 3.0

You should be familiar with the names of different enzymes involved in the replication, transcription and translation of DNA. Even if you don't know, it is easy to make a good guess just by looking at the names. You are asked for an enzyme that will help synthesize a chain of RNA. You can then narrow it down to a choice which includes the word RNA. The two choices are either replicase or polymerase. In producing a strand of RNA, nothing is being replicated. A chain (polymer)of RNA is being made which is complementary but not identical to the strand of DNA. It is easy to conclude that RNA polymerase must be involved (BIO 3.0).

Q 154 B   P2, L6-8, L10-13; D.↔P2, L1-3
The passage states that the myeloma part of the hybridoma provides the immortality needed to clone a large amount of antibody, and that the immune lymphocyte part (which came from the spleen) provides the specificity of the antibody (answer choice **B.**).

Q 155 D   BIO 8.3; B: BIO 7.5
You should be familiar with the function of the spleen from the biology review. The spleen does not *produce* blood cells in the adult.

Q 156 A   P6/7 (#4. and #5.)
Recall that Q154 emphasized the aspect of "antibody specificity" in creating a monoclonal antibody. In the procedure described, individual hybridoma cells are cloned and the clones are tested for the presence of the desired antibody at the end. This makes purification unnecessary since each well contains a different hybridoma cell which will produce daughter cells - all of which will create the same (*mono*clonal) antibody. {Inference: a *well* is an individual compartment or depression in a plastic tray or glass block}

Q 157 B   deduce; P2, L20
The purpose of the procedure is to produce large amounts of a particular antibody. The only cells of concern in cloning the antibody are the hybridoma cells. They are the combination of the optimal characteristics of both spleen and myeloma cells. Myeloma cells or spleen cells by themselves are not useful in cloning antibodies, so the culture medium should inhibit their growth while enhancing hybridoma proliferation.

Q 158 D   deduce; BIO 8.1, 8.2
By injecting a person with an inactivated form of an antigen, an immune response is elicited in which antibodies are produced and memory cells are made that will react quickly in the event of a subsequent infection. This is the process by which vaccines work (= "active" immunity). The antigen is inactivated so as to activate the immune system *without* risking the development of the disease or infection. Injecting the person with the antibody itself may help the person if they have been infected by something displaying the corresponding antigen (= "passive" immunity), but it will not induce the body to produce its own antibodies nor memory cells, so it offers no future protection against a subsequent infection.

Q 159 tests your memory of the definition of enantiomers: they come in pairs and are two <u>non-superimposable</u> mirror images of each other (ORG 2.2). Answer choice **A.** is the only compound which you can draw the mirror image then twist the image to superimpose onto the original molecule.

Q 160 D   BIO 2.2
The question is asking for a feature that *eukaryotes* have that *prokaryotes* (i.e. bacteria) do not have. A cell wall is listed and this is a difference between the two types of cells, however, a cell wall is a feature that the *prokaryote* has that a eukaryote, other than plants and fungi, does not have.

One of the major differences between prokaryotes and eukaryotes is that prokaryotes contain no membrane bound organelles. Therefore, a eukaryote would have lysosomes, while a prokaryote would not.

Q 161 D   BIO 14.2
This question is simple. Only a basic knowledge of genetics is required.

Q 162 tests your memory of a couple of the IR absorption peaks (ORG 14.1). The absolute minimum to memorize are the bands for an alcohol (OH, 3200 - 3650) and that for the carbonyl group (C=O, 1630 - 1780) because these are the two most encountered functional groups in MCAT organic chemistry.

Bottle II has a peak at 1710 (carbonyl) + 3333 - 3500 (hydroxyl) = carboxylic acid (i.e. benzoic acid). Bottle IV has a peak at 3333 so it must be the alcohol. Without doing anything else, there is only one possible answer, **D**.

{*For fun, draw the structures of the four compounds*; allyl, ORG 4.2, add -OH to make it an alcohol; benzoic acid - ORG 8.1; the four carbon ketone 2-butanone (= *methyl ethyl ketone*) and the four carbon aldehyde butyraldehyde (= *butanal*) - ORG 7.1}

Q 163 will see if you have the most basic understanding of a proton NMR (ORG 14.2). Not including the reference peak at zero, there is only one peak! This means two things: (i) each H must be living in an environment which is identical to any other H in the entire molecule (only answer choice **B.** is possible); and (ii) since there is only one peak, to calculate the number of H's n on an adjacent carbon: $n + 1 = 1$. Thus n is zero indicating that each H is attached to a carbon whose neighboring carbon has no attached H's (again, only option **B.** is possible).

GS-3, Passage IV, Questions 164-168

Prelude: you don't need to understand every detail in order to answer these questions correctly. Nonetheless, let's pull out the magnifying glass . . .

Begin by reading the first paragraph. The key words are 'conjugated dienes' and 'electrophilic addition'. A <u>diene</u> is an alkene with two double bonds (i.e. 1,3-buta*diene*; the numbers 1,3 locate the double bonds, but- means 4 carbons, see Reaction I in the problem). <u>Conjugated</u> means there is a single bond between the two double bonds (ORG 7.1). <u>Electrophilic addition</u> is the most important mechanism for you to understand regarding alkenes! {*see* ORG 4.2.1}

Consider the second paragraph and Reaction I. Let's discuss the mechanism. First we need to understand the nature of a double bond: *it is an electron dense area; therefore, the electrons attract positively charged substances = <u>electrophiles</u>*. A classic electrophile is H^+. Thus in a prototypical electrophilic addition reaction a compound like HBr is added to an alkene. The HBr ionizes and the electrophile H^+ adds to the double bond in accordance to **Markovnikoff's rule**. For short we'll call it Mark's rule! Some student's like to memorize Mark's rule as follows: the electrophile or H^+ *prefers* to add to the carbon where most of its buddies (other H's) are! Then the nucleophile (i.e. Br^-) attaches to the carbocation which is *usually* more substituted (i.e. more attached groups which does not include H's); these groups, i.e. alkyl groups, are somewhat electron donating and thus stabilize the carbocation intermediate.

Umm, one question: where the heck is the electrophile in Br_2? After all, it's a diatomic molecule where both atoms are identical. For this we must revert to an analogy . . .

Consider two 5 year old girls, identical twins, walking in a park hand in hand with rather *neutral* facial expressions. Someone pulls out an ice cream cone which is presented to the closer of the two twins. The twin closest to the ice cream begins to smile (a *positive* facial expression), while the other twin realizing she is going to miss out on the treat begins to frown (a rather *negative* expression). An outside force has *induced* polarity in the twins = *an induced dipole*!

When Br_2 approaches a double bond, the polarity changes. The electrons in the double bond repel the electrons in the bond between the bromine atoms making the distribution of electrons among the 'twins' unequal. Thus one Br atom becomes slightly negative (δ^-), while the other becomes slightly positive (δ^+). The δ^+ Br is the electrophile which becomes increasingly attracted to the double bond which in turn continues to repel the Br-Br bond until the electrophile Br attaches while the leaving group Br^- floats away before acting as a nucleophile.

Back to Reaction I: we now know how to create the intermediate. The double bond induces a dipole in Br_2 resulting in one Br atom adding to the carbon with the most H's (*Mark's rule*), leaving a carbocation as an intermediate. Draw the reaction below:

Q 164 B is the only possible answer since it is the only answer with carbocations as intermediates! You should have them in your reaction above.

Q 165 is very nice! It tests your understanding of the following concept: the more stable intermediate requires the <u>smallest</u> activation energy and thus forms a product *faster* (= *the kinetic product*, A), while the less stable intermediate requires <u>more</u> energy (*higher temperature*, i.e. 40 ° C in the problem) to form a product (= *thermodynamic product*, B). {CHM 9.6}

Q 166 is a continuation of the preceding paragraph. The real question is: which intermediate is the most stable? By looking at the two intermediates (Q164, II.), you can see that the compound on the left has a positive charge on a 2° carbon (= *secondary carbocation*), while the compound on the right has a positive charge at the 1° carbon (= *primary carbocation*). Since the secondary carbocation is more stable (ORG 4.2.1, 6.2.1), it must produce compound A. Now simply imagine our nucleophile Br⁻ adding to our secondary carbocation intermediate. Now it's just a matter of nomenclature (ORG 4.1).

Q 167 is a direct definition of a structural isomer (ORG 2.1).

Q 168 is also quick and easy! To begin with, answer choice **B.** is retarded (!) because it's a *five* carbon ring while our reactant is a *six* carbon ring (cyclo*hex*ene). Answer choice **C.** also is illogical since electrophilic addition adds to the double bond! For fun, let's name answer choices **A.** and **D.**: A. is *cis*-1,2-dibromocyclohexane (*cis* tells us the two Br atoms are on the same side of the plane of the cyclohexane molecule), and **D.** is *trans*-1,2-dibromocyclohexane (*trans* tells us the two Br atoms are on opposite sides of the plane of the cyclohexane molecule). Which is more stable? Naturally the electronegative Br atoms would prefer to be as far apart as possible because of <u>electron shell repulsion</u> (i.e. Fig IV.B.12.1 in ORG 12.3.2). The *trans* molecule affords maximum distance between the Br atoms and is thus more stable.

Q 169 D   PoE
The amount of DNA in a haploid organism will certainly affect the organism's phenotype. Recall that a haploid organism does not have a homologous chromosome which could mask a recessive allele (B: BIO 14.2, 15.1).

A bacterium with little DNA is very much different from a human with considerably more DNA. The rate at which meiosis occurs will be affected by the amount of DNA that needs to be replicated and divided.

The length of time *between* meiotic divisions is not likely to be dramatically affected by the amount of DNA. However, any organism, regardless of the amount of DNA present, must be able to reproduce in order to survive. {*Period!*}

Q 170 B   P2, L1-4; B: BIO 16.3
The passage states that the divergence of populations in their DNA content could reduce chromosome pairing in their hybrids and so reduce fertility. The only option consistent with this statement is answer choice **B.**, hybrid inviability (BIO 16.3).

Q 171 A   deduce; P2; cf. BIO 15.5
Option **B.** suggests that sequences in the chromosome will duplicate themselves and then pairing could occur with the repetitive sequences in the homologous chromosome, which is not possible since duplication is a random mutation (BIO 15.5) {*note that the suggestion that "unpaired sequences . . . duplicate" (i.e. mutation) is not the same as replication/duplication using the repetitive sequences as templates*}. Option **C.** suggests a translocation of the unmatched genetic material to allow pairing. However, translocation occurs randomly and could not guarantee that the correct sequence is moved each time. Option **D.** suggests that the chromosome with the unmatched sequence will undergo a deletion. Like translocation and duplication, deletion would occur randomly. Secondarily, a deletion would *rarely* be so large as to delete an entire repetitive sequence. The only reasonable option is answer choice **A.** in which the unmatched sequence can be temporarily moved out of the way (looped).

Q 172 D   P1, L3-5; deduce
The passage states that organisms with high C values (more DNA) reproduce more slowly than organisms with low C values. In the parasite-host relationship, the parasite reproduces much more than the host. Many generations of a parasite may infect a single host (i.e. bacteria vs. humans, ticks vs. dogs, etc.). Therefore, it is reasonable to narrow down the choices to ones in which the parasite is said to have less DNA. Although it is usually true that the parasite is smaller than the host, this is not necessarily caused by the difference in DNA content. In fact, the passage gives an example of two organisms with large differences in C values that are the same size as adults (P1, L5-7). This leaves only option **D.**

Q 173 B   deduce
A species' fitness is ultimately enhanced by an abundance of variation within the gene pool (B: BIO 16.2, 16.3). Varying the numbers and distributions of repetitive sequences affects the genome of the hybrids in different ways, giving the opportunity for new, adaptive combinations. Note that option **A.** is incorrect as the reduction in hybrid viability is not substantial (P2). Option **C.** is incorrect since there is no evidence from either the passage nor the biology review that the amount of DNA has an effect on the fitness of a species (cf. P1, L5-7). Option **D.** is incorrect since the passage describes (P2, P3) that the presence of repetitive

sequences reduces the fertility of the hybrid, somewhat. Thus one would expect that the fertility of the species would be affected even less or, more likely, not at all.

Q 174 C   KW: *bidirectional*
Bidirectional replication suggests that replication will occur in two directions. The only option consistent with this is option **C.** which states that DNA replication will begin on both sides of the origin.

Q 175 C   Ap C
In order to draw any conclusions about what actually caused the bacteria to die, a <u>control group</u> must be used. Both groups of Pol A mutants must be exposed to exactly the same environmental conditions up until the point of exposing the bacteria to UV light. One group is exposed, while the control group is not exposed. Since this is the only difference the bacteria experienced, it can be concluded that the UV light killed the bacteria if the control group survives. If the control group also dies, it would indicate that a different variable, yet to be determined, caused the death of both groups. This is a fundamental principle of true experiments.

Q 176 A   P4; P5
The passage tells you that the Pol A mutants lacked Pol I enzyme, yet they were able to grow normally for several generations. In order for the cells to grow and divide, their DNA would need to be replicated (BIO 2.2, 14.2). Therefore the strongest evidence that the Pol I enzyme is not essential to replication is that the mutants can in fact reproduce.

Q 177 D   P6; ORG 12.2.2; BIO 4.3
TS type *E. coli* have a gene which codes for a Pol III enzyme that becomes nonfunctional only at high temperatures, rendering the cell unable to grow. Pol III enzyme is always produced and present, it is just unable to function at high temperatures. The Pol III enzyme is affected by heat in a way that causes it to stop functioning properly. The loss of an enzyme's tertiary structure will affect its function and can occur at elevated temperatures.

Q 178 C   BIO 1.2.2
This question requires basic knowledge of the process of DNA replication.

Q 179 D   B: BIO 1.2.2; deduce (draw diag.)
A diagram would be helpful here to visualize the circular replication of the chromosome. In the first replication a uniformly normal circular chromosome would replicate producing two molecules that are half normal and half labelled (one parent strand, one new ³H-thymidine

labelled daughter strand). The preceding is the essence of semi-conservative replication (BIO 1.2.2; *see* Passage II and its questions in the GS-3 exam). When this molecule replicates (the second round of replication), the parent strand will be the template on one branch of the replication fork and the labelled strand will be the template on the other branch of the replication fork. The parent (normal) strand will produce another half normal, half labelled molecule. The labelled strand will produce a new molecule in which both strands are labelled (e.g. has twice as much labelled portion as the other daughter molecule).

Q 180 C   KS: 8 divisions; 10×2^n, n=8
In the span of two hours, the bacteria will have divided eight times (8×15 min $= 120$ min $=$ 2 hours). You can think about it like this: in 15 min (#1 = 1st doubling time), the 10 bacteria will all have duplicated, making 20. After another 15 min (#2 = 2nd doubling time), all of those 20 bacteria will have duplicated, making 40. This doubling goes on and on a total of 8 times: #3 = 80, #4 = 160, #5 = 320, #6 = 640, #7 = 1280, #8 = 2560.

Alternatively, there are equations for doubling time and half-lives (cf. PHY 12.4), and you should be familiar with how to use them. For doubling time, $X \times 2^n$, where X is the number originally present and n is the number of doubling times. Thus in Q180 we get:

$$X \times 2^n = 10 \times 2^8 = 10 \times 256 = 2560.$$

For half-lives, $X \times (½)^n$, where X is the number originally present and n is the number of half-lives. {*see* PHY 12.4}

GS-3, Passage VII, Questions 181-185

You must be comfortable with these types of problems because flow diagrams are MCAT classics!

Let's work through an example. Consider Figure 1. The flow chart begins with an unknown compound which is not soluble in water. The compound is then treated with 10% NaOH. If the compound is insoluble in the NaOH then we test the compound in 2,4-DNP (*of course, the mechanism of all these reactions and what 'DNP' stands for are irrelevant!*). Had the compound been soluble in NaOH then Table 1 tells us that the unknown compound must be an organic acid (= *a carboxylic acid or a phenol*). To determine what type of organic acid, Figure 1 shows us that the next step is treatment with 5% sodium bicarbonate, $NaHCO_3$. If the test is positive (i.e. the organic acid is soluble in $NaHCO_3$), then Table 1 tells us the compound must be a carboxylic acid.

Q 181 can be answered without looking at any of the information in the problem! By definition, alkanes (i.e. heptane) are hydrophobic (= *'insoluble in'* or *'afraid of'* water). The other answers are nonsense!

Q 182 tests your ability to use the figure and the table. Follow the flow chart in Figure 1. Water insoluble + 10% NaOH soluble + 5% $NaHCO_3$ soluble = a carboxylic acid (*see the preceding example we worked through*). Then we try 2% $KMnO_4$ (*potassium permanganate*), which Table 1 tells us is the Bayer test. According to Table 1, the Bayer test is positive for alkenes. According to Q182, the Bayer test is negative. Thus we are looking for a carboxylic acid (-COOH) which is not an alkene. '**A.**', which is benzoic acid, is the only possible answer.

Q 183 is asking you to remember the following simple facts: (i) signals on a proton NMR are used to determine the *number* and *types* of hydrogens in a molecule; (ii) an acid can donate a proton (hydrogen); (iii) if the solvent is D_2O instead of H_2O then the acidic proton can be replaced by deuterium instead of another proton; (iv) loss of a proton means loss of a signal. {ORG 14.2.1}

Q 184 is really asking the following question: what determines basicity in an amine? And an even more basic question (*pardon the pun!*), what is a base?

A base accepts protons (CHM 6.2). This means a base must possess a negative or partially negative charge in order to attract a proton. The partial negative charge on an amine is carried by nitrogen (ORG 11.1.1). Clearly, substituents attached to the nitrogen which donate electrons will increase the partial negative charge on N thus increasing its attractiveness to a proton which makes the amine a better base. Conversely, substituents which withdraw electrons from N will decrease its partial negative charge which decreases its attractiveness to a proton which means decreased basicity.

Now the problem is quite simple. The differences between the three aliphatic amines are: **I.** has no electronegative substituent; **II.** has flourine which is the most electronegative element in the periodic table (CHM 2.3F); and **III.** has chlorine which is very much electronegative but not as much as flourine. Thus the order of basicity is: **I.**, the most basic, then **III.** with chlorine helping to withdraw electrons away from N, then **II.**, the weakest base of the three because the electronegative strength of F pulls electrons from N the most.

Q 185 is very, very, very, very easy! The passage tells you and we worked out that a positive $NaHCO_3$ test indicates a carboxylic acid. Answer choice **C.** is the only choice which is a carboxylic acid! Everything else is irrelevant!
{*For interest, its name is propanoic acid* (nomenclature ORG 8.1) *and IR info can be found in* ORG 14.1}

{Please notice how many questions in the preceding passage could have been answered without reading the passage! Though this is certainly not always the case, it does underline an important point: if you are running out of time in any science section on the MCAT, skip reading the passages and go straight to the questions.}

Q 186 C   BIO 1.2
You must be familiar with cellular structures to answer this question.

Q 187 C   BIO 6.1
You must be familiar with the structures of the brain and their functions to answer this question.

Q 188 D   BIO 1.1, 1.2.1
Membrane receptors are <u>proteins</u> which are usually produced by rough endoplasmic reticulum (as opposed to free ribosomes).

Q 189 A   BIO 12.2, 12.3
You must be familiar with the structures of the upper and lower respiratory tracts to answer this question. The larynx comes before the trachea.

Q 190 C   ORG 12.1.2
A pH above the isoelectric point means that the amino acid is in *relatively* basic conditions. A base will accept a proton (H^+) from the amino acid, leaving the amino acid negatively charged.

Q 191 A   P1, L6-8
Information concerning the relative amounts of T and R conformations present before substrate is added is given in the passage.

Q 192 B   deduce; B: BIO 4.1
If a molecule has a high affinity for something, it is likely to be associated with it maximally. The substrate binds more tightly to the R conformation even though the R conformation is present in small amounts because R has a higher affinity for the substrate than T.

Q 193 A   Ap A.3.3; CHM 9.7(FIII.A.9.3)

The graph described would have time along the horizontal axis and the amount of substrate-enzyme complex (amount of substrate added to enzyme) along the vertical axis. The amount of substrate-enzyme complex would increase steadily as more substrate is added until a point at which all enzymes are involved in a substrate-enzyme complex, and any more substrate added will have no effect. The graph would show a steadily increasing line of positive slope which reaches a point at which it levels off into a horizontal line. This curve is called a hyperbole.

Q 194 A   deduce; B: BIO 4.1

The symmetry model describes an instance of something which may be described as positive cooperativity (P2, L2-5; BIO 4.3). The model does not exclude the enzyme from having cofactors, and places no restriction on what the enzyme's function will be. However, the symmetry model does not account for the existence of any other conformations than the two described (P2).

Q 195 B   BIO 4.1, 4.3

You must be familiar with how enzyme function is regulated to answer this question. An allosteric enzyme has a site other than the one for the substrate at which a molecule (not the substrate) that directs the function of the enzyme can bind.

Q 196 C   P1, L5-7; BIO 1.2.2

You must be familiar with the method by which DNA is linked together. You should know that the chain is made by additions to the hydroxyl group of the third carbon in the sugar. Thus if the nucleotide will not accept a bond (= *phosphodiester*; ORG 12.5), then the hydroxyl group at C3 (BIO 1.2.2) must be missing.

Q 197 B   BIO 1.2.2; P2, L1-3

DNA polymerase is the only enzyme listed that functions to build the new chain of complementary DNA.

Q 198 C   BIO 1.2.2

Note the word *deoxy*nucleoside. This should alert you to the fact that you are dealing with DNA and not RNA. The only option listed that is used in RNA but not DNA is **C.**, dUTP.

Q 199 C   F1; P3

The shortest strands of DNA travelled the farthest in the gel, so the first nucleotide added will be at the bottom of the gel. The last nucleotide of the strand will be on the longest piece of

DNA and will be at the top of the gel (P3). You simply need to identify the bottommost and topmost nucleotides. {*Previous knowledge of this stuff is not expected and not required!*}

Q 200 C   KW: *template*; F1

The passage tells you that you read the Sanger gel from bottom to top (P3). From the bottom, the gel reads GTACCGCA. However, the question asks what the sequence of the DNA *template* (BIO 1.2.2) was. The gel will show the sequence of the complementary strand (P3). Therefore, the template strand must be CATGGCGT (BIO 1.2.2).

Q 201 D   deduce

The good news is that in the science sections of the MCAT, thanks to the bell curve, you can get a near perfect score while still making several boo-boos because of questions you don't really understand. Well, the bad news is that this is a very tough question (☹) to keep everyone humble (☺)!

Answer choice **A.** is incorrect since electrophoresis, as described by the passage (P3), is quite necessary as it provides information about the size of the fragments; for example, we would know how far A is from the end of the molecule compared to the nucleotide above and below in the gel (Fig. 1). Answer choice **B.** is incorrect since radioactive treatment is necessary in order to read the products of electrophoresis on the radiogram (P3). Answer choice **C.** is unlikely since adding a step is unlikely to make the procedure faster, moreover, adding a flourescent compound to an established procedure will not make it cheaper!

Finally, P2 describes how all four reactions are carried out in separate reaction mixtures or containers and Figure 1 shows the four different reactions running in four different gels. In so doing, it is clear which fragment contains A, T, G or C at its labelled end. However, if the dideoxynucleoside triphosphates were color labelled, different reactions could occur simultaneously in the same vessel and detected on one gel using the radiogram and then analysing the color of each band (i.e. all red = ddA, green = ddC, etc.) instead of using four different containers and then checking under each ddX as in Figure 1. *Interesting!*

Q 202 C   deduce; B: BIO 11.2

You should be familiar with the different types of muscles and where they are likely to be found (BIO 11.2). Smooth muscles often form the lining of organs such as the stomach which can be filled with some substance and contracts in an <u>involuntary</u> manner. Skeletal muscles are involved in <u>voluntary</u> movements (BIO 11.2). The passage states that the detrusor muscles (and thus the internal urethral sphincter) are controlled in part by parasympathetic neurons, which would indicate a degree of involuntary action (P2, L1-6; P3, L5-7). The external urethral sphincter can be contracted even when the detrusor muscle is strongly contracting, indicating some sort of voluntary control (P2, L6-9). These descriptions fit the functions of the smooth and skeletal muscles for internal and external urethral sphincters, respectively.

Q 203 C   deduce; B: BIO 6.3.1

On a hot day, the body would tend to conserve all the water it can. Thus the bladder would contain less urine than usual. Since the body is trying to resorb water not electrolytes (i.e. ADH, BIO 6.3.1, 6.3.1F) the urine the bladder contains would be more concentrated with solutes (less water present). This corresponds to a small amount of hypertonic urine. {*For the definitions of hypertonic and hypotonic, see* BIO 1.1.1}

Q 204 A   BIO 10.1

You should be familiar with the structures involved in the excretory system from the biology review. However, even if little is initially known, you can infer a lot from information in the passage. The passage states that urine flows through the ureters *to* the bladder (P1). The question is asking what urine flows into *from* the bladder so this eliminates option **B.** The passage discusses the urethra and its sphincters in such a way that it is quite reasonable to conclude that this is the correct answer (P2, L4-9).

Q 205 C   PoE

You should know enough about each of the systems listed so that this question should seem easy. The circulatory system has vessels which are elastic and muscular, indicating that stretching may occur (B: BIO 7.2, 7.3). The respiratory system also involves muscles and stretching (B: BIO 12.3, 12.4). The digestive system includes the stomach, and anyone who has ever eaten too much knows that there is some stretching going on (B: BIO 9.1/2/3/5)! The endocrine system, however, includes glands which secrete different substances into the circulatory system. Its function does not seem to rely on stretch receptors.

Q 206 A   BIO 6.1, 6.1.4; P3, L4-7

This question requires that you know the functions of the cranial nerves. The most important one to be familiar with, the vagus nerve, innervates smooth muscles of internal organs (i.e. the bladder).

Q 207 A   P3, L12-14

The passage clearly shows that when the detrusor muscles contract, the internal sphincter opens, or conversely, the internal sphincter is closed when the detrusor muscles relax.

Q 208 A   BIO 6.3.1

You should know about the excretory system and the hormones which affect it, which would allow you to choose the correct answer immediately. As well, you should also know the functions of different hormones, which would allow you to eliminate those that do not affect the urine (BIO 6.3).

GS-3, Passage XI, Questions 209-214

Yeah! More mechanisms! Let's make some alkenes . . .

Experiment 1 uses isopropyl iodide (= an alk*yl* hal*ide* = 2-iodopropane) and K^+ $^-OCH_2CH_3$ (*recall: alkoxides are strong bases*, ORG 6.2.4) in a classic E2 reaction (ORG 6.2.4). By telling you that the reaction is first order with respect to each of the *two* reagents simply emphasizes the fact that the reaction is second order *overall*, E$\underline{2}$ (CHM 9.3).

Q 209 is answered by the above. Draw the mechanism and E2 product below. The product is propene (= *propylene*).

The above represents the '94% yield'. For fun, draw below how the *minor* product could be formed through either of the two nucleophilic substitution mechanisms (ORG 6.2.3). Either way, this minor product is called ethyl isopropyl ether.

Q 210 is so simple it makes me sad (☹ !). Draw propylene which you created in the preceding mechanism and add the two hydrogens from H_2:

{*see* ORG 4.2.3}

Q 211 tests your respect for $KMnO_4$ as a powerful oxidizing agent. It can add oxygen(s) to reactants. Under abrasive conditions it can cleave the double bond; however, 'cold and dilute' is not abrasive. Thus the product is ethylene glycol (*see* ORG 4.2.2).

Q 212 turns back to the passage. In Experiment II, 1-bromopentane is treated with the strong base KOH. The possible mechanisms to explain the products which they tell us are produced are either: (i) OH$^-$ removes a proton from C-2 (= *the 2nd carbon in 1-pentane*) creating a secondary carbanion intermediate which produces 1-pentene via E2 (12% yield); or (ii) ethanol or ethoxide (*which could be produced in low yield from* ethanol + OH$^-$) simply attacks the δ^+ C-1 kicking out or *substituting* -Br with $-OCH_2CH_3$ creating ethyl pentyl ether via S_N2 (88% yield; *for ether nomenclature and synthesis see* ORG 10.1; S_N2 - ORG 6.2.3).

<u>Q 213</u> asks us to remember 'Mark's rule': alkene + acid ⇒ under ionic conditions (i.e. no: uv, hf, ↑energy/heat), hydrogen adds preferentially to where its buddies are (= *the greatest number of other H's at the double bond* = a simplification of Markovnikoff's rule, *see* ORG 4.2.1). Thus answer choice **B.** is the major product and **A.** is the minor product.

<u>Q 214</u> is an extension of the previous answer. Reaction I abides by Mark's rule producing the Markovnikoff product 2-bromobutane, preferentially. Reaction II uses the same reactants but via a free radical mechanism. By definition (ORG 4.2.1), the anti-Markovnikoff product is produced preferentially (1-bromobutane).

<u>Q 215</u> **B**   **BIO 1.1.2**
Carrier-mediated transport is the only option listed that has a maximum rate at which molecules can be helped to cross the membrane. At this point all of the carrier molecules are operating at their maximum rate and increasing the concentration gradient will have no effect. If the method of transport was simple diffusion, more and more molecules would diffuse as the concentration gradient increased (*see the classic curves*: BIO 1.1.2F). Osmosis is the diffusion of water, and it would increase as the concentration gradient also increased.

<u>Q 216</u> tests you on two points. Firstly, the definition of an isoelectric point: it is the pH at which an amino acid has <u>no net charge</u> (ORG 12.1.2). Therefore, it *cannot* migrate in an electric field (PHY 9.1.3). Secondly, you must look at the structure of lysine (*unless you've already memorized that it is a basic amino acid*, ORG 12.1.2). Notice it has only one acid side group (-COOH) but two basic side groups (-NH₂). Thus overall it is a basic molecule making its isoelectric point, which is related to the pK_a's, also basic (*above a pH of 7*).

<u>Q 217</u> **C**   **Ap A.1.4; 3!=6**
This question is essentially a mathematics problem. It is asking how many different ways a certain number of things can be ordered (permutations). There are three different amino acids and they can be arranged in 3! different ways to create six different molecules (Ap A.1.4):

$$n! = 3! = 3 \times 2 \times 1 = 6.$$

Recall that the tripeptides A-B-C and C-B-A are different since one end has an amino group and the other has a carboxylic acid group (BIO 3.0, ORG 12.1 and 12.2.1).

<u>Q 218</u> **A**   **BIO 14.3**
You must be familiar with the menstrual cycle to answer this question. If you know which hormones the pituitary gland secretes (FSH, LH; BIO 6.3.1F), you can narrow down the choices since the question asks which hormone the ovary secretes. One of the hallmarks of the

follicular phase is that <u>estrogen</u> causes thickening (*proliferation*) of the uterine lining (*endometrium*) [BIO 14.3].

Q 219 provides you 'new' information based on which you are supposed to derive a logical answer. Physically, both **I.** and **III.** should be able to change configurations: chair → boat → second chair. Only **II.** is clearly restrained from free movement.

THE GOLD STANDARD

Understanding

GS-3

The Writing Sample

Explanation: the following includes two different responses to the Writing Sample for Part I in the GS-3 exam. Each essay is followed by a grade and an explanation. For information regarding grading and developing your essay, please refer to Chapter 4, Part 2 in The Gold Standard Text.

In matters of ~~every~~ concience the law of majority is unimportant. For instance, a high school student, greatly susceptible ~~they~~ to peer pressure would choose not to smoke eventhough the majority of his peers feel that it is a desirable thing to do. According to the statement this student should make his choice based on what he believes to be right, regardless of the general ~~certain~~ consesnsus of his peers.

There are some situations in which the law of majority is important in matters of conscrenic. For instance, a politician that believes in firearms can not make a law to force his constituents to carry guns, if they are horrible opposed to such weapons in the first place. Therefore the politician, in doing what he feels is right wouldn't be able to ignore the general ~~consen~~ consensus of the people of his state about firearms because his decision about such a law would affect them as well as him.

~~The~~ Certain circumstances would govern whether the law of ~~any~~ majority is important or not in matters of conscience. If a ~~their~~ person acts in such a way that he can ~~leave~~ live with ~~with~~ and it doesn't have adverse effects on other people who may feel quite differently, then the law of majority is unimportant. If a person's conscience dictates them to act in ways that hurt others, then the consensus of the majority must be taken into account. For instance, a Christian school teacher can't ~~imp~~ force her class that is majority Jewish to sing christmas ssongs ~~because~~ she believes it's the proper thing to do during the holidays. That would antagonize the class, which would have been ~~part of~~ taken into consideration when she wanted to do what's right.

IF YOU NEED MORE SPACE, CONTINUE ON THE NEXT PAGE.

Example of a 2-Level Response

Recall the following regarding a 2-level response:

2 ⇒ The essay completely fails to address adequately one or more of the tasks. There may be recurring mechanical errors (i.e. spelling and grammar). Problems with analysis and organization are typical.

In this case the writer has few mechanical errors which are only occasionally distracting (i.e. P1, L1: *conscience*; P1, L10: *consensus*; P2, L6: *horribly*; etc.). The paper is clearly written. However, the treatment of peer pressure as the law of majority is somewhat of a stretch. More importantly, the fact that there is no serious effort to define the terms provided results in a distortion of the first task and subsequent ambiguity. Always remember the following: providing an example for task 1 is not necessarily the same as providing an <u>explanation of the meaning of the statement</u>.

There is another lesson to keep in mind regarding the first task. Many students (*though it was not done in the preceding essay*) make the mistake of openly agreeing with or opposing the statement provided. The problem comes in the subsequent tasks when you are to provide an example which opposes the statement (task 2) and then resolve the two different perspectives (task 3). Some students end up forgetting the opinion they provided in task 1 and then wind up contradicting themselves in the subsequent tasks. Though it is your prerogative, it is not necessary to provide your opinion for the Writing Sample.

In this essay the examples provided for tasks 2 and 3 are simplistic and barely address the tasks. There is little variation in sentence structure and length. Contractions are used (P3, L14 and L17) which should be avoided in formal writing.

In our democratic society, we have created many laws or rules gained through legislation. These rules are discussed, developed and enacted by elected officials who represent the majority of their constituents. However, the laws produced in this manner may be in conflict with a particular individual's beliefs or values. Thus the statement suggests that when such a conflict is evident, the individual's beliefs superceed the law, rendering the rules of the majority irrelevant.

The statement allows for some dangerous situations. For example, in 1996 many churches frequented by the African-American community were set ablaze by individuals — some of whom were members of racist movements. Both arson and such race-based acts are illegal in America. As in this case, the individuals who acted in defiance of the law of majority claimed they were abiding by their own beliefs and values. Thus they acted with a clear conscience destroying the lives and communities of innocent victims. Such a crime is immoral, unacceptable and - according to the rules of the majority - illegal. Clearly, the law of majority must supercede the conscience of the perpetrators of such a crime.

The dividing line becomes clear. Life, liberty and the pursuit of happiness are the foundations of our Constitution. The concept is both logical and moral. Our conscience should be our guide as we exercise our freedom. However, since our neighbors and fellow Americans share the same rights, someone's conscience should never be used as a reason why someone's Constitutionally protected rights are stripped away. In conclusion, one's conscience should be one's guide but when it interferes with the rights of others, the law of majority becomes more important.

IF YOU NEED MORE SPACE, CONTINUE ON THE NEXT PAGE.

Example of a 5-Level Response

Recall the following regarding a 5-level response:

5 ⇒ All tasks are addressed by the essay. The treatment of the subject is substantial but not as thorough as for a six point essay. While some depth, structure and good vocabulary and sentence control is exhibited, this is at a lower level than for a six point essay.

In this essay all three tasks are explored. The writer demontrates good control of sentence length and structure (esp. P2). The use of sophisticated vocabulary and the reference to the Constitution allows the analysis to be more effective. Ideas flow easily and logically. The writing is clear. There are few mechanical errors which hardly serve as a distraction.

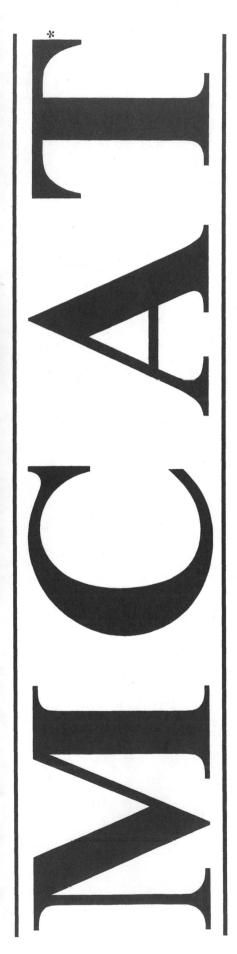

Don't Guess.

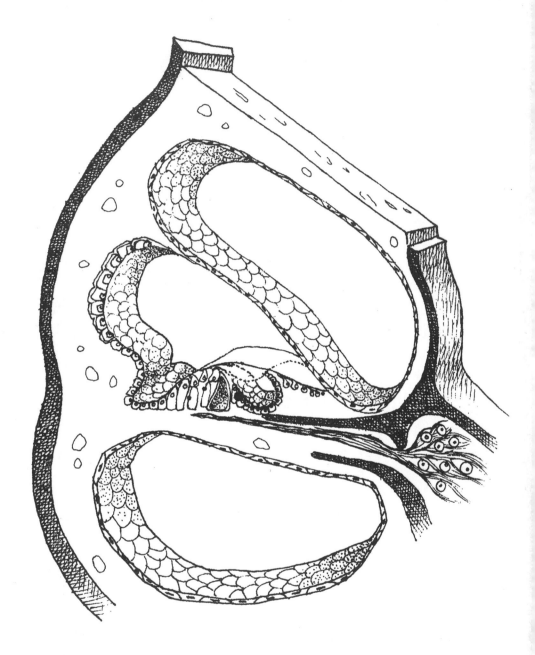

www.MCAT-prep.com

The Only Prep You Need™

Free access to online, timed and interactive Gold Standard tests updated for the new MCAT CBT.